Handbook of
Childhood and
Adolescent Obesity

Issues in Clinical Child Psychology

Series Editor: **Michael C. Roberts,** University of Kansas – Lawrence, Kansas

A continuation Order Plan is available for this series. A continuation order will bring delivery of each new volume immediately upon publication. Volumes are billed only upon actual shipment. For further information please contact the publisher.

Handbook of
Childhood and
Adolescent Obesity

Edited by

Elissa Jelalian
Warren Alpert Medical School of Brown University, Providence, RI, USA

Ric G. Steele
University of Kansas, Lawrence, KS, USA

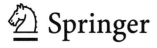 Springer

Editors

Elissa Jelalian, Ph.D.
Warren Alpert Medical School of Brown
  University
Providence, RI
USA
Elissa_Jelalian@brown.edu

Ric G. Steele, Ph.D., ABPP
Clinical Child Psychology Program
University of Kansas
Lawrence, KS
USA
rsteele@ku.edu

ISBN: 978-0-387-76922-6   e-ISBN: 978-0-387-76924-0
DOI: 10.1007/978-0-387-76924-0

Library of Congress Control Number: 2007941929

Printed on acid-free paper

9 8 7 6 5 4 3 2 1

springer.com

Dedications

Contents

SECTION III. RISK FACTORS FOR OBESITY IN CHILDREN AND YOUTH

SECTION IV. INTERVENTIONS

SECTION V. PREVENTION OF PEDIATRIC OBESITY

SECTION VI. FUTURE DIRECTIONS

Section I

Prevalence, Correlates, and Consequences

1

Pediatric Obesity: Trends and Epidemiology

RIC G. STEELE, TIMOTHY D. NELSON, and ELISSA JELALIAN

Pediatric obesity is a prevalent and rapidly increasing problem that poses a serious risk to the health and well-being of the nation's youths. As epidemiological studies have shed light on the severity of the problem, concern about children's weight problems has intensified, leading some to refer to pediatric obesity as a new "epidemic" (American Academy of Pediatrics Committee on Nutrition, 2003). In this context, this chapter will provide an overview of the epidemiology of the epidemic as well as a discussion of emerging trends. We will also briefly introduce important topics such as the correlates and consequences of pediatric obesity, prevention, and intervention, all of which will be explored in greater detail throughout the volume.

Prevalence of Pediatric Overweight

Recent estimates indicate that approximately 17 percent of children and adolescents in the United States are obese (i.e., a Body Mass Index at or above the 95th percentile) (American Medical Association [AMA], 2007), and over 33 percent are either obese or overweight (i.e., a Body Mass Index at or above the 85th percentile (AMA; Centers for Disease Control and Prevention [CDC], 2006; Ogden et al., 2006). Pediatric weight problems affect children of all ages at alarming rates. Reports suggest that about 26 percent of 2- to 5-year-olds are obese or overweight. Among children ages 6 to 11, about 37 percent are overweight or obese. For adolescents between the ages of 12 and 19, the combined overweight and obese rate is estimated

RIC G. STEELE and TIMOTHY D. NELSON • University of Kansas, Lawrence, KS 66045.
ELISSA JELALIAN • Brown University, Providence, RI 02912.

to exceed 34 percent (Ogden et al.). The high prevalence of pediatric obesity parallels the adult obesity epidemic, with over 32 percent of adults being categorized as obese.

Perhaps even more concerning than the current rates of obesity and overweight among children is the significant increase in these conditions over recent years. According to estimates by Ogden et al. (2006), the percentage of children and adolescents who were obese increased by approximately 23 percent between 1999 and 2004, and the percentage of those who were overweight increased more than 19 percent. During this period, the largest increase in pediatric obesity was among children ages 2–5; the rate grew nearly 35 percent. These increases in obesity among young children are especially alarming in light of research suggesting that children who are overweight before age 8 are likely to have more severe obesity as adults (Freedman, Khan, Dietz, Srinivasan & Berenson, 2001).

The recent increases in pediatric obesity rates are part of a larger trend toward escalating weight problems in children over the last 35 years. Data available through the CDC provide a striking depiction of the developing obesity epidemic. Since the early 1970s, obesity rates among children and adolescents of all ages have risen dramatically (CDC, 2006). The largest increase was observed among children between the ages of 6 and 11; the overweight rate went from four percent to 18.8 percent—an increase of 370 percent, (CDC). Similar trends were noted among younger children (178% increase among children ages 2–5) and adolescents (185% increase among adolescents ages 12–19). A recent study by Kim et al. (2006) found that these alarming trends were seen even in infants, with a 73.5 percent increase in overweight infants observed between 1980 and 2001. The sharp rise in obesity rates shows few signs of abating, and some researchers predict that up to half of all children and adolescents in North and South America could be overweight by 2010 (Wang & Lobstein, 2006).

Ethnic and Gender Differences in Pediatric Obesity

Although obesity is on the rise among all demographic groups, prevalence rates differ across gender and ethnic groups. Results from the National Health and Nutrition Examination Survey (NHANES) indicate that non-Hispanic black female children and adolescents had the highest overweight rates and were significantly more likely to be overweight than non-Hispanic white female children and Mexican American female children (Ogden et al., 2006). This trend continues into adulthood, when non-Hispanic black women are more likely than any other subgroup to be obese. Among males, Mexican American children and adolescents had significantly higher overweight rates than non-Hispanic white and non-Hispanic black children and adolescents.

Consequences of Pediatric Obesity

The consequences of pediatric obesity are numerous, and their severity has been realized only in recent years. Serious consequences can be seen in childhood and into adulthood, including increased risk for a variety of physical and psychosocial difficulties. Studies have found that obese and overweight children are at elevated risk for type 2 diabetes, sleep apnea, arthritis, gallstones, and some types of cancer (Ravussin & Swinburn, 1992; Thompson, Edelsburg, Kinsey, & Oster, 1998; Wang & Dietz, 2002). Psychosocial costs include increased risk for negative self-concepts, lower popularity, peer victimization, and lower overall quality of life (Davison & Birch, 2001; Erickson, Robinson, Haydel, & Killen, 2000; Storch, et al., 2007; Thompson & Tantleff-Dunn, 1998; Whitaker, Wright, Pepe, Seidel, & Dietz, 1997). Overweight children are also at risk for obesity into adulthood, which in turn is associated with a number of medical and mental health risks (Freedman et al., 2001). Beyond individual consequences, the costs of the increasing prevalence of obesity to the national health care system promise to be substantial.

In light of the myriad of direct and indirect consequences of pediatric obesity for the individual and the nation, public attention and rhetoric on the subject have escalated recently. The discussion has focused on a number of important topics, including policy issues, prevention efforts, and intervention strategies. Each of these will be explored in greater detail throughout the book, but we offer an overview here as a way of framing some of the most important issues.

Policy Issues

Much of the public discourse about obesity has focused on the role of policy in the current epidemic. Policy issues at the local, state, and national levels have come under scrutiny, and policy changes at the various levels have been proposed to counter the growing obesity problem. At the local level, school lunch options, recess time, and funding for community parks and recreation are often among the topics of debate. At the state level, requirements for physical education and health education are relevant to pediatric obesity (American Academy of Pediatrics Committee on Sports Medicine and Fitness and Committee on School Health, 2000). Nationally, dietary guidelines and physical activity recommendations have been put forth to encourage healthier behaviors among children and adolescents (United States Department of Agriculture, 2005). While there is little agreement among policy-makers and stakeholders on exactly what measures should be taken to curb pediatric weight problems, there is a building consensus that action must be taken and that policy shifts will be an important part of the solution.

Related to the discussion of public policy is the recent focus on the role of American culture in promoting and maintaining unhealthy behaviors. Most pertinent to the obesity epidemic is the notion of a national culture that promotes unhealthy eating behaviors and a largely sedentary lifestyle (Nelson, Neumark-Stzainer, Hannan, Sirard, & Story, 2006). Food manufacturers and fast-food companies have come under increasing political and economic pressures to offer "healthy alternatives" and to reduce the use of unhealthy substances (e.g., trans fats) in their products (Food and Drug Administration, 2003). Similarly, the sedentary lifestyle of many Americans has been cited as a major contributor to obesity, and initiatives to foster a culture of activity have emerged (American Academy of Pediatrics Council on Sports Medicine and Fitness and Council on School Health, 2006).

The ubiquity of unhealthy options in our communities demonstrates the challenge of promoting healthy behaviors in American society. Providing a fitting metaphor for the degree to which convenient yet unhealthy options are integrated into the nation's cultural and economic fabric, *The New York Times* (Santora, 2004) observed that even many of the premier hospitals in the United States have fast-food franchises in their cafeterias. The juxtaposition of healthy ideals and less-than-healthy realities is not limited to hospitals but can also be seen in countless schools across the country. While children may learn the benefits of a healthy diet and vigorous exercise in health class, they often walk out of the classroom only to be confronted with vending machines selling high-sugar soft drinks and recess periods that have been shortened to make way for mandatory test preparation (American Academy of Pediatrics Committee on School Health, 2004; American Academy of Pediatrics Council on Sports Medicine and Fitness and Council on School Health, 2006). The common mixed messages presented to children and adolescents about diet and activity are a target for many reform efforts.

Prevention

As the need for broad measures to address the pediatric obesity epidemic has been recognized, significant attention has been focused on ways to prevent weight problems among children. Although genetics may play a substantial role in many cases of obesity, much can be done in the way of prevention by changing individual behaviors (e.g., diet and exercise) (American Academy of Pediatrics Committee on Nutrition, 2003). Prevention programs may target obesigenic behaviors and aim to facilitate lifelong healthy habits. To date, a majority of such programs have been offered in school settings with the goals of increasing children's physical activity, decreasing sedentary behavior, and improving dietary habits. These efforts have had mixed results.

Beyond more individualistic prevention approaches, prevention efforts are emerging in broader socioecological contexts. Most notable are the recent changes in the public policy and corporate policy arenas that have led to changes in some school breakfast and lunch menus as well as changes in marketing strategies vis-à-vis processed food and fast-food products. These larger contexts of change may reflect a cultural shift toward healthier behaviors spurred on by increasing awareness of the health risks associated with overweight and obesity.

Whether these changes will result in a reversal of current trends in pediatric overweight is not known. Given the scope of the current problem, preventionists will be challenged to be forward-thinking in developing efforts to overcome obstacles to optimal health. Historically, prevention efforts in the United States have often been neglected in favor of later treatment; however, the current epidemic will require a substantial shift toward preventative efforts (American Academy of Pediatrics Committee on Nutrition, 2003).

Intervention

While the need for obesity prevention is clear, intervention will be necessary for the millions of children and adolescents who are already overweight and the millions more who will develop weight problems in the coming years. Fortunately, the treatment of pediatric obesity is a growing area of research, and much important work has already been done (Black & Young-Hyman, 2007). Interventions often employ behavioral or cognitive-behavioral approaches to bring about behavior change with a specific focus on changing diet and exercise habits. Recognizing the role of the family in children's and adolescents' habit formation, many intervention programs incorporate family elements and attempt to use parents as role models for positive behavior change (Germann, Kirschenbaum, & Rich, 2007; Johnston & Steele, 2007).

A plethora of laboratory-based (i.e., efficacy) studies have been conducted, identifying promising intervention strategies for addressing weight problems in children (Becque, Katch, Rocchini, Marks, & Moorhead, 1988; Epstein, Valoski, Kalarchian & McCurley, 1995; Holtz, Smith & Winters, 1999). Fewer examinations of such treatments in "real-world" settings (i.e., effectiveness studies) have been completed (Jelalian, Wember, Bungeroth & Birmaher, 2007); however, such investigations are beginning to emerge in the literature (Johnston & Steele, 2007). Similar to other areas of child treatment, the next step for pediatric obesity intervention research will be to demonstrate effectiveness in typical clinical settings and disseminate effective programs widely (see Clinical Treatment and Services Research Workgroup, 1999 for discussion of efficacy, effectiveness, and dissemination research).

About This Volume

While the statistics describing the pediatric obesity epidemic are sobering, they do not fully convey the costs—physical, psychological, and economic—associated with this problem. Likewise, estimates of prevalence fail to capture the challenges of attempting to reverse these alarming trends. The problem, however, has not gone unnoticed and important research into the causes, correlates, and treatment of pediatric obesity is available. This handbook aims to concisely present relevant parts of that literature and contribute to the discussion about weight problems in children. Furthermore, we hope this volume will encourage further research aimed at addressing the rising pediatric obesity epidemic.

Toward this end, the volume is divided into six sections. The first provides an overview of the prevalence, correlates, and consequences of pediatric obesity, including current and long-term secondary health conditions and associated mental health conditions. Of particular use to policy-makers, administrators, and public health professionals, this section lays the foundation for the scope of the problem as well as the areas of functioning that obesity affects.

The second section focuses on assessment issues related to the onset and maintenance of pediatric obesity. The chapters specifically address definitions and measurement of obesity in children (with particular attention to how these differ from those of adults) as well as assessment of children's and adolescents' dietary practices and eating attitudes and behaviors. We see these chapters as being of particular practical importance to health care providers, educators, and prevention specialists. However, in addition to the practical aspects of this section, the chapters speak to measurement issues that will facilitate further research on evidence-based therapies for children and youths with weight management issues.

Building on appropriate assessment techniques, the third section examines factors that pose specific risks for the development of obesity in children. Of particular interest are chapters that focus on the interaction of physiological and genetic factors with environmental components. Because children from lower-income groups tend to be at increased risk for obesity, Chapter 9 (Goodman) specifically addresses socioeconomic risks for childhood obesity.

Getting to the heart of efforts to curb the growing epidemic, the fourth and fifth sections specifically address issues related to prevention and intervention. They cover practices and programs that have demonstrated efficacy/effectiveness in addressing pediatric overweight. Of particular note, chapters in these sections highlight specific variables that may affect the degree to which interventions are accepted by diverse samples as well as intervention and prevention efforts aimed at various levels of implementation (e.g., home, school, community). A chapter on how public policy has affected obesity brings a public health perspective to the obesity problem and provides a window into how intervention and prevention programs may be incorporated into the social structures of children and adolescents.

The handbook concludes with a section on future directions in pediatric obesity research and practice. Chapters examining innovative or emerging treatment techniques will provide clinicians with novel approaches for their clients and will provide researchers with directions for further study. Overall, the volume provides a comprehensive overview of the multidimensional and complex nature of pediatric obesity, with attention to evaluation, psychosocial and medical correlates, prevention, and intervention strategies; it has information relevant for clinicians, policy-makers, and researchers alike. Specifically, we anticipate that the volume will provide an up-to-date and concise synthesis of rapidly growing prevention and intervention literatures, allowing clinicians to place their practices on a strong research base and policy-makers to move beyond rhetoric and toward evidence-informed decisions in the larger socioecological systems. Further, we expect that the volume will be useful to researchers in identifying important directions for future study while placing new investigations within the context of what we already know about pediatric obesity.

CONCLUSION

The prevalence of pediatric obesity has increased tremendously over the past two decades across all demographic groups and ages. As a result, health-related conditions once thought of as "adult diseases" are becoming more prevalent in children and adolescents, and psychosocial sequelae for children and youths continue to be identified. As detailed throughout this volume, no single factor is responsible for the growing epidemic and the resulting health and mental health consequences; a number of factors at a variety of socioecological levels have contributed independently and in concert with other factors. Solutions to the nation's pediatric obesity epidemic must be similarly multifaceted. This volume is offered with the hope of bringing together clinicians, educators, researchers, administrators, and policy-makers to create such solutions.

REFERENCES

American Academy of Pediatrics Committee on Nutrition. (2003). Prevention of pediatric overweight and obesity. *Pediatrics, 112*, 424–430.

American Academy of Pediatrics Committee on School Health. (2004). Soft drinks in schools. *Pediatrics, 113*, 152–154.

American Academy of Pediatrics Committee on Sports Medicine and Fitness and Committee on School Health. (2000). Physical fitness and activity in schools. *Pediatrics, 105*, 1156–1157.

American Academy of Pediatrics Council on Sports Medicine and Fitness and Council on School Health. (2006). Active healthy living: Prevention of childhood obesity through increased physical activity. *Pediatrics, 117*, 1834–1842.

American Medical Association. (2007). Expert committee recommendations on the assessment, prevention, and treatment of child and adolescent overweight and obesity. Retrieved June 24, 2007 from http://www.ama-assn.org/ama1/pub/upload/mm/433/ped_obesity_recs.pdf

Becque, M. D., Katch, V. L., Rocchini, A. P., Marks, C. R., & Moorhead, C. (1988). Coronary risk incidence of obese adolescents: Reduction by exercise plus diet intervention. *Pediatrics, 81*, 605–612.

Black, M. M., & Young-Hyman, D. (2007). Introduction to the special issue: Pediatric overweight. *Journal of Pediatric Psychology, 32*, 1–5.

Centers for Disease Control and Prevention. (2006). National health and nutrition examination survey: Childhood overweight. Retrieved February 10, 2007, from http://www.cdc.gov/nccdphp/dnpa/obesity/childhood/index.htm.

Clinical Treatment and Services Research Workgroup (CTSRW). (1999). *Bridging science and service: A report by the National Advisory Mental Health Council's clinical treatment and services research workgroup* (NIH Publication #99-4353). Bethesda, MD: National Institutes of Health, National Institute of Mental Health.

Davison, K. K., & Birch, L. L. (2001). Weight status, parent reaction, and self-concept in five-year-old girls. *Pediatrics, 107*, 46–53.

Epstein, L. H., Valoski, A. M., Kalarchian, M. A., & McCurley, J. (1995). Do children lose and maintain weight easier than adults: A comparison of child and parent weight changes from six to ten years. *Obesity Research, 3*, 411–417.

Erickson, S. J., Robinson, T. N., Haydel, K. F., & Killen, J. D. (2000). Are overweight children unhappy? Body mass index, depressive symptoms, and overweight concerns in elementary school children. *Archives of Pediatric and Adolescent Medicine, 154*, 931–935.

Food and Drug Administration. (2003). FDA acts to provide better information to consumers on trans fats. Retrieved February 12, 2007, from http://www.fda.gov/oc/initiatives/transfat/backgrounder.html.

Freedman, D. S., Khan, L. K., Dietz, W. H., Srinivasan, S. R., & Berenson, G. S. (2001). Relationship of childhood overweight to coronary heart disease risk factors in adulthood: The Bogalusa heart study. *Pediatrics, 108*, 712–718.

Germann, J. N., Kirschenbaum, D. S., & Rich, B. H. (2007). Child and parental self-monitoring as determinants of success in the treatment of morbid obesity in low-income minority children. *Journal of Pediatric Psychology, 32*, 52–63.

Holtz, C., Smith, T. M., & Winters, F. D. (1999). Childhood obesity. *Journal of the American Osteopathic Association, 99*, 366–371.

Jelalian, E., Wember, Y. M., Bungeroth, H., & Birmaher, V. (2007). Practitioner review: Bridging the gap between research and clinical practice in pediatric obesity. *Journal of Child Psychology and Psychiatry, 48*, 115–127.

Johnston, C. A., & Steele, R. G. (2007). Treatment of pediatric overweight: An examination of feasibility and effectiveness in an applied clinical setting. *Journal of Pediatric Psychology, 32*, 106–110.

Kim, J., Peterson, K. E., Scanlon, K. S., Fitzmaurice, G. M., Must, A., Oken, E., et al. (2006). Trends in overweight from 1980 through 2001 among preschool-aged children enrolled in a health maintenance organization. *Obesity, 14*, 1107–1112.

Nelson, M. C., Neumark-Stzainer, D., Hannan, P. J., Sirard, J. R., & Story, M. (2006). Longitudinal and secular trends in physical activity and sedentary behavior during adolescence. *Pediatrics, 118*, e1627–e1634.

Ogden, C. L., Carroll, M. D., Curtin, L. R., McDowell, M. A., Tabak, C. J., & Flegal, K. M. (2006). Prevalence of overweight and obesity in the United States, 1999–2004. *Journal of the American Medical Association, 295*, 1549–1555.

Ravussin, E., & Swinburn, B. A. (1992). Pathophysiology of obesity. *Lancet, 340*, 404–408.

Santora, M. (2004, October 26). Burgers for the health professional. *The New York Times*. Retrieved on February 11, 2007, from http://www.nytimes.com/2004/10/26/nyregion/26fast.html.

Storch, E. A., Milsom, V. A., DeBraganza, N., Lewin, A. B., Geffken, G. R., Silverstein, J. H. (2007). Peer victimization, psychosocial adjustment, and physical activity in overweight and at-risk-for-overweight youth. *Journal of Pediatric Psychology, 32*, 80–89.

Thompson, D., Edelsberg, J., Kinsey, K. L., & Oster, G. (1998). Estimated economic costs of obesity to U.S. business. *American Journal of Health Promotion, 13*, 120–127.

Thompson, J. K., & Tantleff-Dunn, S. (1998). Assessment of body image disturbance in obesity. *Obesity Research, 6*, 375–377.

United States Department of Agriculture. (2005). Dietary guidelines for Americans. Retrieved February 12, 2007, from http://www.ncypyramiel.gov/guidelines/index.html.

Wang, G., & Dietz, W. H. (2002). Economic burden of obesity in youths aged 6 to 17 years: 1979–1999. *Pediatrics, 109*, E81.

Wang, Y., & Lobstein, T. (2006). Worldwide trends in childhood overweight and obesity. *International Journal of Pediatric Obesity, 1*, 11–25.

Whitaker, R. C., Wright, J. A., Pepe, M. S., Seidel, K. D., & Dietz, W. H. (1997). Predicting obesity in young adulthood from childhood and parental obesity. *New England Journal of Medicine, 337*, 869–873.

2

Health Consequences of Obesity in Children and Adolescents

PATRICK VIVIER and CHRISTINE TOMPKINS

As discussed in Chapter 1, obesity has become a highly prevalent problem among children and adolescents. This is a major public health crisis, as obesity in childhood and adolescence can have a range of negative health consequences, including heart disease, diabetes, breathing difficulty and orthopedic complications. While the burdens of obesity-related morbidity and mortality may not be fully evident until adulthood, the health burdens of obesity are more often being diagnosed during childhood and adolescence. In this chapter we review the range of health consequences of childhood and adolescent obesity, focusing on the major manifestations.

We begin with a brief review of the health burdens associated with adult obesity and then examine the extent to which overweight children become overweight adults. As will be discussed below, the health burdens of adult obesity are substantial. Therefore, the link between being overweight as a child or adolescent and being obese as an adult is critical. If a large proportion of the children who are currently overweight become obese adults, the public health consequences will be considerable. This link alone should be enough to motivate health care providers and public health officials to undertake the prevention and treatment approaches outlined in subsequent chapters. While the consequences for adults should be sufficient to lead to a focus on childhood obesity, as will be detailed in the remainder of this chapter, we do not have to wait for adulthood to see the toll of childhood and adolescent obesity.

PATRICK VIVIER and CHRISTINE TOMPKINS • Brown University, Providence, RI 02912.

The Health Consequences of Adult Obesity, and Do They Pertain to Children?

The health consequences of adult obesity have been well-established. Obese adults are at greater risk for a range of morbidities, including type 2 diabetes mellitus, stroke, osteoarthritis, some cancers and cardiovascular disease as well as cardiovascular disease risk factors such as dyslipidemia and hypertension (Must et al., 1999). For a number of these conditions, the more obese the patient, the greater the risk of morbidity. Therefore, what matters is not just whether the adult is obese but how obese the adult is. For example, using a referent group of normal-weight (Body Mass Index [BMI] 18.5–24.9) women, Must et al. found the prevalence ratios of high blood pressure for women under 55 were 1.65 for overweight women (BMI 25–29.9), 3.22 for women in the Class 1 obesity category (BMI 30–34.9), 3.9 for women in the Class 2 obesity category (BMI 35–39.9) and 5.45 for women in the Class 3 obesity category (BMI greater than or equal to 40) (Must et al.).

In addition to experiencing greater morbidity, obese adults also have a substantially greater risk of mortality (Hu et al., 2004; Manson et al., 1995). Using data from the Nurses' Health Study, Hu et al. found that compared with those who were lean and physically active, women who were obese and active were at nearly twice the risk for death (1.91 multivariate relative risk of death) and those who were obese and inactive were at more than twice the risk (multivariate relative risk of 2.42). In their analysis of data from the National Health and Nutrition Examination Survey, Fontaine, Redden, Wang, Westfall, and Allison (2003) found that obesity markedly decreased life expectancy. This was particularly evident among white men aged 20 to 30. A 20-year-old white male with severe obesity (BMI greater than 45) was estimated to lose 13 years of life when compared with a white male of optimal weight. Taking into account that the life expectancy would be 78 years without the obesity burden, this represents a 17% reduction in total life expectancy and a 22% reduction in remaining life years (Fontaine et al.).

While the predictive data for morbidity and mortality in obese children and adolescents is emerging, a similar trend can be seen. It has been shown that children and adolescents with higher BMI (greater than 85th percentile for overweight, greater than 95th percentile for obese) are at greater risk for morbidity than their peers at lower BMI percentiles (Reilly, 2005). The Institute of Medicine report on childhood obesity made the ominous statement that obesity could potentially reverse the positive life expectancy trends that have been achieved through the control of infectious diseases (Institute of Medicine, 2005).

ᵓo Overweight Children and Adolescents Become Obese Adults?

Given the morbidity and mortality associated with adult obesity, the ᵇetween childhood obesity and adult obesity is a major concern. ᵇer of studies have found an association between childhood weight ᵓnd adult weight status (Dietz, 1998a; Freedman, Khan, et al., 2004,

2005; Guo et al., 2000; Guo, Roche, Chumlea, Gardner, & Siervogel, 1994; Power, Lake, & Cole, 1997; Togashi et al., 2002; Whitaker, Pepe, Wright, Seidel, & Dietz, 1998; Whitaker, Wright, Pepe, Seidel, & Dietz, 1997; Wright, Parker, Lamont, & Craft, 2001). For example, Power and colleagues found that childhood BMI had a "moderate prediction of adult BMI" in their analysis of 1958 birth cohort in England (Power et al.). In that study 20–30% of the variability in BMI at age 33 was explained by the BMI at age 11 or 16. Whitaker and colleagues found that adolescent obesity was a substantial risk factor for obesity in young adulthood (i.e., ages 20 to 29) (Whitaker et al.). Even after adjustments were made for parental weight status, obese adolescents had 17.5 greater odds than non-obese adolescents of becoming obese young adults. In this study adolescent obesity was a greater risk factor for obesity than obese parents.

There is variation in the extent of the association between childhood weight status and adult weight status. The association varies between studies and within studies depending on factors such as age when the child was obese, race/ethnicity, gender, and extent of the childhood weight problem. For example, in the Whitaker study discussed above, while adolescent obesity was associated with greatly increased odds of adult obesity, this was not the case for obesity in early childhood. Children who were obese at age 1 or 2 had 1.3 greater odds (95% Confidence Interval (CI) : 0.6–3.) of becoming obese as young adults (Whitaker et al., 1998). Thus, early childhood obesity was not an important predictor of adult obesity.

While there is variation in study findings, it is clear that being obese, particularly in adolescence, puts a child at risk for becoming an obese adult. Further, it has been established that childhood weight status is associated with adult morbidity and mortality (Dietz, 1998a, 1998b; Must, 1996; Wright et al., 2001). In a long-term follow-up of the Third Harvard Growth Study, researchers found that being overweight as an adolescent led to an increased rate of diabetes, coronary heart disease, atherosclerosis, hip fracture and gout in adulthood (Dietz, 1998b). For males, being overweight as an adolescent was not only a risk factor for a range of morbidities but also a significant risk factor for adult mortality. The research that established the associations between childhood weight status, adult weight status and adult morbidity/mortality was largely undertaken before the major increase in the prevalence of childhood overweight. If these associations hold, the public health implications will be substantial.

In the remainder of this chapter we examine specific conditions associated with childhood obesity. It is no longer necessary to wait until overweight children enter adulthood to measure the impact of obesity on their health. As will be discussed, a range of obesity-related conditions are now being manifest during the pediatric years.

Cardiovascular Disease and Related Factors

It is clear that obesity during childhood and adolescence has important negative consequences for cardiovascular health (Dietz, 1998a, 1998b; Ebbeling,

Pawlak, & Ludwig, 2002; Must, 1996; Reilly et al., 2003). Specifically, childhood/adolescent obesity is associated with hypertension, dyslipidemia and abnormalities of the coronary arteries. The obesity-related cardiovascular abnormalities have important implications during both childhood and adulthood.

Atherosclerotic changes can be detected in the aorta among children by age 3, with changes noted in coronary arteries by ages 8 to 13 (Freedman, 2002). Obesity is a major risk factor in the development of atherosclerotic lesions. Strong evidence for this being the case in children and adolescents, along with adults, comes from the Bogalusa Heart Study. This is a long-term study of cardiovascular risk factors from birth through 38 years of age in Louisiana. As part of the study, autopsies were performed on young people who died of any cause during the study period. The researchers examined autopsy results for 204 deaths among young people (mean ages in early 20s). A majority of the deaths were caused by accidents or homicides. The researchers wrote, "The extent of atherosclerotic lesions correlated positively and significantly with body-mass index" (Berenson et al., 1998, p. 1652). Conditions known to be associated with childhood/adolescent obesity, such as hypertension and dyslipidemia, were also correlated with atherosclerotic lesions.

Another autopsy study of young people (ages 15 to 34), this one by McGill et al. (2000) also supports the link between obesity and atherosclerotic lesions. As in the Berenson study, obesity-related factors, dyslipidemia and hypertension were also associated with atherosclerotic lesions. A third autopsy study performed on 40 teenagers, aged 13 to 19, found that both visceral fat and age-adjusted waist circumference were associated with intima thickness of the left anterior descending artery; however, there was not an association with BMI (Kortelainen & Sarkioja, 2001).

Imaging studies also provide support for the impact of childhood/adolescent obesity on atherosclerotic changes (Freedman et al., 2004; Oren et al., 2003; Tounian et al., 2001; Woo et al., 2004). The studies have demonstrated that childhood obesity has negative vascular effects, such as intima-media thickness of the carotid artery, arterial wall stiffness, and endothelial dysfunction. These consequences are measurable during the pediatric and adult age periods.

Hypertension is another important cardiovascular disease risk factor associated with childhood/adolescent obesity (Dietz, 1998b; Must, 1996; Must et al., 1999; Reilly et al., 2003). In the Minneapolis Children's Blood Pressure Study, Sinaiko, Donahue, Jacobs, and Prineas (1999) found that initial childhood BMI and increases in BMI during childhood were significantly related to systolic blood pressure in young adulthood. In the Bogalusa Heart Study, adolescent-onset overweight showed adverse effects on systolic and diastolic blood pressure during young adulthood (Srinivasan, Bao, Wattigney, & Berenson, 1996). In addition to leading to a risk of adult hypertension, overweight has a measurable impact on blood pressure during childhood and adolescence. The impact of being overweight on children and adolescents has been demonstrated in a number of studies (Li et al., 2005; Lurbe et al., 1998; Reich et al., 2003; Ribeiro et al., 2005). The effect may be reversible with diet, exercise and weight loss (Ribeiro et al.).

Dyslipidemia is another critical cardiovascular risk factor that is worsened when a person is overweight (Dietz, 1998a, 1998b; Freedman et al., 2004; Garces et al., 2005; Must et al., 1999; Reilly et al., 2003). As with blood pressure changes, the changes in lipid profiles raise concerns about cardiovascular health in both pediatric and adult ages. There is also evidence that diet and exercise can help reverse dyslipidemia (Sung et al., 2002).

In summary, childhood and adolescent obesity has adverse effects on cardiovascular health. These include dyslipidemia, elevated blood pressure and cardiovascular lesions. The negative cardiovascular impact of being overweight is evident during childhood and adolescence. The impact is even more severe in adulthood, particularly when obesity persists. There is encouraging evidence that improvements in diet and exercise can be effective at reversing cardiovascular morbidity.

Type 2 Diabetes Mellitus and Related Conditions

Perhaps the most distressing aspect of the dramatic rise in childhood and adolescent obesity has been the accompanying increase in the prevalence of insulin resistance and type 2 diabetes mellitus, also known as non-insulin-dependent diabetes mellitus (Young, Dean, Flett, & Wood-Steiman, 2000). Once thought of as "adult-onset," diabetes this disease has increased dramatically among children and adolescents (Ludwig & Ebbeling, 2001; Pinhas-Hamiel & Zeitler, 2000; Pontiroli, 2004; Rocchini, 2002; Wei et al., 2003). In some areas, type 2 diabetes is becoming or already is the most common form of diabetes among children or adolescents. This dramatic increase in the prevalence of type 2 diabetes, and the occurrence earlier in life, is alarming.

While the exact mechanism of insulin resistance is unknown, it is thought that obesity, along with other diabetes risk factors, leads to insulin resistance (Daniels, 2006; Ludwig & Ebbeling, 2001). Essentially, as the body's cells become more resistant to insulin, the body tries to over-compensate by producing more insulin. In time, this elevated state of insulin production causes stress on the pancreatic cells, and the body's need for insulin is no longer met. Eventually, glucose levels are no longer normal. Glucose abnormalities usually manifest initially as postprandial (i.e., post-meal) hyperglycemia, but eventually the ability to maintain even fasting glucose levels is impaired. This resultant hyperglycemia and abnormal glucose metabolism result in the diagnosis of type 2 diabetes mellitus.

Important long-term complications of type 2 diabetes include vascular disease that can lead to heart attacks, strokes, kidney disease and failure, blindness, and other health problems. In addition, the hyperinsulinemia associated with type 2 diabetes has been shown to be an independent risk factor for heart disease.

The link between obesity and the development of type 2 diabetes has been clearly demonstrated, including associations with hyperinsulinemia, postprandial hyperglycemia and fasting hyperglycemia (Artz, Haqq, &

Freemark, 2005; Ludwig & Ebbeling, 2001; Misra et al., 2004; Plourde, 2002; Wei et al., 2003). Obesity has also been found to put adolescents at risk for the metabolic syndrome, a combination of obesity, impaired glucose control, dyslipidemia and hypertension (Cook, Weitzman, Auinger, Nguyen, & Dietz, 2003; Ferreira, Twisk, van Mechelen, Kemper, & Stehouwer, 2005; Weiss et al., 2004).

The risks of adult morbidity and mortality from type 2 diabetes are substantial. It has been estimated that men diagnosed with diabetes mellitus at age 40 will lose 11.6 life years and 18.6 quality-adjusted life years (Narayan, Boyle, Thompson, Sorensen, & Williamson, 2003). It has been estimated that a woman diagnosed at the same age will lose 14.3 life years and 22 quality-adjusted life years. How much life will be lost because of the rapidly rising rates of diabetes mellitus among adolescents?

Psychosocial Consequences and Quality of Life

While this topic is discussed elsewhere in this book, its importance cannot be overstated, and it will be discussed briefly here. There has been some controversy regarding the psychological impact of childhood obesity. A substantial number of studies have been undertaken to assess specific psychological issues. The range of methodologies and differences in outcomes of the studies make it difficult to draw simple conclusions about childhood/adolescent obesity and psychological well-being. However, there are enough studies demonstrating the association between obesity and psychological consequences to raise substantial concerns. In their systematic review of the health consequences of childhood obesity, Reilly and colleagues (2003) concluded, "Obese children *are* more likely to experience psychological or psychiatric problems than non-obese children" (Reilly et al., 2003, pp. 748–749). They found that girls were at greater risk (compared to boys) for psychological morbidity and that the risk increased with age (Reilly et al.). Further, the Institute of Medicine report concluded, "Young people are also at risk of developing serious psychosocial burdens related to being obese" (Institute of Medicine, 2005, p. 2).

An important factor in the psychosocial impact of obesity on young people appears to be related to stigmatization (Schwartz & Puhl, 2003). As has been demonstrated in a number of studies, children are less inclined to look favorably on obese peers (Brylinsky & Moore, 1994; Cramer & Steinwert, 1998; Kraig & Keel, 2001; Latner & Stunkard, 2003; Richardson, Goodman, Hastorf, & Dornbusch, 1961; Schwartz & Puhl, 2003). It appears that negative perceptions of children who are overweight begin early in life. Researchers have demonstrated that even preschool children have negative views of overweight children (Cramer & Steinwert, 1998). Making matters worse, some adults, including high school teachers, hold negative views of overweight children (Neumark-Sztainer, Story, & Harris, 1999).

Given the nature of psychosocial issues and quality of life, combined with complexities in the research methodologies employed to assess them, it is difficult to briefly summarize the consequences of childhood/adolescent obesity in these areas. A substantial number of studies make clear that obesity has a negative impact on children and adolescents that goes well beyond physiologic derangements. Further, these negative effects can extend into adulthood.

Orthopedic Complications

Being overweight can stress the skeletal system at any age, but children have the additional vulnerability of skeletal systems that are growing. The immature skeletal system, in particular the open growth plates and more cartilaginous bones, combined with the added weight puts overweight children at risk for orthopedic problems (Dietz, 1998b; Must & Strauss, 1999). For young children, the pressure on their leg bones from their excess weight can cause bowing of the tibia and femur, "analogous to the bowing that occurs when downward pressure is exerted on a flexible stick" (Dietz, p. 522). Blount's disease, a combination of bowing of the tibia and overgrowth of the medial aspect of the tibia, is one of the resulting conditions. Approximately two-thirds of patients with Blount's disease are obese (Dietz, 1998b). Blount's disease, in particular late-onset Blount's disease (children age 4 or older), can require surgical correction (Behrman, Liegman, & Jenson, 2000).

Another important complication of obesity in the pediatric age group is slipped capital femoral epiphysis, when the top of the femur separates at the growth plate. It can be a very serious condition requiring surgical correction and can have long-term complications. Obesity is a significant risk factor for slipped capital femoral epiphysis. It has been postulated that obesity is a risk factor because of the increased pressure at the growth plate from the extra weight (Dietz, 1998b). Another theory is that the condition is related to changes in sex hormone levels among obese adolescents (Behrman et al., 2000). Regardless of the etiology, obesity is an important risk factor.

Additional orthopedic problems, such as structural or pressure patterns in the foot, may also accompany childhood/adolescent obesity (Dowling, Steele, & Baur, 2001, 2004; Riddiford-Harland, Steele, & Storlien, 2000). In addition, obesity may interfere with recovery from orthopedic injuries. Timm, Grupp-Phelan, and Ho (2005) studied patients between 8 and 18 years who went to emergency departments with ankle sprains. They found that children with a BMI greater than or equal to the 85th percentile were more likely to have persistent symptoms six months after their acute injuries. Obese children may also be at greater risk of complications following a leg fracture (Leet, Pichard, & Ain, 2005).

Pulmonary Complications and Breathing Disorders

One of the primary pulmonary conditions that affect the pediatric population is asthma. Asthma is a chronic illness that has potentially life-threatening consequences. Asthma—and its symptoms of coughing and wheezing—is produced by a chronic inflammatory process that entails airway constriction, smooth muscle hypertrophy, and mucous production.

While the cause is unclear, asthma has a higher prevalence in overweight and obese children (Lazarus, Colditz, Berkey, & Speizer, 1997; Li et al., 2003; Must, 1996). Rodriguez, Winkelby, Ahn, Sundquist, and Kraemer (2002) found that children with a BMI greater than the 85th percentile had an increased risk of asthma independent of socioeconomic status, age, sex, ethnicity, and tobacco smoke exposure. Possible causes for increased rates of asthma in overweight and obese children fall into both cause and effect categories. That is, asthma potentially causes children to have decreased physical activity because of difficulty breathing, which may contribute to overweight or obesity. Likewise, one of the treatments for asthma (e.g., oral corticosteroids) is known to have the side effect of weight gain. Asthma may also be an effect of overweight or obesity because of the known presence of chronic inflammation in those with a higher BMI. Whatever the reason, the prevalence and severity of childhood asthma have paralleled the dramatic increase in childhood and adolescent obesity in the last 20 years (Daniels, 2006).

Obstructive sleep apnea is also a concern for obese children and adolescents (Must & Strauss, 1999; Wing et al., 2003). Sleep apnea involves either a lack of effective breathing at nighttime or a lack of breathing altogether. While patients with obstructive sleep apnea tend to snore, sleep apnea is different from simple snoring in that there is usually an accompanying decrease in oxygen saturation. The body responds to this hypoventilation by periodically "waking the brain up" in order to correct the hypoventilation. This results in markedly disordered sleep and daytime sleepiness. There is some evidence that in addition to affecting sleep in obese children, obstructive sleep apnea may have a negative effect on learning and memory (Must & Strauss). If persistent and left untreated, the Pickwickian syndrome—a combination of severe obesity, hypoven tilation, somnolence, polycythemia, right ventricular hypertrophy and eventually heart failure—may develop and can have devastating effects (Must & Strauss).

Other Conditions

A range of other conditions have been associated with obesity beginning in childhood or adolescence. These include neurological problems, specifically pseudotumor cerebri, a condition of increased intracranial pressure (Dietz, 1998b). The symptoms include headaches and visual impairment. In its most severe form it can lead to blindness. Liver abnormalities have also been noted, with obese children being at risk for liver steatosis (Chan et al., 2004; Guzzaloni, Grugni, Minocci, Moro, & Morabito, 2000; Marion, Baker, & Dhawan, 2004). Gallbladder disease is another potential complication of childhood/adolescent obesity (Must & Strauss, 1999). Hematology-related complications have also been suggested. Researchers have found a greater prevalence of iron deficiency and greater treatment-associated complications for overweight children with acute myeloid leukemia compared to children of normal weight (Lange et al., 2005; Pinhas-Hamiel et al., 2003). Gynecologic problems have been reported as well (Dietz; Neville, & Walker, 2005), as have developmental issues, such as poorer gross motor development and endurance performance (Wang & Dietz, 2002).

Health Care Costs

While we have focused on the health consequences of childhood and adolescent obesity, we should at least mention that substantial economic burdens are associated with the obesity epidemic, for both the pediatric and adult age groups. Wang and Dietz (2002) examined the economic costs of obesity-associated diseases in patients ages 6 to 17 by assessing the National Hospital Discharge Survey, 1979–1999 (Wang & Dietz). They found that hospital costs for obesity-associated problems increased from $35 million during 1979–1981 to $127 million during 1997–1999, a threefold increase. Obesity-related conditions among adults have also led to substantial health care costs (Finkelstein, Fiebelkorn, & Wang, 2003; Thorpe, Florence, Howard, & Joski, 2004).

When examining health care costs, one must always consider the indirect costs in addition to the direct costs outlined above. In children and adolescents, it is difficult to measure the indirect costs. In general, indirect costs are measured by premature death, loss of productivity, absenteeism, sick leave, and disability (Lobstein, Baur, & Uauy, 2004). Many of these do not directly apply to children and have thus been difficult to study in children and adolescents. However, with more children being diagnosed as overweight or obese, and being diagnosed at earlier ages, it is not difficult to see how these "indirect costs" will be affected as these children become adults. It is clear that treating obesity-related conditions is a major cost to the health care system, and that cost is growing rapidly.

Treatment and Prevention

The most vital tool in the prevention and treatment of overweight and obesity is their recognition by the primary care provider. If children and adolescents are not properly "diagnosed" as overweight or obese, little can be done to prevent further consequences. The Centers for Disease Control and Prevention (CDC) produced BMI growth charts in 2000, and using these is the most objective way for primary care providers to diagnose overweight and obesity in children and adolescents. Although there is some controversy about using these BMI charts in the diagnosis of obesity, the International Obesity Taskforce considers them reasonable measures of adiposity (Dietz & Robinson, 1998). Children who are at or above 85% for their age on the BMI chart should be regarded as overweight, while children above 95% for their age should be regarded as obese.

After the appropriate diagnosis of overweight or obesity has been made, it is essential to look for the presence of obesity-related diseases (Caprio, 2006). These include the conditions addressed above: hypertension, dyslipidemia, insulin resistance and diabetes, sleep apnea, psychological effects, etc. If present, these secondary diseases should be treated by the primary care physician, or a referral to the appropriate subspecialist should be made.

Identifying overweight and obesity and treating their secondary medical consequences, however, will not end the current public health crisis. It is vitally important that all primary care providers feel comfortable adequately addressing overweight and obesity *prevention* with *all* of their patients. Prevention should address both diet and physical activity. Intensive discussions regarding food preparation, portion size, calorie content, fast food, and soda and juice intake are vital. Further, it is important that the primary care provider discuss behaviors involving eating and mealtime: Do the provider's patients eat while watching the television? Do other distractions to prevent the patients from focusing on their meals and, specifically, their intakes?

Physical activity recommendations should place a priority on routine daily activity outside school as well as reduction in sedentary behaviors such as playing video games and watching television (Robinson, 1999). While exercise has not been shown to significantly affect BMI without concurrent dietary modification, it is nonetheless an important piece of the overweight and obesity puzzle. Recommendations for dietary modification and physical activity should be given to the entire family; it is rare that the child or adolescent is the only family member affected by overweight or obesity.

While several medications and surgical options are specifically geared toward weight reduction, few recommendations guide treatment for children and adolescents (Caprio, 2006). There may be a place for obesity medication and surgery for those with severe medical complications, but it is beyond the scope of this chapter.

SUMMARY

The health consequences of obesity in childhood and adolescence are substantial, affecting multiple organ systems. These health consequences can manifest themselves in childhood, adolescence or adulthood. We are already seeing the effects of the obesity epidemic on morbidity and mortality.

The overweight and obesity epidemic presents a large challenge for health care providers, who are now partially responsible for its remedy. If a reversal of the current trend does not take place soon, devastating effects on our nation's public health will intensify. These include reduction in life expectancy, the presence of more severe and chronic illness, and a tremendous amount of health care expenditures for both direct and indirect costs. It is essential that our government and public health officials continue to make this a priority for our nation's people through continued support of health care providers and direct public education.

REFERENCES

Artz, E., Haqq, A., & Freemark, M. (2005). Hormonal and metabolic consequences of childhood obesity. *Endocrinology Metabolism Clinics of North America, 34,* 643–658.

Behrman, R. E., Liegman, R. M., & Jenson, H. B. (2000). *Nelson textbook of pediatrics* (16th ed.). Philadelphia: W.B. Saunders Company.

Berenson, G. S., Srinivasan, S. R., Bao, W., Newman, W. P., Tracy, R. E., & Wattigney, W. A. (1998). Association between multiple cardiovascular risk factors and atherosclerosis in children and young adults. *New England Journal of Medicine, 338*, 1650–1656.

Brylinsky, J. A., & Moore, J. C. (1994). The identification of body build stereotypes in young children. *Journal of Research in Personality, 28*, 170–181.

Caprio, S. (2006). Treating child obesity and associated medical conditions. *The Future of Children, 16*, 209–224.

Chan, D. F. Y., Li, A. M., Chu, W. C. W., Chan, M. H. M., Wong, E. M. C., Liu, E. K. H., et al. (2004). Hepatic steatosis in obese Chinese children. *International Journal of Obesity, 28*, 1257–1263.

Cook, S., Weitzman, M., Auinger, P., Nguyen, M., & Dietz, W. H. (2003). Prevalence of a metabolic syndrome phenotype in adolescents: Findings from the Third National Health and Nutrition Examination Survey, 1988–1994. *Archives of Pediatric and Adolescent Medicine, 157*, 821–827.

Cramer, P., & Steinwert, T. (1998). Thin is good, fat is bad: How early does it begin? *Journal of Applied Developmental Psychology, 19*, 429–451.

Daniels, S. R. (2006). The consequences of childhood overweight and obesity. *The Future of Children, 16*, 47–67.

Dietz, W. H. (1998a). Childhood weight affects adult morbidity and mortality. *Journal of Nutrition, 128*, 411S–414S.

Dietz, W. H. (1998b). Health consequences of obesity in youth: Childhood predictors of adult disease. *Pediatrics, 101*, 518–525.

Dietz, W. H., & Robinson, T. (1998). Use of BMI as a measure of overweight in children and adolescents. *Journal of Pediatrics, 132*, 191–193.

Dowling, A. M., Steele, J. R., & Baur, L. A. (2001). Does obesity influence foot structure and plantar pressure patterns in prepubescent children? *International Journal of Obesity, 25*, 845–852.

Dowling, A. M., Steele, J. R., & Baur, L. A. (2004). What are the effects of obesity in children on plantar pressure distributions? *International Journal of Obesity and Related Metabolic Disorders, 28*, 1514–1519.

Ebbeling, C. B., Pawlak, D. B., & Ludwig, D. S. (2002). Childhood obesity: Public-health crisis, common sense cure. *Lancet, 360*, 473–482.

Ferreira, I., Twisk, J. W. R., van Mechelen, W., Kemper, H. C. G., & Stehouwer, C. D. A. (2005). Development of fatness, fitness and lifestyle from adolescence to the age of 36 years: Determinants of the metabolic syndrome in young adults: The Amsterdam Growth and Health Longitudinal Study. *Archives of Internal Medicine, 165*, 42–48.

Finkelstein, E. A., Fiebelkorn, I. C., & Wang, G. (2003). National medical spending attributable to overweight and obesity: How much, and who's paying? *Health Affairs, 22*, 219W3–226W3.

Fontaine, K. R., Redden, D. T., Wang, C., Westfall, A. O., & Allison, D. B. (2003). Years of life lost due to obesity. *Journal of the American Medical Association, 289*, 187–193.

Freedman, D. S. (2002). Clustering of coronary heart disease risk factors among obese children. *Journal of Pediatric Endocrinology & Metabolism, 15*, 1099–1108.

Freedman, D. S., Dietz, W. H., Tang, R., Mensah, G. A., Bond, M. G., Urbina, E. M., et al. (2004). The relation of obesity throughout life to carotid intima-media thickness in adulthood: The Bogalusa Heart Study. *International Journal of Obesity, 28*, 159–166.

Freedman, D. S., Khan, L. K., Serdula, M. K., Dietz, W. H., Srinivasan, S. R., & Berenson, G. S. (2004). Inter-relationships among childhood BMI, childhood height, and adult obesity: The Bogalusa Heart Study. *International Journal of Obesity, 28*, 10–16.

Freedman, D. S., Khan, L. K., Serdula, M. K., Dietz, W. H., Srinivasan, S. R., & Berenson, G. S. (2005). Racial differences in the tracking of childhood BMI to adulthood. *Obesity Research, 13*, 928–935.

Garces, C., Gutierrez-Guisado, J., Benavente, M., Cano, B., Viturro, E., Ortega, H., et al. (2005). Obesity in Spanish schoolchildren: Relationship with lipid profile and insulin resistance. *Obesity Research, 13*, 959–963.

Guo, S. S., Huang, C., Maynard, L. M., Demerath, E., Towne, B., Chumlea, W. C., et al. (2000). Body mass index during childhood, adolescence, and young adulthood in relation to adult overweight and adiposity: The Fels longitudinal study. *International Journal of Obesity, 24*, 1628–1635.

Guo, S. S., Roche, A. F., Chumlea, W. C., Gardner, J. D., & Siervogel, R. M. (1994). The predictive value of childhood body mass index values for overweight at age 35y. *American Journal of Clinical Nutrition, 59*, 810–819.

Guzzaloni, G., Grugni, G., Minocci, A., Moro, D., & Morabito, F. (2000). Liver steatosis in juvenile obesity: Correlations with lipid profile, hepatic biochemical parameters and glycemic and insulinemic responses to an oral glucose tolerance test. *International Journal of Obesity, 24*, 772–776.

Hu, F. B., Willet, W. C., Li, T., Stampfer, M. J., Colditz, G. A., & Manson, J. E. (2004). Adiposity as compared with physical activity in predicting mortality among women. *New England Journal of Medicine, 351*, 2694–2703.

Institute of Medicine. (2005). *Preventing childhood obesity*. Washington, DC: The National Academies Press.

Kortelainen, M. L., & Sarkioja, T. (2001). Visceral fat and coronary pathology in male adolescents. *International Journal of Obesity, 25*, 228–232.

Kraig, K. A., & Keel, P. K. (2001). Weight-based stigmatization in children. *International Journal of Obesity, 25*, 1661–1666.

Lange, B. J., Gerbing, R. B., Feusner, J., Skolnik, J., Sacks, N., Smith, F. O., et al. (2005). Mortality in overweight and underweight children with acute myeloid leukemia. *Journal of the American Medical Association, 293*, 203–211.

Latner, J. D., & Stunkard, A. J. (2003). Getting worse: The stigmatization of obese children. *Obesity Research, 11*, 452–456.

Lazarus, R., Colditz, G., Berkey, C. S., & Speizer, F. E. (1997). Effects of body fat on ventilatory function in children and adolescents: Cross-sectional findings from a random population sample of school children. *Pediatric Pulmonology, 24*, 187–194.

Leet, A. I., Pichard, C. P., & Ain, M. C. (2005). Surgical treatment of femoral fractures in obese children: Does excessive body weight increase the rate of complications? *Journal of Bone and Joint Surgery, 87*, 2609–2613.

Li, A. M., Chan, D., Wong, E., Yin, J., Nelson, E. A. S., & Fok, T. F. (2003). The effects of obesity on pulmonary function. *Archives of Diseases in Children, 88*, 361–363.

Li, A. Q., Zhao, Z. I., Zhang, L. L., Lu, F. H., Yan, Z. H., Li, Y. Y., et al. (2005). Overweight influence on circadian variation of ambulatory blood pressure in Chinese adolescents. *Clinical and Experimental Hypertension, 27*, 195–201.

Lobstein, T., Baur, L., & Uauy, R. (2004). Obesity in children and young people: A crisis in public health. *Obesity Reviews, 5*, 4–85.

Ludwig, D. S., & Ebbeling, C. B. (2001). Type 2 diabetes mellitus in children: Primary care and public health considerations. *Journal of the American Medical Association, 286*, 1427–1430.

Lurbe, E., Alvarez, V., Liao, Y., Tacons, J., Cooper, R., Cremades, B., et al. (1998). The impact of obesity and body fat distribution on ambulatory blood pressure in children and adolescents. *American Journal of Hypertension, 11*, 418–424.

Manson, J. E., Willett, W. C., Stampfer, M. J., Colditz, G. A., Hunter, D. J., Hankinson, S. E., et al. (1995). Body weight and mortality among women. *New England Journal of Medicine, 333*, 677–685.

Marion, A. W., Baker, A. J., & Dhawan, A. (2004). Fatty liver disease in children. *Archives of Disease in Childhood, 89*, 648–652.

McGill, H. C., McMahan, A., Zieske, A. W., Sloop, G. D., Walcott, J. V., Troxclair, D. A., et al. (2000). Associations of coronary heart disease risk factors with the intermediate lesion of atherosclerosis in youth: The Pathobiological Determinants of Atherosclerosis in Youth (PDAY) Research Group. *Arteriosclerosis, Thrombosis, and Vascular Biology, 20*, 1998–2004.

Misra, A., Vikram, N. K., Arya, S., Pandey, R. M., Dhingra, V., Chatterjee, A., et al. (2004). High prevalence of insulin resistance in postpubertal Asian Indian children is associated with adverse truncal body fat patterning, abdominal adiposity and excess body fat. *International Journal of Obesity, 28*, 1217–1226.

Must, A. (1996). Morbidity and mortality associated with elevated body weight in children and adolescents. *American Journal of Clinical Nutrition, 63*, 445S–447S.

Must, A., Spadano, J., Coakley, E. H., Fields, A. E., Colditz, G., & Dietz, W. H. (1999). The disease burden associated with overweight and obesity. *Journal of the American Medical Association, 282*, 1523–1529.

Must, A., & Strauss, R. S. (1999). Risks and consequences of childhood and adolescent obesity. *International Journal of Obesity and Related Metabolic Disorders, 23*, S2–S11.

Narayan, K. M. V., Boyle, J. P., Thompson, T. J., Sorensen, S. W., & Williamson, D. F. (2003). Lifetime risk for diabetes mellitus in the United States. *Journal of the American Medical Association, 290*, 1884–1890.

Neumark-Sztainer, D., Story, M., & Harris, T. (1999). Beliefs and attitudes about obesity among teachers and school health care providers working with adolescents. *Journal of Nutritional Education, 31*, 3–9.

Neville, K. A., & Walker, J. L. (2005). Precocious pubarche is associated with SGA, prematurity, weight gain, and obesity. *Archives of Disease in Childhood, 90*, 258–261.

Oren, A., Vos, L. E., Uiterwaal, C. S. P. M., Gorissen, W. H. M., Grobbee, D. E., & Bots, M. L. (2003). Change in body mass index from adolescence to young adulthood and increased carotid intima-media thickness at 28 years of age: The atherosclerosis risk in young adults study. *International Journal of Obesity, 27*, 1383–1390.

Pinhas-Hamiel, O., Newfield, R. S., Koren, I., Agmon, A., Lilos, P., & Phillip, M. (2003). Greater prevalence of iron deficiency in overweight and obese children and adolescents. *International Journal of Obesity, 27*, 416–418.

Pinhas-Hamiel, O., & Zeitler, P. (2000). "Who is the wise man?—The one who foresees consequences:" Childhood obesity, new associated comorbidity and prevention. *Preventive Medicine, 31*, 702–705.

Plourde, G. (2002). Impact of obesity on glucose and lipid profiles in adolescents at different age groups in relation to adulthood. *BMC Family Practice, 3*, 18.

Pontiroli, A. E. (2004). Type 2 diabetes mellitus is becoming the most common type of diabetes in school children. *Acta Diabetologica, 41*, 85–90.

Power, C., Lake, J. K., & Cole, T. (1997). Body mass index and height from childhood to adulthood in the 1958 British birth cohort. *American Journal of Clinical Nutrition, 66*, 1094–1101.

Reich, A., Muller, G., Gelbrich, G., Deutscher, K., Godicke, R., & Kiess, W. (2003). Obesity and blood pressure-results from the examination of 2365 schoolchildren in Germany. *International Journal of Obesity, 27*, 1459–1464.

Reilly, J. J. (2005). Descriptive epidemiology and health consequences of childhood obesity. *Best Practice and Research Clinical Endocrinology and Metabolism, 19*, 327–341.

Reilly, J. J., Methven, E., McDowell, Z. C., Hacking, B., Alexander, D., Stewart, L., et al. (2003). Health consequences of obesity. *Archives of Disease in Childhood, 88*, 748–752.

Ribeiro, M. M., Silva, A. G., Santos, N. S., Guazzelle, I., Matos, L. N. J., Trombetta, I. C., et al. (2005). Diet and exercise training restore blood pressure and vasodilatory responses during physiological maneuvers in obese children. *Circulation, 111*, 1915–1923.

Richardson, S. A., Goodman, N., Hastorf, A. H., & Dornbusch, S. M. (1961). Cultural uniformity in reaction to physical disabilities. *American Sociologic Review, 26*, 241–247.

Riddiford-Harland, D. L., Steele, J. R., & Storlien, L. H. (2000). Does obesity influence foot structure in prepubescent children? *International Journal of Obesity, 24*, 541–544.

Robinson, T. N. (1999). Reducing children's television viewing to prevent obesity: A randomized controlled trial. *Journal of the American Medical Association, 282*, 1561–1567.

Rocchini, A. P. (2002). Childhood obesity and a diabetes epidemic. *New England Journal of Medicine, 346*, 854–855.

Rodriguez, M. A., Winkleby, M. A., Ahn, D., Sundquist, J., & Kraemer, H. C. (2002). Identification of population subgroups of children and adolescents with high asthma prevalence: findings from the Third National Health and Nutrition Examination Survey. *Archives of Pediatrics and Adolescent Medicine, 156*, 269–275.

Schwartz, M. B., & Puhl, R. (2003). Childhood obesity: A societal problem to solve. *Obesity Reviews, 4*, 57–71.

Sinaiko, A. R., Donahue, R. P., Jacobs, D. R., Jr., & Prineas, R. J. (1999). Relation of weight and rate of increase in weight during childhood and adolescence to body size, blood pressure, fasting insulin, and lipids in young adults: The Minneapolis Children's Blood Pressure Study. *Circulation, 99,* 1471–1476.

Srinivasan, S. R., Bao, W., Wattigney, W. A., & Berenson, G. S. (1996). Adolescent overweight is associated with adult overweight and related multiple cardiovascular risk factors: The Bogalusa Heart Study. *Metabolism, 45,* 235–240.

Sung, R. Y. T., Yu, C. W., Chang, S. K. Y., Mo, S. W., Woo, K. S., & Lam, C. W. K. (2002). Effects of dietary intervention and strength training on blood lipid level in obese children. *Archives of Disease in Childhood, 86,* 407–410.

Thorpe, K. E., Florence, C. S., Howard, D. H., & Joski, P. (2004). The impact of obesity on rising medical spending: Higher spending for obese patients is mainly attributable to treatment for diabetes and hypertension. *Health Affairs, 23,* 480W4–486W4.

Timm, N. L., Grupp-Phelan, J., & Ho, M. L. (2005). Chronic ankle morbidity in obese children following an acute ankle injury. *Archives of Pediatric and Adolescent Medicine, 159,* 33–36.

Togashi, K., Masuda, H., Rankinen, T., Tanaka, S., Bouchard, C., & Kamiya, H. (2002). A 12-year follow-up study of treated obese children in Japan. *International Journal of Obesity, 26,* 770–777.

Tounian, P., Aggoun, Y., Dubern, B., Varille, V., Guy-Grand, B., Sidi, D., et al. (2001). Presence of increased stiffness of the common carotid artery and endothelial dysfunction in severely obese children: A prospective study. *Lancet, 358,* 1400–1404.

Wang, G., & Dietz, W. H. (2002). Economic burden of obesity in youths aged 6 to 17 years: 1979–1999. *Pediatrics, 109,* e81.

Wei, J. N., Sung, F. C., Lin, C. C., Lin, R. S., Chiang, C. C., & Chuang, L. M. (2003). National surveillance for type 2 diabetes mellitus in Taiwanese children. *Journal of the American Medical Association, 290,* 1345–1350.

Weiss, R., Dziura, J., Burgert, T. S., Tabmorlane, W. V., Taksali, S. E., Yeckel, C. W., et al. (2004). Obesity and the metabolic syndrome in children and adolescents. *New England Journal of Medicine, 350,* 2362–2374.

Whitaker, R. C., Pepe, M. S., Wright, J. A., Deidel, K. D., & Dietz, W. H. (1998). Early adiposity rebound and the risk of adult obesity. *Pediatrics, 101,* e5.

Whitaker, R. C., Wright, J. A., Pepe, M. S., Seidel, K. D., & Dietz, W. H. (1997). Predicting obesity in young adulthood from childhood and parental obesity. *New England Journal of Medicine, 337,* 869–873.

Wing, Y. K., Hui, S. H., Pak, W. M., Ho, C. K., Cheung, A., Li, A. M., et al. (2003). A controlled study of sleep related disordered breathing in obese children. *Archives of Disease in Childhood, 88,* 1043–1047.

Woo, K. S., Chook, P. L., Yu, C. W., Sung, R. Y. T., Qiao, M., Leung, S. S. F., et al. (2004). Overweight in children is associated with arterial endothelial dysfunction and intima-media thickening. *International Journal of Obesity, 28,* 852–857.

Wright, C. M., Parker, L., Lamont, D., & Craft, A. W. (2001). Implications of childhood obesity for adult health: Findings from thousand families cohort study. *British Medical Journal, 323,* 1280–1284.

Young, T. K., Dean, H. J., Flett, B., & Wood-Steiman, P. (2000). Childhood obesity in a population at high risk for type 2 diabetes. *Journal of Pediatrics, 136,* 365–369.

3

Psychosocial Factors Related to Obesity in Children and Adolescents

MEG H. ZELLER and AVANI C. MODI

As outlined in Chapter 2, the long-term medical consequences of obesity are well-documented, with precursors for adult disease becoming increasingly prevalent in overweight youth. It is asserted, however, that the greater immediate and observable costs of pediatric obesity are psychosocial (Dietz, 1998). The purpose of this chapter is to review the known psychosocial correlates of pediatric obesity derived from the empirical literature. These psychosocial correlates cross a number of domains and environments that are central to understanding healthy child and adolescent development. We have organized the chapter to reflect specific psychosocial factors within the family and peer environments and then psychosocial functioning at the individual level. Throughout the chapter and in our summary, we discuss the implications of these data for weight management treatment as well as important directions for future research.

Psychosocial Functioning in the Family Environment

We are only beginning to understand the parental and familial psychosocial characteristics that typify the obesigenic family environment. This is surprising given the compelling empirical evidence supporting family-based intervention, which identifies parental behavior as a key component of effective treatment (Epstein, Valoski, Wing, & McCurley,1994; Golan, Weizman, Apter, & Fainaru, 1998; Wrotniak, Epstein, Paluch, & Roemmich, 2004). As is discussed in Chapter 12, pediatric obesity is linked to family

MEG H. ZELLER and AVANI C. MODI • Cincinnati Children's Hospital Medical Center, Cincinnati, OH 45229.

socioeconomic and demographic factors. Further, it is well-established that parental obesity holds strong predictive power in the development and persistence of obesity in the child and adolescent years, arguably the result of a gene-environment interaction. These important data describe a broad context of familial correlates and risk factors for pediatric obesity. As detailed below, there is increasing evidence that additional psychosocial factors characterize the family environment of obese youth.

Maternal Distress

Two groups of researchers examined parental psychological functioning in clinical samples of obese children and adolescents, and they found that a remarkable percentage of mothers (28–50%) reported clinically significant levels of psychological distress (Epstein, Myers, & Anderson, 1996; Zeller, Saelens, Roehrig, Kirk, & Daniels, 2004). These mothers did so at higher rates than mothers of nonoverweight youth, (Zeller et al., 2007). In contrast, the prevalence of clinically significant paternal distress was within normative base rates (Epstein, Klein, & Wisniewski, 1994b; Zeller et al., 2007). These data are concerning, as maternal psychopathology is known to disrupt parenting and the parent-child relationship and can lead to poor physical and psychological health outcomes in children (Beardslee, Versage, & Gladstone, 1998; Burke, 2003). It is therefore not surprising that maternal distress has been linked to pediatric obesity treatment outcomes. For example, higher maternal distress was associated with poorer child weight loss (Epstein, Wisniewski, & Weng, 1994), and although maternal distress improved during active family-based weight management treatment, these gains were not maintained post-treatment (Epstein, Paluch, Gordy, Saelens, & Ernst, 2000). In contrast, we documented that higher maternal distress does not predict attrition from treatment (Zeller, Kirk, et al., 2004). One could therefore hypothesize that a mother may keep her family in treatment when she is distressed because she likely benefits from the support and structure provided. However, this distress may reduce the effectiveness of parenting skills she needs to support her child in adopting a healthier lifestyle. Future research should examine the links between maternal distress and parenting and determine whether maternal distress is typical of families with obese youth who are not accessing care.

Family Functioning

Several groups of researchers have examined the family functioning of obese youth. Family functioning, or the family emotional climate, is typically defined by dimensions such as support, conflict, cohesion, and control (Kronenberger & Thompson, 1990). Within the broader pediatric literature, high levels of familial cohesion and support and low levels of conflict are documented protective factors for child/adolescent adjustment and the management of pediatric chronic illness (Drotar, 1997; Wysocki, 1993).

Several community-based studies have examined parental perceptions of the family emotional climates of obese youth as compared with those of nonobese youth. The data suggest either no group differences (Klesges et al., 1992; Stradmeijer, Bosch, Koops, & Seidell, 2000) or evidence of more problematic family functioning for obese youth (Davis, Rovi, & Johnson, 2005; Mendelson, White, & Schliecker, 1995; Wilkins, Kendrick, Stitt, Stinett, & Hammarlund, 1998; Young-Hyman, Tanofsky-Kraff, Yanovski, & Yanovski, 2004; Zeller et al., 2007). For example, in an African American sample, parents of obese children perceived lower levels of cohesion among family members than families of nonobese children did but similar levels of conflict and control (Young-Hyman et al.). In contrast, mothers of overweight youth reported higher control within the family environment than mothers of nonoverweight youth (Wilkins et al.). Within clinical samples, parents reported lower cohesion than instrument norms when treatment was started (Banis et al., 1988). In a recent study (Zeller et al.), mothers (but not fathers) of obese youth in a clinical sample characterized their family functioning as higher in interpersonal conflict and lacking in cohesion and structure (i.e., Family Environment Scale (FES); Conflicted factor) relative to mothers of nonoverweight youth.

Within the published pediatric literature, there is minimal evidence on whether family functioning plays a role in pediatric weight management treatment outcomes. We were able to locate one study that documented poorer treatment outcomes for children whose parents characterized the family environment as more disorganized and chaotic than for obese youth with fewer of these family characteristics (Kirschenbaum, Harris, & Tomarken, 1984).

Similar trends suggestive of impairment have emerged when investigators have asked overweight youth about their family environments. For example, adolescent perceptions of lower family cohesion were associated with higher weight status for girls, although not for boys (Mendelson et al., 1995). Alternately, Mellin and colleagues demonstrated that adolescent perceptions of higher family "connectedness" may function as a protective factor, as it was associated with better psychosocial health. Further, adolescents who reported higher family connectedness were also more likely to engage in healthier behaviors including breakfast eating; higher fruit and vegetable consumption; and, for boys, less television time (Mellin, Neumark-Sztainer, Story, Ireland, & Resnick, 2002).

Recognizing that important work has documented the associations of maternal feeding style (e.g., control/restriction) with overweight in youth (Birch & Fisher, 2000; Francis & Birch, 2005), researchers only recently have begun to examine the family emotional climate specifically at mealtimes. We recently reported that compared with the mealtimes of families of nonoverweight youth, the family mealtimes of obese youth were characterized by mothers being more challenging behaviorally and both fathers and mothers perceiving mealtimes as less positive in terms of family interactions (Zeller et al., 2007). Two recent studies have used in-home mealtime observational coding strategies to capture family interaction patterns. Moens, Braet, and Soetens (2007) observed that parents of overweight children were more likely to use maladaptive control strategies and less supportive behaviors at mealtimes than parents of nonoverweight youth. Similarly, Jacobs and Fiese (2006) observed that having parents who had a difficult time managing meals, assigning roles, and responding to emotions distinguished a group of children with asthma who were overweight from those who were not. These studies provide initial evidence of the utility and potential importance of naturalistic and objective observational methodologies to examine mealtime family functioning in an obese pediatric population.

Parenting Practices

While there is a broad literature describing how specific parenting attitudes and practices influence child behavior and psychosocial adjustment, we know very little about the parenting practices of caregivers of obese youth. As is discussed in Chapter 10, specific parental feeding strategies (e.g., feeding restriction, discouragement to eat) have been associated with increased energy intake and body mass in young children (Birch & Fisher, 1998; Johnson & Birch, 1994). However, the small literature describing more global parenting practices is less definitive. Positive parenting practices, also referred to as authoritative parenting, are typically defined by a blend of warmth, involvement and monitoring of activities; control that is firm yet flexible; and consistent discipline that is not harsh. In contrast, authoritarian parenting is characterized by low warmth, high and coercive control, and harsh discipline. Permissive parenting lacks warmth, monitoring, control, and discipline. Both authoritarian and permissive styles are associated with more negative outcomes in children (e.g., behavior, social competence) in the general population (Kotchick & Forehand, 2002). Within the obesity literature, Gable and Lutz (2000) documented that parents of obese youth did not differ from parents of nonobese youth in their self-perceptions of parenting practices (e.g., authoritative, authoritarian). Agras, Hammer, McNicholas, and Kraemer (2004) recently found that there were no predictive relationships between parents' reports of their parenting practices and obesity development in their children from preschool to middle childhood. Most recently, however, Stein and colleagues (Stein, Epstein, Raynor, Kilanowski, & Paluch, 2005) demonstrated that change in a child's perception of parenting style, specifically greater perceived father acceptance (i.e., warmth), was associated with better weight management outcomes.

Summary and Implications

Taken together, this small family literature does not present a consistent psychosocial profile for families of obese youth. This is likely because of the use of different informants, different instruments, or different scoring of the same instrument (e.g., Family Environment Scale [Moos & Moos, 1994]) across existing studies. This has resulted in potentially disparate dimensions of family functioning and parenting practices from which to draw conclusions. Further well-designed and controlled research is critically needed. In addition, we lack a thorough understanding of how family factors may relate to pediatric weight treatment outcomes. For example, family conflict and lower parental warmth are risk factors associated with poorer adherence to treatments for other pediatric chronic medical conditions such as cystic fibrosis (DeLambo, Ievers-Landis, Drotar, & Quittner, 2004) and diabetes (Davis et al., 2001; Lewin et al., 2006). However, there remains a need to develop consistent and context-specific assessment tools for obesity in the areas of family functioning and parenting skills. With these tools it is highly likely that we can better identify the family-based psychosocial factors that promote adherence to more healthful eating and activities.

Psychosocial Functioning in the Peer Environment

Peer relations are central to children's healthy social and emotional development. Poor peer relations in childhood result in considerable risk for internalized symptoms, low self-concept and peer rejection in adolescence (Hymel, Rubin, Rowden, & LeMare, 1990; Morison & Masten, 1991; Rubin, Chen, McDougall, Bowker, & McKinnon, 1995) as well as greater psychopathology and poorer life adaptation (e.g., school/job performance, interpersonal relations) in adulthood (Bagwell, Newcomb, & Bukowski, 1998). Unfortunately, both anecdotal and growing empirical evidence support the idea that one significant psychosocial correlate of pediatric obesity involves problematic social interactions and interpersonal relations with peers.

When obese youth have been asked directly about their experiences within the peer environment, they have described stigmatization and victimization. Obese children and adolescents, relative to their nonoverweight peers, reported more name-calling, teasing about their appearances (Neumark-Sztainer, Story, & Faibisch, 1998; Pierce & Wardle 1997; Storch et al., 2006; Thompson et al., 2007) and weight-related criticism while they were physically active (Faith, Leone, Ayers, Heo, & Pietrobelli, 2002). Obese adolescents reported more victimization by peers than adolescents of average weight (Janssen, Craig, Boyce, & Pickett, 2004; Pearce, Boergers, & Prinstein, 2002). The nature of this victimization was consistent with gender differences reported in the broader developmental literature (Crick & Grotpeter, 1995) in which obese boys reported more overt physical victimization (e.g., being hit and kicked), whereas girls reported more relational victimization (e.g., damage or control of friendships). Storch and colleagues (Storch et al.) have recently advanced the literature by demonstrating a cross-sectional association between overweight and obese youth reports of greater peer victimization and greater internalizing and externalizing symptomatology. Further, greater peer victimization was associated with lower levels of physical activity, which was explained in part by depressive symptoms and greater loneliness. Thus, links between peer victimization, psychological adjustment, and lifestyle behaviors are suggested.

Researchers have also entered the peer environment and asked peers about friendships, social interactions, and social acceptance patterns and then examined whether these patterns are affected by child/adolescent weight status. While investigators have reported no differences in obese and nonobese children and adolescents' levels of peer acceptance (Baum & Forehand, 1984; Phillips & Hill, 1998), a majority of data support group differences in a number of peer domains. For example, children who were overweight *received* and *initiated* more negative interactions with peers than nonoverweight children did (Baum & Forehand). In a more recent study, Janssen and colleagues reported that obese adolescents were not only victims of verbal bullying by peers but also perpetrators of this type of aggression (Janssen et al., 2004).

Recent findings drawn from a large epidemiological sample from the National Longitudinal Study of Adolescent Health (Strauss & Pollack, 2003) documented that obese adolescents were much less likely to be nominated by their peers as a "friend" relative to normal-weight adolescents, and had friends who were less popular themselves. The number of friendship nominations was related to degree of overweight in a dose-dependent manner. This social marginalization was most prominent for non-Hispanic whites and females in particular, with smaller effects for Hispanic/Latino and African American adolescents. In general, the adolescents who had more friends reported watching fewer hours of TV and were involved in more school-based clubs and sporting activities.

Parents recognize the social difficulties their obese offspring face. In both community-based and clinical studies that utilized the Child Behavior Checklist (CBCL) (Achenbach & Rescorla, 2001) or the Behavior Assessment System for Children (BASC) (Reynolds & Kamphaus, 1992), parents reported that their obese children or adolescents were experiencing significant social problems compared with nonobese children or adolescents (Braet, Mervielde, & Vandereycken, 1997) or instrument norms (Banis et al., 1988; Epstein, Klein, et al., 1994; Young-Hyman, Schlundt, Herman-Wenderoth, & Bozylinski, 2003; Zeller, Saelens, et al., 2004).

Certainly, the literature that describes children's attitudes about physical appearance and body type suggests the peer environment is not accepting of obesity. In hypothetical peer paradigms, investigators have shown that children and adolescents will choose negative attributes ("ugly," "lazy," "sad," "poor leader") to describe an obese "peer" (Bell & Morgan, 2000; Hill & Silver, 1995; Latner & Stunkard, 2003). Further, youth will rank obese "peers" as the "least liked" as compared with "peers" portrayed with observable physical conditions or disabilities (e.g., crutches, wheelchair, amputated limbs, craniofacial anomaly) as well as "peers" who are not overweight (Latner & Stunkard).

There is further empirical evidence that peer relations affect treatment outcomes. Epstein and colleagues indicated that mothers' reports of higher social problems in children were predictive of weight increase at two-year follow-ups, with greater social problems being related to a greater weight increase (Epstein, Wisniewski, et al., 1994). In a later study, improvements in child overweight status were positively associated with improvements in child psychological adjustment, including decreased social problems and increased social competence (Myers, Raynor, & Epstein, 1998). Researchers have also documented that peer social support incorporated into the weight management intervention is beneficial for weight loss and maintenance for both adults (Wing & Jeffery, 1999) and adolescents (Jelalian & Mehlenbeck, 2002).

Summary and Implications

The peer environment provides a rich context to understand psychosocial consequences of pediatric obesity. Whether obese youth themselves, their peers or their parents are asked about the topic, it is evident that obese children and adolescents struggle in the peer domain. It is likely that the negative attitudes children hold regarding obesity and physical appearance set the stage for stigmatization, victimization, and rejection. However, there is also preliminary evidence that obese youth may exhibit behaviors that are not conducive to positive peer interactions. To date, no studies have tracked the peer relations of obese youth over time; however, the impact of negative peer relations on psychosocial adjustment and, potentially, the development of healthful behaviors is likely both short- and long-term. Understanding these trajectories of psychosocial risk for obese youth and their role in obesity development is an important area for future research.

Psychosocial Functioning at the Individual Level

Health-Related Quality of Life

Research examining the health-related quality of life (HRQOL) of obese youth has dramatically increased in the past five years. HRQOL is a useful outcome tool to assess the impact of a particular condition or disease on the daily functioning of individuals. It is defined as the physical, emotional, and social well-being of a person based on that person's own perspective (Schipper, Clinch, & Olweny 1996). HRQOL measures, such as the PedsQL™ (Pediatric Quality of Life Inventory) (Varni, Seid, & Kurtin, 2001) and the Child Health Questionnaire (Landgraf, Abetz, & Ware, 1996), allow for cross-disease comparisons, while disease- or condition-specific instruments measure aspects of daily functioning that are specific to particular diseases (e.g., asthma, cancer, obesity).

Investigators measuring HRQOL in obese children and adolescents have documented significant impairments in daily functioning relative to nonobese youth or instrument norms (Fallon et al., 2005; Friedlander, Larkin, Rosen, Palermo, & Redline, 2003; Ravens-Sieberer, Redegeld, & Bullinger, 2001; Schwimmer, Burwinkle, & Varni, 2003; Stern et al., 2007; Swallen, Reither, Haas, & Meier, 2005; Wake, Salmon, Waters, Wright, & Hesketh, 2002; Williams, Wake, Hesketh, Maher, & Waters, 2007; Zeller & Modi, 2006; Zeller, Roehrig, Modi, Daniels, & Inge, 2006). When investigators have examined HRQOL across the weight spectrum, the results suggest HRQOL decreases with increasing weight. For example, in a community-based Australian sample, higher BMI was associated with lower PedsQL child self reports and parent proxy scores (Williams et al., 2005). Obese and overweight youth differed from nonoverweight youth most in the social and physical subdomains. Within a sample of treatment-seeking obese youth (BMI greater than or equal to the 95th percentile), higher BMI was associated with lower parent proxy Psychosocial and Physical Health PedsQL scores (Schwimmer et al.). Finally, adolescents presenting for bariatric surgery, and thus at extreme levels of obesity (BMI greater than or equal to 40), have exhibited the greatest global impairments in HRQOL reported to date (Zeller et al., 2006).

These preliminary HRQOL studies primarily utilized generic measures of HRQOL to examine how obesity compares to other diseases. For example, Ravens-Sieberer and colleagues (Ravens-Sieberer et al., 2001), using the generic German KINDL (Ravens-Sieberer & Bullinger, 1998), found that children and adolescents with obesity reported poorer HRQOL in psychological well-being, self-esteem, friends, family, and school domains than children with asthma and atopic dermatitis. Similarly, Schwimmer and colleagues demonstrated that overweight Hispanic and white youth reported significant HRQOL impairments on the PedsQL, with scores of the overweight group similar to those of youth diagnosed with cancer (Schwimmer et al., 2003).

A series of recent studies broadened the scope of HRQOL research by examining predictors of HRQOL for obese youth. For example, we documented that poorer HRQOL was strongly linked to depressive symptoms and lower perceived social support in obese youth seeking treatment (Zeller & Modi, 2006a). There is also preliminary evidence suggesting the relationship between BMI and HRQOL may vary by race, with higher BMI scores being related to lower HRQOL for white adolescents than African American adolescents (Fallon et al., 2005). Looking within the subpopulation of adolescents with extreme obesity (BMI greater than or equal to 40) who were seeking treatment, we documented that African American teens reported less impact of weight on their body esteem and physical day-to-day lives than white adolescents (Zeller et al., 2005).

To date, researchers have had to rely on generic HRQOL measures, known to lack the specificity and sensitivity of disease-specific measures (Quittner, Davis, & Modi, 2003). Kolotkin and colleagues recently developed a weight-related HRQOL measure for adolescents, the Impact of Weight on Quality of Life-Kids (IWQOL-Kids) (Kolotkin et al., 2006). This measure consists of four domains (Physical Comfort, Body Esteem, Social Life, and Family Relations) and a total score, which have solid psychometric properties. Given the increase of intervention research for children and adolescents with obesity, weight-related HRQOL may be a good outcome measure, as it takes into account the child's own perspective of his/her functioning as it relates to obesity status. Furthermore, the Food and Drug Administration (FDA) has recently begun developing a road map on the use of patient-reported outcomes as both primary and secondary outcome measures in clinical trials, with a focus on utilizing well-validated items and measures that encompass HRQOL (Revicki et al., 2000).

Internalizing symptoms

A relatively large cross-sectional literature documents depressive and/ or internalizing (e.g., depression/anxiety) symptomatology in overweight and obese youth within both clinical (Braet et al., 1997; Britz et al., 2000; Epstein, Klein, et al., 1994; Erermis et al., 2004; Sheslow, Hassink, Wallace, & DeLancey, 1993; Zeller, Saelens, et al., 2004) and nonclinical samples (Erermis et al., Isnard et al., 2003; Tanofsky-Kraff et al., 2004). In contrast, data also suggest depressive symptomatology is not a consistent correlate of obesity in youth (Goodman & Whitaker, 2002; Lamertz, Jacobi, Yassouridis, Arnold, & Henkel, 2002; Young-Hyman et al., 2003; Zeller & Modi, 2006).

There are a number of important caveats, however. First, across this literature, obese youth most typically exhibit subclinical or average depressive or internalizing symptomatology, with only a small subset of youth having a clinically significant range of symptoms or meeting diagnostic criteria for a depressive disorder. For example, we (Zeller & Modi, 2006) recently reported that only 11% of obese children and adolescents in a clinical sample reported depressive symptoms in the clinical range on the Children's Depression Inventory (Kovacs, 1992), a rate consistent with a 10% prevalence rate of depressive symptoms in a nonclinical community sample of youth (Dubois, Felner, Bartels, & Silverman, 1995).

Second, symptomatology rates vary depending on the informant and method of assessment. For example, mothers described greater depressive and internalizing symptomatology in their offspring than obese youth reported themselves (Tanofsky-Kraff et al., 2004; Zeller, Saelens, et al., 2004).

Finally, as previously mentioned, maternal distress is an important correlate of pediatric obesity in clinical samples that was shown to be the strongest predictor of poorer psychological adjustment in obese children and adolescents relative to other youth factors (e.g., degree of overweight, gender, race, age) (Epstein et al., 1996; Zeller, Saelens, et al., 2004). Given these findings, and the general support that mothers' reports on child adjustment may be biased by maternal distress (Renouf & Kovacs, 1994; Sanger, MacLean, & Van Slyke, 1992), exclusive reliance on mothers' report in clinical settings may be problematic.

There is growing and compelling evidence regarding the important links between depressive symptomatology, obesity development, and obesity persistence. Depressive symptomatology in both childhood (Pine, Goldstein, Wolk, & Weissman, 2001) and adolescence (Richardson et al., 2003) was implicated as a risk factor for the development of obesity in adulthood. Furthermore, obese adolescents who had higher levels of depressive symptoms were more likely to persist in their obesity over time (Goodman & Whitaker, 2002; Mustillo et al., 2003). Links between depressive symptoms and failed treatment outcomes have also been demonstrated. Depressive symptoms were associated with poor adherence to weight management intervention for African American adolescent females (White et al., 2004). We demonstrated that depressive symptoms were predictors of attrition from a pediatric weight management program for both African American and white youth (Zeller, Kirk, et al., 2004). Thus, depressive symptomatology may be a critically important correlate for further study.

Whether anxiety is a specific psychosocial correlate of pediatric obesity remains unknown. Few researchers have targeted this question, and existing data are inconclusive. For example, within community-based samples overweight youth did not differ from nonoverweight youth in anxiety symptoms (Tanofsky-Kraff et al., 2004), although they were described as reporting significantly higher rates of anxiety symptoms than instrument norms (Isnard et al., 2003). Similarly, Britz and colleagues (Britz et al., 2000) reported that obese adolescents enrolled in an inpatient weight loss program had a higher lifetime prevalence of anxiety disorders based on structured diagnostic interviews than community-based obese or nonobese control groups, who did not differ in prevalence rates. To the contrary, Lamertz and colleagues (Lamertz et al., 2002) reported an adolescent's likelihood of meeting criteria for anxiety disorders was no higher if that adolescent was obese or nonobese.

Externalizing symptoms

Relative to other domains of psychosocial functioning, behavior disorders that are more externalizing in nature (e.g., aggression, oppositional behavior) have been less frequently studied in overweight and obese youth, likely because of the lower prevalence of these behaviors. However, several studies that utilized the CBCL provide data regarding externalizing behaviors. Investigators documented in both clinical and nonclinical samples of obese youth that mother-reported externalizing or aggressive symptoms were in the nonclinical range compared with instrument norms (Epstein, Klein, et al., 1994; Zeller, Saelens, et al. 2004) although at rates higher than those of non-treatment-seeking obese and/or nonobese age-mates (Braet et al., 1997; Erermis et al., 2004; Tanofsky-Kraff et al., 2004; Tershakovec, Weller, & Gallagher, 1994; Young-Hyman et al., 2003).

When researchers have examined the impact of externalizing symptoms longitudinally, links were suggested with obesity's development and persistence. There have been two longitudinal studies, both of which utilized community samples and semi-structured diagnostic interviews. Mustillo and colleagues reported that meeting diagnostic criteria for oppositional defiant disorder was associated with obesity in childhood as well as persistent obesity in adolescence (Mustillo et al., 2003). Pine and colleagues linked meeting diagnostic criteria for conduct disorder in adolescence to the development of obesity in young adulthood (Pine, Cohen, Brook, & Coplan, 1997).

Self-esteem

The stigmatization associated with obesity has long been assumed to have a negative impact on self-esteem in obese youth. However, it remains unclear whether low self-esteem is a consistent correlate of pediatric obesity or whether that depends on how self-esteem is defined (e.g., global or domain-specific). Further, there is evidence that self-esteem may vary by age, gender, and/or race. For example, cross-sectional studies have demonstrated that obese youth report lower global self-esteem (Banis et al., 1988; Kimm et al., 1997; Phillips & Hill, 1998) as well as comparable self-esteem relative to nonobese age-mates (Kaplan & Wadden, 1986; Mendelson & White, 1985; Wadden, Foster, Brownell, & Finley, 1984) and instrument norms (Kimm, Sweeney, Janosky, & MacMillan, 1991; Sheslow et al., 1993; Young-Hyman et al., 2003). However, investigators who have tapped the unique subdomains of self-esteem (Harter, 1985, 1988) have reported more consistent findings that suggest specific areas of impairment. For example, obese children and adolescents have reported lower self-perceptions of athletic competence, social acceptance, and/or physical appearance relative to non-overweight children and adolescents or instrument norms (Braet et al., 1997; French, Perry, Leon, & Fulkerson, 1996; Israel & Ivanova, 2002; Kimm et al., 1997; Phillips & Hill, 1998; Young-Hyman et al., 2003).

Comprehensive reviews of the cross-sectional literature have suggested that overweight adolescents may be at greater risk for self-esteem difficulties than younger school-age children (French, Story, & Perry, 1995; Miller & Downey, 1999). Certainly longitudinal designs have supported this trend. For example, it was demonstrated that persistent obesity from middle childhood to adolescence was associated with decreasing self-esteem, particularly for non-Hispanic white and Hispanic females as compared with African American females (Brown et al., 1998; Strauss, 2000). In addition, improved self-esteem was associated with change in degree of overweight and participation in a weight loss camp (Walker, Gately, Berwick, & Hill, 2003) and clinical trial (Jelalian & Mehlenbeck, 2002).

Summary and Implications

While the very early literature characterized obese children as "fundamentally unhappy and maladjusted" (Bruch, 1941), the present and growing empirical literature proves more equivocal. While high rates of diagnosable psychopathology are not the norm for obese children or adolescents, some youth appear at greater risk for depressive symptomatology and lower self-esteem. It is clear, however, that obese youth, particularly those seeking treatment, experience significant impairments in HRQOL.

Summary and Future Directions

The present chapter provided a summary of the psychosocial correlates of pediatric obesity. As we have outlined, our current knowledge is informed by what Friedman and Brownell (1995) characterized as "first generation" studies. These studies identify what the correlates or consequences are for obesity in the pediatric population by utilizing largely cross-sectional designs. Clearly this generation of literature speaks to obesity affecting specific psychosocial domains, such as HRQOL and peer relations. However, the current literature suggests that obese children and their families are heterogeneous, with psychosocial difficulties not being a universal characteristic for these youth.

The second generation of studies must identify risk and resilience factors that affect psychosocial functioning within the obese population. For example, within the past 10 years, researchers have begun to examine whether psychosocial risk (e.g., self-esteem, HRQOL) varies by racial/ethnic group. Although data describing the psychosocial adjustment of African American youth is increasing (Brown et al., 1998; Fallon et al., 2005; Strauss, 2000; Young-Hyman et al., 2003, Zeller & Modi, 2006), with few exceptions, there are limited psychosocial data regarding Hispanic (Schwimmer et al., 2003; Strauss, 2000; Strauss & Pollack, 2003), Asian (Xie et al., 2005), or Native American youth, known to be at considerable risk for obesity.

Researchers have also begun to assess the relative risk of comorbid medical conditions on psychosocial functioning. For example, researchers demonstrated a cumulative negative impact on HRQOL for obese youth who also had sleep-disordered breathing (Crabtree, Varni, & Gozal, 2004; Schwimmer et al., 2003). This additive negative effect on HRQOL was not evident for other obesity-related comorbidities, including asthma, type 2 diabetes, Blount's disease, polycystic ovary syndrome, nonalcoholic fatty liver disease, fasting hyperinsulinemia, and dyslipidemia. However, using an asthma-specific HRQOL measure, Blandon and colleagues (Blandon Vijil, del Rio Navarro, Berber Eslava, & Sienra Monge, 2004) reported that children with both asthma and obesity reported lower scores than those with asthma who were normal or overweight. These data suggest that comorbidities affecting respiratory functioning may further impair the HRQOL of children with obesity. Therefore, a closer look at obese youth with comorbid medical conditions is necessary, as they may be at heightened psychosocial risk.

Psychosocial research in obesity has grown tremendously in the past decade; however, several additional areas warrant attention. First, recent data have implicated difficult temperaments in young children in the development of obesity by middle childhood (Agras et al., 2004) as well as in adulthood (Pulkki-Raback, Elovainio, Kivimaki, Raitakari, & Keltikangas-Jarvinen, 2005). Second, there is increasing evidence of an association between retrospectively reporting adverse childhood experiences, including child abuse and neglect, and being obese in adulthood (Felitti 1991; Grilo et al., 2005; Williamson, Thompson, Anda, Dietz, & Felitti, 2002). There is a need for prospective studies that explore the role of adverse childhood experiences and the resulting post-traumatic symptoms in the development of obesity. Third, the degree of obesity has increased at an alarming rate (Jolliffe, 2004), making severely obese adolescents a new population for which there is notable concern and limited understanding (Inge, Zeller, Lawson, & Daniels, 2005). A first glance at this unique population, specifically those seeking bariatric surgery, suggests significant global impairments in HRQOL and higher rates of clinical-range depressive symptoms, which is in sharp contrast to what has been described to date (Zeller, Kirk, et al. 2006). Fourth, even though obesity is a developmental phenomenon, we are severely lacking prospective longitudinal studies, which are vital to the advancement of the field. The cross-sectional nature of our current knowledge limits the ability to draw causal or directional conclusions. Do psychosocial factors at the family, peer, or individual level contribute to obesity's persistence or progression in adolescence and adulthood?

Finally, the Strategic Plan for NIH (National Institutes of Health) Obesity Research (U.S. Department of Health and Human Services, 2004) has called for prospective observational research to identify the potentially modifiable behavioral and environmental factors that contribute to obesity development and persistence in childhood and adolescence. There are likely psychosocial factors within the individual and environment that function as barriers to successful weight management. Treatment barriers in other pediatric medical conditions are both context- and family-specific (Modi & Quittner, 2006), thus calling for individualized intervention. The identification of these psychosocial barriers is critical to the development of more efficacious treatment paradigms.

REFERENCES

Achenbach, T. M., & Rescorla, L. A. (2001). *Manual for ASEBA school-age forms & profiles*. Burlington, VT: University of Vermont, Research Center for Children, Youth, & Families.

Agras, W. S., Hammer, L. D., McNicholas, F., & Kraemer, H. C. (2004). Risk factors for childhood overweight: A prospective study from birth to 9.5 years. *Pediatrics, 145*, 20–25.

Bagwell, C. L., Newcomb, A. F., & Bukowski, W. M. (1998). Preadolescent friendship and peer rejection as predictors of adult adjustment. *Child Development, 69*, 140–153.

Banis, H. T., Varni, J. W., Wallander, J. L., Korsch, B. M., Jay, S. M., Adler, R., et al. (1988). Psychological and social adjustment of obese children and their families. *Child: Care, Health and Development, 14*, 157–173.

Baum, C. G., & Forehand, R. (1984). Social factors associated with adolescent obesity. *Journal of Pediatric Psychology, 9*, 293–302.

Beardslee, W. R., Versage, E. M., & Gladstone, T. R. (1998). Children of affectively ill parents: A review of the past 10 years. *Journal of the American Academy of Child and Adolescent Psychiatry, 37*, 1134–1141.

Bell, S. K., & Morgan, S. B. (2000). Children's attitudes and behavioral intentions toward a peer presented as obese: Does a medical explanation for the obesity make a difference? *Journal of Pediatric Psychology, 25*, 137–145.

Birch, L. L., & Fisher, J. O. (1998). Development of eating behaviors among children and adolescents. *Pediatrics, 101*, 539–549.

Birch, L. L., & Fisher, J. O. (2000). Mothers' child-feeding practices influence daughters' eating and weight. *American Journal of Clinical Nutrition, 71*, 1054–1061.

Blandon Vijil, V., del Rio Navarro, B., Berber Eslava, A., & Sienra Monge, J. J. (2004). Quality of life in pediatric patients with asthma with and without obesity: A pilot study. *Allergologia et Immunopathologia, 32*, 259–264.

Braet, C., Mervielde, I., & Vandereycken, W. (1997). Psychological aspects of childhood obesity: A controlled study in a clinical and nonclinical sample. *Journal of Pediatric Psychology, 22*, 59–71.

Britz, B., Siegfried, W., Ziegler, A., Lamertz, C., Herpertz-Dahlmann, B. M., Remschmidt, H., et al. (2000). Rates of psychiatric disorders in a clinical study group of adolescents with extreme obesity and in obese adolescents ascertained via a population based study. *International Journal of Obesity, 24*, 1707–1414.

Brown, K. M., McMahon, R. P., Biro, F. M., Crawford, P., Schreiber, G. B., Similo, S. L., et al. (1998). Changes in self-esteem in black and white girls between the ages of 9 and 14 years. The NHLBI Growth and Health Study. *Journal of Adolescent Health, 23*, 7–19.

Bruch, H. (1941). Obesity in childhood and personality development. *American Journal of Orthopsychiatry, 11*, 467–475.

Burke, L. (2003). The impact of maternal depression on familial relationships. *International Review of Psychiatry, 15*, 243–255.

Crabtree, V. M., Varni, J. W., & Gozal, D. (2004). Health-related quality of life and depressive symptoms in children with suspected sleep-disordered breathing. *Sleep, 27*, 1131–1138.

Crick, N. R., & Grotpeter, J. K. (1995). Relational aggression, gender, and social-psychological adjustment. *Child Development, 66*, 710–722.

Davis, C. L., Delamater, A. M., Shaw, K. H., La Greca, A. M., Eidson, M. S., Perez-Rodriguez, J. E., et al. (2001). Parenting styles, regimen adherence, and glycemic control in 4- to 10-year-old children with diabetes. *Journal of Pediatric Psychology, 26*, 123–129.

Davis, E. M., Rovi, S., & Johnson, M. S. (2005). Mental health, family function and obesity in African-American women. *Journal of the National Medical Association, 97*, 478–482.

DeLambo, K. E., Ievers-Landis, C. E., Drotar, D., & Quittner, A. L. (2004). Association of observed family relationship quality and problem-solving skills with treatment adherence in older children and adolescents with cystic fibrosis. *Journal of Pediatric Psychology, 29*, 343–353.

Dietz, W. H. (1998). Health consequences of obesity in youth: Childhood predictors of adult disease. *Pediatrics, 101*, 518–525.

Drotar, D. (1997). Relating parent and family functioning to the psychological adjustment of children with chronic health conditions: What have we learned? What do we need to know? *Journal of Pediatric Psychology, 22*, 149–165.

Dubois, D. L., Felner, R. D., Bartels, C. L., & Silverman, M. M. (1995). Stability of self-reported depressive symptoms in a community sample of children and adolescents. *Journal of Clinical Child Psychology, 24*, 386–396.

Epstein, L. H., Klein, K. R., & Wisniewski, L. (1994). Child and parent factors that influence psychological problems in obese children. *International Journal of Eating Disorders, 15*, 151–158.

Epstein, L. H., Myers, M. D., & Anderson, K. (1996). The association of maternal psychopathology and family socioeconomic status with psychological problems in obese children. *Obesity, 4*, 65–74.

Epstein, L. H., Paluch, R. C., Gordy, C. C., Saelens, B. E., & Ernst, M. M. (2000). Problem solving in the treatment of childhood obesity. *Health Psychology, 68*, 717–721.

Epstein, L. H., Valoski, A. M., Wing, R. R., & McCurley, J. (1994). Ten-year outcomes of behavioral family-based treatment for childhood obesity. *Health Psychology, 13*, 373–383.

Epstein, L. H., Wisniewski, L., & Weng, R. (1994). Child and parent psychological problems influence child weight control. *Obesity, 2*, 509–515.

Erermis, S., Cetin, N., Tamar, M., Bukusoglu, N., Akdeniz, F., & Goksen, D. (2004). Is obesity a risk factor for psychopathology among adolescents? *Pediatrics International, 46*, 296–301.

Faith, M. S., Leone, M. A., Ayers, T. S., Heo, M., & Pietrobelli, A. (2002). Weight criticism during physical activity, coping skills, and reported physical activity in children. *Pediatrics, 110*, e23.

Fallon, E. M., Tanofsky-Kraff, M., Norman, A. C., McDuffie, J. R., Taylor, E. D., Cohen, M. L., et al. (2005). Health-related quality of life in overweight and nonoverweight black and white adolescents. *Journal of Pediatrics, 147*, 443–450.

Felitti, V. J. (1991). Long-term medical consequences of incest, rape, and molestation. *Southern Medical Journal, 84*, 328–331.

Francis, L. A. & Birch, L. L. (2005). Maternal influences on daughters' restrained eating behavior. *Health Psychology, 24*, 548–554.

French, S. A., Perry, C. L., Leon, G. R., & Fulkerson, J. A. (1996). Self-esteem and change in body mass index over 3 years in a cohort of adolescents. *Obesity, 4*, 27–33.

French, S. A., Story, M., & Perry, C. L. (1995). Self-esteem and obesity in children and adolescents: A literature review. *Obesity, 3*, 479–490.

Friedlander, S. L., Larkin, E. K., Rosen, C. L., Palermo, T. M., & Redline, S. (2003). Decreased quality of life associated with obesity in school-aged children. *Archives of Pediatric and Adolescent Medicine, 157*, 1206–1211.

Friedman, M. A., & Brownell, K. D. (1995). Psychological correlates of obesity: Moving to the next research generation. *Psychological Bulletin, 117*, 3–20.

Gable, S., & Lutz, S. (2000). Household, parent, and child contributions to childhood obesity. *Family Relations, 49*, 293–300.

Golan, M., Weizman, A., Apter, A., & Fainaru, M. (1998). Parents as exclusive agents of change in the treatment of childhood obesity. *American Journal of Clinical Nutrition, 67*, 1130–1135.

Goodman, E., & Whitaker, R. C. (2002). A prospective study of the role of depression in the development and persistence of adolescent obesity. *Pediatrics, 110*, 497–504.

Grilo, C. M., Masheb, R. M., Brody, M., Toth, C., Burke-Martindale, C. H., & Rothschild, B. S. (2005). Childhood maltreatment in extremely obese male and female bariatric surgery candidates. *Obesity, 13*, 123–130.

Harter, S. (1985). *The self-perception profile for children.* Denver, CO: University of Denver, Department of Psychology, Unpublished manuscript.

Harter, S. (1988). *The Self-perception profile for adolescents.* Denver. CO: University of Denver, *Department of Psychology.* Unpublished manuscript.

Hill, A. J., & Silver, E. K. (1995). Fat, friendless and unhealthy: 9-year old children's perception of body shape stereotypes. *International Journal of Obesity, 19*, 423–430.

Hymel, S., Rubin, K. H., Rowden, L., & LeMare, L. (1990). Children's peer relationships: Longitudinal prediction of internalizing and externalizing problems from middle to late childhood. *Child Development, 61*, 2004–2021.

Inge, T. H., Zeller, M. H., Lawson, M. L., & Daniels, S. R. (2005). A critical appraisal of evidence supporting bariatric surgical approach to weight management for adolescents. *Journal of Pediatrics, 147*, 10–19.

Isnard, P., Michel, G., Frelut, M. L., Vila, G., Falissard, B., Naja, W., et al. (2003). Binge eating and psychopathology in severely obese adolescents. *International Journal of Eating Disorders, 34*, 235–243.

Israel, A. C., & Ivanova, M. Y. (2002). Global and dimensional self-esteem in preadolescent and early adolescent children who are overweight: Age and gender differences. *International Journal of Eating Disorders, 31*, 424–429.

Jacobs, M. P., & Fiese, B. H. (2007). Family mealtime interactions and overweight children with asthma: Potential for compounded risks? *Journal of Pediatric Psychology, 32*, 64–68.

Janssen, I., Craig, W. M., Boyce, W. F., & Pickett, W. (2004). Associations between overweight and obesity with bullying behaviors in school-aged children. *Pediatrics, 113*, 1187–1194.

Jelalian, E., & Mehlenbeck, R. (2002). Peer-enhanced weight management treatment for overweight adolescents: Some preliminary findings. *Journal of Clinical Psychology in Medical Settings, 9*, 15–23.

Johnson, S. L., & Birch, L. L. (1994). Parents' and children's adiposity and eating style. *Pediatrics, 94*, 653–661.

Jolliffe, D. (2004). Extent of overweight among US children and adolescents from 1971 to 2000. *International Journal of Obesity and Related Metabolic Disorders, 28*, 4–9.

Kaplan, K. M., & Wadden, T. A. (1986). Childhood obesity and self-esteem. *Journal of Pediatrics, 109*, 367–370.

Kimm, S. Y., Barton, B. A., Berhane, K., Ross, J. W., Payne, G. H., & Schreiber, G. B. (1997). Self-esteem and adiposity in black and white girls: The NHLBI Growth and Health Study. *Annals of Epidemiology, 7*, 550–560.

Kimm, S. Y., Sweeney, C. G., Janosky, J. E., & MacMillan, J. P. (1991). Self-concept measures and childhood obesity: A descriptive analysis. *Journal of Developmental and Behavioral Pediatrics, 12*, 19–24.

Kirschenbaum, D. S., Harris, E. S., & Tomarken, A. J. (1984). Effects of parental involvement in behavioral weight loss therapy for preadolescents. *Behavior Therapy, 15*, 485–500.

Klesges, R. C., Haddock, C. K., Stein, R. J., Klesges, L. M., Eck, L. H., & Hanson, C. L. (1992). Relationship between psychosocial functioning and body fat in preschool children: A longitudinal investigation. *Journal of Consulting and Clinical Psychology, 60*, 793–796.

Kolotkin, R. L., Zeller, M., Modi, A. C., Samsa, G. P., Polanichka Quinlan, N., Yanovski, J. A., et al. (2006). Assessing weight-related quality of life in adolescents. *Obesity, 14*, 448–457.

Kotchick, B. A., & Forehand, R. (2002). Putting parenting in perspective: A discussion of the contextual factors that shape parenting practices. *Journal of Child and Family Studies, 11*, 255–269.

Kovacs, M. (1992). *Children's depression inventory.* North Tonawanda, NY: Multi-Health Systems.

Kronenberger, W. G., & Thompson, R. J. (1990). Dimensions of family functioning in families with chronically ill children: A higher order factor analysis of the Family Environment Scale. *Journal of Clinical Child Psychology, 19*, 380–388.

Lamertz, C. M., Jacobi, C., Yassouridis, A., Arnold, K., & Henkel, A. W. (2002). Are obese adolescents and young adults at higher risk for mental disorders? A community survey. *Obesity, 10*, 1152–1160.

Landgraf, J., Abetz, L., & Ware, J. E. (1996). *Child Health Questionnaire (CHQ): A user's manual.* Boston: The Health Institute, New England Medical Center.

Latner, J. D. & Stunkard, A. J. (2003). Getting worse: The stigmatization of obese children. *Obesity, 11*, 452–456.

Lewin, A. B., Heidgerken, A. D., Geffken, G. R., Williams, L. B., Storch, E. A., Gelfand, K. M., et al. (2006). The relation between family factors and metabolic control: The role of diabetes adherence. *Journal of Pediatric Psychology, 31*, 174–183.

Mellin, A. E., Neumark-Sztainer, D., Story, M., Ireland, M., & Resnick, M. D. (2002). Unhealthy behaviors and psychosocial difficulties among overweight adolescents: The potential impact of familial factors. *Journal of Adolescent Health, 31*, 145–153.

Mendelson, B. K., & White, D. R. (1985). Development of self-body-esteem in overweight youngsters. *Developmental Psychology, 21*, 90–96.

Mendelson, B. K., White, D. R., & Schliecker, E. (1995). Adolescent's weight, sex, and family functioning. *International Journal of Eating Disorders, 17*, 73–79.

Miller, C. T., & Downey, K. T. (1999). A meta-analysis of heavyweight and self-esteem. *Personality and Social Psychology Review, 3*, 68–84.

Modi, A. C., & Quittner, A. L. (2006). Barriers to treatment adherence for children with cystic fibrosis and asthma: What gets in the way? *Journal of Pediatric Psychology, 31*, 846–858.

Moens, E., Braet, C., & Soetens, B. (2007). Observation of family functioning at mealtime: A comparison between families of children with and without overweight. *Journal of Pediatric Psychology, 32*, 52–63.

Moos, R. H., & Moos, B. S. (1994). *Family Environment Scale manual: Development, applications, research*, 3rd ed. Palo Alto, CA: Consulting Psychological Press.

Morison, P., & Masten, A. S. (1991). Peer reputation in middle childhood as a predictor of adaptation in adolescence: A seven-year follow-up. *Child Development, 62*, 991–1007.

Mustillo, S., Worthman, C., Erkanli, A., Keeler, G., Angold, A., & Costello, E. J. (2003). Obesity and psychiatric disorder: Developmental trajectories. *Pediatrics, 111*, 851–859.

Myers, M. D., Raynor, H. A., & Epstein, L. H. (1998). Predictors of child psychological changes during family-based treatment for obesity. *Archives of Pediatric and Adolescent Medicine, 152*, 855–861.

Neumark-Sztainer, D., Story, M., & Faibisch, L. (1998). Perceived stigmatization among overweight African-American and Caucasian adolescent girls. *Journal of Adolescent Health, 23*, 264–270.

Pearce, M. J., Boergers, J., & Prinstein, M. J. (2002). Adolescent obesity, overt and relational peer victimization, and romantic relationships. *Obesity, 10*, 386–393.

Phillips, R. G., & Hill, A. J. (1998). Fat, plain, but not friendless: Self-esteem and peer acceptance of obese pre-adolescent girls. *International Journal of Obesity and Related Metabolic Disorders, 22*, 287–293.

Pierce, J. W., & Wardle, J. (1997). Cause and effect beliefs and self-esteem of overweight children. *Journal of Child Psychology and Psychiatry and Allied Disciplines, 38*, 645–650.

Pine, D. S., Cohen, P., Brook, J., & Coplan, J. D. (1997). Psychiatric symptoms in adolescence as predictors of obesity in early adulthood: A longitudinal study. *American Journal of Public Health, 87*, 1303–1310.

Pine, D. S., Goldstein, R. B., Wolk, S., & Weissman, M. M. (2001). The association between childhood depression and adulthood body mass index. *Pediatrics, 107*, 1049–1056.

Pulkki-Raback, L., Elovainio, M., Kivimaki, M., Raitakari, O. T., & Keltikangas-Jarvinen, L. (2005). Temperament in childhood predicts body mass in adulthood: The cardiovascular risk in Young Finns study. *Health Psychology, 24*, 307–315.

Quittner, A. L., Davis, M. A., & Modi, A. C. (2003). Health-related quality of life in pediatric populations. In M. Roberts (Ed.), *Handbook of pediatric psychology* (pp. 696–709). New York: Guilford Publications.

Ravens-Sieberer, U., & Bullinger, M. (1998). Assessing health-related quality of life in chronically ill children with the German KINDL: First psychometric and content analytical results. *Quality of Life Research, 7*, 399–407.

Ravens-Sieberer, U., Redegeld, M., & Bullinger, M. (2001). Quality of life after in-patient rehabilitation in children with obesity. *International Journal of Obesity and Related Metabolic Disorders, 25,* S63–S65.

Renouf, A. G., & Kovacs, M. (1994). Concordance between mothers' reports and children's self-reports of depressive symptoms: A longitudinal study. *Journal of the American Academy of Child and Adolescent Psychiatry, 33,* 208–216.

Revicki, D. A., Osoba, D., Fairclough, D., Barofsky, I., Berzon, R., Leidy, N. K., et al. (2000). Recommendations on health-related quality of life research to support labeling and promotional claims in the United States. *Quality of Life Research, 9,* 887–900.

Reynolds, C. R., & Kamphaus, R. W. (1992). *Behavior assessment system for children: Manual.* Circle Pines, MN: American Guidance Service.

Richardson, L. P., Davis, R., Poulton, R., McCauley, E., Moffitt, T. E., Caspi, A., et al. (2003). A longitudinal evaluation of adolescent depression and adult obesity. *Archives of Pediatric and Adolescent Medicine, 157,* 739–745.

Rubin, K. H., Chen, X., McDougall, P., Bowker, A., & McKinnon, J. (1995). The waterloo longitudinal project: Predicting internalizing and externalizing problems in adolescence. *Developmental Psychopathology, 7,* 751–764.

Sanger, M. S., MacLean, W. E., & Van Slyke, D. A. (1992). Relation between maternal characteristics and child behavior ratings. Implications for interpreting behavior checklists. *Clinical Pediatrics, 31,* 461–466.

Schipper, H., Clinch, J. J., & Olweny, C. L. (1996). Quality of life studies: Definitions and conceptual issues. In B. Spilker (Ed.), *Quality of life and pharmacoeconomics in clinical trials* (2nd ed., pp. 11–23). Philadelphia: Lippincott-Raven.

Schwimmer, J. B., Burwinkle, T. M., & Varni, J. W. (2003). Health-related quality of life of severely obese children and adolescents. *Journal of the American Medical Association, 289,* 1813–1819.

Sheslow, D., Hassink, S., Wallace, W., & DeLancey, E. (1993). The relationship between self-esteem and depression in obese children. *Annals of the New York Academy of Sciences, 699,* 289–291.

Stein, R. I., Epstein, L. H., Raynor, H. A., Kilanowski, C. K., & Paluch, R. A. (2005). The influence of parenting change on pediatric weight control. *Obesity, 13,* 1749–1755.

Stern, M., Mazzeo, S. E., Gerke, C. K., Porter, J. S., Bean, M. K., & Laver, J. H. (2007). Gender, ethnicity, psychosocial factors, and quality of life among severely overweight, treatment-seeking adolescents. *Journal of Pediatric Psychology, 32,* 90–94.

Storch, E. A., Milsom, V. A., DeBraganza, N., Lewin, A. B., Geffken, G. R., & Silverstein, J. H. (2007). Peer victimization, psychosocial adjustment, and physical activity in overweight and at-risk-for-overweight youth. *Journal of Pediatric Psychology, 32,* 80–89.

Stradmeijer, M., Bosch, J., Koops, W., & Seidell, J. (2000). Family functioning and psychosocial adjustment in overweight youngsters. *International Journal of Eating Disorders, 27,* 110–114.

Strauss, R. S. (2000). Childhood obesity and self-esteem. *Pediatrics, 105,* e15.

Strauss, R. S., & Pollack, H. A. (2003). Social marginalization of overweight children. *Archives of Pediatric and Adolescent Medicine, 157,* 746–752.

Swallen, K. C., Reither, E. N., Haas, S. A., & Meier, A. M. (2005). Overweight, obesity, and health-related quality of life among adolescents: The National Longitudinal Study of Adolescent Health. *Pediatrics, 115,* 340–347.

Tanofsky-Kraff, M., Yanovski, S. Z., Wilfley, D. E., Marmarosh, C., Morgan, C. M., & Yanovski, J. A. (2004). Eating-disordered behaviors, body fat, and psychopathology in overweight and normal-weight children. *Journal of Consulting and Clinical Psychology, 72,* 53–61.

Tershakovec, A. M., Weller, S. C., & Gallagher, P. R. (1994). Obesity, school performance and behaviour of black, urban elementary school children. *International Journal of Obesity and Related Metabolic Disorders, 18,* 323–327.

Thompson, J. K., Shroff, H., Herbozo, S., Cafri, G., Rodriguez, J., & Rodriguez, M. (2007). Relations among multiple peer influences, body dissatisfaction, eating disturbance, and self-esteem: A comparison of average weight, at risk of overweight, and overweight adolescent girls. *Journal of Pediatric Psychology, 32,* 24–29.

U.S. Department of Health and Human Services, National Institutes of Health. (2004). *Strategic plan for NIH obesity research.* NIH publication No. 04-5493.

Varni, J. W., Seid, M., & Kurtin, P. S. (2001). PedsQL 4.0: Reliability and validity of the Pediatric Quality of Life Inventory version 4.0 generic core scales in healthy and patient populations. *Medical Care, 39*, 800–812.

Wadden, T. A., Foster, G. D., Brownell, K. D., & Finley, E. (1984). Self-concept in obese and normal-weight children. *Journal of Consulting and Clinical Psychology, 52*, 1104–1105.

Wake, M., Salmon, L., Waters, E., Wright, M., & Hesketh, K. (2002). Parent-reported health status of overweight and obese Australian primary school children: A cross-sectional population survey. *International Journal of Obesity and Related Metabolic Disorders, 26*, 717–724.

Walker, L. L. M., Gately, P. J., Berwick, B. M., & Hill, A. J. (2003). Children's weight loss camps: Psychological benefit or jeopardy? *International Journal of Obesity, 27*, 748–754.

White, M. A., Martin, P. D., Newton, R. L., Walden, H. M., York-Crowe, E. E., Gordon, S. T., et al. (2004). Mediators of weight loss in a family-based intervention presented over the internet. *Obesity, 12*, 1050–1059.

Wilkins, S. C., Kendrick, O. W., Stitt, K. R., Stinett, N., & Hammarlund, V. A. (1998). Family functioning is related to overweight in children. *Journal of the American Dietetics Association, 98*, 572–574.

Williams, J., Wake, M., Hesketh, K., Maher, E., & Waters, E. (2005). Health-related quality of life of overweight and obese children. *Journal of the American Medical Association, 293*, 70–76.

Williamson, D. F., Thompson, T. J., Anda, R. F., Dietz, W. H., & Felitti, V. (2002). Body weight and obesity in adults and self-reported abuse in childhood. *International Journal of Obesity and Related Metabolic Disorders, 26*, 1075–1082.

Wing, R. R., & Jeffery, R. W. (1999). Benefits of recruiting participants with friends and increasing social support for weight loss and maintenance. *Journal of Consulting and Clinical Psychology, 67*, 132–138.

Wrotniak, B. H., Epstein, L. H., Paluch, R. A., & Roemmich, J. N. (2004). Parent weight change as a predictor of child weight change in family-based behavioral obesity treatment. *Archives of Pediatric and Adolescent Medicine, 158*, 342–347.

Wysocki, T. (1993). Associations among teen-parent relationships, metabolic control, and adjustment to diabetes in adolescents. *Journal of Pediatric Psychology, 18*, 441–452.

Xie, B., Chou, C. P., Spruijt-Metz, D., Liu, C., Xia, J., Gong, J., et al. (2005). Effects of perceived peer isolation and social support availability on the relationship between body mass index and depressive symptoms. *International Journal of Obesity, 29*, 1137–1143.

Young-Hyman, D., Schlundt, D. G., Herman-Wenderoth, L., & Bozylinski, K. (2003). Obesity, appearance, and psychosocial adaptation in young African American children. *Journal of Pediatric Psychology, 28*, 463–472.

Young-Hyman, D., Tanofsky-Kraff, M., Yanovski, S., & Yanovski, J. (2004). Contribution of family environment to weight and body size dissatisfaction in overweight children and adolescents [Abstract].*Obesity, 12S*, A81.

Zeller, M. H., Kirk, S., Claytor, R., Khoury, P., Grieme, J., Santangelo, M., et al. (2004). Predictors of attrition from a pediatric weight management program. *Journal of Pediatrics, 144*, 466–470.

Zeller, M. H., & Modi, A. C. (2006). Predictors of health-related quality of life in obese youth. *Obesity, 14*, 122–130.

Zeller, M. H., Modi, A. C., Loux, T., Bell, S., Roehrig, H., Haromon, C., et al. (2005). Health-related quality of life in adolescent extreme obesity [Abstract]. *Obesity, 13S*, A70.

Zeller, M. H., Reiter-Purtill, J., Modi, A. C., Gutzwiller, J., Vannatta, K., & Davies, W. H. (2007). A controlled study of critical parent and family factors in the obesigenic environment. *Obesity, 15*,126–136.

Zeller, M. H., Roehrig, H. R., Modi, A. C., Daniels, S. R., & Inge, T. H. (2006). Health-related quality of life and depressive symptoms in adolescents with extreme obesity presenting for bariatric surgery. *Pediatrics, 117*, 1155–1161.

Zeller, M. H., Saelens, B. E., Roehrig, H., Kirk, S., & Daniels, S. (2004). Psychological adjustment of obese youth presenting for weight management treatment. *Obesity, 12*, 1576–1586.

4

Binge Eating Among Children and Adolescents

MARIAN TANOFSKY-KRAFF

With the alarming increase in pediatric obesity[1] (Ogden et al., 2006), it is imperative that correlates and predictors of excessive weight gain be identified and targeted for decreasing the vast number of youths struggling with overweight. While genetics plays an enormous role in determining body weight, other physiologic, social, psychological, and behavioral factors have a substantial impact as well. This chapter focuses specifically on binge eating, defined as overeating while experiencing a lack of control over what or how much is being eaten (American Psychiatric Association [APA], 2000). Relatively recent evidence suggests that binge eating may play a significant role in the development and maintenance of obesity.

This chapter will begin with an overview of binge eating in adults, with a focus on the putative diagnosis of binge eating disorder. A discussion of the challenge involved in measuring binge eating among youths will follow. Cross-sectional data on binge eating among adolescents will then be reviewed, followed by the corresponding literature including child samples. Since a number of studies have combined participants in middle childhood (6–12 years) with adolescents (13–17 years), for the purposes of this chapter, all studies including individuals younger than 10 years will

MARIAN TANOFSKY-KRAFF • Uniformed Services University of the Health Sciences and National Institute of Child Health and Human Development, Bethesda, MD 20892.

This research was supported by the Intramural Research Program of the NIH, grant ZO1-HD-00641 (NICHD, NIH) to Dr. J. Yanovski.

[1]Current Centers for Disease Control and Prevention terminology indicates that children with a Body Mass Index (BMI, kg/m^2) greater than or equal to the 85th percentile are "at risk for overweight" and that those with a BMI greater than or equal to the 95th percentile are "overweight" (Ogden et al., 2002). For the purposes of the present chapter, the terms "overweight" and "obese" are used interchangeably and refer to BMI greater than or equal to the 95th percentile unless otherwise indicated.

be included in sections focusing on children. Prospective studies analyzing the outcomes and predictors of binge eating will be presented. The final section will address directions and challenges for future research. Throughout this chapter, only studies that defined binge eating as including a sense of "loss of control" while overeating will be addressed. Studies that equate the construct of binge eating with overeating *without* assessing whether a loss of control is experienced will not be reviewed. Furthermore, data regarding binge eating should be considered as in the absence of purging or nonpurging compensatory behaviors. A caveat, however, is that a number of epidemiologic studies do not discriminate binge eating in conjunction with compensatory behaviors from binge eating in the absence of such behaviors.

Binge Eating Disorder in Adults

Although binge eating in obese adults was first described in 1959 (Stunkard, 1959), it was not until 35 years later that the proposed criteria for binge eating disorder (BED) were outlined in the Diagnostic and Statistical Manual of Mental Disorders (DSM-IV) (APA, 1994). BED is characterized by recurrent episodes of binge eating (overeating while experiencing a sense of loss of control regarding what or how much one is eating) accompanied by dysfunctional eating behaviors and marked distress regarding binge eating (Table 4.1). People with BED do not regularly engage in inappropriate compensatory behaviors, such as self-induced vomiting, excessive exercise, fasting, or laxative/diuretic use (APA, 2000). As a result, BED is often associated with excess body weight and obesity (Yanovski, Nelson, Dubbert, & Spitzer, 1993).

As many as 20–30% of adults attending specialized weight loss clinics and approximately 3–5% of the obese subset of the general population meet criteria for BED (Spitzer et al., 1991; Spitzer, Yanovski, Wadden, et al., 1993). Of note, the estimate is lower when clinical interviews are used in assessment (Kashubeck-West, Mintz, & Saundersam, 2001). BED seems

Table 4.1. Research Criteria for Binge Eating Disorder

A. Recurrent episodes of binge eating occur. An episode of binge eating is characterized by both of the following:
  (1) Eating, in a discrete period of time (e.g., within any two-hour period), an amount of food that is definitely larger than most people would eat in a similar period of time under similar circumstances.
  (2) A sense of lack of control over eating during the episode (e.g., a feeling that one cannot stop eating or control what or how much one is eating).
B. The binge eating episodes are associated with three (or more) of the following:
  (1) Eating much more rapidly than normal.
  (2) Eating until feeling uncomfortably full.
  (3) Eating large amounts of food when not feeling physically hungry.
  (4) Eating alone because of being embarrassed by how much one is eating.
  (5) Feeling disgusted with oneself, depressed, or very guilty after overeating.
C. Marked distress regarding binge eating is present.
D. The binge eating occurs, on average, at least two days a week for six months.
E. The binge eating is not associated with the regular use of inappropriate compensatory behaviors (e.g., purging, fasting, excessive exercise) and does not occur exclusively during the course of anorexia nervosa or bulimia nervosa.

to be equally prevalent in minority populations; a 1998 study found an overall BED prevalence rate of 1.5% in a biracial cohort of young adults (2.9% in the obese subset), with similar rates among African American women, white women, and white men and somewhat lower rates among African American men (Smith, Marcus, Lewis, Fitzgibbon, & Schreiner, 1998). By contrast, a community study found African American women to engage in recurrent binge eating more frequently than white women (Striegel-Moore, Wilfley, Pike, Dohm, & Fairburn, 2000).

BED is associated with a number of health complications and psychosocial problems. Adults with BED suffer from higher levels of disabilities, poorer quality of life, and poorer physical health than obese adults without an eating disorder (de Zwaan et al., 2002; Johnson, Spitzer, & Williams, 2001), and they have eating- and weight-related psychopathology at levels similar to those of people with bulimia nervosa (Masheb & Grilo, 2000; Wilfley et al., 2000). Women with BED have significantly more physical symptoms (e.g., headaches, menstrual problems) and indicators of poor health (e.g., limited ability to conduct usual activities, difficulty sleeping) than normal controls after co-occurring psychiatric disorders have been controlled for (Johnson et al.). Moreover, BED has been associated with social impairment and poor interpersonal functioning (Crow, Stewart Agras, Halmi, Mitchell, & Kraemer, 2002; Johnson et al.; Steiger, Gauvin, Jabalpurwala, Seguin, & Stotland, 1999; Wilfley, Wilson, & Agras, 2003). Finally, recurrent binge eating in obese people has been consistently associated with Axis I psychiatric disorders and Axis II personality disorders (Mussell et al., 1996, Wilfley et al.; Yanovski et al., 1993). Studies have found that as many as 75% of BED patients report a lifetime history of a psychiatric disorder (Marcus, 1995; Yanovski et al.).

Recurrent binge eating is a predictor of inappropriate weight gain and obesity in adults. In a community sample of individuals with bulimia nervosa and BED, Fairburn and colleagues (Fairburn, Cooper, Doll, Norman, & O'Connor, 2000) found that participants with BED gained an average of $4.2 \pm 9.8 \, kg$ over five years, while those with bulimia nervosa gained less weight $(3.3 \pm 10.8 \, kg)$ over the same time period. At follow-up, significantly more participants with BED met criteria for obesity (BMI $\geq 30 \, kg/m^2$) than those with bulimia nervosa. Of the BED group, the proportion of individuals with obesity increased from 22% at baseline to 39% at follow-up (Fairburn et al.). These findings are notable but should be interpreted cautiously since individuals without an eating disorder were not included in the study as a means of comparison. Nevertheless, among treatment-seeking samples, some studies have shown that people with BED have poorer responses to obesity treatment or more rapidly regain lost weight following treatment than those without an eating disorder (Sherwood, Jeffery, & Wing, 1999; Yanovski & Sebring, 1994). While some data suggest that BED and subthreshold BED may remit without treatment (Fairburn et al.), results from a longitudinal study of people meeting full criteria for BED found that the disorder tends to persist until treated (Crow, 2002).

A number of retrospective studies of individuals with BED have suggested that the initiation of binge eating episodes occurs well before adulthood. The mean recalled age of first binge episode ranged from 10.6

to 16 years across studies (Abbott et al., 1998; Binford, Pederson-Mussell, Peterson, Crow, & Mitchell, 2004; Grilo & Masheb, 2000; Marcus, Moulton, & Greeno, 1995; Mussell et al., 1995; Spurrell, Wilfley, Tanofsky, & Brownell, 1997), with one study reporting that almost 6% of the sample recalled first binge eating at age 5 or younger (Spurrell et al.). Such findings have prompted a number of researchers to examine binge eating behaviors in children and adolescents. Given the dramatic rise in pediatric obesity over the past three decades (Ogden et al., 2006), an increase in binge eating among youths is a reasonable hypothesis.

What is Binge Eating in Children and Adolescents?

To date, a relatively small literature on binge eating among youths exists. This lack of research may be due, in part, to the possibility that childhood binge eating may differ from such behaviors in adults or that construct explanations in adult measures (which are often adapted for child use) do not resonate with children. Most eating-disordered behaviors are difficult to assess, particularly among younger children, who may be manifesting only the early signs of eating disorders. Furthermore, children may be unaware of their emotional experiences, particularly with regard to the experience of loss of control over eating. Thus, an overarching challenge presented to researchers and clinicians is how to assess eating patterns given that children are not often aware of their emotional experiences during eating episodes and may find it difficult to understand and report them (Maloney, McGuire, & Daniels, 1988). Indeed, it has been suggested that the DSM-IV-TR (APA, 2000) does not adequately account for binge eating behaviors among children (Marcus & Kalarchian, 2003).

Differences in the prevalence rates, correlates and outcomes of binge eating among youths are likely affected by the methods used to assess binge eating and may have an important influence on study results, particularly among younger children. To date, most studies have used single-item surveys, self-report questionnaires, or parents' reports of their children's behaviors; a minority of cases have used interview methodology. Comparisons of these methods suggest that responses differ based upon the type of measure used and the particular respondent. Among samples of non-treatment-seeking children and adolescents of all weight strata, comparisons of self-reports of binge eating to parents' reports of their children's binge eating (Johnson, Grieve, Adams, & Sandy, 1999; Steinberg et al., 2004) and child self-reports to child interview methodology (Field, Taylor, Celio, & Colditz, 2004; Tanofsky-Kraff et al., 2003) have found that the identification of binge eating presence is inconsistent across measures. Furthermore, parents' reports of their children's binge eating have demonstrated poor concordance with interviews with children (Tanofsky-Kraff, Yanovski, & Yanovski, 2005). Similarly low levels of agreement between self-reports of binge eating and interview methods were revealed in a study of obese 10- to 16-year-olds seeking inpatient weight loss treatment (Decaluwe & Braet, 2004). Although interview-based methodologies, as opposed to self-report questionnaires, are recommended and considered the optimal means to assess binge eating behaviors among adults (Bryant-Waugh, Cooper, Taylor, & Lask, 1996; Wilfley, Schwartz, Spurrell, & Fairburn, 1997), it remains unclear whether this recommendation holds true for children.

Until a clear phenotype of binge eating among youths is defined and an optimal mode of assessment is determined, it is suggested that pediatric clinicians consider the following guideline. If feasible, multiple assessments should be administered to both the child and the parent. Ideally, interview methods, including probes to explicate the concept of loss of control while eating, are recommended. Furthermore, it may be useful to ask families about constructs that may be associated with binge eating, such as eating in response to both negative and positive emotions, eating in the absence of hunger or past satiation, and the individual child's feelings about his or her eating patterns.

Prevalence and Correlates of Binge Eating in Adolescence

Epidemiologic Studies

A number of large studies, including school and community adolescent samples using survey measures, have reported high rates of binge eating in the absence of full-syndrome BED, ranging from approximately 6% to almost 40% (Croll, Neumark-Sztainer, Story, & Ireland, 2002; French et al., 1997; Greenfeld, Quinlan, Harding, Glass, & Bliss, 1987; Johnson, Rohan, & Kirk, 2002; Neumark-Sztainer, Story, Resnick, & Blum, 1997). Although several studies have reported few or no differences between girls and boys or among racial and ethnic groups, Croll and colleagues found females to be twice as likely as males to report binge eating (25.6% versus 12.5%), with binge eating most common among Hispanic females (Croll et al., 2002). The former finding was supported by a survey of nontreatment-seeking 13- to 19-year-olds in which 45% of females and 16% of males reported binge eating (Greenfeld et al.). By contrast, Field and colleagues found no significant gender difference with regard to the prevalence of binge eating but did find Hispanic boys twice as likely as white boys to report binge eating (Field, Colditz, & Peterson, 1997b). Using a questionnaire to assess binge eating in African American and white male and female teenagers, Johnson et al. (2002) found that binge eating was most commonly reported by African American males. However, in two multiracial cohorts of adolescent females, substantial differences in binge eating based on ethnicity or race were not detected (Field, Colditz, & Peterson, 1997a; French et al.). Studies specifically examining the prevalence of full-syndrome BED in non-treatment-seeking teenagers report that few meet criteria for full-syndrome BED (Johnson, Kirk, & Reed, 2001; Stice & Agras, 1998). Making use of interview methodology, Stice and Agras found that only 4% report binge eating.

The prevalence of binge eating has also been studied in relation to sexual orientation. French and colleagues found a relationship between sexual orientation and binge eating; male homosexual and female heterosexual adolescents were more likely to report binge eating than heterosexual males and homosexual females, respectively (French, Story, Remafedi,

Resnick, & Blum, 1996). In another study examining sexual orientation, Austin et al. (2004) replicated these findings in males and also reported that compared with heterosexual females, "mostly heterosexual" girls (individuals who defined themselves as neither heterosexual nor bisexual but somewhere in between) were more likely to binge eat.

Correlates of Binge Eating

Regardless of demographic variables, adolescents who report binge eating are more likely to manifest disordered eating cognitions, depressive symptoms, poor family and social functioning, and emotional stress than those who do not (French et al., 1997; Johnson et al., 2002; Ledoux, Choquet, & Manfredi, 1993; Neumark-Sztainer, & Hannan, 2000; Steiger, Puentes-Neuman, & Leung, 1991). Furthermore, cross-sectional data suggest that binge eating is associated with overweight in adolescents. A school-based study of 7th- through 12th-graders found that overweight participants self-report binge eating more frequently than do their normal-weight peers (Neumark-Sztainer et al., 1997). Similar findings have been reported in a number of studies; older and heavier teens report a higher prevalence of binge eating than their younger and leaner counterparts (Ackard, Neumark-Sztainer, Story, & Perry, 2003; Field et al., 1997a). The association between binge eating, overweight and sex remains unclear. In a study by Field et al. (1997b), overweight was associated with binge eating in girls but not boys, while Ackard et al. reported a relationship between binge eating and obesity among boys but not girls.

Treatment-Seeking Overweight Adolescents

Although few non-treatment-seeking adolescents meet full criteria for BED, the prevalence of BED among treatment-seeking obese teens has been reported by three studies. Among a sample of 51 girls aged 14–16 years, 30% manifested "unequivocal binge-eating" by interview assessing the BED criteria (Berkowitz, Stunkard, & Stallings, 1993). Decaluwe and Braet (2003) reported that only 1% of 196 boys and girls (10–16 years) seeking either inpatient or outpatient weight loss treatment met full BED criteria based upon their responses to the Eating Disorder Examination (EDE) (Fairburn & Cooper, 1993) adapted for children (Bryant-Waugh et al., 1996). In a more recent study of 12- to 17-year-old severely obese teens, not only did 6.3% meet criteria for BED according to their EDE interviews, but participants with BED suffered from eating-related and psychological distress at levels similar to those of adults with the disorder (Glasofer et al., 2007).

Findings from studies that did not assess for full BED criteria suggest that subthreshold binge eating (fewer than two binge episodes per week over six months) among overweight adolescents appears to be substantial, with estimates ranging from 20% (Isnard et al., 2003) to approximately 35% (Decaluwe, Braet, & Fairburn, 2001) in weight loss treatment-seeking samples. Studies of adolescents seeking weight loss treatment have found that those who report subthreshold binge eating have greater eating-related distress, anxiety, and depressive symptomatology and poorer self-esteem than those who do not report any binge eating (Berkowitz et al., 1993; Decaluwe, & Braet, 2003; Decaluwe et al.; Glasofer et al., 2007; Goossens, Braet and Decaluwe, 2007; Isnard et al.). In contrast to non-treatment samples, BMI differences between binge eaters and non-binge eaters have generally not been found (Berkowitz et al.; Decaluwe, Braet, & Fairburn, 2003; Glasofer et al., 2007; Goossens et al., 2007; Isnard et al. 2003), with the exception of the Decaluwe and Braet study (2003). Of the studies examining both sexes, again only Decaluwe and Braet reported a significant difference, with binge eating more common among girls than boys.

Binge Eating in Young Children

Fewer studies of binge eating have been conducted with young children, particularly among non-treatment-seeking samples. A recent study of 6-year-old children living in Germany found that 2% of children engaged in binge eating, according to their parents' responses to a survey administered at well-child visits (Lamerz et al., 2005). Among a nonclinical sample of girls aged 7–13 years assessed by questionnaire, 10.4% reported binge eating behaviors (Maloney, McGuire, Daniels, & Specker, 1989). In a large survey-based study of boys and girls (9–14 years), Field et al. (1999) found that the prevalence of monthly binge eating among girls increased linearly with age; only 0.4% of 9-year-olds endorsed binge eating, but 3.6% of 14-year-olds did. None of these investigations assessed for the full DSM-IV-TR (APA, 2000) criteria for BED. One study making use of interview methodology (EDE adapted for children) found that among non-treatment-seeking overweight (BMI greater than or equal to the 85th percentile for age, sex and race) (Frisancho, 1990) and nonoverweight children aged 6–13 years, none met full criteria for BED (Tanofsky-Kraff et al., 2004). However, in the month prior to assessment, 6.3% reported engaging in binge episodes and 3.1% reported experiencing loss of control (LOC) while eating, although the amount of food ingested was not unambiguously large. Those with binge/LOC eating were heavier, had more adiposity and endorsed greater disordered eating cognitions than children who endorsed overeating episodes without LOC or no episodes (Tanofsky-Kraff et al.). In the studies that examined body weight, a relationship consistently emerged between overweight and the likelihood that children endorsed either binge eating or LOC eating (Field et al., 1999; Lamerz et al.; Tanofsky-Kraff et al.).

Not surprisingly, therefore, a number of researchers examining binge eating have focused specifically on samples of overweight children. Studying non-treatment-seeking overweight (BMI greater than or equal to the 85th percentile for age, sex and race) (Frisancho, 1990) children (6–10 years), Morgan et al. (2002) found that 5.3% of the sample met criteria for BED according to self-report questionnaires and that those experiencing LOC while eating over the past six months were heavier and had greater body fat than children not experiencing LOC. Moreover, children reporting LOC had higher anxiety, more depressive symptoms, and increased body dissatisfaction than overweight children without LOC. With the use of interview methodology with a sample of overweight (BMI greater than or equal to the 85th percentile for age, sex and race) (Frisancho)

6- to 13-year-olds, none of whom were seeking treatment, 29.5% reported LOC eating at least once in their lifetimes, but none met criteria for BED (Tanofsky-Kraff, Faden, Yanovski, Wilfley, & Yanovski, 2005). While differences were found between children with and without LOC — the former group had greater disordered eating cognitions, ineffectiveness, negative self-esteem, and parent-reported externalizing problems — no differences were detected between groups with regard to BMI or adiposity.

Only one study has specifically examined binge eating among children in the laboratory (Mirch et al., 2006). A sample of overweight children (6–12 years), all of whom demonstrated evidence of insulin resistance and were seeking medication weight loss treatment, were administered the Questionnaire of Eating and Weight Patterns (Spitzer, Yanovski, & Marcus, 1993) – Adolescent Version (Johnson et al., 1999) to determine the presence of binge eating. Children endorsing binge eating over the six months prior to assessment became hungrier sooner following a preload, reported a greater desire to eat, and ingested more energy during a laboratory test meal than children who did not endorse binge eating (Mirch et al.). Such findings suggest that binge eating among young children may be an observable behavior that is distinct among a subset of overweight youths. Research is required to determine whether similar results would emerge among healthy-weight and older children who endorse binge eating.

Outcome of Youths who Binge Eat

Weight Loss Treatment

The pediatric literature examining binge eating in relation to weight loss treatment outcome is limited. Epstein and colleagues found no significant changes in binge eating behaviors following family-based behavioral weight loss treatment for 8- to 12-year-olds (Epstein, Paluch, Saelens, Ernst, & Wilfley, 2001). By contrast, in a sample of obese youths (7–17 years) taking part in an inpatient non-diet healthy lifestyle program focusing on healthy eating, moderate exercise, and cognitive-behavioral treatment, the mean frequency of binge eating episodes was significantly lower at both post-treatment and 14-month follow-up (Braet, Tanghe, Decaluwe, Moens, & Rosseel, 2004). One recent study examined the impact of LOC eating on weight loss achieved during a family-based behavioral program for 8- to 13-year-olds (Levine, Ringham, Kalarchian, Wisniewski, & Marcus, 2006). Following treatment, children reporting LOC experienced similar weight loss to those not reporting LOC. These preliminary data suggest that weight loss treatment may not have an adverse impact on young binge eaters and that LOC eating may not affect weight loss outcome.

Prospective Research

Perhaps of greatest concern is the finding that children and adolescents who self-report binge eating episodes tend to experience increased weight and fat gain over time compared with youths who do not report binge eating. In a large study of boys and girls (9–14 years), Field et al. (2003) found that binge eating, as assessed by survey reports, was an independent predictor of weight gain among boys. As assessed by an adapted version of the EDE, binge eating was a predictor of elevated weight gain (Stice, Cameron, Killen, Hayward, & Taylor, 1999) and obesity onset (Stice, Presnell, & Spangler, 2002) among adolescent girls followed over a four-year period. However, this finding was not replicated in a third study (Stice, Presnell, Shaw, & Rohde, 2005). Finally, in a study of 146 children aged 6–12 at baseline, all of whom were overweight or at risk for overweight because of a family history of obesity (Whitaker, Wright, Pepe, Seidel, & Dietz, 1997), binge eating at baseline was a predictor of additional increases in body fat mass four years later (Tanofsky-Kraff et al., 2006). Taken together, these data point to the role that binge eating during youth may play in the development or maintenance of obesity. Additional research is required to determine whether early binge eating increases the risk for other adverse conditions such as full-syndrome eating disorders, other psychiatric disturbance, or additional health consequences above and beyond those associated with obesity.

A number of researchers have examined potential predictive factors for the development of binge eating with the aim of identifying targets for early prevention. To date, a limited number of studies have been published. In a five-year prospective study of 216 mothers and their children, Stice and colleagues annually assessed the development of overeating in children at ages 2 through 5 years by asking mothers to respond to the question "Does your child enjoy eating certain foods so much that it appears that he/she has difficulty stopping?" (Stice, Agras, & Hammer, 1999). The researchers found that 33.8% of the children began overeating at some point during the study and that overeating increased annually, with the highest percentage of the emergence of overeating in any one-year period being 17.6%. Furthermore, a number of factors predicted an increased hazard for the emergence of overeating, including: factors related to maternal eating behaviors such as "heightened restraint" and "drive for thinness," mothers' BMI, parental overweight history, and infant (first month of life) BMI and sucking duration.

Studies among older youths have examined child and adolescent attitudes and behaviors in the prediction of binge eating. In a prospective investigation of adolescent boys and girls (10–15 years), Field et al. (2002) examined the emergence of unhealthy behaviors including smoking, alcohol intoxication, and binge eating and purging. While the three behaviors were associated with one another prospectively, the construct "weight concerns" was predictive of the emergence of binge eating as well as smoking and drinking alcohol to a state of inebriation. Furthermore, among a sample of ninth-grade girls, dieting was found to be predictive of binge eating onset over a four-year interval (Stice, Killen, Hayward, & Taylor, 1998). Including a number of weight- and shape-related variables in addition to measures of depressive and anxiety symptoms, anger, self-esteem, and social support, Stice et al. (2002) prospectively studied 13- to 17-year-old girls over a two-year period. Binge eating onset was predicted by increased dieting, pressure to be thin, modeling of eating disturbances, appearance overvaluation, body dissatisfaction, depressive symptoms, emotional eating, BMI, low self-esteem, and social support with 92% accuracy. In summary, weight- and body-related attitudes and behaviors of parents of young children and teens may be important factors in targeting the prevention of binge eating onset.

Future Research and Challenges

Because of inconsistent findings regarding factors that predict binge eating in children and adolescents as well as methods to qualitatively define the construct of binge eating in pediatric samples, continued research within these areas is required. A number of topics in need of further exploration are broadly described below.

Clarify and Conceptualize Binge Eating in Children

A better understanding of what constitutes binge eating among youths may produce more consistent findings across studies and help target children in need of intervention for overweight or more severe eating disturbance. Researchers typically base measures that assess disturbed eating patterns upon adult versions that contain probes relevant to adults with binge eating but not necessarily to children. In particular, the construct and experience of "loss of control" requires further investigation, particularly given that some children may not understand the concept, nor may they comfortably admit to feeling "out of control" or "unable to stop" once having started eating. As such, exploratory research is required to capture the qualitative aspects of aberrant eating episodes described by children. Analyzing a number of behavioral, physical, and emotional variables potentially surrounding aberrant eating episodes has been suggested as one method to elucidate eating patterns among overweight individuals (Tanofsky-Kraff & Yanovski, 2004). Such methods may be especially germane to studying children's eating episodes and may provide a child-specific phenotype that is reflective of adult binge eating.

Research should also focus on the importance of the criterion of a "large amount of food given the context" to describe binge episodes in children. Some data already suggest that the experience of LOC among youths, as opposed to episode size, may be the more salient factor associated with emotional distress and body composition (Morgan et al., 2002; Tanofsky-Kraff et al., 2004, 2005). Furthermore, because nutritional needs change in growing children, quantifying whether a given amount of food is unambiguously large given the age and sex of a child as well as the context of the eating episode is not only challenging but often disputable. In taking a conservative approach such as that required in administering the EDE (Fairburn & Cooper, 1993), if an amount of food described during an episode is not unambiguously large, researchers will often code the amount as "not large." Therefore, the quantity of food that constitutes "binge" episodes in children is often not much larger than an amount of food considered "not unambiguously large."

In a 2003 review of the literature on binge eating in children and adolescents, Marcus and Kalarchian proposed provisional BED research

Table 4.2. Provisional Research Criteria for Diagnosing Binge Eating Disorder in Children (Marcus & Kalarchian, 2003)

A. Recurrent episodes of binge eating. An episode of binge eating is characterized by both of the following:
1. Food seeking in absence of hunger (e.g., after a full meal).
2. A sense of lack of control over eating (e.g., endorse that, "When I start to eat, I just can't stop").
B. Binge episodes are associated with one or more of the following:
1. Food seeking in response to negative affect (e.g., sadness, boredom, restlessness).
2. Food seeking as a reward.
3. Sneaking or hiding food.
C. Symptoms persist over a period of three months.
D. Eating is not associated with the regular use of inappropriate compensatory behaviors (e.g., purging, fasting, excessive exercise) and does not occur exclusively during the course of anorexia nervosa or bulimia nervosa.

criteria for children 14 years and younger (Table 4.2). Supporting some data among child samples (Morgan et al., 2002; Tanofsky-Kraff et al., 2004), criterion A1 of their proposed diagnosis removes the requirement of a "large amount of food" being ingested in the definition of a binge, but the experience of LOC is retained. Inclusion of a new requirement of eating "in absence of hunger" (criterion A1) has been suggested as a potentially significant construct in body weight among young children (Faith et al., 2006; Fisher & Birch, 2002). Using a feeding paradigm, Fisher and Birch examined eating in the absence of hunger among 5-year-old girls at baseline and again two years later. Not only was eating in the absence of hunger a stable trait among girls over time, but girls who ate in the absence of hunger were significantly more likely to be overweight than girls who did not eat in the absence of hunger. Of criterion B, the first symptom, "food seeking in response to negative affect," has been studied in young children. Among 5-year-old girls, Carper and colleagues reported evidence of emotional disinhibition of eating in 25% of the sample (Carper, Orlet Fisher, & Birch, 2000). In Stice and colleagues' study of the emergence of eating disturbance during the first five years of life (Stice, Agras et al. 1999), criterion B3, "sneaking or hiding food," was examined. Secretive eating was assessed based upon mothers' responses to the question "Does your child hide any favorite food in his/her room or elsewhere in the house?" During the five-year period, 18.1% of children experienced the emergence of secretive eating. Furthermore, heightened maternal disinhibition, hunger, body dissatisfaction, and bulimic symptoms as well as elevated maternal BMI and paternal history of overweight were predictors of an increased hazard for the emergence of secretive eating (Stice, Agras et al., 1999). Finally, two recent studies report that loss of control and binge eating are associated with eating in response to negative emotions during middle childhood and adolescence (Goossens et al., 2007; Tanofsky-Kraff et al., 2007). Further data is required to assess the significance and impact of emotional and secretive eating as well as criterion B2, "food seeking as a reward" during childhood.

Only one study has tested Marcus and Kalarchian's provisional criteria (Shapiro, Hammer, Woolson, & Bullik, 2007). A brief measure designed specifically to assess the proposed criteria was administered to 55 children (aged 5–13 years) seeking weight loss treatment. The authors diagnosed 30% of the sample with BED. Since similar rates of BED are reported in treatment-seeking adults (Spitzer et al., 1991; Spitzer, Yanovski, & Wadden et al. 1993), these preliminary findings may suggest that Marcus and Kalarchian's provisional criteria for BED are more suitable for children with binge eating problems than those proposed in the DSM-IV-TR (APA, 2000). In summary, researchers should continue to think broadly in creating novel methods to capture the construct of aberrant eating in young children.

Role of Dieting

A common conviction is that binge eating manifests in response to excessive dietary restriction. Restraint theory, which has gained significant support among researchers and clinicians, posits that dietary restriction increases the risk for the onset of binge eating and bulimic pathology (Polivy, & Herman, 1985). While a review of dieting among children and adolescents is beyond the scope of this chapter, a number of studies have reported relationships between dietary restraint and binge (Stice et al., 1998, 2002) and LOC eating (Tanofsky-Kraff et al., 2005). However, findings across retrospective studies of adults with BED (Abbott et al., 1998; Grilo & Masheb, 2000, Marcus et al., 1995, Spurrell et al., 1997) and overweight children (Tanofsky-Kraff et al., 2005) that examine the age when the onset of dieting and binge eating occurs report that a significant number of individuals recall binge eating before they made attempts at dieting for weight loss. Future studies of pediatric binge eating exploring theoretical pathways other than restraint theory are warranted.

CONCLUSION

The emerging literature provides evidence that the prevalence of pediatric binge eating is substantial and appears to be associated with elevated psychological distress and overweight. Similar to binge eating disorder among adults, binge eating among youths does not appear to discriminate between races, ethnicity, or sex. Given the inconsistencies of findings across studies, further research is required to elucidate the construct of binge eating during childhood and adolescence. Nevertheless, since reported binge eating during childhood and adolescence is likely a risk factor for continued excessive weight gain, interventions targeting binge eating may serve as a viable approach toward reducing the current obesity epidemic (Yanovski, 2003).

REFERENCES

Abbott, D. W., de Zwaan, M., Mussell, M. P., Raymond, N. C., Seim, H. C., Crow, S. J., et al. (1998). Onset of binge eating and dieting in overweight women: Implications for etiology, associated features and treatment. *Journal of Psychosomatic Research, 44*, 367–374.

Ackard, D. M., Neumark-Sztainer, D., Story, M., & Perry, C. (2003). Overeating among adolescents: Prevalence and associations with weight-related characteristics and psychological health. *Pediatrics, 111*, 67–74.

American Psychiatric Association (Ed.). (1994). *Diagnostic and statistical manual of mental disorders (4th ed)*. Washington, DC: Author.

American Psychiatric Association. (2000). *Diagnostic and statistical manual of mental disorders DSM-IV-TR*. Washington, DC: Author.

Austin, S. B., Ziyadeh, N., Kahn, J. A., Camargo, C. A., Jr., Colditz, G. A., & Field, A. E. (2004). Sexual orientation, weight concerns, and eating-disordered behaviors in adolescent girls and boys. *Journal of the American Academy of Child and Adolescent Psychiatry, 43*, 1115–1123.

Berkowitz, R., Stunkardm, A. J., & Stallings, V. A. (1993). Binge-eating disorder in obese adolescent girls. *Annals of New York Academy of Sciences, 699*, 200–206.

Binford, R. B., Pederson-Mussell, M., Peterson, C. B., Crow, S. J., & Mitchell, J. E. (2004). Relation of binge eating age of onset to functional aspects of binge eating in binge eating disorder. *International Journal of Eating Disorders, 35*, 286–292.

Braet, C., Tanghe, A., Decaluwe, V., Moens, E., & Rosseel, Y. (2004). Inpatient treatment for children with obesity: Weight loss, psychological well-being, and eating behavior. *Journal of Pediatric Psychology, 29*, 519–529.

Bryant-Waugh, R. J., Cooper, P. J., Taylor, C. L., & Lask, B. D. (1996). The use of the eating disorder examination with children: A pilot study. *International Journal of Eating Disorders, 19*, 391–397.

Carper, J. L., Orlet Fisher, J., & Birch, L. L. (2000). Young girls' emerging dietary restraint and disinhibition are related to parental control in child feeding. *Appetite, 35*, 121–129.

Croll, J., Neumark-Sztainer, D., Story, M., & Ireland, M. (2002). Prevalence and risk and protective factors related to disordered eating behaviors among adolescents: Relationship to gender and ethnicity. *Journal of Adolescent Health, 31*, 166–175.

Crow, S. (2002). Does binge eating disorder exist? Paper presented at the Eating Disorders Research Society, Charleston, South Carolina.

Crow, S. J., Stewart Agras, W., Halmi, K., Mitchell, J. E., & Kraemer, H. C. (2002). Full syndromal versus subthreshold anorexia nervosa, bulimia nervosa, and binge eating disorder: A multicenter study. *International Journal Eating Disorders, 32*, 309–318.

Decaluwe, V., & Braet, C. (2003). Prevalence of binge-eating disorder in obese children and adolescents seeking weight-loss treatment. *International Journal of Obesity Related Metabolic Disorders, 27*, 404–409.

Decaluwe, V., & Braet, C. (2004). Assessment of eating disorder psychopathology in obese children and adolescents: Interview versus self-report questionnaire. *Behavior Research and Therapy, 42*, 799–811.

Decaluwe, V., Braet, C., & Fairburn, C. G. (2001). Binge eating in obese children and adolescents. *International Journal of Eating Disorders, 33*, 78–84.

Decaluwe, V., Braet, C., & Fairburn, C. G. (2003). Binge eating in obese children and adolescents. *International Journal of Eating Disorders, 33*, 78–84.

de Zwaan, M., Mitchell, J., Howell, L., Monson, N., Swan-Kremeier, L., Roerig, J., et al. (2002). Two measures of health-related quality of life in morbid obesity. *Obesity Research, 10*, 1143–1151.

Epstein, L. H., Paluch, R. A., Saelens, B. E., Ernst, M. M., & Wilfley, D. E. (2001). Changes in eating disorder symptoms with pediatric obesity treatment. *Journal of Pediatrics, 139*, 58–65.

Fairburn, C., & Cooper, Z. (1993). The eating disorder examination (12th ed). In: Fairburn, C. G. and Wilson, G. T. (eds) Binge eating, nature, assessment and treatment (317–360), New York, Guilford, 1999.

Fairburn, C., Cooper, Z., Doll, H., Norman, P., & O'Connor, M. (2000). The natural course of bulimia nervosa and binge eating disorder in young women. *Archives of General Psychiatry, 57*, 659–665.

Faith, M. S., Berkowitz, R. I., Stallings, V. A., Kerns, J., Storey, M., & Stunkard, A. J. (2006). Eating in the absence of hunger: A genetic marker for childhood obesity in prepubertal boys? *Obesity, 14*, 131–138.

Field, A. E., Austin, S. B., Frazier, A. L., Gillman, M. W., Camargo, C. A., Jr, & Colditz, G. A. (2002). Smoking, getting drunk, and engaging in bulimic behaviors: In which order are the behaviors adopted? *Journal of the American Academy of Child and Adolescent Psychiatry, 41*, 846–853.

Field, A. E., Austin, S. B., Taylor, C. B., Malspeis, S., Rosner, B., Rockett, H. R., et al. (2003). Relation between dieting and weight change among preadolescents and adolescents. *Pediatrics, 112*, 900–906.

Field, A. E., Camargo, C. A., Jr, Taylor, C. B., Berkey, C. S., Frazier, A. L., Gillman, M. W., et al. (1999). Overweight, weight concerns, and bulimic behaviors among girls and boys. *Journal of the American Academy of Child and Adolescent Psychiatry, 38*, 754–760.

Field, A. E., Colditz, G. A., & Peterson, K. E. (1997a). Racial differences in bulimic behaviors among high school females. *Annal of New York Academy of Sciences, 817*, 359–360.

Field, A. E., Colditz, G. A., & Peterson, K. E. (1997b). Racial/ethnic and gender differences in concern with weight and in bulimic behaviors among adolescents. *Obesity Research, 5*, 447–454.

Field, A. E., Taylor, C. B., Celio, A., & Colditz, G. A. (2004). Comparison of self-report to interview assessment of bulimic behaviors among preadolescent and adolescent girls and boys. *International Journal of Eating Disorders, 35*, 86–92.

Fisher, J. O., & Birch, L. L. (2002). Eating in the absence of hunger and overweight in girls from 5 to 7y of age. *American Journal of Clinical Nutrition, 76*, 226–231.

French, S. A., Story, M., Neumark-Sztainer, D., Downes, B., Resnick, M., & Blum, R. (1997). Ethnic differences in psychosocial and health behavior correlates of dieting, purging, and binge eating in a population-based sample of adolescent females. *International Journal of Eating Disorders, 22*, 315–322.

French, S. A., Story, M., Remafedi, G., Resnick, M. D., & Blum, R. W. (1996). Sexual orientation and prevalence of body dissatisfaction and eating disordered behaviors: A population-based study of adolescents. *International Journal of Eating Disorders, 19*, 119–126.

Frisancho, A. R. (1990). *Anthropometric standards for the assessment of growth and nutritional status.* Ann Arbor, Michigan: The University of Michigan Press.

Glasofer, D. R., Tanofsky-Kraff, M., Eddy, K. T., Yanovski, S. Z., Theim. K., Mirch, M., et al. (2007). Binge eating in overweight treatment-seeking adolescents. *Journal of Pediatric Psychology, 32*, 95–105.

Goossens, L., Braet, C., & Decaluwe, V. (2007). Loss of control over eating in obese youngsters. *Behaviour Research and Therapy, 45(1)*, 1–9.

Greenfeld, D., Quinlan, D. M., Harding, P., Glass, E., & Bliss, A. (1987). Eating behavior in an adolescent population. *International Journal of Eating Disorders, 6*, 99–111.

Grilo, C. M., & Masheb, R. M. (2000). Onset of dieting vs binge eating in outpatients with binge eating disorder. *International Journal of Obesity and Related Metabolic Disorders, 24*, 404–409.

Isnard, P., Michel, G., Frelut, M. L., Vila, G., Falissard, B., Naja, W., et al. (2003). Binge eating and psychopathology in severely obese adolescents. *International Journal of Eating Disorders, 34*, 235–243.

Johnson, J. G., Spitzer, R. L., & Williams, J. B. (2001). Health problems, impairment and illnesses associated with bulimia nervosa and binge eating disorder among primary care and obstetric gynaecology patients. *Psychological Medicine, 31*, 1455–1466.

Johnson, W. G., Grieve, F. G., Adams, C. D., & Sandy, J. (1999). Measuring binge eating in adolescents: Adolescent and parent versions of the questionnaire of eating and weight patterns. *International Journal of Eating Disorders, 26*, 301–314.

Johnson, W. G., Kirk, A. A., & Reed, A. E. (2001). Adolescent version of the questionnaire of eating and weight patterns: Reliability and gender differences. *International Journal of Eating Disorders, 29*, 94–96.

Johnson, W. G., Rohan, K. J., & Kirk, A. A. (2002). Prevalence and correlates of binge eating in white and African American adolescents. *Eating Behaviors, 3*,179–189

Kashubeck-West, S., Mintz, L. B., Saundersam, K. J. (2001). Assessment of eating disorders in women. *The Counseling Psychologist, 29*, 662–694.

Lamerz, A., Kuepper-Nybelen, J., Bruning, N., Wehle, C., Trost-Brinkhues, G., Brenner, H., et al. (2005). Prevalence of obesity, binge eating, and night eating in a cross-sectional field survey of 6-year-old children and their parents in a German urban population. *Journal of Child Psychology and Psychiatry, 46*, 385–393.

Ledoux, S., Choquet, M., & Manfredi, R. (1993). Associated factors for self-reported binge eating among male and female adolescents. *Journal of Adolescence, 16*, 75–91.

Levine, M. D., Ringham, R. M., Kalarchian, M. A., Wisniewski, L., & Marcus, M. D. (2006). Overeating among seriously overweight children seeking treatment: Results of the children's eating disorder examination. *International Journal of Eating Disorders, 39*, 135–140.

Maloney, M. J., McGuire, J., Daniels, S. R., & Specker, B. (1989). Dieting behavior and eating attitudes in children. *Pediatrics, 84*, 482–489.

Maloney, M. J., McGuire, J. B., & Daniels, S. R. (1988). Reliability testing of a children's version of the Eating Attitude Test. *Journal of the American Academy of Child and Adolescent Psychiatry, 27*, 541–543.

Marcus, M. D. (1995). Introduction — binge eating: Clinical and research directions. *Addictive Behaviors, 20*, 691–693.

Marcus, M. D., & Kalarchian, M. A. (2003). Binge eating in children and adolescents. *International Journal of Eating Disorders, 34*(Suppl), 47–57.

Marcus, M. D., Moulton, M. M., & Greeno, C. G. (1995). Binge eating onset in obese patients with binge eating disorder. *Addictive Behaviors, 20*, 747–755.

Masheb, R. M., & Grilo, C. M. (2000). Binge eating disorder: A need for additional diagnostic criteria. *Comprehensive Psychiatry, 41*, 159–162.

Mirch, M. C., McDuffie, J. R., Yanovski, S. Z., Schollnberger, M., Tanofsky-Kraff, M., Theim, K. R., et al. (2006). Effects of binge eating on satiation, satiety, and energy intake of overweight children. *American Journal of Clinical Nutrition, 84*, 732–738.

Morgan, C., Yanovski, S., Nguyen, T., McDuffie, J., Sebring, N., Jorge, M., et al. (2002). Loss of control over eating, adiposity, and psychopathology in overweight children. *International Journal of Eating Disorders, 31*, 430–441.

Mussell, M. P., Mitchell, J. E., de Zwaan, M., Crosby, R. D., Seim, H. C., & Crow, S. J. (1996). Clinical characteristics associated with binge eating in obese females: A descriptive study. *International Journal of Obesity and Related Metabolic Disorders, 20*, 324–331.

Mussell, M. P., Mitchell, J. E., Weller, C. L., Raymond, N. C., Crow, S. J., & Crosby, R. D. (1995). Onset of binge eating, dieting, obesity, and mood disorders among subjects seeking treatment for binge eating disorder. *International Journal of Eating Disorders, 17*, 395–401.

Neumark-Sztainer, D., & Hannan, P. J. (2000). Weight-related behaviors among adolescent girls and boys: Results from a national survey. *Archives of Pediatric and Adolescent Medicine, 154*, 569–577.

Neumark-Sztainer, D., Story, M., French, S. A., Hannan, P. J., Resnick, M. D., & Blum, R. W. (1997). Psychosocial concerns and health-compromising behaviors among overweight and nonoverweight adolescents. *Obesity Research, 5*, 237–249.

Neumark-Sztainer, D., Story, M., Resnick, M. D., & Blum, R. W. (1997). Psychosocial concerns and weight control behaviors among overweight and nonoverweight Native American adolescents. *Journal of the American Dietetic Association, 97*, 598–604.

Ogden, C. L., Carroll, M. D., Curtin, L. R., McDowell, M. A., Tabak, C. J., & Flegal, K. M. (2006). Prevalence of overweight and obesity in the United States, 1999–2004. *Journal of the American Medical Association, 295*, 1549–1555.

Ogden, C. L., Kuczmarski, R. J., Flegal, K. M., Mei, Z., Guo, S., Wei, R., et al. (2002). Centers for Disease Control and Prevention 2000 growth charts for the United States: Improvements to the 1977 National Center for Health Statistics version. *Pediatrics, 109*, 45–60.

Polivy, J., & Herman, C. P. (1985). Dieting and binging: A causal analysis. *American Psychologist, 40*, 193–201.

Shapiro, J. R., Woolson, S. L., Hamer, R. M., Kalarchian, M. A., Marcus, M. D., & Bulik, C. M. (2007). Evaluating binge eating disorder in children: Development of the children's binge eating disorder scale (C-BEDS). *International Journal of Eating Disorder, 40(1)*, 82–89.

Sherwood, N. E., Jeffery, R. W., & Wing, R. R. (1999). Binge status as a predictor of weight loss treatment outcome. *International Journal of Obesity and Related Metabolic Disorders, 23,* 485–493.

Smith, D., Marcus, M., Lewis, C., Fitzgibbon, M., & Schreiner, P. (1998). Prevalence of binge eating disorder, obesity, and depression in a biracial cohort of young adults. Annals of Behavioral Medicine, 20, 227–232.

Spitzer, R., Devlin, M., Walsh, B. T., Hasin, D., Wing, R., Marcus, M., et al. (1991). Binge eating disorder: To be or not to be in DSM-IV. *International Journal of Eating Disorders, 10,* 627–629.

Spitzer, R. L., Yanovski, S., Wadden, T., Wing, R., Marcus, M. D., Stunkard, A., et al. (1993). Binge eating disorder: Its further validation in a multisite study. *International Journal of Eating Disorders, 13,* 137–153.

Spitzer, R. L., Yanovski, S. Z., & Marcus, M. D. (1993). *The questionnaire on eating and weight patterns-revised (QEWP-R).* New York: New York State Psychiatric Institute.

Spurrell, E. B., Wilfley, D. E., Tanofsky, M. B., & Brownell, K. D. (1997). Age of onset for binge eating: Are there different pathways to binge eating? *International Journal of Eating Disorders, 21,* 55–65.

Steiger, H., Gauvin, L., Jabalpurwala, S., Seguin, J. R., & Stotland, S. (1999). Hypersensitivity to social interactions in bulimic syndromes: Relationship to binge eating. *Journal of Consulting and Clinical Psychology, 67,* 765–775.

Steiger, H., Puentes-Neuman, G., & Leung, F. Y. (1991). Personality and family features of adolescent girls with eating symptoms: Evidence for restricter/binger differences in a nonclinical population. *Addictive Behaviors, 16,* 303–314.

Steinberg, E., Tanofsky-Kraff, M., Cohen, M. L., Elberg, J., Freedman, R. J., Semega-Janneh, M., et al. (2004). Comparison of the child and parent forms of the Questionnaire on Eating and Weight Patterns in the assessment of children's eating-disordered behaviors. *International Journal of Eating Disorders, 36,* 183–194.

Stice, E., & Agras, W. S. (1998). Predicting onset and cessation of bulimic behaviors during adolescence: A longitudinal grouping analysis. *Behavior Therapy, 29,* 257–276.

Stice, E., Agras, W. S., & Hammer, L. D. (1999). Risk factors for the emergence of childhood eating disturbances: A five-year prospective study. *International Journal of Eating Disorders, 25,* 375–387.

Stice, E., Cameron, R. P., Killen, J. D., Hayward, C., & Taylor, C. B. (1999). Naturalistic weight-reduction efforts prospectively predict growth in relative weight and onset of obesity among female adolescents. *Journal of Consulting and Clinical Psychology, 67,* 967–974.

Stice, E., Killen, J. D., Hayward, C., & Taylor, C. B. (1998). Age of onset for binge eating and purging during late adolescence: A 4-year survival analysis. *Journal of Abnormal Psychology, 107,* 671–675.

Stice, E., Presnell, K., Shaw, H., & Rohde, P. (2005). Psychological and behavioral risk factors for obesity onset in adolescent girls: A prospective study. *Journal of Consulting and Clinical Psychology, 73,* 195–202.

Stice, E., Presnell, K., & Spangler, D. (2002). Risk factors for binge eating onset in adolescent girls: A 2-year prospective investigation. *Health Psychology, 21,* 131–138.

Striegel-Moore, R. H., Wilfley, D. E., Pike, K. M., Dohm, F. A., & Fairburn, C. G. (2000). Recurrent binge eating in black American women. *Archives of Family Medicine, 9,* 83–87.

Stunkard, A. J. (1959). Eating patterns and obesity. *Psychiatry Quarterly, 33,* 284–295.

Tanofsky-Kraff, M., Cohen, M. L., Yanovski, S. Z., Cox, C., Theim, K. R., Keil, M., et al. (2006). A prospective study of psychological predictors of body fat gain among children at high risk for adult obesity. *Pediatrics, 117,* 1203–1209.

Tanofsky-Kraff, M., Faden, D., Yanovski, S. Z., Wilfley, D. E., & Yanovski, J. A. (2005). The perceived onset of dieting and loss of control eating behaviors in overweight children. *International Journal of Eating Disorders, 38,* 112–122.

Tanofsky-Kraff, M., Morgan, C. M., Yanovski, S. Z., Marmarosh, C., Wilfley, D. E., & Yanovski, J. A. (2003). Comparison of assessments of children's eating-disordered behaviors by interview and questionnaire. *International Journal of Eating Disorders, 33,* 213–224.

Tanofsky-Kraff, M., Theim, K. R., Yanovski, S. Z., Bassett, A. M., Burns, N. P., Ranzenhofer, L. M., et al. (2007). Validation of the emotional eating scale adapted for use in children and adolescents (EES-C). *International Journal of Eating Disorders, 40,* 232–240.

Tanofsky-Kraff, M., & Yanovski, S. Z. (2004). Eating disorder or disordered eating? Non-normative eating patterns in obese individuals. *Obesity Research, 12,* 1361–1366.

Tanofsky-Kraff, M., Yanovski, S. Z., Wilfley, D. E., Marmarosh, C., Morgan, C. M., & Yanovski, J. A. (2004). Eating disordered behaviors, body fat, and psychopathology in overweight and normal weight children. *Journal of Consulting and Clinical Psychology, 72,* 53–61.

Tanofsky-Kraff, M., Yanovski, S. Z., & Yanovski, J. A. (2005). Comparison of child interview and parent reports of children's eating disordered behaviors. *Eating Behaviors, 6,* 95–99.

Whitaker, R. C., Wright, J. A., Pepe, M. S., Seidel, K. D., & Dietz, W. H. (1997). Predicting obesity in young adulthood from childhood and parental obesity. *New England Journal of Medicine, 337,* 869–873.

Wilfley, D., Wilson, G., & Agras, W. (2003). The clinical significance of binge eating disorder. *International Journal of Eating Disorders, 34*(Suppl), 96–106.

Wilfley, D. E., Friedman, M. A., Dounchis, J. Z., Stein, R. I., Welch, R. R., & Ball, S. A. (2000). Comorbid psychopathology in binge eating disorder: Relation to eating disorder severity at baseline and following treatment. *Journal of Consulting and Clinical Psychology, 68,* 641–649.

Wilfley, D. E., Schwartz, M. B., Spurrell, E. B., & Fairburn, C. G. (1997), Assessing the specific psychopathology of binge eating disorder patients: Interview or self-report? *Behavior Research and Therapy, 35,* 1151–1159.

Yanovski, S. Z. (2003). Binge eating disorder and obesity in 2003: Could treating an eating disorder have a positive effect on the obesity epidemic? *International Journal of Eating Disorders, 34*(Suppl), 117–120.

Yanovski, S. Z., Nelson, J. E., Dubbert, B. K., & Spitzer, R. L. (1993). Association of binge eating disorder and psychiatric comorbidity in obese subjects. *American Journal of Psychiatry, 150,* 1472–1479.

Yanovski, S. Z., & Sebring, N. G. (1994). Recorded food intake of obese women with binge eating disorder before and after weight loss. *International Journal of Eating Disorders, 15,* 135–150.

Section II

Assessment of Pediatric Obesity and Contributing Conditions

5

The Definition and Assessment of Childhood Overweight: A Developmental Perspective

CHERMAINE TYLER and GINNY FULLERTON

Overweight has become a serious public health problem not only in the United States but also in countries around the world. The problem has even begun to affect children and adolescents in recent years. This represents a change from the previous decade, when overweight was a health concern for adults. Given the scale of the problem, it is important to establish a clear definition of "overweight" in children as well as an understanding of the techniques used to assess the problem.

Though it does not seem a difficult endeavor, establishing an accurate definition of "overweight" for children is challenging. A number of concerns must be addressed, including arguments for delineating excess weight from excess adipose tissue when defining the problem. Morbidity and mortality are also important to consider before labeling a child as obese. Given that these issues are complex and will likely take considerable time and resources to resolve, it is important that those challenged with the task of classifying and assessing overweight in children have some understanding of how these factors relate to defining "overweight."

This chapter will present the most widely used definitions of "overweight" in children, focusing on the relevance of these definitions for both

CHERMAINE TYLER and GINNY FULLERTON • Baylor College of Medicine, Houston, TX 77030.

health care professionals and researchers. In addition, assessment of overweight using measures of Body Mass Index (BMI) and adiposity will be presented, establishing best practices and strategies for individual and group assessment. Finally, the term "obesity" and the problems with classifying a child with this label will be presented, as the term is often used alternately with overweight or in cases of significant overweight.

Overweight or Obese?

It is quite common to use the terms "overweight" and "obese" interchangeably in reference to children. Though this is often accepted, the terminology can be confusing, especially when one is attempting to compare overweight/obesity in children with the same problems in adults, as the definitions are distinctive for adults. The terms actually refer to different problems (Foreyt & St. Jeor, 1997). "Overweight" refers to excess body weight, including fat and lean body mass, bones, and water, while "obesity" refers to excess body fat. The most common definitions for "overweight" in children use BMI reference points.

The Centers for Disease Control and Prevention (CDC) defines "overweight" in children as having a BMI at or above the 95th percentile for age and gender (Ogden, Flegal, Carroll, & Johnson, 2002). The World Health Organization (WHO) also endorses these reference data (World Health Organization, 1995) for worldwide use in classifying children as overweight. The definition established by the International Obesity Taskforce (IOTF) uses age- and gender-specific BMI cut points to determine overweight (Cole, Bellizzi, Flegal, & Dietz, 2000). There are differences in these definitions, with the CDC classification based on data obtained from children in the United States and the IOTF definition derived from data on children from a number of countries. The latter classification was established to provide a more accurate classification system for use outside the United States and to develop a strategy that maps onto the adult criteria of a BMI of 25 for overweight and 30 for obese. Though distinctive from "over weight", the label "at-risk for overweight" refers to childern between the 85th and 95th percentiles for age and gender (Ogden et al.). Weights of children in this category are generally monitored, and depending on family medical history, the children themselves may be viewed by health care and research professionals as having the same needs as overweight children (Dietz & Robinson, 2005).

The classification of obesity is not as clear. The CDC does not specify a means for categorizing obesity, while the IOTF has a cut point that corresponds to the adult classification of a BMI at or above 30. Without an established definition, BMI percentile cut points are often used in research studies examining weight status and associated consequences in children and adolescents. The inconsistency in defining "child obesity" complicates explaining how obesity relates to both adiposity and health problems. The Expert Committee on the Assessment, Prevention and Treatment of Child and Adolescent Overweight and Obesity (the Expert Committee) has, however, made recommendations that clarify the classification of children as overweight and obese (American Medical Association [AMA], 2007). It proposes that a BMI percentile greater than 95 be used to define "child obesity" and that a BMI percentile between the 85 and 95 be used to define "child overweight." The latter would replace the term "at-risk for overweight."

The associations between overweight/obesity and health problems such as type 2 diabetes, cardiovascular disease, and orthopedic problems have been well-documented for adults (National Institutes of Health, 1998). However, there is evidence that higher BMI percentiles (greater than the 99th percentile) in children are associated with increased health risks as well as excess adiposity (Barlow & Dietz, 1998; Freedman, Mei, Srinivasan, Berenson, & Dietz, 2007). Endocrine and cardiovascular abnormalities are among the most well-documented health factors associated with overweight in children; these include insulin resistance, hypertension, and hyperlipidemia (Dietz, 1998; Freedman et al.). Other health conditions seen more frequently in overweight compared to normal weight children include sleep apnea, gallbladder disease, elevated liver enzymes, pseudotumor cerebri, polycystic ovarian disease, and orthopedic problems (Dietz). These problems are especially concerning given that health complications associated with BMI continue to rise as the rates of overweight children increase (Muntner, He, Cutler, Wildman, & Whelton, 2004; Wang & Dietz, 2002). Nevertheless, the paucity of longitudinal data from epidemiological studies precludes unified agreement on child obesity's relation to adult disease (Chinn, 2006; Daniels et al., 2005).

It is well-accepted that childhood obesity relates to adulthood overweight/obesity (Must, Jacques, Dallal, Bajema, & Dietz, 1992; Freedman, Khan, et al., 2005). Although some data indicate that higher BMI percentiles in children are associated with greater levels of childhood adiposity (Freedman et al., 2007), unfortunately, there is no best practice for measuring excess body fat in children (Freedman, Ogden, Berenson, & Horlick, 2005). Because obesity refers to excess body fat, it is important to have such a measure when making a diagnosis of obesity. There are methods that have been reliably used to assess fat in children, but they are not often accessible to clinicians or researchers (Fu et al., 2003). Given the limitations in assessing adiposity, BMI has been used as a proxy for classifying children as obese.

Because there is an association between child BMI and body fatness (Freedman et al., 2007; Barlow & Dietz, 1998), guidelines have been established to direct clinicians in using a BMI to diagnose obesity in children (Barlow & Dietz). Generally, a BMI greater than the 95th percentile has been used as the indication that a child should receive further assessment. In the guidelines for treatment, clinicians are urged to use their clinical judgment to determine a child's level of obesity (Barlow & Dietz). Finding a comorbid condition such as high blood pressure, elevated cholesterol, or orthopedic problems for a child classified as at-risk for overweight may lead to a child being treated similarly to those classified as obese. Freedman et al. have also recommended using a BMI at or above the 99th percentile as a marker of significant obesity in children. Clinicians or health care providers collaborating with physicians who make these diagnoses may use similar terminology to facilitate clear communication with other providers as well as the patient and family. This also allows those involved in treating the patient to determine a degree of weight loss that justifies changing the diagnosis from obesity to overweight.

Researchers, however, typically work with groups of individuals. In epidemiological and clinical research, it is often necessary to determine changes either in prevalence rates over time or in terms of magnitude of difference between groups. Measuring change requires a standard method for classifying all participants that accounts for differences in age and gender of groups. A standardized BMI (or BMI z-score) statistically adjusts for these factors. The use of a BMI z-score allows one to directly compare children of different ages and genders. Given that a number of data sets were used to derive the IOTF cut points, it is not possible to derive BMI z-scores for use in comparisons across age groups or genders (Cole et al., 2000). The CDC provides values (Kuczmarski et al., 2000) that are to be used to calculate BMI z-scores, which allows for the comparison of weights among large heterogeneous groups across time. In addition, when researchers are describing a particular study population, it is important that they utilize terms that are readily identifiable, and both the CDC and IOTF classifications provide a means for doing so. Given the differences in the definitions, however, it is important that the system used to group participants is clearly stated and that any additional terminology be defined to ensure that cross-study comparisons can be made.

It is worth noting that the CDC and IOTF classification systems yield variable prevalence rates in a given population, with a child being classified as overweight in one system but not the other. A number of studies have been conducted to determine how the systems differ from a given population to another. In one such study, the IOTF and WHO (WHO: $\geq$ 85th percentile = overweight; $\geq$ 95th percentile = obese) classification systems were compared, yielding similar prevalence rates for overweight and obesity across participants (Wang & Wang, 2002). Nevertheless, there were some discrepancies, as the WHO classification yielded higher rates for children younger than 10 and lower rates for older adolescents. These comparisons were conducted for child populations in three countries, including the United States. The results point to the importance of fully describing the classification system used as well as the sample being studied, as age may vary the diagnosis from one system to another.

Assessment

Measurement of children for the purposes of classifying them as overweight or obese represents an important aspect of obtaining an accurate definition. Small deviations from accuracy can result in erroneous classification. Given the health implications and possible social stigma that come with overweight and especially obesity, it is important that those involved in classifying children as overweight be well-informed of the correct measurement methods.

Most people think of weight when overweight is mentioned. However, additional measurements, such as height, gender, and age, are needed to obtain an assessment of BMI. This provides a means for determining the extent to which a person's weight exceeds a normative value for his or her age and gender. This is especially important for children because, unlike adults, they are growing, and rates of growth differ depending on gender and age. Given adiposity's relation to overweight, some description of these methods is also presented.

Body Mass Index

In general, Body Mass Index is the standard measurement used to describe a child's (age 2 or older) or adolescent's weight status (Cole, Faith, Pietrobelli, & Heo, 2005). BMI is a ratio of weight to height assessed with the equation weight (kg) divided by height squared (m²). The anthropometric measurements of height and weight are first taken, and to ensure the accuracy of measurements, duplicate assessment of both is recommended, with a third taken if the first two significantly differ (Daniels, Khoury, & Morrison, 2000). The BMI is calculated using a mean of the heights and weights obtained. Though the calculation is presented, many web sites not only calculate BMI from provided heights and weights but also plot it on CDC growth charts (e.g., *http:// www.cdc.gov/nccdphp/ dnpa/bmi/index.htm*). When the CDC classification system is used, BMI is plotted on a BMI chart that in children is standardized by gender and age. Plotting the BMI yields a percentile, and this is used to classify a child's weight status (i.e., BMI greater than or equal to the 95th percentile is overweight). The percentile represents the percentage of children of the same age and gender whose BMIs are lower than the participant's.

For example, a 10-year, 6-month-old boy who is 4'6" tall and weighs 95 pounds would have a BMI of 22.9, calculated as follows:

[95lbs / (54in * 54in)] * 703 (used for conversion to metric)
(95 / 2916) * 703
.033 * 703 = 22.9 BMI.

Plotting the boy's BMI on the CDC growth chart indicates his BMI is at the 95th (overweight) percentile for age and gender. A girl of the same age with the same BMI would be at the 93rd (at risk of being overweight) percentile for age and gender. Using the IOTF classification, both the boy and girl would be classified as overweight. An example of 16-year, 6-month-old boys and girls indicates that a boy weighing 88.64 kg with a height of 177.8 cm would have a BMI of 28:

[88.64 kg / (1.78 m * 1.78 m)]
88.64 / 3.168 = 28.

This boy's BMI would be at the 95th percentile (overweight), but a girl of the same age would have to have a BMI of 30.2 (e.g., 75 kg, 157.5 cm) to be at the 95th percentile (overweight). The boy would be overweight and the girl obese if IOTF cut points were used. These examples indicate how variability in gender, height, weight, BMI, and classification system can affect the weight classification of a child.

BMI Z-score

Age norms are used to convert BMI into a z-score that can be compared with children of various ages and genders. The BMI z-score represents a child's BMI in a standard, normal distribution with a mean of 0 and a standard deviation of 1. The calculation of the BMI z-score is done using a skewness parameter (L), mean (M), and standard deviation (S), which are available on the CDC's National Center for Health Statistics (2000) web site (*http://www.cdc.gov/nchs/about/major/nhanes/growth-charts/datafiles.htm*), and is as follows:

$$zBMI=\{[(X/M)^L]-1\}/(L*S)$$

A BMI z-score obtained through these *LMS* parameters can be used to ascertain the corresponding BMI percentile for age. For example, a female of age 134.5 months (rounded to the nearest half-point according to CDC guidelines) weighing 68.9 kg with a height of 150.2 cm would have a BMI of 30.5. In order to calculate a z-score, the LMS parameters are obtained from CDC BMI-for-age growth charts ($L = -2.03$, $M = 17.57$, $S = 0.14$) and substituted in the above formula, resulting in a zBMI of 2.29. This z-score corresponds to the 98.9th percentile of a standard normal distribution.

Excess Adiposity

Although BMI is often used to classify children as obese, it is not a direct measure of body fatness. Children are growing and the rates vary with age, so it is difficult to determine a standard measure of adiposity. Though BMI z-score may be correlated with adiposity on a single occasion, it is not the best measure of change in body composition (Cole et al., 2005). Given that obesity refers to excess body fat, a more precise assessment of obesity would include a measure of adipose tissue. There are several methods of assessing adiposity, each with advantages and limitations:

Dual-Energy X-ray Absorptiometry (DXA). The complex methodology of DXA scanning that was originally intended for bone density measurement allows for assessment of bone mineral, lean, and fat tissue masses as two x-ray beams traverse the body. DXA analyses can be used to evaluate whole body composition estimates or regional measurements. DXA has been shown to be a valid and reliable measure of adiposity in children and adolescents (Daniels et al., 2000; Freedman et al., 2005) and is often used as a reference technique for other measures of adiposity (Daniels et al., 2000; Pietrobelli, 2004). Given the high reproducibility of this procedure, it is becoming more widely used (Freedman et al., 2005). However, despite the sensitivity and accuracy of DXA, it tends to be more costly and therefore less practical in some settings (Eisenmann, Heelan, & Welk, 2004).

Bioelectrical Impedance Analysis (BIA). BIA involves measuring the body's resistance to an imperceptible electrical current. This is based on the concept that adipose tissue offers more resistance to the passage of an electrical current than tissue rich in water and electrolytes. BIA is a useful method of estimating adiposity, although some studies have found poor correlations between BIA and other methods (Eisenmann, Heelan, & Welk, 2004). One of the weaknesses of this method is that composition estimates vary across measurement conditions (position, time of day, and room temperature). However, its ease of use, reasonable accuracy, and low cost make BIA a practical consideration for body composition assessment.

Triceps Skinfold Thickness. According to National Health and Nutrition Examination Survey (NHANES) recommendations, triceps skinfold thickness should be measured on a child's right upper arm with the child standing upright. Triceps skinfold thickness is a suitable and feasible measure of percent body fat in children (Pietrobelli, 2004) and can be used for comparisons using reference data with children of the same age and gender (McDowell, Fryar, Hirsch, & Ogden, 2005). However, accuracy is greatly dependent upon the skills of the examiner, and there is a high degree of variability between assessors (Freedman et al., 2005). The 2007 recommendations of the Expert Committee actually advise against the use of this measure for obesity assessment in children (AMA, 2007). It is a challenge to assess triceps skinfold in children who are heavier, and given that the measurement is to ensure an accurate obesity diagnosis, it is a problem that those most likely to need the additional assessment are the most difficult to measure.

Waist Circumference. Waist circumference is a useful tool for assessing abdominal adipose tissue, or visceral fat (Brambilla et al., 2006). It is relatively convenient and easy to measure, correlated with BMI, and associated with obesity-related risks (Higgins, Gower, Hunter, & Goran, 2001; Zhu et al., 2002). As is the case for triceps skinfold thickness, percentiles for this measure can be obtained from CDC reference data (McDowell et al., 2005). Waist circumference has been demonstrated to be a useful measure of fat distribution in children and adolescents (Daniels et al., 2000), and it is associated with adverse health effects in overweight and normal-weight children and adolescents across different ethnic groups (Goran & Gower, 1999). The report of the 2007 Expert Committee does not recommend the assessment for an obesity diagnosis, though there is no advice against its use (AMA, 2007). Body composition varies during pubertal development (Himes et al., 2004), and there is greater abdominal fat deposition as age increases (Daniels et al. 2000). Therefore, this may not be an optimal measure for comparing children in different stages of pubertal development.

SUMMARY

Those working to diagnose children as overweight/obese have a number of choices to make before arriving at the appropriate classification. "Overweight" means just that: a weight in excess of what is normal for a given age and gender. "Obese" refers to having excess body fat. There are standard definitions from the CDC (BMI for age and gender greater than or equal to the 95th percentile) and IOTF (age- and gender-specific cut points) for overweight, and both rely on the use of BMI, which is a calculation that determines the relationship between weight and height. Identifying the system to be used for classification is necessary because the CDC and IOTF classification systems can yield different diagnoses for some children, as shown in the examples presented. In addition, there is the problem of differentiating between overweight and obese, and there is no definitive answer as to who should be classified as obese. The IOTF provides a cut point for classifying a child as obese. Though the CDC offers no criteria for classifying children as obese, many physicians who rely on the CDC growth charts for classification refer to children as obese. However, the American Medical Association's Expert Committee on Child and Adolescent Overweight and Obesity (AMA, 2007) recently recommended a modification of the CDC classification system that lowers the BMI percentile necessary for a classification of overweight (BMI percentile greater than or equal to 85 to less than 95) and includes a classification of obesity (BMI percentile greater than or equal to 95). Generally, obesity diagnoses have been based on the diagnosis of a comorbid weight-related disease or health problem; however, most have not relied on a secondary assessment of body fat. Fortunately, there is new evidence to support the relationship between child BMI and excess body fat, though additional data are needed to firmly support this assertion.

Identifying BMI first requires accurate height and weight measurements, as slight discrepancies in these measures can result in inaccuracies in classification. Though there is an equation for calculating BMI, a number of online sources are available for obtaining an individual BMI (e.g., *http://www.cdc.gov/nccdphp/dnpa/bmi/index.htm*). Obesity, however, refers to excess adiposity, so it would seem necessary to provide some measure of body fat, however, crude it is. Adiposity measures were presented, but many are not generally available for use.

Given that overweight is a relatively new phenomenon in children, there is a great deal of disagreement among experts regarding which definition should be used or why. The controversy over defining "overweight" in children stems partly from the lack of sufficient long-term evidence of related health problems (Chinn, 2006). Given that the classification systems are based on data from different countries, there is also the concern that definitions lose their meaning when applied to different populations. Despite these concerns, most would agree that the problem is growing, regardless of how it is defined. Long-term studies that assess the consequences of overweight for children over time will provide the best evidence for an appropriate assessment.

REFERENCES

American Medical Association. (2007). Expert committee recommendations on the assessment, prevention, and treatment of child and adolescent overweight and obesity. Retrieved April 25, 2008 from http://www.ama-assn.org/ama1/pub/upload/mm/433/ped_obesity_recs.pdf.

Barlow, S. E., & Dietz, W. H. (1998). Obesity evaluation and treatment: Expert committee recommendations. *Pediatrics, 102,* Retrieved from http://pediatrics.aappublications.org/cgi/content/full/102/3/e29.

Brambilla, P., Bedogni, G., Moreno, L. A., Goran, M. I, Gutin, B., Fox, K. R, et al. (2006). Crossvalidation of anthropometry against magnetic resonance imaging for the assessment of visceral and subcutaneous adipose tissue in children. *International Journal of Obesity, 30,* 23–30.

Chinn, S. (2006). Definitions of childhood obesity: Current practice. *European Journal of Clinical Nutrition, 60,* 1189–1194.

Cole, T. J., Bellizzi, M. C., Flegal, K. M., & Dietz, W. H. (2000). Establishing a standard definition for child overweight and obesity worldwide: International survey. *British Medical Journal, 320,* 1–6.

Cole, T. J., Faith, M. S., Pietrobelli, A., & Heo, M. (2005). What is the best measure of adiposity change in growing children: BMI, BMI%, BMI z-score or BMI centile? *European Journal of Clinical Nutrition, 59,* 419–425.

Daniels, S. R., Arnett, D. K., Eckel, R. H., Gidding, S. S., Hayman, L. L., Kumanyika, S., et al. (2005). Overweight in children and adolescents pathophysiology, consequences, prevention, and treatment. *Circulation, 111,* 1999–2012.

Daniels, S. R., Khoury, P. R., & Morrison, J. A. (2000). Utility of different measures of body fat distribution in children and adolescents. *American Journal of Epidemiology, 152,* 1179–1184.

Dietz, W. (1998). Health consequences of obesity in youth: Childhood predictors of adult disease. *Pediatrics, 101(Suppl),* 518–525.

Dietz, W. H., & Robinson, T. N. (2005). Overweight children and adolescents. *The New England Journal of Medicine, 352,* 2100–2109.

Eisenmann, J. C., Heelan, K. A., & Welk, G. J. (2004). Assessing body composition among 3- to 8-year-old children: Anthropometry, BIA, and DXA. *Obesity Research, 12,* 1633–1640.

Foreyt, J. P., & St. Jeor, S. T. (1997). Definitions of obesity and healthy weight. In S.T. St. Jeor (Ed.), *Obesity assessment tools, methods, interpretations. A reference case: The RENO Diet-Heart Study* (pp. 47–56). New York, NY: Chapman & Hall.

Freedman, D. S., Khan, L. K., Serdula, M. K., Dietz, W. H., Srinivasan, S. R., & Berenson, G. S. (2005). The relation of childhood BMI to adult adiposity: The Bogalusa Heart Study. *Pediatrics, 115,* 22–27.

Freedman, D. S., Mei, A., Srinivasan, S. R., Berenson, G. S., & Dietz, W. H. (2007). Cardiovascular risk factors and excess adiposity among overweight children and adolescents: The Bogalusa Heart Study. *The Journal of Pediatrics, 150,* 12–17.

Freedman, D. S., Ogden, C. L., Berenson, G. S., & Horlick, M. (2005). Body mass index and body fatness in childhood. *Current Opinion in Clinical Nutrition and Metabolic Care, 8,* 618–623.

Fu, W. P. C., Lee, H. C., Ng, C. J., Tay, Y-K. D., Kau, C. Y., Seow, C. J., et al. (2003). Screening for childhood obesity: International *vs* population-specific definition. Which is more appropriate? *International Journal of Obesity, 27,* 1121–1126.

Goran, M. I., & Gower, B. A. (1999). Relation between visceral fat and disease risk in children and adolescents. *American Journal of Clinical Nutrition, 70*(Suppl.), 149–156.

Higgins, P. B., Gower, B. A., Hunter, G. R., & Goran, M. I. (2001). Defining health-related obesity in prepubertal children. *Obesity Research, 9,* 233–240.

Himes, J. H., Obarzanek, E., Baranowski, T., Wilson, D. M., Rochon, J., & McClanahan, B. S. (2004). Early sexual maturation, body composition, and obesity in African-American girls. *Obesity Research, 12,* 64S–72S.

Kuczmarski, R. J., Ogden, C. L., Guo, S. S., Grummer-Strawn, L. M., Flegal, K. M., Mei, Z., et.al. (2000). 2000 CDC Growth Charts for the United States: Methods and development. *Vital Health Statistics, 11,* 1–190.

McDowell, M. A., Fryar, C. D., Hirsch, R., & Ogden, C. L. (2005). Anthropometric reference data for children and adults: U.S. population, 1999–2002. *Advance Data, 7,* 1–5.

Muntner, P., He, J., Cutler, J. A., Wildman, R. P., & Whelton, P. K. (2004). Trends in blood pressure among children and adolescents. *Journal of the American Medical Association, 291,* 2107–2113.

Must, A., Jacques, P. F., Dallal, G. E., Bajema, C. J., & Dietz, W. H. (1992). Long-term morbidity and mortality of overweight adolescents: A follow-up of the Harvard Growth Study of 1922 to 1935. *The New England Journal of Medicine, 327,* 1350–1355.

National Center for Health Statistics. (2000). *CDC Growth Charts: United States.* Retrieved December 21, 2006, from http://www.cdc.gov/nchs/about/major/nhanes/growth-charts/datafiles.htm

National Institutes of Health. (1998). Clinical guidelines on the identification, evaluation, and treatment of overweight and obesity in adults: The evidence report. *Obesity Research, 6*(Suppl.), 51–209.

Ogden, C. L., Flegal, K. M., Carroll, M. D., & Johnson, C. L. (2002). Prevalence and trends in obesity among US children and adolescents, 1999–2000. *Journal of the American Medical Association, 288,* 1728–1732.

Pietrobelli, A. (2004). Outcome measurements in paediatric obesity prevention trials. *International Journal of Obesity, 28,* S86–S89.

The World Health Organization. (1995). *Physical status: The use and interpretation of anthropometry, report of the WHO expert committee.* (WHO technical report series; 854). Geneva: World Health Organization.

Wang, D., & Dietz, G. H. (2002). Economic burden of obesity in youths aged 6 to 17 years: 1979–1999. *Pediatrics, 10,* Retrieved from 81-DOI: 10.1542/peds.109.5.e81.

Wang, Y., & Wang, J. Q. (2002). A comparison of international references for the assessment of child and adolescent overweight and obesity in different populations. *European Journal of Clinical Nutrition, 56,* 973–982.

Zhu, S., Wang, Z., Heshka, S., Heo, M., Faith, M. S., & Heymsfield, S. B. (2002). Waist circumferance and obesity-associated risk factors among caucasians in NHANES III: Clinical action thresholds. *American Journal of Clinical Nutrition 76,* 743–749.

6

Diet Assessment in Children and Adolescents

NANCY E. SHERWOOD

Although increases in obesity prevalence over the last few decades have been dramatic in all age groups, trends among youths have been particularly alarming. The prevalence of childhood overweight has almost doubled in the past two decades in the United States (CDC, National Center for Health Statistics [NCHS, 2004]). The emergence of childhood obesity as a serious public health problem underscores the need for dietary assessment tools that are not only reliable and valid but also feasible to administer across multiple settings and age ranges and with diverse populations. Accurate dietary assessment is critical for monitoring the nutritional status of children, examining associations between diet and health, and identifying dietary intake patterns and eating behaviors that are associated with unhealthy weight and weight gain over time. Such information is critical for developing intervention messages and behavioral targets for obesity prevention and treatment programs and for evaluating their effectiveness.

As others have documented, there is no "one-size-fits-all" dietary assessment tool appropriate for all research and clinical applications, and there is always a trade-off with the choice of any diet assessment methodology (Goran, 1998; Rockett, Wolf, & Colditz, 1995). Moreover, the measurement of energy and nutrient intake in children and adolescents is further complicated by a variety of factors, including reliance on a third person (e.g., adult caregiver, teacher) to report a child's intake during the preschool years, cognitive abilities, motivation, and reporting biases (e.g., underreporting and overreporting) influenced by developmental stage and other factors (e.g., weight status). The goal of this chapter is to review the variety of dietary assessment methods available,

NANCY E. SHERWOOD • Health Partners Foundation, Minneapolis, MN 55440.

evidence regarding their reliability and validity for different age groups (preschool-aged children, school-aged children, and adolescents), and the advantages and disadvantages of each approach. Dietary assessment methods reviewed include food records, dietary recalls, food frequencies, brief approaches, and observation largely focused on specific aspects of the diet (e.g., fruit and vegetable intake). This chapter builds on several recent, comprehensive reviews of the dietary assessment literature (Livingstone, Robson, & Wallace, 2004; McPherson, Hoelscher, Alexander, Scanlon, & Serdula, 2000; Rockett et al.; Serdula, Alexander, Scanlon, & Bowman, 2001) and incorporates data from more recently published validation studies. PubMed searches using relevant keywords (e.g., "diet," "nutrition," "children," "adolescents," "validation studies") and reference lists from key articles were used to obtain relevant literature. The chapter concludes with a brief discussion of factors to consider when choosing the best measure for a particular purpose and study population.

Food Records

A food record is a written account of the food and beverages consumed by an individual during a specified time period, ranging from one to seven days. A child and/or an adult caregiver records details about food and beverages consumed each day, including brand names, mixed-dish ingredients, food preparation methods, and portion size estimates. Protocols for food record completion may also include instructions and scales for weighing food items. Respondents are instructed to, and ideally do, record information at the time of consumption to reduce error caused by forgetting; however, little information is available regarding actual participant behavior, and respondents may vary with respect to when they complete food records.

Keeping an accurate food record requires skills that can challenge children and their adult caregivers, including reading, writing, basic math, estimation of portion size, the ability to understand nutrition labels, compliance, and the motivation to keep a food record, particularly over multiple days. Despite these challenges, food records have been shown to have high correlations with "gold standard" validation techniques such as doubly labeled water and are often chosen as a validation standard to compare other dietary assessment methods against (McPherson et al., 2000). A single food record can be used to estimate group means but is inadequate to predict individual-level health outcomes. Completion of multiple-day food records requires a high degree of participant cooperation and motivation. A "pre-coded" food diary (PFD) is an alternative to the food record that may reduce participant burden. The PFD uses lists of foods and provides household measures and photographs for portion size estimation. The PFD eliminates the need for detailed recording of food intake; participants indicate how many units of each food item they consumed during the correct time span (Lillegaard & Andersen, 2005).

A potential disadvantage of either method of record-keeping is that it may lead to an "intervention" effect, with respondents modifying intake as a result of dietary intake self-monitoring.

Preschool-Aged Children

Limited data regarding the validity of food records in preschool-aged children are available. A comprehensive literature review conducted by Serdula et al. (2001) revealed only two studies, with one using doubly labeled water (Davies, Coward, Gregory, White, & Mills, 1994) and the other using diet history as the validation standard (Harbottle & Duggan, 1993). Mean energy intake from food records underestimated energy intake by 3%, with food records underestimating mean energy intake by about 7% in comparison to diet history. Building on the work suggesting that the weighed food record shows evidence of validity, a more recent study provides an estimate of the number of days of food records necessary to accurately rank 6- to 24-month-old children. The estimated numbers of days of food records necessary to assess intake of energy, protein, fat, and carbohydrate with an acceptable degree of accuracy were five, four, four, and three, respectively, with only two days of weight food record collection necessary for reliably assessing consumption of specific micronutrients (e.g., calcium, phosphorus, iron) (Lanigan, Wells, Lawson, Cole, & Lucas, 2004). No information is available regarding factors that may influence the validity of parent-completed food records for preschool children (e.g., weight status of parents and/or children, demographic characteristics).

School-Aged Children

A review by McPherson et al. (2000) summarized findings from six studies examining the validity of the food record among school-aged children. Correlations between food record and validation standard nutrient intakes ranged from 0.52 to 0.71, and differences in mean energy intake ranged from 28% below to 31% above the validation standard. Crawford, Obarzanek, Morrison, and Sabry (1994) examined the comparative advantage of 3-day food records over 24-hour recall and 5-day food frequency, using unobtrusive school lunch observation as the validation standard in a group of 9- and 10-year-old girls. Examination of energy and specific macronutrient intakes showed different ranges and median percentage absolute errors for each method (e.g., the median difference between the diet assessment method and the validation standard). Percentage absolute error ranges favored the 3-day food record (12–22% for the 3-day food record, 20–33% for the 5-day food frequency method, and 19–39% for the 24-hour recall), and the percentage of missing foods and phantom foods also favored the 3-day food record. These data informed the choice to use the 3-day food record as the dietary assessment method for the National Heart Lung and Blood Institute (NHLBI) Growth and Health Study.

A more recent study of 9-year-old children compared energy intake (EI) assessed from a pre-coded food diary with energy expenditure (EE) measured by a validated position-and-movement monitor, the ActiReg® (Lillegaard & Andersen, 2005). Results showed that on average, the PFD underestimated EI by 18% compared with EE measured by the ActiReg®. The correlation between EI and EE was 0.28 ($p < 0.05$). Comparison of underreporters and overreporters did not show any systematic misreporting related to macronutrients, specific foods and beverages (e.g., chocolate, sweets, soft drinks with sugar), or child BMI.

Adolescents

Very few studies have examined the validity of the food record specifically in adolescents. Green et al. (Green, Allen, & O'Connor, 1998) compared adolescents' reports of folate and vitamin B-12 intake on a weighed food record against serum micronutrient levels collected one week prior to completion of the food record. Correlations between recorded folate intake and serum folate were 0.65; between recorded folate intake and red blood cell folate, 0.5; and between recorded vitamin B-12 and serum B-12, 0.32. Studies examining the validity of food records by age suggest that underreporting on the dietary record increases with age (Bjorntorp, 1992). In a study comparing differences in the magnitude of underreporting bias by age, 12-year olds underestimated energy intake by 14%, and 15- to 18-year-olds underestimated energy intake via the food record by 24% (Livingstone et al., 1992). Research also suggests that overweight adolescents are more likely to underestimate food intake than nonoverweight adolescents (Livingstone et al.).

24-Hour Diet Recall

Food recalls are semistructured interviews conducted by trained professionals that require children to remember what and how much they ate during a specific time period, typically the previous day. Accurately responding to a food recall requires abstract thinking and good memory skills. The 24-hour Diet Recall (24hDR) provides an estimate of total previous-day nutrient intake by prompting a child and/or an adult caregiver to talk about all of the foods and beverages consumed during the previous day. The 24hDR incorporates a detailed description of food and beverages, including brand names, mixed-dish ingredients, and food preparation methods. Portion sizes are also estimated with different methods, including two- or three-dimensional food models. The multiple pass technique, during which an interviewer asks respondents about the previous day's food and beverage consumption several times (i.e., passes through the day) increases accuracy and reduces the likelihood of underreporting.

Respondents to 24hDR can include children, adult caregivers, or a combination. By about age 8 or 9, children are thought to be able to accurately respond to a 24hDR (Livingstone, Robson, & Wallace, 2004). Children younger than age 9 typically need adult caregiver assistance to provide accurate dietary information because of limited reading skills, adult caregiver control of food availability, and meal provision (Frank, 1994; McPherson et al., 2000). Although assistance and information provided by adult caregivers are often included to increase the accuracy of children's diet recalls, some questions have been raised about potential ways adult caregivers may either provide biased information or negatively influence a child's report of intake (Sobo & Rock, 2001). Factors affecting the accuracy of parent/guardian-assisted child reports include children's concern about parental judgment regarding amount of food consumed and specific types of food, social desirability on the part of the parent, and lack of knowledge due to the fact that children often eat breakfast, lunch, and after-school snacks outside the home.

Similar to the food record, a single 24 hDR can be appropriate for estimating group nutrient intake means when conducted within a random sample population; however, multiple recalls are needed to accurately estimate usual individual intake and to predict individual-level health outcomes (McPherson et al., 2000). Given the significant interindividual and intraindividual variation in food intake, Nelson et al. (Nelson, Black, Morris, & Cole, 1989) estimated that 10 days of recall would be required to achieve a 0.9 correlation between measured and actual average intake. The participant and researcher burdens associated with this high number of recalls make it highly unlikely to occur. Three 24 hDRs (including one weekend day) have become the standard used in dietary intervention studies with children if resources are available (van Horn et al., 1993). Disadvantages of diet recalls include: expense due to the need for highly trained personnel, the multiple days of assessment needed to attain some level of reliability (Nelson et al.), and the expensive software needed to elicit the foods consumed and convert this detailed information into food servings and nutrients consumed (Baranowski et al., 2002).

Although implementation of quality control procedures adds to the expense of the 24 hDR, adequate quality control protocols are critical for obtaining accurate and consistent data both between different interviewers and over the duration of a study (Shaffer et al., 2004). Recommendations for enhancing quality control include: performing quality control procedures during training and practicing prior to data collection and throughout the data collection period, developing a quality control interview checklist and procedures for addressing interview protocol violations, and developing criteria for inclusion of interviews in data analysis. Shaffer et al. also recommend audio-recording all interviews to avoid knowledge of which interviews have been selected for quality control, as such knowledge may influence interviewer behavior.

Preschool-Aged Children

A comprehensive review of the literature by Serdula et al. (2001) identified 12 studies that evaluated the validity of food recalls estimating the dietary intake of preschool-aged children. No validation studies published after this review were located. Serdula and colleagues reported that 24 hDR's both overestimated and underestimated intake, depending on the validation standard, but generally relative differences between 24 hDR energy intake and the validation standard were within 10–15%. Serdula et al. noted that parents of preschool-aged children show a tendency toward better recollection of main meal items than snacks and desserts and a tendency to omit food items. Too few studies regarding the effect of sex, ethnicity, weight status, and age on recall validity have been conducted to permit any conclusions. Based on an evaluation of one-week test-retest reliability of a 24-hour Dietary Recall completed by parents of preschool children (3- to 5-year-olds), Treiber et al. (1990) estimate that four to seven 24-hour Dietary Recalls may need to be administered for obtaining an estimate of usual nutrient intake for preschool-aged children.

School-Aged Children and Adolescents

Examination of the validity of the 24 hDR has been examined extensively and reviewed in school-aged children (Livingstone et al., 2004; McPherson et al., 2000; Montgomery et al., 2005; Shaffer et al., 2004; Vereecken, Covents, Matthys, & Maes, 2005; Weber et al., 2004). Studies have varied in their use of a validation standard (e.g., food record, direct observation), time frame for the recall (e.g., entire previous day, specific meals only), and whether children's reports were supported by keeping a food record and/or obtaining parent input. These methodological differences make it difficult to make definitive conclusions about the validity and reliability of the dietary recall (McPherson et al.). Although the consensus appears to be that children's reports of dietary intake are not perfect and can both overestimate and underestimate, intake data from dietary recalls are generally comparable to diet records and superior to food frequency questionnaires. Previous reviews have called for systematic research to understand the various influences on reporting accuracy, including study method difference and the impact of age, race/ethnicity, and Body Mass Index. Shaffer et al. have conducted a series of studies to examine some of these influences and have found that using the prior 24 hours as the target period yielded better performance than using the previous day (Baxter, Smith, Litaker, Guinn, et al., 2004) and that interview format (e.g., open, meal, and time interview formats) influences reporting accuracy (Baxter et al., 2003), with the open format appearing to result in lower intrusion rates and overall inaccuracy (Baxter et al.).

A recent advance in adaptation of the 24 hDR for children is the use of interactive multimedia to facilitate children's self-report of their dietary intake in a potentially more cost-effective manner. The use of interactive multimedia approaches to diet assessment has the potential to engage children, graphically display food, and manipulate food images to estimate portion size (Baranowski et al., 2002; Morris, Owen, & Fraser, 1994). As of this writing, two platforms have been developed and have preliminary validation data, the Food Intake Recording Software System

(FIRSSt) (Baranowski et al. 2002) and the Young Adolescent's Nutrition Assessment on Computer (YANA-C). FIRSSt uses interactive multimedia to assist children's self-report of diet by simulating a multiple-pass 24 hDR. Baranowski and colleagues conducted a study of 138 fourth-grade students to evaluate the validity of the FIRSSt in comparison to observation of school lunch and a 24-hour dietary recall conducted by a dietitian. A six-group design systematically varying sequence of self-report (FIRSSt vs 24 hDR), observation of school lunch, and hair sample as a bogus pipeline manipulation was used. Matches, intrusions, and omissions of school lunch consumption observations were used to measure accuracy. The FIRSSt was less accurate than a dietitian-conducted 24 hDR for lunch consumed the previous day; however, the FIRSSt improved in performance for all-day assessments when compared with the 24 hDR.

Vereecken and colleagues (Vereecken et al., 2005) evaluated the relative validity and acceptability of the computerized 24 hDR, the Young Adolescent's Nutrition Assessment on Computer. Food and nutrient intakes assessed with YANA-C were compared with food records (study 1; n=136 11- to 14-year-old students) and 24 hDR interviews (study 2; n=101). Spearman correlations for energy and nutrient intakes ranged between 0.44 and 0.79 for study 1 and between 0.44 and 0.86 for study 2. The YANA-C overestimated nutrient and energy intakes in comparison with the food record but not in comparison with the interview. Both the FIRSSt and the YANA-C appear to be promising methods of collecting detailed dietary information from young adolescents when staff resources are low relative to the standard interviewer-administered 24 hDR.

Food Frequency Questionnaires

Food frequency questionnaires provide estimates of usual food intake by asking respondents to report frequency of consumption and often portion size for a defined list of foods and beverages. Respondents are asked to report their usual intake over a defined period of time ranging from the previous day to the past year. Food frequency questionnaires can be self-administered or completed with individual or group assistance. The food frequency questionnaire (FFQ) was designed to measure typical food intake patterns and not necessarily to provide accurate quantitative measures of individual energy intake (Goran, 1998). Advantages of the food frequency questionnaire include ease of administration, low cost, and opportunity to assess intake over an extended time period (Subar, 2004). Disadvantages include greater measurement error and less specificity relative to other dietary assessment methods (Subar). Goran and others have also pointed out that food frequencies need to be modified to reflect portion sizes typically consumed by youths. A major flaw of the FFQ pointed out by Kristal et al. (Kristal, Peters, & Potter, 2005) in their article "Is It Time to Abandon the Food Frequency Questionnaire?" is that it may lead to inaccurate conclusions regarding diet and disease associations. Specifically, they cite research showing that diet and cancer associations detected when dietary assessment based on dietary biomarkers or food records is used are not observed when FFQs are used. Kristal et al. provide several recommendations for improving food frequency-type measures, including 1) using computerized assessment to overcome some barriers to the traditional print FFQ, 2) measuring dietary behavior (e.g., type of bread (whole grain or not) consumed) instead of nutrients only; and 3) collecting real-time food-use information with computer-aided technologies. The latter may not be applicable for younger children but could be useful for older children and adolescents. McPherson et al. (2000) also point out that FFQ validation studies should include multiple measures of the validation standard (e.g., food records, diet recalls) over the referent period for the FFQ (e.g., six months).

Preschool-Aged Children

The Serdula et al. (2001) comprehensive review of the literature on dietary assessment in preschool children concluded that although FFQs appear to overestimate energy intake in this age group, they may be better at ranking individuals with respect to their usual dietary intake amounts for specific foods/nutrients. For example, energy intake was overestimated by a food frequency questionnaire in comparison to total energy expenditure as measured by double-labeled water in a sample of 4- to 6-year-old children (Kaskoun, Johnson, & Goran, 1994). A food frequency questionnaire also produced estimates of energy intake higher than those obtained from 24-hour dietary recalls in a sample of preschool children (Treiber et al., 1990). Data published since the Serdula et al., 2001 review are consistent with this conclusion. Parrish, Marshall, Krebs, Rewers, and Norris (2003) evaluated the validity of a previous-year FFQ in a sample of 68 1- to 3-year-old children. Validation standards included three or four 24-hour dietary recalls for all children and nutrient biomarkers derived from plasma from approximately half of the children. Correlations between the FFQ and the average of the recalls ranged from 0.08 for total energy intake to 0.42 for vitamin C. Correlations between the FFQ and biological measures ranged from 0.01 for retinol to 0.51 for Vitamin C. Consistent with prior work, the FFQ overestimated energy intake in comparison to the diet recall data, and caloric intake as measured by the FFQ was almost 70% higher on average than caloric intake derived from the diet recall data. No information is available regarding potential factors associated with bias (e.g., demographic characteristics, weight status) in food frequency measures for preschool-aged children.

Andersen, Lande, Trygg, and Hay (2004) examined the validity of a 39-item semi-quantitative FFQ (SFFQ) in a sample of 187 families with a 2-year-old child. Parents completed the SFFQ close to their child's second birthday, and one to two weeks later they completed a seven-day weighed food record. In contrast to Parrish et al. (2003), the SFFQ over estimated energy intake by 7%. The SFFQ generated higher median values than the weighed food record for nine out of 16 nutrients. Parents who completed the SFFQ tended to underreport typical unhealthy foods such as cake, soft drinks, and sweets but tended to overreport more healthy foods such as fruit, vegetables, and potatoes.

Klohe et al. (2005) developed a 191-item FFQ to assess foods consumed by Hispanic, African American, and white 1- to 3-year-olds and evaluated test-retest reliability using a 3- to 4-week interval and validity using a 3-day diet measure derived from a single 24-hour diet recall and 2 days of diet records. Test-retest correlations ranged from 0.5 to 0.9 for different food categories. The mean percentage of participants correctly classified in the same quartile by both FFQ and 3-day diet measure was 36%, with the correct classification rate improving to 78% if the criteria are modified so that participants are within one quartile for both measures. Correlations between food group servings on the FFQ and the 3-day diet measure ranged from 0.1 for starchy vegetables to 0.69 for sweetened beverages, with an average validity correlation of 0.4.

School-Aged Children and Adolescents

Consistent with data for preschool children, a comprehensive review conducted by McPherson et al. (2000) concluded that FFQs tend to overestimate food intake for school-aged children and adolescents. Overestimation of food intake may occur when: 1) FFQs use adult portions to estimate child intake, 2) child completion is compared to parent completion is for younger children, and 3) a single 24-hour diet recall is used as the validation standard. Data suggest that the first administration of an FFQ tends to result in higher levels of food intake than subsequent administrations (McPherson et al.; Metcalf et al., 2003). Data published since the 2000 McPherson et al. review are consistent with these trends. Wilson and Lewis (2004) examined the validity of the Block98 FFQ in a sample of 61 4- to 9-year-old girls using 3-day diet records as the comparison standard. The Block98 FFQ was completed by a trained interviewer and a parent, with input from the child as appropriate. The Block98 FFQ overestimated intake of energy, protein, carbohydrate, and fat in comparison to the 3-day food records, and nutrients assessed by the two methods were moderately correlated (range: $r=0.40$ to 0.55).

Numerous food frequency questionnaires to assess the diets of children and adolescents have been developed and evaluated (Bertoli et al., 2005; Lietz, Barton, Longbottom, & Anderson, 2002; Vereecken & Maes, 2003; Watson, Collins, Dibley, Garg, & Sibbritt, 2003; Wilson & Lewis, 2004), but the Youth/Adolescent Questionnaire (YAQ) is one of the most widely used and systematically validated and provides a good example of the observed patterns of validation data. The YAQ is a self-administered food frequency questionnaire developed for 9- to 18-year-olds. It was based on the validated Nurses' Health Study food frequency questionnaire and was developed to reflect the eating habits of this age group. One-year test-retest reliability estimates range from 0.39 for meats to 0.57 for soda; (Rockett et al., 1995) mean reproducibility was higher for girls than for boys. Validity of the YAQ was examined by comparing the average of three 24-hour diet recalls administered over the course of a year with the average of two YAQs completed at the beginning and end of this time period. Energy-adjusted correlation coefficients between the YAQ and the diet recalls ranged from 0.21 for sodium to 0.54 for folate. After correction for within-person error, the average correlation coefficient was 0.54.

Energy intake estimated from the YAQ has also been validated against the criterion total energy expenditure (TEE) by doubly labeled water (DLW) (Perks et al., 2000). Twenty-three boys and 27 girls (8.6 to 16.2 years of age) completed the YAQ within one year of measurement of TEE. Energy intake by the YAQ and energy expenditure by DLW were similar (p = 0.91). Misreporting of estimated energy intake on the YAQ ranged from a 6.65 milli–Joule/day (mJ/d) overestimation to a 6.39 mJ/d underestimation. When within-subject CVs of repeated measures of the DLW and YAQ methods were used, 25 of the 50 subjects were deemed to have misreported their energy intake. The discrepancy in energy intake (YAQ – TEE) was related to body weight ($r = -0.25$, $P = 0.077$) and percentage body fat ($r = -0.24$, $P = 0.09$). Logistic regression analyses showed that boys with a higher body fat percentage were more likely to underreport energy intake than girls with a higher body fat percentage. These data suggest that the YAQ provides an accurate estimation of mean energy intake for a group but may be less accurate at the individual level.

Cullen and Zakeri (2004) evaluated the reliability and validity of the YAQ in a sample of 89 low-income seventh- and eighth-grade African American and Hispanic youths. Three-week test-retest reliability estimates ranged from 0.19 for percent dietary intake from fat to 0.72 for total energy intake. Validity correlations between the YAQ administered at time 1 and the average of up to six food records ranged from 0.02 for high-fat vegetables to 0.23 for regular vegetables; validity correlations after correcting for the intraclass correlation coefficient-related reliability of the food records ranged from 0.13 for percent energy from fat to 0.36 for regular vegetables.

Brief Approaches

A variant of the food frequency questionnaire is the use of screeners for specific foods or food groups, e.g., fruits and vegetables (Linneman et al., 2004; Edmunds & Ziebland 2002; Buzzard et al., 2001), beverages (Marshall et al., 2003), and macronutrients or nutrients, e.g., fat intake (Dennison, Jenkins & Rockwell, 2000; Smith et al., 2001) and calcium intake (Taylor & Goulding, 1998; Jensen et al., 2004). The advantages of such questionnaires include ease of administration, low cost, and ability to tailor questions to the specific nutritional and behavioral targets of an intervention. Brief food frequency questionnaires appear, however, to have many of the limitations noted above for their lengthier counterparts.

An alternative to the traditional paper-and-pencil food frequency questionnaire is a picture-sort approach (Kumanyika et al., 1996; Yaroch et al., 2000).

Advantages of the picture-sort approach include its novel/engaging process and reduction in literacy demand; these advantages are particularly appealing for dietary assessment in children. Yaroch and colleagues examined the validity and reliability of a modified picture-sort food frequency questionnaire in a sample of 22 low-income, overweight African American adolescent girls. The picture-sort was administered twice during a two-week period and evaluated using the average of three dietary recalls collected within the same time period. Similar to observed patterns with paper-and-pencil questionnaires, the first administration of the picture-sort yielded higher values for energy and nutrient intake than the second. Validity correlations with the diet recall data ranged from 0.32 (protein) to 0.87 (saturated fat); test-retest correlations were low (range 0.28–0.36). Sherwood et al. (Sherwood, Story, Neumark-Sztainer, Adkins & Davis, 2003) developed a similar card-sorting food preference and frequency task for use with younger girls. Preliminary data examining the validity of the picture-sort approach for assessing dietary intake are promising, but further validation work in this area is warranted.

Direct Observation

Direct observation of meals is often considered a "gold standard" for evaluating the validity of other dietary assessment tools. Advantages of direct observation include the facts that it does not rely on a subject's memory, is an unbiased estimate of a subject's intake, and can be practical and economical under certain conditions (Baglio et al., 2004). Direct observation of dietary intake is typically conducted during structured school or group activities such as school lunches. The observer(s) watches subjects during a defined period of time and take notes on amounts consumed, traded or given away, spilled, and not eaten. Despite its intuitive appeal, direct observation is not a "perfect" measure of dietary intake, and factors such as variations in food type and portion size (Gittelsohn, Shankar, Pokhrel & West, 1994) and observer variability may affect accuracy (Baglio et al.). Recommendations for enhancing interobserver variability include assessment of interobserver reliability during training and throughout data collection and retraining of observers as needed (Baglio et al.).

Social Desirability

An understudied, but important, aspect of ensuring accurate reports of dietary intake is measurement of social desirability. Socially desirable responding may lead to inaccurate conclusions regarding the efficacy of dietary interventions, as intervention-related bias in self-reports of diet have been observed (Harnack et al., 2004). Two strategies for detecting socially desirable responding and/or enhancing reporting accuracy are the use of paper-and-pencil social desirability measures (Baxter, Smith, Litaker, Baglio, et al., 2004) and the use of the bogus pipeline procedure (Baranowski

et al., 2002). Klesges and colleagues (Klesges et al., 2004) adapted the
"Lie Scale" from the Revised Children's Manifest Anxiety Scale (Reynolds & Page
1983) to measure social desirability in a sample of preadolescent African
American girls taking part in an obesity prevention study. Social desirability
was found to bias reports of diet and confound associations between Body
Mass Index and energy intake. Baranowski et al. (2002) used a bogus pipeline method to reduce socially desirable responding in their evaluation of the
FIRSSt diet recall. A bogus pipeline informs children that there is another
method for ascertaining the truth of their self-report. The bogus pipeline in
the Baranowski et al. study was a hair sample; participants were told that
the researchers would be able to tell some of what they ate from a chemical
analysis of their hair. Participants who provided hair samples had a
statistically significantly higher percent agreement between the 24 hDRs
and observation but lower concordance on portion size estimates. Those
providing hair samples also had a marginally significantly lower omission
rate when the FIRSSt and the 24 hDR were compared. These data underscore the need for further work to both understand and reduce the impact
of socially desirable responding in dietary assessment.

Conclusions and Recommendations

Reviews of the literature evaluating dietary assessment methods for
use with children and adolescents can be disheartening, as no single
approach captures recent or "usual" dietary intake perfectly and each
assessment method has unique strengths and weaknesses. The purpose,
logistics, and resource constraints must be considered when choosing a
dietary intake assessment measure (Serdula et al., 2001). Table 1 provides
an overview of the diet assessment methods reviewed in this chapter, their
indications, and issues to consider when implementing each measure.
The following questions can be used to guide the process of choosing diet
assessment tools:

1. What is the purpose of the study (e.g., intervention, prospective
   observational study), and is dietary/nutrient intake a primary or
   secondary outcome variable?
2. Are group-level or individual-level data of most interest? A focus
   on individual-level outcomes would indicate the need for multiple
   measures (e.g., multiple days of food records or diet recalls).
3. What are the most relevant aspects of dietary intake for a particular
   study (e.g., total energy intake, macronutrients, consumption of
   specific foods/beverages), and what level of detail of nutrient/food
   analysis is needed? For example, a focus on specific foods/bever-
   ages may require a less comprehensive dietary intake measure than
   a study for which an estimate of total energy intake is needed.
4. What are the characteristics of the target population (e.g., age, cognitive ability, literacy level, race/ethnicity, socioeconomic status,
   weight status), and how might this affect participants' ability to
   accurately complete the measure of interest and/or report their
   dietary intake in a valid and reliable manner?

5. Given that the ability to make direct comparisons with other published studies is important, what diet assessment measures have been used previously for this type of question in this specific population?
6. What modifications may need to be made to tailor the instrument to the study population? (e.g., Does the measure include unique foods/beverages consumed by participants?)
7. Do parents/caregivers need to provide or supplement dietary intake information provided by children?
8. What are the time, budget, and staffing constraints of the project?
9. How could assessment of portion size be enhanced (e.g., photographs, food models, food scales)?
10. What quality control methods should be used to ensure the accuracy of the data (e.g., inter-rater reliability)?
11. What methods could be used to address social desirability biases for a given study (e.g., bogus pipeline, paper-and-pencil measure to detect response patterns that may affect the validity of the data provided)?

Consideration of the above questions will assist the reader in choosing the measure(s) that will meet the diet assessment goals of a project in a cost-effective manner. Because the instrument choice for a given study always represents a compromise between accuracy and feasibility, interpretation of study results should take into account the known biases observed in previous validation work for the specific dietary intake measures utilized, including response patterns associated with weight status.

Future research to enhance dietary assessment methods in children and adolescents is clearly warranted. Prominent among dietary assessment issues worthy of examination are documenting and understanding reporting biases associated with specific methods (e.g., 24 hDR, FFQ), study populations (age group, race/ethnicity, weight status), and study designs (e.g., observational studies, intervention studies). Consistent use of quality control methods and strategies to reduce socially desirable response biases is also encouraged. In addition, Rockett, Berkey, and Colditz (2003) recommend that diet assessment instruments should have the versatility to study new nutrients that have gained significance through scientific research, new foods (e.g., ready-made foods) as well as adolescents' growing discretionary spending on meals and snacks outside the home, new portion sizes, and other factors including fast food, family dinners, and binge drinking.

REFERENCES

Andersen, L. F., Lande, B., Trygg, K., & Hay, G. (2004). Validation of a semi-quantitative food-frequency questionnaire used among 2-year-old Norwegian children. *Public Health Nutrition, 7*, 757–764.

Baglio, M. L., Baxter, S. D., Guinn, C. H., Thompson, W. O., Shaffer, N. M., & Frye, F. H. (2004). Assessment of interobserver reliability in nutrition studies that use direct observation of school meals. *Journal of the American Dietetic Association, 104*, 1385–1392.

Baranowski, T., Islam, N., Baranowski, J., Cullen, K. W., Myres, D., Marsh, T., et al. (2002). The food intake recording software system is valid among fourth-grade children. *Journal of the American Dietetic Association, 102,* 380–385.

Baxter, S. D., Smith, A. F., Guinn, C. H., Thompson, W. O., Litaker, M. S., Baglio, M. L., et al. (2003). Interview format influences the accuracy of children's dietary recalls validated with observations. *Nutrition Research, 23,* 1537–1546.

Baxter, S. D., Smith, A. F., Litaker, M. S., Baglio, M. L., Guinn, C. H., & Shaffer, N. M. (2004). Children's social desirability and dietary reports. *Journal of Nutrition Education and Behavior, 36,* 84–89.

Baxter, S. D., Smith, A. F., Litaker, M. S., Guinn, C. H., Shaffer, N. M., Baglio, M. L., et al. (2004). Recency affects reporting accuracy of children's dietary recalls. *Annals of Epidemiology, 14,* 385–390.

Bertoli, S., Petroni, M. L., Pagliato, E., Mora, S., Weber, G., Chiumello, G., et al. (2005). Validation of food frequency questionnaire for assessing dietary macronutrients and calcium intake in Italian children and adolescents. *Journal of Pediatric Gastroenterology and Nutrition, 40,* 555–560.

Bjorntorp, P. (1992). Abdominal fat distribution and the metabolic syndrome. *Journal of Cardiovascular Pharmacology, 20*(Suppl. 8), 526–528.

Buzzard, I. M., Stanton, C. A., Figueiredo, M., Fries, E. A., Nicholson, R., Hogan, C. J., et al. (2001). Development and reproducibility of a brief food frequency questionnaire for assessing the fat, fiber, and fruit and vegetable intakes of rural adolescents. *Journal of the American Dietetic Association, 101,* 1438–1446.

Centers for Disease Control and Prevention (CDC), National Center for Health Statistics (NCHS). (2004). Statistics NCHS. Prevalence of overweight among children and adolescents: United States, 1999–2002. Retrieved July 5, 2006, from http://www.cdc.gov/nchs/products/pubs/pubd/hestats/overwght99.htm.

Crawford, P. B., Obarzanek, E., Morrison, J., & Sabry, Z. I. (1994). Comparative advantage of 3-day food records over 24-hour recall and 5-day food frequency validated by observation of 9- and 10-year-old girls. *Journal of the American Dietetic Association, 94,* 626–630.

Cullen, K. W., & Zakeri, I. (2004). The youth/adolescent questionnaire has low validity and modest reliability among low-income African-American and Hispanic seventh- and eighth-grade youth. *Journal of the American Dietetic Association, 104,* 1415–1419.

Davies, P. S., Coward, W. A., Gregory, J., White, A., & Mills, A. (1994). Total energy expenditure and energy intake in the preschool child: A comparison. *The British Journal of Nutrition, 72,* 13–20.

Dennison, B. A., Jenkins, P. L., & Rockwell, H. L. (2000). Development and validation of an instrument to assess child dietary fat intake. *Preventive Medicine, 31,* 214–224.

Edmunds, L. D., & Ziebland, S. (2002). Development and validation of the Day in the Life Questionnaire (DILQ) as a measure of fruit and vegetable questionnaire for 7–9 year olds. *Health Education Research, 17,* 211–220.

Frank, G. C. (1994). Environmental influences on methods used to collect dietary data from children. *The American Journal of Clinical Nutrition, 59*(Suppl. 1), 207S–211S.

Gittelsohn, J., Shankar, A. V., Pokhrel, R. P., & West, K. P., Jr. (1994). Accuracy of estimating food intake by observation. *Journal of the American Dietetic Association, 94,* 1273–1277.

Goran, M. I. (1998). Measurement issues related to studies of childhood obesity: Assessment of body composition, body fat distribution, physical activity, and food intake. *Pediatrics, 101,* 505–518.

Green, T. J., Allen, O. B., & O'Connor, D. L. (1998). A three-day weighed food record and a semiquantitative food-frequency questionnaire are valid measures for assessing the folate and vitamin B-12 intakes of women aged 16 to 19 years. *The Journal of Nutrition, 128,* 1665–1671.

Harbottle, L., & Duggan, M. B. (1993). Dietary assessment in Asian children-a comparison of the weighed inventory and diet history methods. *European Journal of Clinical Nutrition, 47,* 666–672.

Harnack, L., Himes, J. H., Anliker, J., Clay, T., Gittelsohn, J., Jobe, J. B., et al. (2004). Intervention-related bias in reporting of food intake by fifth-grade children participating in an obesity prevention study. *American Journal of Epidemiology, 160,* 1117–1121.

Jensen, J. K., Gustafson, D., Boushey, C. J., Auld, G., Bock, M. A., Bruhn, C. M., et al. (2004). Development of a food frequency questionnaire to estimate calcium intake of Asian, Hispanic, and white youth. *Journal of the American Dietetic Association,* 104, 762–769.

Kaskoun, M. C., Johnson, R. K., & Goran, M. I. (1994). Comparison of energy intake by semiquantitative food-frequency questionnaire with total energy expenditure by the doubly labeled water method in young children. *The American Journal of Clinical Nutrition,* 60, 43–47.

Klesges, L. M., Baranowski, T., Beech, B., Cullen, K., Murray, D. M., Rochon, J., et al. (2004). Social desirability bias in self-reported dietary, physical activity and weight concerns measures in 8- to 10-year-old African-American girls: Results from the Girls Health Enrichment Multisite Studies (GEMS). *Preventive Medicine,* 38, S78–S87.

Klohe, D. M., Clarke, K. K., George, G. C., Milani, T. J., Hanss-Nuss, H., & Freeland-Graves, J. (2005). Relative validity and reliability of a food frequency questionnaire for a triethnic population of 1-year-old to 3-year-old children from low-income families. *Journal of the American Dietetic Association,* 105, 727–734.

Kristal, A. R., Peters, U., & Potter, J. D. (2005). Is it time to abandon the food frequency questionnaire? *Cancer Epidemiology, Biomarkers & Prevention,* 14, 2826–2828.

Kumanyika, S., Tell, G. S., Fried, L., Martel, J. K., Chinchilli, V. M., et al. (1996). Picture-sort method for administering a food frequency questionnaire to older adults. *Journal of the American Dietetic Association,* 96, 137–144.

Lanigan, J. A., Wells, J. C., Lawson, M. S., Cole, T. J., & Lucas, A. (2004). Number of days needed to assess energy and nutrient intake in infants and young children between 6 months and 2 years of age. *European Journal of Clinical Nutrition,* 58, 745–750.

Lietz, G., Barton, K. L., Longbottom, P. J., & Anderson, A. S. (2002). Can the EPIC food-frequency questionnaire be used in adolescent populations? *Public Health Nutrition,* 5, 783–789.

Lillegaard, I. T., & Andersen, L. F. (2005). Validation of a pre-coded food diary with energy expenditure, comparison of under-reporters v. acceptable reporters. *The British Journal of Nutrition,* 94, 998–1003.

Linneman, C. K., Hessler, K., Nanney, S., Steger-May, K., Huynh, A., & Haire-Joshu, D. (2004). Parents are accurate reporters of their preschoolers' fruit and vegetable consumption under limited conditions. *Journal of Nutrition Education and Behavior,* 36, 305–308.

Livingstone, M. B., Prentice, A. M., Coward, W. A., Strain, J. J., Black, A. E., Davies, P. S., et al. (1992). Validation of estimates of energy intake by weighed dietary record and diet history in children and adolescents. *The American Journal of Clinical Nutrition,* 56, 29–35.

Livingstone, M. B., Robson, P. J., & Wallace, J. M. (2004). Issues in dietary intake assessment of children and adolescents. *The British Journal of Nutrition,* 92(Suppl. 2), S213–S222.

Marshall, T. A., Eichenberger Gilmore, J. M., Broffitt, B., Levy, S. M., & Stumbo, P. J. (2003). Relative validation of a beverage frequency questionnaire in children ages 6 months through 5 years using 3-day food and beverage diaries. *Journal of the American Dietetic Association,* 103, 714–720.

McPherson, R. S., Hoelscher, D. M., Alexander, M., Scanlon, K. S., & Serdula, M. K. (2000). Dietary assessment methods among school-aged children: Validity and reliability. *Preventive Medicine,* 31, S11–S33.

Metcalf, P. A., Scragg, R. K., Sharpe, S., Fitzgerald, E. D., Schaaf, D., & Watts, C. (2003). Short-term repeatability of a food frequency questionnaire in New Zealand children aged 1–14 y. *European Journal of Clinical Nutrition,* 57, 1498–1503.

Montgomery, C., Reilly, J. J., Jackson, D. M., Kelly, L. A., Slater, C., Paton, J. Y., et al. (2005). Validation of energy intake by 24-hour multiple pass recall: Comparison with total energy expenditure in children aged 5–7 years. *The British Journal of Nutrition,* 93, 671–676.

Morris, J. M., Owen, G. S., & Fraser, M. D. (1994). Practical issues in multimedia user interface design for computer-based instruction. In S. Reisman (Eds.), *Multimedia computing, preparing for 21st century* (pp. 225–286). Harrison, PA: Idea Group Publishing.

Nelson, M., Black, A. E., Morris, J. A., & Cole, T. J. (1989). Between- and within-subject variation in nutrient intake from infancy to old age: Estimating the number of days required to rank dietary intakes with desired precision. *The American Journal of Clinical Nutrition, 50*, 155–167.

Parrish, L. A., Marshall, J. A., Krebs, N. F., Rewers, M., & Norris, J. M. (2003). Validation of a food frequency questionnaire in preschool children. *Epidemiology, 14*, 213–217.

Perks, S. M., Roemmich, J. N., Sandow-Pajewski, M., Clark, P. A., Thomas, E., Weltman, A., et al. (2000). Alterations in growth and body composition during puberty. IV. Energy intake estimated by the youth-adolescent food-frequency questionnaire: Validation by the doubly labeled water method. *The American Journal of Clinical Nutrition, 72*, 1455–1460.

Reynolds, C. R., & Page, K. D. (1983). National normative and reliability data for the revised children's manifest anxiety scale. *School Psychology Review, 12*, 324–326.

Rockett, H. R., Berkey, C. S., Colditz, G. A. (2003). Evaluation of dietary assessment instruments in adolescents. *Current Opinion in Clinical Nutrition and Metabolic Care, 6*, 557–562.

Rockett, H. R., Wolf, A. M., & Colditz, G. A. (1995). Development and reproducibility of a food frequency questionnaire to assess diets of older children and adolescents. *Journal of the American Dietetic Association, 95*, 336–340.

Serdula, M. K., Alexander, M. P., Scanlon, K. S., & Bowman, B. A. (2001). What are preschool children eating? A review of dietary assessment. *Annual Review of Nutrition, 21*, 475–498.

Shaffer, N. M., Baxter, S. D., Thompson, W. O., Baglio, M. L., Guinn, C. H., & Frye, F. H. (2004). Quality control for interviews to obtain dietary recalls from children for research studies. *Journal of the American Dietetic Association, 104*, 1577–1585.

Sherwood, N. E., Story, M., Neumark-Sztainer, D., Adkins, S., & Davis, M. (2003). Development and implementation of a visual card-sorting technique for assessing food and activity preferences and patterns in African American girls. *Journal of the American Dietetic Association, 103*, 1473–1479.

Smith, K. W., Hoelscher, D. M., Lytle, L. A., Dwyer, J. T., Nicklas, T. A., Zive, M. M., et al. (2001). Reliability and validity of the Child and Adolescent Trial for Cardiovascular Health (CATCH) Food Checklist: A self-report instrument to measure fat and sodium intake by middle school students. *Journal of the American Dietetic Association, 101*, 635–647.

Sobo, E. J., & Rock, C. L. (2001). "You ate all that!" caretaker-child interaction during children's assisted dietary recall interviews. *Medical Anthropology Quarterly, 15*, 222–244.

Subar, A. F. (2004). Developing dietary assessment tools. *Journal of the American Dietetic Association, 104*, 769–770.

Taylor, R. W., & Goulding, A. (1998). Validation of a short food frequency questionnaire to assess calcium intake in children aged 3 to 6 years. *European Journal of Clinical Nutrition, 52*, 464–465.

Treiber, F. A., Leonard, S. B., Frank, G., Musante, L., Davis, H., Strong, W. B., et al. (1990). Dietary assessment instruments for preschool children: Reliability of parental responses to the 24-hour recall and a food frequency questionnaire. *Journal of the American Dietetic Association, 90*, 814–820.

van Horn, L. V., Stumbo, P., Moag-Stahlberg, A., Obarzanek, E., Hartmuller, V. W., Farris, R. P., et al. (1993). The Dietary Intervention Study in Children (DISC): Dietary assessment methods for 8- to 10-year-olds. *Journal of the American Dietetic Association, 93*, 1396–1403.

Vereecken, C. A., Covents, M., Matthys, C., & Maes, L. (2005). Young adolescents' nutrition assessment on computer (YANA-C). *European Journal of Clinical Nutrition, 59*, 658–667.

Vereecken, C. A., & Maes, L. (2003). A Belgian study on the reliability and relative validity of the health behavior in school-aged children food-frequency questionnaire. *Public Health Nutrition, 6*, 581–588.

Watson, J. F., Collins, C. E., Dibley, M. J., Garg, M. G., & Sibbritt, D. (2003). Design considerations in the development of a food-frequency questionnaire for school-aged children. *Asia Pacific Journal of Clinical Nutrition, 12*, S24.

Weber, J. L., Lytle, L., Gittelsohn, J., Cunningham-Sabo, L., Heller, K., Anliker, J. A., et al. (2004). Validity of self-reported dietary intake at school meals by American Indian children: The Pathways Study. *Journal of the American Dietetic Association, 104*, 746–752.

Wilson, A. M., & Lewis, R. D. (2004). Disagreement of energy and macronutrient intakes estimated from a food frequency questionnaire and 3-day diet record in girls 4 to 9 years of age. *Journal of the American Dietetic Association, 104*, 373–378.

Yaroch, A. L., Resnicow, K., Davis, M., Davis, A., Smith, M., & Kahn, L. K. (2000). Development of a modified picture-sort food frequency questionnaire administered to low-income, overweight, African-American adolescent girls. *Journal of the American Dietetic Association, 100*, 1050–1056.

7

Development of Eating Patterns

**VICKY PHARES, JESSICA CURLEY,
and ARIZ ROJAS**

As can be seen throughout this book, childhood and adolescent obesity is of great concern. Obesity during childhood and adolescence has been associated with physical, behavioral, and academic difficulties (Anderson & Butcher, 2006; Datar & Sturm, 2006). This chapter will discuss developmental patterns related to normative eating habits as well as eating patterns associated with problematic eating. Given that the behavioral correlates of eating habits and nutrition begin at birth, this chapter will cover eating patterns from infancy through adolescence. Because issues outside the family (such as the school environment and media) are also related to the development of eating patterns, they will be discussed briefly. The primary focus of this chapter, however, will be the influences of the family on the development of eating patterns.

Infancy

The extant literature on early childhood feeding patterns has largely focused on food refusal and failure to thrive but to a lesser extent on obesity (Woolston, 1987; Woolston & Szydlo, 2004). This finding is particularly surprising given that the incidence of infant and childhood obesity has increased dramatically over the years (Kim et al., 2006; Ogden et al., 2006). According to the Centers for Disease Control and Prevention, the latest update of the National Health and Nutrition Examination Survey (NHANES) estimates the prevalence of childhood obesity at 19%, higher than in previous years (CDC, 2006). Given this trend, it is imperative for

---

VICKY PHARES, JESSICA CURLEY, and ARIZ ROJAS • University of South Florida, Tampa, FL 33620.

researchers, clinicians, and pediatricians to understand the developmental progression of obesity across the life span as well as to identify the factors that contribute to overweight status in infants.

Nutrition

Adequate nutrition is of utmost importance for the growing infant (World Health Organization, 2006b). During the first six months of life, the infant's primary source of nutrition is through breast milk or formula. Within the United States, approximately 14.2% of infants are exclusively breast-fed (i.e., only breast milk—no water, solids, or other liquids) during the first six months of life. However, a larger percentage of mothers (41.5%) continue breast-feeding at six months but may supplement feeding with water, formula, or other liquids (CDC, 2007). The World Health Organization (WHO, 2006a) recommends that complementary feeding (e.g., solid foods) be supplemental to breast milk and introduced no earlier than 6 months of age, although the American Academy of Pediatrics (AAP) is somewhat more liberal and suggests 4–6 months (AAP, 1998). Introduction of solid foods before this time period may result in overfeeding (Morin, 2004) and place the infant at risk for obesity. When infants are overfed, they are susceptible to obesity of simple excessive caloric intake (Woolston & Szydlo, 2004).

The same is true for fruit juices. According to the AAP (2001), fruit juices should not be introduced until 6 months of age, as they offer no additional nutritional benefit if provided earlier. Excessive consumption of fruit juice has been associated with malnutrition (including over nutrition), diarrhea, and tooth decay (AAP).

In summary, careful attention should be given to an infant's nutritional intake. Selection of inappropriate formulas and early introduction of solid foods and juices may place an infant at unnecessary risk for obesity. The sections that follow will identify risk factors for obesity and highlight practices, such as breast-feeding, that serve preventative functions.

Risk for Obesity

Feeding Practices. The largest controversy to date has centered on breast- versus formula-feeding. Proponents of breast-feeding implicate that it reduces the risk of infant and childhood obesity (Dewey, 2003; Gillman et al., 2001, Lande et al., 2003). On the other hand, some cite equivocal evidence for the protective effect of breast-feeding (Butte, 2001). Lande and colleagues found that mothers who breast-fed their infants had lower consumption of foods with high carbohydrates and fat as well as lower intake of sugar-sweetened drinks. In turn, their infants' caloric intake was 10% lower than non-breast-fed infants and their water intake was higher. Similar results were reported by Taveras et al. (2004), who indicated that for each additional month of breast-feeding, maternal restriction of dietary intake was reduced by 10%. This finding may sound counterintuitive, but high restriction of intake is detrimental to infant self-regulation. Mothers who breast-fed for at least six months in the study were less likely to restrict their children's food intake at one year. The authors conjecture that care givers who bottle-feed may be more observant of remaining formula and force infants to feed, leading to overfeeding.

A large systematic review of the literature on infant feeding was conducted by Owen, Martin, Whincup, Smith, and Cook (2005), who used odds ratios of obesity within a fixed effects model to compare breast-fed infants with formula-fed infants. The authors confirmed that breast-feeding was associated with decreased risk for obesity. In addition, the association was stronger when breast-feeding was prolonged. A similar finding was reported by Taveras et al. (2004), who found that a longer period of breast-feeding was associated with decreased restriction of food intake, which serves as a protective factor for obesity. As such, the WHO recommends that infants be breast-fed for the first six months of life in order to secure optimal growth and development. After six months, the WHO suggests the introduction of safe foods and continued breast-feeding for two or more years (WHO, 2002).

Regardless of whether an infant is breast- or bottle-fed, it is important for parents and medical professionals to monitor the infant's weight gain. As mentioned previously, infant weight gain is largely attributed to infant feeding practices during the first several months of life. When infants are overfed and subsequently overweight during the first four months of life, they are at significantly greater risk for developing obesity in childhood (Stettler, Zemel, Kumanyika, & Stallings, 2002). Specifically, Stettler and colleagues found that rapid weight gain during the first four months of life predicted obesity at age 7 independently from weight at birth and at age 1. An astonishing 100 grams of weight increase per month was associated with a 30% increased risk for overweight status at age 7. Since it has been established that formula and other milks accelerate weight gain in infants (Kramer et al., 2004), it is imperative that weight gain be evaluated early in life. Sowan and Stember (2000) recommend monthly weight checks for infants with Body Mass Index percentiles above the 75th percentile.

As a final point, energy intake and sucking behavior are also predictive of infants' risk for obesity (Stunkard, Berkowitz, Schoeller, Macslin, & Stallings, 2004). In a study of 78 mothers and their infants, Stunkard et al. were interested in determining predictors of obesity during the first two years of life. Results showed that regardless of prior body weight, energy intake or daily caloric intake (as measured by weight of food and/or milk/formula) predicted greater weight gain at all time points (i.e., 6–24 months). However, greater energy intake may have resulted in part from sucking behavior. Like energy intake, number of sucks at three months predicted weight gain at all time points. In addition, sucking behavior differentiated infants at high and low risk for obesity (as measured by maternal BMI). That is, infants at high risk had a substantially higher rate of sucking than low-risk infants. Thus, the rate of sucking and amount of nourishment that is relinquished to the infant may place him or her at additional risk for obesity.

Taken together, there is ample evidence to suggest that breast-feeding serves protective value in decreasing the risk of obesity in infants and children. Breast-feeding has the ability to regulate infant weight gain, which teaches the infant self-regulation and reduces the risk of infant and childhood obesity. Further research is needed to elucidate the relationship between infant sucking behavior and subsequent weight gain.

Parental Characteristics. While feeding practices and patterns contribute significantly to infant risk for obesity, parental characteristics also play a role. Sowan and Stember (2000) analyzed a sample of 630 infants and their families, who were recruited from the multisite National Institutes of Health Infant Growth Study. Results from this prospective, longitudinal study identified several parental factors that put infants at risk for excessive weight gain. Logistic regression models isolated maternal age, pre-pregnancy weight, pregnancy weight, and smoking as significant predictors of overweight status in infants. Paternal characteristics were not predictive of risk for obesity. Specifically, maternal age at birth was predictive of infants' excessive weight gain at 10 months, with the odds of obesity increasing from 20–40% with each five-year increment in maternal age. Likewise, maternal pre-pregnancy weight predicted obesity at seven months, with an increase in risk of 20–30% for each 25-pound increment in maternal weight; however, weight gain during pregnancy only predicted infant weight at one month, with a 10% increase in risk for every 5-pound increase in pregnancy weight gain. Finally, prenatal smoking was associated with infants' excessive weight gain only at seven months. Similarly, Lande et al. (2003) found that mothers who smoked were less likely to breast-feed their infants. Thus, maternal factors may interact with feeding practices and place the infant at additional risk for obesity.

Cultural preferences for infant body size may also place infants at risk for obesity. In a study of 240 low-income mothers from diverse racial backgrounds, Worobey and Lopez (2005) asked mothers to rate their infants' body sizes, select the ideal infant body size, and disclose their attitudes about feeding practices. Results indicated that Mexican mothers *perceived* their infants as leanest, followed by other Hispanic mothers, black mothers and then white mothers, who perceived their infants as heaviest. However, the reverse was true for preferred weight. That is, Mexican mothers *preferred* heavier infants, whereas white mothers preferred leaner infants. The authors speculate that because Hispanic/Latina mothers find heavier infants desirable, they may be more likely to encourage feeding and even overfeed their infants. Overall, these results have important implications for cultural preferences and infant feeding practices.

Finally, it is important to note the contribution of parental psychopathology to overweight status in infants. In particular, maternal depressive symptomatology has been linked to disrupted feeding practices (McLearn, Minkovitz, Strobino, Marks, & Hou, 2006). As part of the National Evaluation of Healthy Steps for Young Children study, 4874 mothers completed measures of parenting practices and depressive symptomatology, which were analyzed by McLearn et al. Notably, mothers with depressive symptoms (17.8%) were more likely to discontinue breast-feeding than mothers without depressive symptoms. Furthermore, mothers with such symptoms were more likely to engage in less-than-optimal feeding practices, such as incorporating cereal and juices for their 2- to 4-month-old infants. However, this finding was not significant after adjusted regression models. These results suggest that mothers with depressive symptomatology are less likely to carry out behaviors that require active engagement, such as breast-feeding (McLearn et al.), and may place their infants at risk for additional problems.

Overall, the number of infants with unhealthy weight gains is increasing exponentially, raising concerns about psychological and medical problems (e.g., cardiovascular disease and juvenile diabetes). Multiple factors contribute to the developmental progression of overweight status in infants, including the early termination of breast-feeding, complementary feeding, and the premature introduction of fruit juices and drinks. Furthermore, feeding practices, cultural preferences, and parental characteristics influence an infant's BMI, caloric intake, and energy expenditure. These issues continue to be relevant in early childhood and during the preschool years.

Early Childhood/Preschool Years

In the early childhood and preschool years, a transition is made from describing the process of food intake as *feeding* to describing it as *eating* (Nicholls, 2004). This change in terminology is due to preschool children's increased self-sufficiency to feed themselves instead of completely relying on a caregiver, as is the case in infancy. However, preschool children's caregivers and the environments in which they reside greatly influence the development of their eating patterns. For preschool children, eating occurs as a result of the interaction of social, cultural, and environmental factors as they begin to learn when and how much to eat (Birch, 1991). Even in these early years children may show characteristics and symptoms of disordered eating that could lead to eating disorders or obesity.

Eating Patterns

So what may lead to the development of these disorders in preschool children? We will first look at several factors that are shown to differentiate between normative and problem eating patterns in the early years. These factors include nutrient intake, meal frequency and duration, portion sizes, and bite size and chew rates.

Nutrient Intake. Sherry (2005) reviewed six strategies set forth by the CDC for the prevention of overweight and chronic disease in the pediatric population. One of these strategies was to increase fruit and vegetable consumption and other sources of important nutrients. In a longitudinal study of over 7000 preschoolers, an additional increase of fruits and vegetables each day was found to decrease children's odds of becoming overweight (Conrey et al., 2004). While Gillis and Gillis (2005) found that both obese and nonobese youths were not consuming an adequate nutrient intake, obese youths consumed a higher rate of needed energy than non-obese youths. Even with this greater overall intake, obese youths were not receiving an appropriate amount of important nutrients, including calcium and Vitamin D. Therefore, measures to improve nutrient intake in all youths need to be taken. Kranz, Siega-Riz, and Herring (2004) and Knol, Haughton and Fitzhugh (2005) agreed that nutrient intake needs to be improved and sugar and fat intake decreased in pediatric populations, as these measures should help alleviate the growing prevalence of obesity in children.

While youths' nutrition has somewhat improved in the past decades, there is still a great need for increased nutrition in preschool children (Kranz et al., 2004). As Cockroft, Durkin, Masding, and Cade (2005) found, preschoolers' nutrient intake differed depending on their environments and demographic variables such as their schools and highest educational level of their households. Thus, a child's environment has been found to play a large role in eating behaviors and will be discussed further.

Meal Frequency and Duration.   Meal frequency and duration have been shown to be influential factors in the development of increased weight and obesity. In a sample of 5- and 6-year-olds, Toschke, Kuchenhoff, Koletzko, and von Kries (2005) found that the prevalence of obesity decreased when the number of meals the children consumed decreased. This association between increased daily meal frequency and obesity in children was found independent of other risk factors for obesity. In a longitudinal study of preschool children, Nakao, Aoyama, and Suzuki (1990) found that shorter meal duration was the factor most strongly associated with weight and BMI. This finding supported previous research that found larger bites, more rapid eating pace, and shorter meals were associated with obese children's eating patterns rather than nonobese children's (Drabman, Cordua, Hammer, Jarvie, & Horton, 1979).

Portion Sizes.   The sizes of the portions a child consumes during meals are as important as the number of meals a child eats per day in the prevention of obesity. Sherry (2005) discussed decreasing portion sizes as a strategy in preventing pediatric overweight. As children reach the preschool years, they are much more influenced by portion sizes and tend to eat more when the portions are larger (Mrdjenovic & Levitsky, 2005). They also begin to consume substantially more snacks, desserts, and soft drinks. This increased consumption may be related to preschool children's increased self-sufficiency and ability to make their own food choices. Fisher, Rolls, and Birch (2003) further discussed how increases in portion sizes stimulate increased food consumption. However, they found that when preschool children were allowed to serve themselves, they consumed significantly less than when served a large portion by an adult. Therefore, parents and caregivers need to be educated about appropriate portion sizes in order to hinder the development of overweight and obesity in children at a very young age. Future research should examine interventions for preventing pediatric overweight including reducing portion sizes and allowing children to serve themselves.

Sherry (2005) found that preschoolers increased their consumption of a variety of foods, particularly unhealthy ones. Nicklaus, Chabanet,

Boggio, and Issanchou (2005) found that energy intake greatly increased in the preschool years, but restriction of food variety was also characteristic at this age. Higher energy intake was related to higher Body Mass Index in preschoolers. Preschoolers who had experienced a longer duration of breast-feeding during infancy showed a greater variety of food consumption, including healthier foods. This finding further supported the positive effects of breast-feeding that were discussed in the infancy section of this chapter.

Bite Size and Frequency. Bite size and bite frequency or chew rates have been shown to differ between obese and nonobese preschool children. Fisher et al. (2003) found that when children were served large-portion lunches, their average bite size was significantly larger than when they were served reference-portion lunches. In addition, mean bite size was positively related to BMI, in that heavier children took larger bites. Drabman et al. (1979) examined bite and chew rates of normal vs overweight preschool children and found that overweight children showed a higher rate of fewer chews per bite and higher bite rates.

Environmental Factors and Influences

Because preschool children are largely influenced by and reliant on their parents and other caregivers, the environment in which they are raised plays a large role in the development of healthy or destructive eating patterns.

Parents and Caregivers. Many researchers have studied how parents and other caregivers instill and support certain eating behaviors in children at a very young age. From both genetic (Faith, 2005) and home environmental influences (Lindsay, Sussner, Kim, & Gortmaker, 2006), parents play a role in the development of their children's food- and physical-activity-related behaviors. This section will focus primarily on environmental factors, such as specific parental behaviors that have been found to be associated with normative and detrimental eating patterns.

Because parents serve as models for their children's eating behaviors, it is important that they are educated on what constitutes healthy eating patterns (Bish, Regis, & Gottesman, 2005; Vereecken, Keukelier, & Maes, 2004). The educational level of parents has been found to be related to their own eating behaviors, which are in turn related to their children's eating behaviors, such that parents with a lower occupational status consume fewer fruits and vegetables and more soft drinks than parents with a higher occupational status (Vereecken et al.). Thus, there is a need for parents to be educated, through interventions in their homes or their children's schools, about appropriate food choices, portions, and behaviors to teach and model for themselves and their children (Harvey-Berino & Rourke, 2003; Lindsay et al., 2006).

Lewinsohn et al. (2005) discussed the importance of paying attention to the quality of parent-child interactions in order to understand etiologies in feeding and eating behaviors. Some studies have looked at parental verbal behaviors that have had positive influences on preschool children's eating patterns. Iannotti, O'Brien, and Spillman (1994) found that mothers' verbal encouragements, rationales, and actions, instead of negative consequences or punishment, were most successful in getting African American preschoolers to eat healthier foods. Likewise, Vereecken et al. (2004) found that verbal praise was a significant predictor of getting preschool children to consume more vegetables. On the other hand, some studies have discussed parental behaviors that have had negative consequences on preschoolers' eating patterns. Sanders, Patel, le Grice, and Shepherd (1993) looked at the interactions of parents with toddlers and preschoolers with and without feeding difficulties. Parents of children with feeding disorders displayed more negative and coercive behaviors, such as aversive instruction and negative eating-related comments. In addition, Vereecken et al. found that parents' permissiveness and use of food as a reward increased preschoolers' consumption of unhealthy foods, such as soft drinks and sweets. Also, it was found that maternal restriction of snack food intake predicted greater snack food intake in preschool girls (Fisher & Birch, 1999). These negative parental behaviors and responses may further put children at risk for developing detrimental eating patterns and possible obesity. Therefore, as Patrick, Nicklas, Hughes, and Morales (2005) found, a positive and authoritative feeding style by parents proved most advantageous in the development of healthy eating patterns in their children, including increased consumption of fruits, vegetables, and dairy products. Thus, an authoritative parenting style has been found to be associated with positive eating patterns across developmental stages.

Schools and Neighborhoods.   As mentioned above, there is a growing need to encourage and educate parents, caregivers, and children on how to engage in healthy eating patterns and practices. Because children and families exist within a broader system of influences, such as their schools and communities, some researchers have expanded their resources to implement interventions in these areas. Zakus (1982) stated the importance of intervening in schools when children are young and having school programs that target activity and nutritional education become integral to the system. Fuller, Keller, Olson, and Plymale (2005) highlighted several practices and interventions targeted at preschoolers to help them learn about nutritious eating, including offering smaller portions of new foods along with food that the child likes, making food fun (e.g., pieces of fruit arranged to look like a smiley face), using star charts for rewarding the child's attempt to taste a new food, and being a good role model. In addition, Cason (2001) described a preschool nutrition program based on the theory of multiple intelligences so that children's physical, emotional, and social needs were addressed. Results showed significant improvements in preschoolers' healthy snack identification; frequency of fruit, vegetable, dairy, and meat consumption; and willingness to taste different foods.

Other environmental factors, such as neighborhoods and proximity to fast-food restaurants, have been studied. Burdette and Whitaker (2004) recently explored the relationship between overweight, low-income preschool children and their proximity to fast-food restaurants and playgrounds and the safety of their neighborhoods. As Adair and Popkin (2005) said, the globalization of fast-food restaurants is affecting children's eating patterns cross-culturally. However, other countries do not seem to be affected at the same rate as the United States. Therefore, there is an increased need in the United States to research and implement effective strategies to prevent and treat children's negative eating patterns at a young age.

Middle Childhood and Adolescence

As children move from early childhood into middle childhood and adolescence, they tend to gain more independence in many aspects of their lives, including food-related choices. The research on eating behaviors in middle childhood and adolescence tends to focus on the ways in which youths eat and the factors that are associated with their eating behaviors.

Eating Patterns

There are a number of continuities in eating patterns from early childhood to middle childhood to adolescence. Preschool children who showed greater variety in their food choices were more likely to have greater variety in their food choices in childhood, adolescence, and even early adulthood (Nicklaus, Boggio, Chabanet, & Issanchou, 2005). Regulation of intake is another area of study in middle childhood and adolescence. As children move from early to middle childhood, their regulation of intake changes, as does their food responsiveness. One study with a community sample found that children's responsiveness to food (i.e., desire for eating) and their enjoyment of food increase with age (Wardle, Guthrie, Sanderson, & Rapoport, 2001). Conversely, their satiety responsiveness (e.g., reducing food intake after a snack) decreased with age. Another study found that after being exposed to strong smells of desirable food and being allowed to eat a small amount of appetizing food, normal-weight children decreased their intake of food, whereas children who were overweight showed no decrease in intake (Jansen et al., 2003). Thus, it appears that intake after exposure to food cues is less regulated in children with weight problems than in those without weight problems. A related concept, eating in the absence of hunger, has been shown to be significantly more frequent in prepubertal boys who were at high risk for obesity than in boys who were at low risk for obesity (Faith et al., 2006). This pattern was not found in girls.

Individual characteristics, such as stress and impulsivity, have been linked to eating behaviors in children and adolescents. For example, higher rates of stress were associated with more unhealthy eating and with using eating as a coping mechanism in elementary-school-aged children (Jenkins, Rew, & Sternglanz, 2005). Notably, Hispanic/Latino/Latina American children showed the highest rates of using food as a coping mechanism, with African American children and white American children showing lower rates. Regarding impulsivity, obese children showed lower rates of inhibitory control than normal-weight children (Nederkoorn, Braet, VanEijs, Tanghe, & Jansen, 2006). In addition, obese children with more eating binges showed higher rates of impulsivity than did obese children with fewer eating binges (Nederkoorn et al.). There is growing evidence that impulsivity plays a role in obesity in adults as well (Davis, Levitan, Smith, Tweed, & Curtis, 2006).

In addition to these individually based factors that are related to eating patterns, a number of environmental factors and influences are related to children's and adolescents' eating patterns. Most notably, parents, the media, and the school environment can be related to eating patterns in youths.

Environmental Factors and Influences

Parents and Caregivers. Although children and adolescents are more able to show independence in eating patterns and food choices than are infants and toddlers, parents continue to influence eating patterns throughout childhood and adolescence. It is well-established that offspring of obese parents are at risk for the development of obesity themselves (Benton, 2004; Davison, Francis, & Birch, 2005; Wu & Suzuki, 2006). In addition to the genetic linkages, research on children and adolescents in this area focuses on a number of interrelated behavioral factors within families, including parental modeling, parental control/restriction, and family meals.

Overall, it appears that parental modeling has a significant association with children's and adolescents' eating behaviors. Children's and parents' behaviors are significantly related for weight control (Keery, Eisenberg, Boutelle, Neumark-Sztainer, & Story, 2006), intake of healthy food, intake of unhealthy food, and eating motivations (Brown & Ogden, 2004). Thus, parents who model appropriate eating habits can likely increase their children's healthy eating habits.

Conversely, parental control and restriction of children's and adolescents' intake are often associated with poorer dietary outcomes. It appears that parental control, especially parental overcontrol, of a child's food intake is associated with poor self-regulation in the child that is further associated with overweight status in the child (Brown & Ogden, 2004; Faith, Scanlon, Birch, Francis, & Sherry, 2004). Thus, Brown & Ogden argued that parents can have a better impact on their children's eating behaviors by serving as positive role models rather than by trying to control their children's dietary intake.

Related to the opportunity to model parental eating, it appears that having family meals together is associated with healthier eating in children and adolescents. In a community sample of children and young adolescents, Taveras et al. (2005) found that higher frequency of family meals was associated with lower rates of overweight and obesity. Similarly, other studies have found that adolescents who reported higher rates of having meals with their families were less likely to show disordered eating, such as binge eating (Neumark-Sztainer, Wall, Story, & Fulkerson, 2004). Benton (2004) found that having an emotionally healthy atmosphere during a meal was associated with children and adolescents eating in a healthier manner. Thus, part of the suggestion for having family meals together is predicated on the notion that the parents can provide a positive atmosphere in which to share the family meal and that parents can model healthy eating behaviors.

In addition to this research, there are findings from obesity prevention and treatment programs that can help with understanding parents' role in the development of eating behaviors in children and adolescents. When comparing the results of a treatment for obese children that focused on either the child only or the parents only, superior results were found for children's weight loss in the parent-only group, and these results remained after seven years (Golan & Crow, 2004). In addition, obese children who participated in a weight control program showed better long-term results when they perceived higher rates of acceptance from their fathers (Stein, Epstein, Raynor, Kilanowski, & Paluch, 2005). Thus, parents can clearly be active agents of change in their children's weight control, and focusing on families can be an effective way to intervene in childhood and adolescent obesity and even to prevent it (Kitzmann & Beech, 2006; Lindsay et al., 2006).

Involvement with Media and Other Technology. In addition to parental influences in the development of children's and adolescents' eating behaviors, there has been a great deal of attention to how exposure to the media and involvement with other technologies influence children's eating behaviors and food intake. The majority of research has focused on television viewing and computer usage. Within the United States and internationally, there is consistent evidence that higher rates of television viewing are associated with higher BMI scores in children and adolescents (Arluk, Branch, Swain, & Dowling, 2003; Janssen et al., 2005). Although the mechanisms are not well-understood, it appears that metabolic rate does not differ between television and other sedentary activities that are not associated with obesity, such as reading or resting, so it appears that metabolic rate does not explain the link between television viewing and higher BMI by itself (Cooper, Klesges, DeBon, Klesges, & Shelfton, 2006). Children's television programming is often full of commercials that focus on unhealthy food choices (Albon, 2005), and the more that children are exposed to advertisements about unhealthy foods, the higher their BMI (Lobstein & Dibb, 2005). Thus, it may be that the information children and adolescents are exposed to on television, in combination with the lack of physical activity during television viewing, may be at least one of the reasons for these consistent findings.

There is equivocal evidence as to the relationship between BMI and computer usage. Some studies have found an association between higher rates of BMI and more time on the computer (Arluk et al., 2003), whereas other studies have not found a significant relationship (Janssen et al., 2005). Perhaps the types of activities being completed on the computer (such as homework in a word processing program that does not expose the child to advertisements vs surfing the web and being exposed to advertisements that are similar in content to those on television) may help explain some of the variations in these findings. Clearly, further research is needed on this topic.

Overall, there is clear evidence that television viewing is associated with unhealthy weight gain in children and adolescents. Based on a review of overweight and obesity prevalence in children in 34 countries, Janssen et al. (2005) highlighted the need to decrease children's television viewing and to increase their participation in physical activities.

Schools. There is growing public awareness of the importance of providing healthy food choices for children and adolescents in their schools. Adolescents often mention that convenience, availability, time, and cost were factors that influenced their food choices at school (Kubik, Lytle, & Fulkerson, 2005). Given that children and adolescents can often make their own choices about eating at school (e.g., eating a healthy lunch from the cafeteria or buying chips and cookies out of a vending machine), an increasing number of school districts are trying to provide only healthy food and beverages in vending machines on campus (Kubik et al.). (See Chapters 11 and 16 for further discussion of food choices on school campuses.)

There is surprisingly little research on the role of peers and friends in relation to the development of eating behaviors, but there are indications that children's and adolescents' eating behaviors are associated with the eating behaviors of those with whom they spend time. Benton (2004) found that peers can serve as role models for children and adolescents to try new and different types of foods. In focus groups, adolescents often acknowledged that social support from their peers and friends to eat in a healthy manner often influenced their choice of healthy foods (Kubik et al., 2005). Overall, schools and peers appear to have a potential influence on the development of children's and adolescents' eating behaviors, but there is more research in the area of family influences than in the area of the school setting.

SUMMARY

Overall, there are a number of influences on the development of eating behaviors in children and adolescents. Beginning in the prenatal environment and continuing through early childhood, middle childhood, and adolescence, factors inside as well as outside the family can influence the development of eating behaviors. Many preventionists (e.g., Benton, 2004) argue that having healthy parental role models in families where family members share nutritious meals together in an emotionally supportive environment would go a long way toward helping children and adolescents develop healthy eating behaviors.

REFERENCES

Adair, L. S., & Popkin, B. M. (2005). Are child eating patterns being transformed globally? *Obesity Research, 13*, 1281–1299.

Albon, D. J. (2005). Approaches to the study of children, food and sweet eating: A review of the literature. *Early Child Development and Care, 175*, 407–417.

American Academy of Pediatrics, Committee on Nutrition. (1998). Supplemental foods for infants. In R. E. Kleinman (Ed.), *Pediatric nutrition handbook*, (4th ed., pp. 43–53). Elk Grove Village, IL: American Academy of Pediatrics.

American Academy of Pediatrics, Committee on Nutrition. (2001). The use and misuse of fruit juice in pediatrics. *Pediatrics, 107*, 1210–1213.

Anderson, P. M., & Butcher, K. F. (2006). Childhood obesity: Trends and potential causes. *The Future of Children, 16,* 19–45.

Arluk, S. L., Branch, J. D., Swain, D. P., & Dowling, E. A. (2003). Childhood obesity's relationship to time spent in sedentary behavior. *Military Medicine, 168,* 583–586.

Benton, D. (2004). Role of parents in the determination of the food preferences of children and the development of obesity. *International Journal of Obesity, 28,* 858–869.

Birch, L. L. (1991). Obesity and eating disorders: A developmental perspective. *Bulletin of Psychonomic Society, 29,* 265–272.

Bish, B., Regis, K., & Gottesman, M. M. (2005). Educating parents about portion sizes for preschoolers. *Journal of Pediatric Health Care, 19,* 54–59.

Brown, R., & Ogden, J. (2004). Children's eating attitudes and behaviour: A study of the modeling and control theories of parental influence. *Health Education Research, 19,* 261–271.

Burdette, H. L., & Whitaker, R. C. (2004). Neighborhood playgrounds, fast food restaurants, and crime: Relationships to overweight preschool children. *Preventive Medicine, 38,* 57–63.

Butte, N. F. (2001). The role of breastfeeding in obesity. *Pediatric Clinics of North America, 48,* 189–198.

Cason, K. L. (2001). Evaluation of a preschool nutrition education program based on the theory of multiple intelligences. *Journal of Nutrition Education, 33,* 161–164.

Centers for Disease Control and Prevention. (2006). *Prevalence of overweight among children and adolescents: United States, 2003–2004.* http://www.cdc.gov/nchs/products/pubs/pubd/hestats/overweight/overwght_child_03.htm. Cited 8 Feb 2008.

Centers for Disease Control and Prevention. (2007). *2005 National Immunization Survey: Table 3: Any and exclusive breastfeeding rates by age among children born in 2004.* http://www.cdc.gov/breastfeeding/data/NIS_data/data_2004.htm. Cited 10 Feb 2008.

Cockroft, J. E., Durkin, M., Masding, C., & Cade, J. E. (2005). Fruit and vegetable intakes in a sample of pre-school children participating in the "Five for All" project in Branford. *Public Health Nutrition, 8,* 861–869.

Conrey, E. J., Welsh, J., Sherry, B., Rockett, H., Mehrle, D., & Grummer-Strawn, L. (2004). Association between overweight low-income preschoolers and fruit and vegetable consumption. *American Journal of Epidemiology, 159,* S75.

Cooper, T. V., Klesges, L. M., DeBon, M., Klesges, R. C., & Shelton, M. L. (2006). An assessment of obese and non obese girls' metabolic rate during television viewing, reading, and resting. *Eating Behaviors, 7,* 105–114.

Datar, A., & Sturm, R. (2006). Childhood overweight and elementary school outcomes. *International Journal of Obesity, 30,* 1449–1460.

Davis, C., Levitan, R. D., Smith, M., Tweed, S., & Curtis, C. (2006). Associations among overeating, overweight, and attention deficit/hyperactivity disorder: A structural equation modeling approach. *Eating Behaviors, 7,* 266–274.

Davison, K. K., Francis, L. A., & Birch, L. L. (2005). Reexamining obesigenic families: Parents' obesity-related behaviors predict girls' change in BMI. *Obesity Research, 13,* 1980–1990.

Dewey, K. G. (2003). Is breastfeeding protective against child obesity? *Journal of Human Lactation, 19,* 9–18.

Drabman, R. S., Cordua, G. D., Hammer, D., Jarvie, G. J., & Horton, W. (1979). Developmental trends in eating rates of normal and overweight preschool children. *Child Development, 50,* 211–216.

Faith, M. S. (2005). Development and modification of child food preferences and eating patterns: Behavior genetics strategies. *International Journal of Obesity, 29,* 549–556.

Faith, M. S., Berkowitz, R. I., Stallings, V. A., Kerns, J., Storey, M., & Stunkard, A. J. (2006). Eating in the absence of hunger: A genetic marker for childhood obesity in prepubertal boys? *Obesity Research, 14,* 131–138.

Faith, M. S., Scanlon, K. S., Birch, L. L., Francis, L. A., & Sherry, B. (2004). Parent-child feeding strategies and their relationships to child eating and weight status. *Obesity Research, 12,* 1711–1722.

Fisher, J. O. & Birch, L. L. (1999). Restricting access to foods and children's eating. *Appetite, 32,* 405–419.

Fisher, J. O., Rolls, B. J., & Birch, L. L. (2003). Children's bite size and intake of an entrée are greater with large portions than with age-appropriate or self-selected portions. *The American Journal of Clinical Nutrition, 77,* 1164–1170.

Fuller, C., Keller, L., Olson, J., & Plymale, A. (2005). Helping preschoolers become healthy eaters. *Journal of Pediatric Healthcare, 19,* 178–182.

Gillis, L. & Gillis, A. (2005). Nutrition inadequacy in obese and non-obese youth. *Canadian Journal of Dietetic Practice and Research, 66,* 237–242.

Gillman, M. W., Rifas-Shiman, S. L., Camargo, C. A., Jr., Berkey, C. S., Frazier, A. L., Rockett, H. R. et al. (2001). Risk of overweight among adolescents who were breast-fed as infants. *Journal of the American Medical Association, 285,* 2461–2467.

Golan, M., & Crow, S. (2004). Targeting parents exclusively in the treatment of childhood obesity: Long-term results. *Obesity Research, 12,* 357–361.

Harvey-Berino, J., & Rourke, J. (2003). Obesity prevention in preschool Native-American children: A pilot study using home visiting. *Obesity Research, 11,* 606–611.

Iannotti, R. J., O'Brien, R. W., & Spillman, D. M. (1994). Parental and peer influences on food consumption of preschool African-American children. *Perceptual and Motor Skills, 79,* 747–752.

Jansen, A., Theunissen, N., Slechten, K., Nederkoorn, C., Boon, B., Mulkens, S., et al. (2003). Overweight children overeat after exposure to food cues. *Eating Behaviors, 4,* 197–209.

Janssen, I., Katzmarzyk, P. T., Boyce, W. F., Vereecken, C., Mulvihill, C., Roberts, C., et al. (2005). Comparison of overweight and obesity prevalence in school-aged youth from 34 countries and their relationships with physical activity and dietary patterns. *Obesity Reviews, 6,* 123–132.

Jenkins, S. K., Rew, L., & Sternglanz, R. W. (2005). Eating behaviors among school-age children associated with perceptions of stress. *Issues in Comprehensive Pediatric Nursing, 28,* 175–191.

Keery, H., Eisenberg, M. E., Boutelle, K., Neumark-Sztainer, D., & Story, M. (2006). Relationships between maternal and adolescent weight-related behaviors and concerns: The role of perception. *Journal of Psychosomatic Research, 61,* 105–111.

Kim, J., Peterson, K. E., Scanlon, K. S., Fitzmaurice, G. M., Must, A., Oken, E., et al. (2006). Trends in overweight from 1980 through 2001 among pre-school-aged children enrolled in a health maintenance organization. *Obesity, 14,* 1107–1112.

Kitzmann, K. M., & Beech, B. M. (2006). Family-based interventions for pediatric obesity: Methodological and conceptual challenges from family psychology. *Journal of Family Psychology, 20,* 175–189.

Knol, L. L., Haughton, B., & Fitzhugh, E. C. (2005). Dietary patterns of young, low-income US children. *Journal of the American Dietetic Association, 105,* 1765–1773.

Kramer, M. S., Guo, T., Platt, R. W., Vanilovich, I., Sevkovskaya, Z., Dzikovich, I., et al. (2004). Feeding effects on growth during infancy. *The Journal of Pediatrics, 145,* 600–605.

Kranz, S., Siega-Riz, A. M., & Herring, A. H. (2004). Changes in diet quality of American preschoolers. *American Journal of Public Health, 94,* 1525–1530.

Kubik, M. Y., Lytle, L., & Fulkerson, J. A. (2005). Fruits, vegetables, and football: Findings from focus groups with alternative high school students regarding eating and physical activity. *Journal of Adolescent Health, 36,* 494–500.

Lande, B., Andersen, L., Veierød, M. B., Bærug, A., Johansson, L., Trygg, K. U., et al. (2003). Breast-feeding at 12 months of age and dietary habits among breast-fed and non-breast-fed infants. *Public Health Nutrition, 7,* 495–503.

Lewinsohn, P. M., Holm-Denoma, J. M., Gau, J. M., Joiner, T. E., Striegel-Moore, R., Bear, P., & Lamoureux, B. (2005). Problematic eating and feeding behaviors of 36-month-old children. *International Journal of Eating Disorders, 38,* 208–219.

Lindsay, A. C., Sussner, K. M., Kim, J., & Gortmaker, S. (2006). The role of parents in preventing childhood obesity. *Future Child, 16,* 169–186.

Lobstein, T., & Dibb, S. (2005). Evidence of a possible link between obesogenic food advertising and child overweight. *Obesity Reviews, 6,* 203–208.

McLearn, K., Minkovitz, C. S., Strobino, D. M., Marks, E., & Hou, W. (2006). Maternal depressive symptoms at 2 to 4 months post partum and early parenting practices. *Archives of Pediatrics and Adolescent Medicine, 160,* 279–284.

Morin, K. H. (2004). Infant nutrition. *The American Journal of Maternal Child Nursing, 29,* 313–317.

Mrdjenovic, G., & Levitsky, D. A. (2005). Children eat what they are served: The imprecise regulation of energy intake. *Appetite, 44,* 273–282.

Nakao, H., Aoyama, H., & Suzuki, T. (1990). Development of eating behavior and its relation to physical growth in normal weight preschool children. *Appetite, 14,* 45–57.

Nederkoorn, C., Braet, C., VanEijs, Y., Tanghe, A., & Jansen, A. (2006). Why obese children cannot resist food: The role of impulsivity. *Eating Behaviors, 7,* 315–322.

Neumark-Sztainer, D., Wall, M., Story, M., & Fulkerson, J. A. (2004). Are family meal patterns associated with disordered eating behaviors among adolescents? *Journal of Adolescent Health, 35,* 350–359.

Nicholls, D. (2004). Eating problems in childhood and adolescence. In J. K. Thompson (Ed.), *Handbook of eating disorders and obesity* (pp. 635–655). Hoboken, NJ: Wiley.

Nicklaus, S., Boggio, V., Chabanet, C., & Issanchou, S. (2005). A prospective study of food variety seeking in childhood, adolescence, and early adult life. *Appetite, 44,* 289–297.

Nicklaus, S., Chabanet, C., Boggio, V., & Issanchou, S. (2005). Food choices at lunch during the third year of life: Increase in energy intake but decrease in variety. *Acta Paediatrica, 94,* 1023–1029.

Ogden, C. L., Carroll, M. D., Curtin, L. R., McDowell, M. A., Tabak, C. J., & Flegal, K. M. (2006). Prevalence of overweight and obesity in the United States, 1999–2004. *Journal of the American Medical Association, 295,* 1549–1555.

Owen, C. G., Martin, R. M., Whincup, P. H., Smith, C. D., & Cook, D. G. (2005). Effect of infant feeding on the risk of obesity across the life course: A quantitative review of published evidence. *Pediatrics, 115,* 1367–1377.

Patrick, H., Nicklas, T. A., Hughes, S. O., & Morales, M. (2005). The benefits of authoritative feeding style: Caregiver feeding styles and children's food consumption patterns. *Appetite, 44,* 243–249.

Sanders, M. R., Patel, R. K., le Grice, B., & Shepherd, R. W. (1993). Children with persistent feeding difficulties: An observational analysis of the feeding interactions of problem and non-problem eaters. *Health Psychology, 12,* 64–73.

Sherry, B. (2005). Food behaviors and other strategies to prevent and treat pediatric overweight. *International Journal of Obesity, 29,* S116–S126.

Sowan, N. A., & Stember, M. L. (2000). Parental risk factors for infant obesity. *The American Journal of Maternal Child Nursing, 25,* 234–241.

Stein, R. I., Epstein, L. H., Raynor, H. A., Kilanowski, C. K., & Paluch, R. A. (2005). The influence of parenting change on pediatric weight control, *Obesity Research, 13,* 1749–1755.

Stettler, N., Zemel, B. S., Kumanyika, S., & Stallings, V. A. (2002). Infant weight gain and childhood overweight status in a multicenter, cohort study. *Pediatrics, 109,* 194–199.

Stunkard, A. J., Berkowitz, R. I., Schoeller, D., Maislin, G., & Stallings, V. A. (2004). Predictors of body size in the first 2 years of life: A high-risk study of human obesity. *International Journal of Obesity, 28,* 503–513.

Taveras, E. M., Rifas-Shiman, S. L., Berkey, C. S., Rockett, H. R. H., Field, A. E., Frazier, A. L., Colditz, G. A., & Gillman, M. W. (2005). Family dinner and adolescent overweight. *Obesity Research, 13,* 900–906.

Taveras, E. M., Scanlon, K. S., Birch, L., Rifas-Shiman, S. L., Rich-Edwards, J. W., & Gillman, M. W. (2004). Association of breastfeeding with maternal control of infant feeding at age 1 year. *Pediatrics, 114,* 577–583.

Toschke, A. M., Kuchenhoff, H., Koletzko, B., & von Kries, R. (2005). Meal frequency and childhood obesity. *Obesity Research, 13,* 1932–1938.

Vereecken, C. A., Keukelier, E., & Maes, L. (2004). Influence of mother's educational level on food parenting practices and food habits of young children. *Appetite, 43,* 93–103.

Wardle, J., Guthrie, C. A., Sanderson, S., & Rapoport, L. (2001). Development of the children's eating behaviour questionnaire. *Journal of Child Psychology and Psychiatry, 42,* 963–970.

Woolston, J. L. (1987). Obesity in infancy and early childhood. *American Academy of Child and Adolescent Psychiatry, 26,* 123–126.

Woolston, J. L. & Szydlo, D. (2004). Infant and childhood obesity. In J. M. Wiener & M. K. Dulcan (Eds.), *The american psychiatric publishing textbook of child and adolescent psychiatry* (pp. 659–669). Washington, DC: American Psychiatric Publishing.

World Health Organization. (2002). *Infant and young child nutrition: Global strategy on infant and young child feeding.* Retrieved August 23, 2006 from http://www.who.int/nutrition/topics/infantfeeding_recommendation/en/index.html.

World Health Organization. (2006a). *Complementary feeding.* Retrieved August 23, 2006 from http://www.who.int/nutrition/topics/complementary_feeding/en/index.html.

World Health Organization. (2006b). *Nutrition: challenges.* Retrieved August 23, 2006 from http://www.who.int/nutrition/challenges/en/index.html.

Worobey, J., & Lopez, M. I. (2005). Perceptions and preferences for infant body size by low-income mothers. *Journal of Reproductive and Infant Psychology, 23,* 303–308.

Wu, Q., & Suzuki, M. (2006). Parental obesity and overweight affect the body-fat accumulation in the offspring: The possible effect of a high-fat diet through epigenetic inheritance. *Obesity Reviews, 7,* 201–208.

Zakus, G. E. (1982). Obesity in children and adolescents: Understanding and treating the problem. *Social Work in Health Care, 8,* 11–29.

Section III

Risk Factors for Obesity in Children and Youth

8

Physiological Mechanisms Impacting Weight Regulation

DAVID FIELDS and PAUL HIGGINS

Within the framework of body weight regulation, the first law of thermodynamics (i.e., the Law of Conservation of Energy - "Energy cannot be created nor destroyed, it simply is transferred from one form to another") concisely and eloquently identifies the basic paradigm of body weight regulation, and is described by the equation below:

$$\text{Energy intake} + \text{Energy expenditure} = \pm \text{ Body weight}$$

Therefore, the regulation of body weight is a balance between food intake and energy expenditure, where excess calories are stored as extra pounds and a deficit between intake and expenditure results in weight loss.

This chapter serves as a link between the treatment literature that might be recommended at a clinic, and the physiologic mechanisms underlying weight regulation. With this end in mind, we have chosen to present the chapter in two parts—with the first looking at the control of energy expenditure and the second looking at the physiology of appetite regulation. The section on control of energy expenditure will focus on a distinct aspect of physical activity—spontaneous free-living energy expenditure—and attempt to answer the basic question of why it is so hard for some people to be physically active. The section on the physiology of appetite regulation will focus on signaling pathways (both neural-peptides and hormones) originating from three distinct regions: a) adipose tissue, b) gastrointestinal system and pancreas, and c) the central nervous system.

DAVID FIELDS • University of Oklahoma Health Science Center, Oklahoma City, OK 73104.
PAUL HIGGINS • Southwest Foundation for Biomedical Research, San Antonio, TX 78245.

After reading this chapter on the "physiological mechanisms impacting weight regulation," it is our hope that mental health professionals can then knowledgeably apply the treatment literature to achieve for the greatest effect for their clients. As a result of reading this chapter, it is our hope that some principles underlying the previously described prevention programs (Chapter 4) will be more meaningful, consequently giving psychologists a greater understanding of why some programs *should* be more effective than others or why it is more difficult for *some* children to lose weight than others.

CONTROL OF ENERGY EXPENDITURE

The three chief components of energy expenditure are the resting metabolic rate, the thermic effect of food, and activity related thermogenesis. The resting metabolic rate is the energy expended at rest in a post-absorptive state. Resting metabolic rate is the largest energy consumer, comprising approximately 65 percent of the total calories expended per day, and is predominately determined by body size—specifically non-fat or fat-free mass (organ tissue and muscle tissue mass) (Deriaz, Fournier, Tremblay, Despres, & Bouchard, 1992). The thermic effect of food is the energy expended during digestion and the assimilation of foodstuffs. The thermic effect of food comprises approximately 15 percent of total daily calorie expenditure and is dependent upon the macronutrient composition of the foods consumed (Hill, DiGirolamo, & Heymsfield, 1985). Activity related thermogenesis is both the energy expended during exercise (purposeful movement) with the intent of improving health, and nonexercise-related activities (Levine, Eberhardt, & Jensen, 1999; Levine, Schleusner, & Jensen, 2000). Activity related thermogenesis comprises approximately 25 percent of total daily calorie expenditure and varies highly from person to person—partly because of the high degree of nonexercise activity (Donahoo, Levine, & Melanson, 2004; Levine & Kotz, 2005).

While neuron-endocrine control of energy intake has been studied at length, little attention has been given to the central control of energy expenditure. The inter-individual variation in the face of excess energy intake is highly varied with changes in spontaneous physical activity inversely related to increased body weight, and this relationship differs between obese and normal weight individuals (Levine et al., 1999; Levine & Kotz, 2005). It has been reported that normal weight individuals sit less and have a greater amount of spontaneous physical activity as compared to their obese counterparts, and that the relationship remains unchanged even after weight gain in normal weight individuals and weight loss in obese individuals (Levine et al.; Levine & Kotz).

Data is emerging to suggest that physical activity is centrally controlled and regulated. In one study, 16 nonobese adults were fed 1,000 kcal/day more than what was needed to maintain their body weight for eight weeks (Levine et al., 1999). On average, of the 1,000 excess calories, 432 kcal/day were stored as fat while the remaining 544 kcal/day were lost or *burned off* through increased spontaneous physical activity, the thermic effect of food, and through resting metabolic rate. Of particular note, spontaneous physical activity was predictive of the level of fat mass gained—this is to say that those who gained the least amount of fat mass were those with the greatest increases in spontaneous physical activity (Levine et al.).

In another study, the posture (i.e., standing and sitting) and physical activity of 20 obese and normal weight sedentary subjects were studied continually for 10 days (Levine et al., 2005). Subjects that were obese remained seated for 164 minutes longer and stood upright or ambulated 152 minutes less, in comparison with the normal weight group (Levine et al.). To further clarify the impact of excess energy intake and the subsequent changes in posture and spontaneous physical activity, with an interest in understanding the role of physiologic mechanisms in physical activity, Levine and colleagues enrolled 16 of the original 20 subjects in a follow-up study. Seven obese subjects were put on a controlled weight-loss program for two months while nine normal weight subjects were put on a controlled overfeeding program for two months. As a result, the obese group lost an average of 18 pounds while the lean group gained nine pounds (Levine et al.). Spontaneous physical activity, specifically the postural allocation (i.e., time spent sleeping, sitting, and standing) was analyzed both pre- and post-weight loss/gain. Though no significant differences were found, a trend for the obese subjects to sit more and ambulate less after weight loss—as compared to pre-weight loss—was observed. The normal weight subjects sat less and ambulated more as compared to their pre-weight gain (Levine et al.). Interestingly, the obese post-weight loss and lean post-weight gain groups maintained their original spontaneous physical activity. Taken together, these results suggest that individuals tend to defend a *pre-set* body weight and imply that spontaneous physical activity may be physiologically regulated. Interestingly, evidence of a pre-set body weight that is physiologically regulated through alterations in spontaneous physical activity is observed across different species (Dulloo, 2002; Jones, Bellingham, & Ward, 1990; Kemnitz et al., 1993; Mabry & Campbell, 1975; Robin, Boucontet, Chillet, & Groscolas, 1998).

Spontaneous physical activity represents a vast resource of untapped expendable energy that, until recently, was poorly understood and appreciated (Levine, 2004). By better understanding this phenomenon and the impact of regulatory factors affecting and potentially controlling it, clinicians may be able to improve weight loss recommendations and regimens.

At first glance, one may be skeptical of the impact of spontaneous physical activity on body weight regulation, but in a recent study, spontaneous physical activity was shown to play a significant role in the control of body weight regulation (Lanningham-Foster, Nysse, & Levine, 2003). Lanningham-Foster and colleagues reported that the mechanization of common everyday tasks—such as washing dishes by hand vs. using a dishwasher, washing clothes by hand vs. using a washing machine, stair climbing vs. taking the elevator, walking/riding a bicycle to work vs. driving—saves an individual, on average, a total of 111 kcal/day (Lanningham-Foster et al.). This translates into an extra 3,330 kcal/month, 39,960 kcal/year, or (in other words) 11.4 pounds of saved calories a year (Lanningham-Foster et al.). To avoid transferring these energy savings into weight gain, they must be compensated by either a decrease in food intake or an increase in other forms of physical activity. Similarly, the built environment infringes upon our ability to regulate body weight. Factors such as the availability of sidewalks, bike paths, parks, and recreational areas—all within the context of a safe environment—impede physical activity and must be taken into account if intervention programs are to be effectively implemented, especially in inner city urban areas (Levine & Kotz, 2005). It is likely that modernization has played a significant role in the recent obesity trends that are now observed.

Numerous studies have examined genetic influences on physical activity (Bouchard, Malina, & Perusse, 1997; Lauderdale et al., 1997; Maia, Thomis, & Beunen, 2002; Perusse, Leblanc, & Bouchard, 1988; Perusse, Tremblay, Leblanc, & Bouchard, 1989; Simonen et al., 2002, 2003), with a recent study using sophisticated methodology to measure physical activity (doubly labeled water) (Franks et al. 2005). In this study, 100 monozygotic twin pairs had their total energy expenditures and resting metabolic rates measured. It was concluded that the degree of familial resemblance in physical activity patterns is predominately explained by their shared environment rather than by genetic factors (Franks et al.). However, Bouchard et al. (1990), in a classic twin over-feeding study, showed that excess caloric intake resulted in an increase in spontaneous physical activity, with the relationship modulated by genetic factors. In this study, 12 male twin pairs were fed 1,000 kcal/day more than they needed for 12 weeks. Although the range of weight gain was large (4.3 to 13.3 kg) between pairs, weight gain within each pair was similar. They concluded that the similarity within twin pairs in response to the overfeeding is evidence of a large genetic contribution to weight regulation. Obviously, further work is required to substantiate the role of genetics and physiologic mechanisms in the regulation of spontaneous physical activity.

Evidence for Specific Gene Variants and Systemic Mediators in the Control of Physical Activity

It was commonly thought that energy balance-related peptides such as ghrelin, melanin concentrating hormone, leptin, and orexin controlled only the food intake side of the equation. However, evidence is emerging to show a role for these agents in the regulation of spontaneous physical activity. Of these peptides, ghrelin—which is predominately released from the stomach (see below)—and melanin concentrating hormone are believed to decrease spontaneous physical activity (Ahima, Bjorbaek, Osei, & Flier, 1999; Tschop, Smiley, & Heiman, 2000). Some evidence suggests that leptin, cocaine amphetamine-regulated transcript, and orexin may increase spontaneous physical activity (Ahima et al.; Kristensen et al., 1998; Wortley, Chang, Davydova, Fried, & Leibowitz, 2004).

A recent study explored the effect of genes that code for neuropeptide-Y, cocaine and amphetamine-regulated transcript, agouti-related protein, pro-opiomelanocortin, and several of their receptors on physical activity (Loos et al., 2005). Only the melanocortin-4 receptor gene showed a significant association with a three-day record of physical activity (Loos et al.). Others have shown associations between variants in specific genes, such as those coding for the angiotensin-converting enzyme (Winnicki et al., 2004), the calcium sensing receptor (Lorentzon, Lorentzon, Lerner & Nordstrom, 2001), aromatase (Salmen et al., 2003), and physical activity, however much these data are equivocal and require further substantiation. Hence, it is premature to conclusively draw associations between physical activity and specific gene variants, especially when so many factors other than genetics affect physical activity (social, psycho-social, built environment, and familial issues, to name a few).

Of all the neuropeptides associated with physical activity regulation, orexin has come under the greatest scrutiny. Orexin (also known as hypocretin) is a neuropeptide synthesized in the lateral hypothalamus, whose function seems to alter spontaneous physical activity based upon the energy balance status of the body, and appears to exert this effect by acting upon centers in the hypothalamic paraventricular nucleus (de Lecea et al., 1998; Kalra et al., 1999). In mice, the absence of orexin results in a decrease in physical activity and higher prevalence of obesity, while the injection of orexin directly into the paraventricular nucleus increases spontaneous physical activity in a dose-dependent fashion (Christ et al., 2002). Juxtaposed, a constant state of obesity will elevate orexin levels and result in a *down regulation* or decreased sensitivity of orexin receptors in the paraventricular nucleus region of the hypothalamus, resulting in decreased spontaneous physical activity (Novak, Kotz, & Levine, 2006). Taken together, results from these studies suggest that physical activity may have a neuro-endocrine component. In conclusion, we should never lose sight of the fact that the maintenance of body weight is not simple. On the contrary, it is the sum of many factors affecting both energy expenditure and energy intake.

Practical Application

For a clinician, the mantra for weight regulation is elementary: *move more* and try to *eat less*. From much of the work described above, spontaneous physical activity is an important and readily pliable component of the total daily energy expenditure that can be augmented in children. In general, exercise *per se should not be overemphasized*. Rather, patients should focus on increasing energy expenditure via other means. For example, they should stand when talking on the phone or, even better, walk while they talk—take the one or two flight of stairs instead of the elevator, park a little further out at the mall instead of trying to find a parking place by the door, stand while they talk when taking a coffee break, take the batteries out of the TV remote control, tap their foot while they work, go to the bathroom down the hallway instead of around the corner when taking bathroom breaks, and the possible scenarios can go on and on. Some examples for children may include: matching every hour of television or computer time with an hour of play or activity time; standing while playing video games;

playing organized sports; enrolling in youth sweat programs; purchasing toys that are human-powered instead of battery-operated; removing televisions and computers from the bedroom; making movement fun by setting specific goals for steps taken using a pedometer; encouraging parental participation in activity/games. The concept that small changes in common every day life can be an effective tool to control body weight compared to a structured four-times-a-week exercise program is not intuitive. The average time spent sitting for a lean (407 minutes/day) vs. obese (571 minutes/day) individual differs substantially (Levine et al., 2005; Ravussin, 2005). A *targeted approach* toward increasing movement could reduce weight gain in individuals at risk of obesity, and precipitate weight loss in the overweight and obese. If an obese person were to substitute the 164 minutes a day standing instead of sitting, as they currently do, they would expend an additional ~352 kcal/day (Levine et al.; Ravussin). An increase of this magnitude would be considerably helpful in combating the escalating rise in obesity and would fall within the World Health Organization's recommendation of an additional 200 kcal/day of energy expenditure to reduce the obesity burden (*World Health Organization*, 1997).

PHYSIOLOGY OF APPETITE REGULATION

Our emotions, learned behaviors, social environment, built environment (e.g., side walks, playgrounds, well-lit and safe recreational fields), and genes impact how much we eat or do not eat. Ultimately, all of these factors are integrated and processed through highly complex sensing systems in the central nervous system. These sensing systems receive signals from peripheral locations throughout the body and from neighboring regions of the brain. In particular, a portion of the hypothalamus known as the arcuate nucleus appears to be an important component of the control center for the interpretation and integration of the myriad of signals balancing energy intake and energy storage (Stanley, Wynne, McGowan, & Bloom, 2005). Thus, the hypothalamus receives feedback from both the circulation and from other parts within the brain. After interpreting these signals, the hypothalamus influences food intake and components of energy expenditure. These energy-balancing signals are considered to be of three distinct types based upon the location in which they originated:

1) Postprandial. These signals are generated during and after meal consumption. In general, these signals are peptides that come from the gastrointestinal tract and pancreas. Some interact with receptors on neurons in the gut that convey signals to the hindbrain and ultimately to the hypothalamus. For the most part, these peptides encourage us to stop eating or to reduce food intake. In addition, neural signals can be triggered by the stretching of the intestine in the presence of food.
2) Adipose depots. These signals are also hormonal and are produced and secreted from the adipose tissue. These signals interact directly

Table 8.1. Physiology of food intake regulation

Signaling agent	Site of production	Effect on food intake
Adiponectin	Adipose tissue	↓(?)
Agouti-related peptide	CNS	↑
↓-melancortin stimulating hormone	CNS	↓
Bombesin	Intestine	↓
Cannabinoids	CNS	↓
Cholecystokinin	Intestine / CNS	↑
Ghrelin	Stomach	↓
Glucagon-like peptide 1	Intestine / CNS	↓
Insulin	Pancreas	↓
Leptin	Adipose tissue	↓
Neuropeptide Y	CNS	↑
Obestatin	Stomach	↓
Opioid	CNS	↑
Pancreatic polypeptide	Pancreas / intestine	↓
Peptide YY	Intestine	↓
Resistin	Adipose	↓(?)

Central nervous system (CNS)

with the hypothalamus. Many of these signals have been shown to reduce appetite and increase energy expenditure in animals.

3) Central regulators. Numerous signals act within the brain itself. Some act to alter energy intake while others alter expenditure. Many peripheral regulators operate, at least in part, via these signals. Central regulators are typically in the form of neuro-transmitting peptides.

The sum of these signals helps determine feelings of hunger and consequently determine the volume of food consumed and the duration of the meal. An overview of these regulators is presented in Table 8.1. Although several of these molecules have been discussed above in regard to their role in energy expenditure in the proceeding sections, we will briefly introduce some of the major molecules that encompass these three categories and define their specific roles in appetite regulation. We hope that the reader will gain an appreciation for the complexity of appetite regulation and an understanding of the roles of some of the important regulators. The research summarized below will include data from human and animal models—predominantly rodent—of energy intake regulation.

Postprandial Signals

Insulin. Insulin is secreted rapidly after a meal in response to rising concentrations of glucose in the blood. In addition to its direct metabolic effects on glucose and lipid metabolism, evidence also suggests that insulin acts in the central nervous system to reduce food intake (Air, Benoit, Blake Smith, Clegg, & Woods, 2002; Air, & Strowski et al., 2002). When exogenous insulin is administered centrally to animals (rodents and primates), they reduce their food intake in a dose-dependent manner (Ikeda et al., 1986; Woods, Lotter, McKay, & Porte, 1979). Receptors for insulin are abundant in the mammalian brain, and insulin from the peripheral circulation is likely to interact with these receptors (Marks, Porte, Stahl, & Baskin, 1990). The specific pathway upon which insulin acts on food intake remains unclear, although this potent metabolic hormone is considered a long-term down-regulator of food intake—at least in healthy individuals (Woods, Decke, & Vasselli, 1974).

Pancreatic polypeptide. Pancreatic polypeptide is made and secreted by cells in the pancreas and gastrointestinal tract. Pancreatic polypeptide levels are diurnal and are typically higher in the morning than at night and rise in tandem with food intake (Track, McLeod, & Mee, 1980). As can be predicted from secretory patterns, peripheral infusions of pancreatic ploypeptide tend to reduce food intake in rodents and in normal weight humans. However, its utility in overweight and obese humans is not known. Indeed, obese rodents appear to be more resistant to its appetite suppressing effects compared to their lean counterparts (McLaughlin & Baile, 1981). When taken together, recent evidence does not suggest a major role for pancreatic polypeptide in short-term food intake (Schmidt et al., 2005), although its role in long-term energy balance cannot be ruled out (Koska, DelParigi, de Courten, Weyer, & Tataranni, 2004).

Glucagon-like peptide-1. Glucagon-like peptide-1 (GLP-1) is a peptide hormone manufactured and secreted from a group of cells known as L-cells, located in the intestine. However, GLP-1 is also manufactured in the central nervous system. GLP-1 is also rapidly produced during a meal and is secreted into the portal circulation where it has a number of physiologic actions. The appetite-suppressing effect of GLP-1 is well-documented in various animal models and its receptors are present in the brain (Badman & Flier, 2005). It seems that GLP-1 infusion has a small affect on food intake in humans (Verdich et al., 2001), however chronically low circulating levels could affect energy balance over extended periods of time (Stanley et al., 2005). Because GLP-1 is an important regulator of glucose homeostasis, analogs of the molecule are being tested as potential antidiabetic drugs, in addition to its potential beneficial effect on the regulation of food intake (Turton et al., 1996).

Peptide YY. Peptide YY is also produced from the L-cells of the intestines, particularly in the latter portions of the gut. It has received much attention over the few past years. Early studies showed that peptide YY secretion increased with food intake, and infusions of the peptide were shown to reduce food intake in humans and rodents (Batterham et al., 2002; Challis et al., 2003). Much excitement ensued as peptide YY came to be considered one of the most important regulators of food intake discovered to date. The peptide has been shown to reduce food intake for long periods after intravenous administration, and can cross the blood-brain barrier. Consequently, it has a direct effect on the arcuate nucleus (Batterham et al.). Nevertheless, recent studies have questioned its utility as a weight loss and appetite-reducing drug (Tschop et al., 2004) and further studies are required to conclusively assess the potential of this intriguing peptide.

Bombesin. Bombesin is produced in the intestines and its concentrations increase following food intake, suggesting, in accord with the peptides described above, that it has a role in reducing food intake (Gibbs et al., 1979). Bombesin was found to reduce food intake in normal weight women, but interestingly not in obese women (Yamada, Wada, Santo-Yamada & Wada, 2002). Further research is being conducted on this peptide.

Cholecystokinin. Cholecystokinin is produced in many parts of the intestine, including the duodenum and jejunum. It is also produced in the central nervous system and has neurotransmitter-like properties in this location. Among its many effects, cholecystokinin acts to reduce food intake and meal duration (Kissileff, Pi-Sunyer, Thornton, & Smith, 1981). However, it is rapidly cleared from the circulation and its effects are relatively short in duration. Furthermore, rodents treated with cholecystokinin have been shown to compensate for reduced meal time intake by increasing meal frequency (West, Fey, & Woods, 1984). Little is known about the roles of cholecystokinin in long-term food intake and energy balance regulation and current data remain inconclusive.

Ghrelin. Ghrelin *increases* food intake, as opposed to the other postprandial molecules discussed above. Ghrelin is highest during fasting, and lowest during food intake, and has been shown to be a potent appetite stimulator, hence, ghrelin is considered a "hunger hormone" (Cummings et al., 2001). It is produced predominantly in the stomach and appears to have several modes of action and interaction with central nervous system signals (Date et al., 2002; Faulconbridge, Cummings, Kaplan, & Grill, 2003; Nakazato et al., 2001). Intravenous injection of ghrelin increases hunger, and consequently food intake in normal weight humans and those with cancer (Neary et al., 2004). Ghrelin may be an important peptide in body weight regulation, and is consequently a potential anti-obesity drug target. However, its specific role in the etiology of obesity is yet to be fully understood.

Obestatin. Discovered only very recently, obestatin is a peptide very similar to ghrelin that is also produced and secreted by the stomach (Zhang et al., 2005). Interestingly, its function on appetite directly opposes that of ghrelin. Although a very close relative of ghrelin, obestatin was shown to reduce food intake in rats (Zhang et al.). Receptors for the peptide were shown to be present in the hypothalamus, indicating a potential site of action for its appetite suppressing effects. This novel peptide finding further illustrates the complexities and subtleties of the interplay among the signals governing food intake. Furthermore, its discovery highlights the fact that there may be many more important, as yet, undiscovered molecules in this system.

Signals from Adipose Depots

Leptin. Leptin was the first of a host of factors discovered to be produced and secreted from fat cells (adipocytes), and heralded the recognition of adipose tissue as an active endocrine tissue rather than a storage depot for triglycerides. Leptin is central to the signaling of long-term energy stores. Concentrations rise and fall with rising and falling fat stores, and signal the brain that energy stores within the body are high or low. Leptin can cross from the circulation into the brain, and acts predominantly in the arcuate nucleus (Zhang et al., 1994). Mice that are purposely generated to lack either the gene that codes for leptin, or for the gene that codes for its receptor, overeat and become obese (Badman & Flier, 2005). However, chronic energy imbalance due to leptin deficiency in humans is rare (Montague et al., 1997). Given that obese individuals have higher concentrations of leptin than their normal-weight counterparts, leptin deficiency is not the cause of obesity in and of itself (Stanley et al., 2005). However, a lack of sensitivity or resistance to the effects of leptin may play a role in weight gain. Alternatively, weight gain or its cause(s) may result in leptin resistance, but unfortunately the answers to these questions are still not clear.

Adiponectin. Adiponectin is another peptide produced from adipose tissue that is found in the circulation. It has been shown to increase after fasting in rodents. Apart from its role in glucose metabolism, it has been suggested that adiponectin exerts other effects on energy balance (Stanley et al., 2005). Lower concentrations of adiponectin are found in obese individuals (Hu, Liang, & Spiegelman, 1996) and seems to increase with weight loss (Hotta et al., 2001), hence suggesting a role in the signaling of long-term energy homeostasis.

Resistin. Resistin is also produced by adipose tissue and secreted into the circulation and, as its name suggests, seems to induce cellular resistance to insulin. In addition, higher resistin concentrations seem to be present in obese states, although this is not generally accepted (Kusminski, McTernan, & Kumar, 2005). Hence, the role for resistin in energy balance is presently unclear.

Central Regulators

Neuropeptide Y. Neuropeptide Y molecules share structural similarity with pancreatic polypeptide and peptide YY, and are present in high concentrations in the aforementioned arcuate nucleus. It is the most potent appetite stimulator found to date. Hence, as expected, neuropeptide Y increases with fasting and decreases after food intake (Kalra, Dube, Sahu, Phelps, & Kalra, 1991), and when chronically administered to rats, neuropeptide Y causes obesity (Zarjevski, Cusin, Vettor, Rohner-Jeanrenaud, & Jeanrenaud, 1993). Despite this, mice lacking the gene for neuropeptide Y have normal body weight (Bannon et al., 2000), suggesting a large degree of compensation among these systems, as described below.

Opioids. Opioids are a class of molecules that bind to the opioid receptors in the central nervous system and elicit feelings of euphoria. Regardless of the status of energy balance, certain foods (typically those that are highly palatable) are capable of eliciting increased caloric consumption. While the precise nature of these pathways is complex, endogenous opioids such as ß-endorphin and others acting via κ-opioid receptors are involved in increasing food intake in the presence of sweet tasting foods

(Hayward, Pintar, & Low, 2002; Wilding, 2002). The effects of these opioids on long-term energy balance have yet to be elucidated, but they are highly likely to be involved in the mediation of the way in which certain foods stimulate appetite and increase intake.

Melanocortins. The melanocortin system comprises two important antagonistic agents that act at a single receptor. Agouti-related protein, together with α-melanocyte stimulating hormone, acts through the melanocortin-4 receptor in the arcuate nucleus to regulate food intake (Wilding, 2002). Agouti-related protein increases appetite, while α-melanocyte stimulating hormone decreases appetite. Agouti-related protein is able to stimulate appetite by inhibiting the action of α-melanocyte stimulating hormone at the melanocortin-4 receptor (Wilding).

Endocannabinoids. The appetite-stimulating effects of *Cannabis Sativa's* naturally occurring compound δ9-tetrahydrocannabinol are well-known. Two receptors have been found for δ9-tetrahydrocannabinol, one of which (the CB1 receptor) is the most abundant in the brain (Di Marzo & Matias, 2005). Endogenous cannabinoids were discovered in the 1990s and are derivatives of the common polyunsaturated fatty acid—arachidonic acid. Stimulators of CB1 potently increase appetite, while antagonists to the receptor decrease food intake, including the consumption of highly palatable foods. Recent research indicates a broader role for the endocannabinoid system in energy balance because the system has also been found to be active in the gastrointestinal tract and in fat tissue (Di Marzo & Matias). Research is being conducted to manipulate this system for the treatment of obesity.

Interactions among Signals

It is important to note that these signals do not operate independently and many interact and intercompensate in their respective energy-balancing functions. Examples of these interactions are described below.

Leptin has been shown to inhibit the activity of neuropeptide Y and agouti-related protein neurons in the arcuate nucleus, and reduce levels of these central appetite stimulators (Stanley et al., 2005). Hence, in the presence of high leptin concentrations (sufficient energy stores), leptin will act via these regulators and others to reduce food intake and maintain body weight. Insulin may exert its effects on food intake via similar pathways in the arcuate nucleus. Insulin infused centrally into rats was shown to stop the typical neuropeptide Y increase that accompanies food restriction (Schwartz et al., 1992). Insulin's actions here may, in part, contribute to its overall satiating effect. In a similar fashion, peripherally infused pancreatic polypeptide reduces ghrelin formation in the stomach, and neuropeptide Y production in the hypothalamus of the brain, and could explain its satiating effect (Stanley et al.).

Data from rodent gene knock-out studies have strongly suggested the interdependent and compensatory nature of the energy-balancing signal. For example, rodents who have no neuropeptide Y have normal body weight (Bannon et al., 2000), and rodents lacking ghrelin have normal intakes of food (Wortley et al., 2004). These findings suggest that when one compo-nent of this large multifaceted signal is absent, other parts are altered in an attempt to compensate.

Nutrients Affecting Food Intake

Several nutrients are also thought to regulate appetite. These include glucose and fatty acids. Hunger is typically experienced during periods of low blood sugar. Although this could be attributable to the lower levels of insulin also experienced in this state, glucose sensitive neurons are present in the hypothalamus, potentially directly implicating glucose as a satiating factor (Wilding, 2002). Low levels of fatty acids may be involved in decreasing food intake, as suggested by rodent studies designed to reduce levels of fatty acids (Loftus et al., 2000). The relative importance of nutri-ent signaling in the overall picture of appetite regulation remains to be determined.

Practical Application

Decreasing food and energy intake via low calorie diets has been used in adults but requires comprehensive medical supervision when applied in children (Druce & Bloom, 2006). However, more subtle approaches, such as reducing the food portion sizes consumed by children, may represent an appropriate form of intervention. Food portion sizes have been increasing in the United States over the past 30 years (Young & Nestle, 2002). Studies indicate that higher portion sizes encourage increased energy consumption in children four years of age and older (Rolls, Engell, & Birch, 2000). Indeed it has been suggested that a large component of a child's eating behaviors prior to age four are self-regulated—governed by their own internal cues (Rolls et al.). This self-regulation seems to be less well-maintained after this age (Rolls et al.). Hence, reducing portion sizes and encouraging children to stop eating when they feel full, rather than encouraging them to "clean their plates," may help to promote a healthy body weight (Ello-Martin, Ledikwe, & Rolls, 2005). In addition, it has been shown that when children are allowed to serve themselves, they consume significantly less food (Orlet Fisher, Rolls, & Birch, 2003). In short, reducing portion sizes and allowing children to determine their own intake may be important strategies for promoting a healthy body weight in childhood.

A complete understanding of the systems regulating food intake will undoubtedly lead to a myriad of drug treatment options in the future. However, two promising agents have already been developed. A brief intro-duction to these agents is presented below.

GLP-1 analogs have been developed for use as antidiabetic drugs and may also have potential in the treatment of obesity. As with many intestinal hormones, enzymatic breakdown in the periphery heavily reduces their half-life and hence, their efficacy. Exogenous GLP-1 has been shown to exert a small but dose dependent effect in reducing food intake (Verdich et al., 2001). However, the long-term efficacy of GLP-1 and its analogs on the maintenance of body weight is yet to be determined. Analogs resistant to breakdown will likely improve the potential therapeutic use of glucagon-like peptide-1 for weight loss.

Manipulation of the endo-cannabinoid system using Rimonabant has been an effective weight-loss agent with additional beneficial side effects, including reductions in serum lipids (Gelfand & Cannon, 2006a, 2006b). Rodent studies have shown that Rimonabant reduces food intake and promotes weight loss (Di Marzo et al., 2001). In the human trials conducted to date, similar encouraging findings were reported (Gelfand & Cannon). In addition, improvements in serum lipids and other markers of the metabolic syndrome were improved in obese individuals treated with the drug. However, side effects included nausea and depression. As a result, this agent has not received FDA approval for use in the United States.

In general, determination of the safety and utility of drug agents based on appetite-regulating molecules will require more study. Obviously, lifestyle intervention—particularly physical activity promotion and monitoring of food portion sizes—are the most safe and practical approaches in children and adolescents.

SUMMARY

We have described portions of a large and complexly coordinated signal from the central energy storage depot of the body, the organs involved in food energy digestion and absorption, and the central nervous system. It should be noted that several other classes of signaling molecules, such as corticosteroids and cytokines, were deemed outside the scope of this chapter and were not discussed. This multifaceted signal ultimately arrives at the control center—i.e., the arcuate nucleus of the hypothalamus, cerebral cortex, and brain stem—for interpretation and subsequent regulation of energy balance. Much of this emerging science has yet to be established, and although it may seem like there is inconsistency among studies, the complexity of these signaling pathways cannot be understated. Many of the molecules comprising this signal share structural similarity and, in some cases, are coded for by the same gene, yet have different or conflicting functions. Furthermore, we have yet to understand many of the interactions amongst these signals, their relative importance, and the consequences of their deregulation. This understanding will lead to better treatment and prevention tactics, and help to ameliorate the growing burden of obesity and its related disorders.

REFERENCES

Ahima, R. S., Bjorbaek, C., Osei, S., & Flier, J. S. (1999). Regulation of neuronal and glial proteins by leptin: Implications for brain development. *Endocrinology, 140,* 2755–2762.

Air, E. L., Benoit, S. C., Blake Smith, K. A., Clegg, D. J., & Woods, S. C. (2002). Acute third ventricular administration of insulin decreases food intake in two paradigms. *Pharmacology Biochemistry and Behavior, 72,* 423–429.

Air, E. L., Strowski, M. Z., Benoit, S. C., Conarello, S. L., Salituro, G. M., Guan, X. M., et al. (2002). Small molecule insulin mimetics reduce food intake and body weight and prevent development of obesity. *Nature Medicine, 8*, 179–183.

Badman, M. K., & Flier, J. S. (2005). The gut and energy balance: Visceral allies in the obesity wars. *Science, 307*, 1909–1914.

Bannon, A. W., Seda, J., Carmouche, M., Francis, J. M., Norman, M. H., Karbon, B., et al. (2000). Behavioral characterization of neuropeptide y knockout mice. *Brain Research, 868*, 79–87.

Batterham, R. L., Cowley, M. A., Small, C. J., Herzog, H., Cohen, M. A., Dakin, C. L., et al. (2002). Gut hormone pyy(3–36) physiologically inhibits food intake. *Nature, 418*, 650–654.

Bouchard, C., Malina, R., & Perusse, L. (1997). *Genetics of fitness and physical performance*. Champaign, IL: Human Kinetics.

Bouchard, C., Tremblay, A., Despres, J. P., Nadeau, A., Lupien, P. J., Theriault, G., et al. (1990). The response to long-term overfeeding in identical twins. *New England Journal of Medicne, 322*, 1477–1482.

Challis, B. G., Pinnock, S. B., Coll, A. P., Carter, R. N., Dickson, S. L., & O'Rahilly, S. (2003). Acute effects of pyy3–36 on food intake and hypothalamic neuropeptide expression in the mouse. *Biochemical and Biophysical Research Communications, 311*, 915–919.

Christ, C. Y., Hunt, D., Hancock, J., Garcia-Macedo, R., Mandarino, L. J., & Ivy, J. L. (2002). Exercise training improves muscle insulin resistance but not insulin receptor signaling in obese zucker rats. *Journal of Applied Physiology, 92*, 736–744.

Cummings, D. E., Purnell, J. Q., Frayo, R. S., Schmidova, K., Wisse, B. E., & Weigle, D. S. (2001). A preprandial rise in plasma ghrelin levels suggests a role in meal initiation in humans. *Diabetes, 50*, 1714–1719.

Date, Y., Murakami, N., Toshinai, K., Matsukura, S., Niijima, A., Matsuo, H., et al. (2002). The role of the gastric afferent vagal nerve in ghrelin-induced feeding and growth hormone secretion in rats. *Gastroenterology, 123*, 1120–1128.

de Lecea, L., Kilduff, T. S., Peyron, C., Gao, X., Foye, P. E., Danielson, P. E., et al. (1998). The hypocretins: Hypothalamus-specific peptides with neuroexcitatory activity. *Proceedings of the National Academy of Sciences of the United States of America, 95*, 322–327.

Deriaz, O., Fournier, G., Tremblay, A., Despres, J. P., & Bouchard, C. (1992). Lean-body-mass composition and resting energy expenditure before and after long-term overfeeding. *American Journal of Clinical Nutrition, 56*, 840–847.

Di Marzo, V., Goparaju, S. K., Wang, L., Liu, J., Batkai, S., Jarai, Z., et al. (2001). Leptin-regulated endocannabinoids are involved in maintaining food intake. *Nature, 410*, 822–825.

Di Marzo, V., & Matias, I. (2005). Endocannabinoid control of food intake and energy balance. *Nature Neuroscience, 8*, 585–589.

Donahoo, W. T., Levine, J. A., & Melanson, E. L. (2004). Variability in energy expenditure and its components. *Current Opinion in Clinical Nutrition and Metabolic Care, 7*, 599–605.

Druce, M., & Bloom, S. R. (2006). The regulation of appetite. *Archives of Disease in Childhood, 91*, 183–187.

Dulloo, A. G. (2002). Biomedicine. A sympathetic defense against obesity. *Science, 297*, 780–781.

Ello-Martin, J. A., Ledikwe, J. H., & Rolls, B. J. (2005). The influence of food portion size and energy density on energy intake: Implications for weight management. *American Journal of Clinical Nutrition, 82*(Suppl. 1), 236S–241S.

Faulconbridge, L. F., Cummings, D. E., Kaplan, J. M., & Grill, H. J. (2003). Hyperphagic effects of brainstem ghrelin administration. *Diabetes, 52*, 2260–2265.

Franks, P. W., Ravussin, E., Hanson, R. L., Harper, I. T., Allison, D. B., Knowler, W. C., et al. (2005). Habitual physical activity in children: The role of genes and the environment. *American Journal of Clinical Nutrition, 82*, 901–908.

Gelfand, E. V., & Cannon, C. P. (2006a). Rimonabant: A cannabinoid receptor type 1 blocker for management of multiple cardiometabolic risk factors. *Journal of the American College of Cardiology, 47*, 1919–1926.

Gelfand, E. V., & Cannon, C. P. (2006b). Rimonabant: A selective blocker of the cannabinoid cb1 receptors for the management of obesity, smoking cessation and cardiometabolic risk factors. *Expert Opinion on Investigational Drugs, 15*, 307–315.

Gibbs, J., Fauser, D. J., Rowe, E. A., Rolls, B. J., Rolls, E. T., & Maddison, S. P. (1979). Bombesin suppresses feeding in rats. *Nature, 282*, 208–210.

Hayward, M. D., Pintar, J. E., & Low, M. J. (2002). Selective reward deficit in mice lacking beta-endorphin and enkephalin. *The Journal of Neuroscience, 22*, 8251–8258.

Hill, J. O., DiGirolamo, M., & Heymsfield, S. B. (1985). Thermic effect of food after ingested versus tube-delivered meals. *American Journal of Physiology, 248*(3 Pt 1), E370–E374.

Hotta, K., Funahashi, T., Bodkin, N. L., Ortmeyer, H. K., Arita, Y., Hansen, B. C., et al. (2001). Circulating concentrations of the adipocyte protein adiponectin are decreased in parallel with reduced insulin sensitivity during the progression to type 2 diabetes in rhesus monkeys. *Diabetes, 50*, 1126–1133.

Hu, E., Liang, P., & Spiegelman, B. M. (1996). Adipoq is a novel adipose-specific gene dysregulated in obesity. *The Journal of Biological Chemistry, 271*, 10697–10703.

Ikeda, H., West, D. B., Pustek, J. J., Figlewicz, D. P., Greenwood, M. R., Porte, D., Jr., et al. (1986). Intraventricular insulin reduces food intake and body weight of lean but not obese zucker rats. *Appetite, 7*, 381–386.

Jones, L. C., Bellingham, W. P., & Ward, L. C. (1990). Sex differences in voluntary locomotor activity of food-restricted and ad libitum-fed rats. Implications for the maintenance of a body weight set-point. *Comparative Biochemistry and Physiology, 96*, 287–290.

Kalra, S. P., Dube, M. G., Pu, S., Xu, B., Horvath, T. L., & Kalra, P. S. (1999). Interacting appetite-regulating pathways in the hypothalamic regulation of body weight. *Endocrine Reviews, 20*, 68–100.

Kalra, S. P., Dube, M. G., Sahu, A., Phelps, C. P., & Kalra, P. S. (1991). Neuropeptide y secretion increases in the paraventricular nucleus in association with increased appetite for food. *Proceedings of the National Academy of Sciences of the United States of America, 88*, 10931–10935.

Kemnitz, J. W., Weindruch, R., Roecker, E. B., Crawford, K., Kaufman, P. L., & Ershler, W. B. (1993). Dietary restriction of adult male rhesus monkeys: Design, methodology, and preliminary findings from the first year of study. *Journal of Gerontology, 48*, B17–B26.

Kissileff, H. R., Pi-Sunyer, F. X., Thornton, J., & Smith, G. P. (1981). C-terminal octapeptide of cholecystokinin decreases food intake in man. *American Journal of Clinical Nutrition, 34*, 154–160.

Koska, J., DelParigi, A., de Courten, B., Weyer, C., & Tataranni, P. A. (2004). Pancreatic polypeptide is involved in the regulation of body weight in pima Indian male subjects. *Diabetes, 53*, 3091–3096.

Kristensen, P., Judge, M. E., Thim, L., Ribel, U., Christjansen, K. N., Wulff, B. S., et al. (1998). Hypothalamic cart is a new anorectic peptide regulated by leptin. *Nature, 393*(6680), 72–76.

Kusminski, C. M., McTernan, P. G., & Kumar, S. (2005). Role of resistin in obesity, insulin resistance and type ii diabetes. *Clinical Science (Lond), 109*, 243–256.

Lanningham-Foster, L., Nysse, L. J., & Levine, J. A. (2003). Labor saved, calories lost: The energetic impact of domestic labor-saving devices. *Obesity Research, 11*, 1178–1181.

Lauderdale, D. S., Fabsitz, R., Meyer, J. M., Sholinsky, P., Ramakrishnan, V., & Goldberg, J. (1997). Familial determinants of moderate and intense physical activity: A twin study. *Medicine Science in Sports and Exercise, 29*, 1062–1068.

Levine, J. A. (2004). Nonexercise activity thermogenesis (neat): Environment and biology. *American Journal of Phyiology and Endocrinology and Metabolism, 286*, E675–E685.

Levine, J. A., Eberhardt, N. L., & Jensen, M. D. (1999). Role of nonexercise activity thermogenesis in resistance fat gain in humans. *Science, 283*, 212–214.

Levine, J. A., & Kotz, C. M. (2005). Neat - non-exercise activity thermogensis - egocentric & geocentric environmental factors vs. Biological regulation. *Acta Physiologica Scandinavica, 184*, 309–318.

Levine, J. A., Lanningham-Foster, L. M., McCrady, S. K., Krizan, A. C., Olson, L. R., Kane, P. H., et al. (2005). Interindividual variation in posture allocation: Possible role in human obesity. *Science, 307*(5709), 584–586.

Levine, J. A., Schleusner, S. J., & Jensen, M. D. (2000). Energy expenditure of non-exercise activity. *American Journal of Clinical Nutrition, 72,* 1451–1454.

Loftus, T. M., Jaworsky, D. E., Frehywot, G. L., Townsend, C. A., Ronnett, G. V., Lane, M. D., et al. (2000). Reduced food intake and body weight in mice treated with fatty acid synthase inhibitors. *Science, 288*(5475), 2379–2381.

Loos, R. J., Rankinen, T., Tremblay, A., Perusse, L., Chagnon, Y., & Bouchard, C. (2005). Melanocortin-4 receptor gene and physical activity in the quebec family study. *International Journal of Obesity (Lond), 29,* 420–428.

Lorentzon, M., Lorentzon, R., Lerner, U. H., & Nordstrom, P. (2001). Calcium sensing receptor gene polymorphism, circulating calcium concentrations and bone mineral density in healthy adolescent girls. *European Journal of Endocrinology, 144,* 257–261.

Mabry, P. D., & Campbell, B. A. (1975). Potentiation of amphetamine-induced arousal by food deprivation: Effect of hypothalamic lesions. *Physiology and Behavior, 14,* 85–88.

Maia, J. A., Thomis, M., & Beunen, G. (2002). Genetic factors in physical activity levels: A twin study. *American Journal of Preventive Medicine, 23*(Suppl. 2), 87–91.

Marks, J. L., Porte, D., Jr., Stahl, W. L., & Baskin, D. G. (1990). Localization of insulin receptor mrna in rat brain by in situ hybridization. *Endocrinology, 127,* 3234–3236.

McLaughlin, C. L., & Baile, C. A. (1981). Obese mice and the satiety effects of cholecystokinin, bombesin and pancreatic polypeptide. *Physiology and Behavior, 26,* 433–437.

Montague, C. T., Farooqi, I. S., Whitehead, J. P., Soos, M. A., Rau, H., Wareham, N. J., et al. (1997). Congenital leptin deficiency is associated with severe early-onset obesity in humans. *Nature, 387*(6636), 903–908.

Nakazato, M., Murakami, N., Date, Y., Kojima, M., Matsuo, H., Kangawa, K., et al. (2001). A role for ghrelin in the central regulation of feeding. *Nature, 409*(6817), 194–198.

Neary, N. M., Small, C. J., Wren, A. M., Lee, J. L., Druce, M. R., Palmieri, C., et al. (2004). Ghrelin increases energy intake in cancer patients with impaired appetite: Acute, randomized, placebo-controlled trial. *The Journal of Clinical Endocrinology and Metabolism, 89,* 2832–2836.

Novak, C. M., Kotz, C. M., & Levine, J. A. (2006). Central orexin sensitivity, physical activity, and obesity in diet-induced obese and diet-resistant rats. *American Journal of Physiology and Endocrinology and Metabolism, 290,* E396–E403.

Orlet Fisher, J., Rolls, B. J., & Birch, L. L. (2003). Children's bite size and intake of an entree are greater with large portions than with age-appropriate or self-selected portions. *American Journal of Clinical Nutrition, 77,* 1164–1170.

Perusse, L., Leblanc, C., & Bouchard, C. (1988). Familial resemblance in lifestyle components: Results from the canada fitness survey. *Canadian Journal of Public Health, 79,* 201–205.

Perusse, L., Tremblay, A., Leblanc, C., & Bouchard, C. (1989). Genetic and environmental influences on level of habitual physical activity and exercise participation. *American Journal of Epidemiology, 129,* 1012–1022.

Ravussin, E. (2005). Physiology. A neat way to control weight? *Science, 307*(5709), 530–531.

Robin, J. P., Boucontet, L., Chillet, P., & Groscolas, R. (1998). Behavioral changes in fasting emperor penguins: Evidence for a "refeeding signal" linked to a metabolic shift. *American Journal of Physiology, 274*(3 Pt 2), R746–R753.

Rolls, B. J., Engell, D., & Birch, L. L. (2000). Serving portion size influences 5-year-old but not 3-year-old children's food intakes. *Journal of the American Diatetic Association, 100,* 232–234.

Salmen, T., Heikkinen, A. M., Mahonen, A., Kroger, H., Komulainen, M., Pallonen, H., et al. (2003). Relation of aromatase gene polymorphism and hormone replacement therapy to serum estradiol levels, bone mineral density, and fracture risk in early postmenopausal women. *The Annals of Medicine, 35*, 282–288.

Schmidt, P. T., Naslund, E., Gryback, P., Jacobsson, H., Holst, J. J., Hilsted, L., et al. (2005). A role for pancreatic polypeptide in the regulation of gastric emptying and short-term metabolic control. *The Journal of Clinical Endocrinology and Metabolism, 90*, 5241–5246.

Schwartz, M. W., Sipols, A. J., Marks, J. L., Sanacora, G., White, J. D., Scheurink, A., et al. (1992). Inhibition of hypothalamic neuropeptide y gene expression by insulin. *Endocrinology, 130*, 3608–3616.

Simonen, R. L., Perusse, L., Rankinen, T., Rice, T., Rao, D. C., & Bouchard, C. (2002). Familial aggregation of physical activity levels in the quebec family study. *Medicine and Science in Sports and Exercise, 34*, 1137–1142.

Simonen, R. L., Rankinen, T., Perusse, L., Rice, T., Rao, D. C., Chagnon, Y., et al. (2003). Genome-wide linkage scan for physical activity levels in the quebec family study. *Medicine and Science in Sports and Exercise, 35*, 1355–1359.

Stanley, S., Wynne, K., McGowan, B., & Bloom, S. (2005). Hormonal regulation of food intake. *Physiological Reviews, 85*, 1131–1158.

Track, N. S., McLeod, R. S., & Mee, A. V. (1980). Human pancreatic polypeptide: Studies of fasting and postprandial plasma concentrations. *Canadian Journal of Physiology and Pharmacology, 58*, 1484–1489.

Tschop, M., Castaneda, T. R., Joost, H. G., Thone-Reineke, C., Ortmann, S., Klaus, S., et al. (2004). Physiology: Does gut hormone pyy3–36 decrease food intake in rodents? *Nature, 430*(6996),

Tschop, M., Smiley, D. L., & Heiman, M. L. (2000). Ghrelin induces adiposity in rodents. *Nature, 407*(6806), 908–913.

Turton, M. D., O'Shea, D., Gunn, I., Beak, S. A., Edwards, C. M., Meeran, K., et al. (1996). A role for glucagon-like peptide-1 in the central regulation of feeding. *Nature, 379*(6560), 69–72.

Verdich, C., Flint, A., Gutzwiller, J. P., Naslund, E., Beglinger, C., Hellstrom, P. M., et al. (2001). A meta-analysis of the effect of glucagon-like peptide-1 (7–36) amide on ad libitum energy intake in humans. *The Journal of Clinical Endocrinology and Metabolism, 86*, 4382–4389.

West, D. B., Fey, D., & Woods, S. C. (1984). Cholecystokinin persistently suppresses meal size but not food intake in free-feeding rats. *American Journal of Physiology, 246*(5 Pt 2), R776–R787.

Wilding, J. P. (2002). Neuropeptides and appetite control. *Diabetic Medicine, 19*, 619–627.

Winnicki, M., Accurso, V., Hoffmann, M., Pawlowski, R., Dorigatti, F., Santonastaso, M., et al. (2004). Physical activity and angiotensin-converting enzyme gene polymorphism in mild hypertensives. *American Journal of Medical Genetics, 125*, 38–44.

Woods, S. C., Decke, E., & Vasselli, J. R. (1974). Metabolic hormones and regulation of body weight. *Psychological Reviews, 81*, 26–43.

Woods, S. C., Lotter, E. C., McKay, L. D., & Porte, D., Jr. (1979). Chronic intracerebroventricular infusion of insulin reduces food intake and body weight of baboons. *Nature, 282*(5738), 503–505.

World Health Organization. (1997). *Obesity: Preventing and managing the global epidemic.* Geneva: WHO.

Wortley, K. E., Chang, G. Q., Davydova, Z., Fried, S. K., & Leibowitz, S. F. (2004). Cocaine- and amphetamine-regulated transcript in the arcuate nucleus stimulates lipid metabolism to control body fat accrual on a high-fat diet. *Regulatory Peptides, 117*, 89–99.

Yamada, K., Wada, E., Santo-Yamada, Y., & Wada, K. (2002). Bombesin and its family of peptides: Prospects for the treatment of obesity. *European Journal of Pharmacology, 440*(2–3), 281–290.

Young, L. R., & Nestle, M. (2002). The contribution of expanding portion sizes to the US obesity epidemic. *American Journal of Public Health, 92*, 246–249.

Zarjevski, N., Cusin, I., Vettor, R., Rohner-Jeanrenaud, F., & Jeanrenaud, B. (1993). Chronic intracerebroventricular neuropeptide-y administration to normal rats mimics hormonal and metabolic changes of obesity. *Endocrinology, 133*, 1753–1758.

Zhang, Y., Proenca, R., Maffei, M., Barone, M., Leopold, L., & Friedman, J. M. (1994). Positional cloning of the mouse obese gene and its human homologue. *Nature, 372*(6505), 425–432.

Zhang, J. V., Ren, P. G., Avsian-Kretchmer, O., Luo, C. W., Rauch, R., Klein, C., et al. (2005). Obestatin, a peptide encoded by the ghrelin gene, opposes ghrelin's effects on food intake. *Science, 310*(5750), 996–999.

9

Socioeconomic Factors Related to Obesity in Children and Adolescents

ELIZABETH GOODMAN

This chapter will explore socioeconomic risks for the development and persistence of overweight and obesity among children and adolescents. These factors are part of the social environment in which the developing child is immersed. In childhood and adolescence, health and development are inextricably linked. However, although the influence of the social environment on the developing child has been the subject of research for decades, research into the process by which the social world (and in particular its structuring) influences health is explored less well (Adler et al., 1994; Anderson & Armstead, 1995; Bradley & Corwyn, 2002; Williams, 1990). It is especially important to understand how social hierarchies influence children's health and well-being, because children do not have a voice in the political process that shapes their socioeconomic context.

Understanding socioeconomic risks for obesity is critical because so many children and adolescents live in lower socioeconomic environments. U.S. census data indicates that nearly one in six children under the age of 18 years live in poverty. Data from The National Longitudinal Study of Adolescent Health revealed that seven out of every 10 teens live in a home without a college-educated parent; for one in 10, no parent in the home completed high school or received a GED. Lower socioeconomic status represents a pervasive environmental exposure that may be, as Cassel said, "capable of changing human resistance in important ways and making

ELIZABETH GOODMAN • Floating Hospital for Children at Tufts-New England Medical Center and the Tufts University School of Medicine, Boston, MA 02111.

subsets of people more or less susceptible to these ubiquitous agents in our environment" (Cassel, 1976, p. 108). Thus, many young people are developing in a low social status environment that influences both their psychological and physiological functioning.

The prevalence of low socioeconomic status has a profound ability to influence obesity and related morbidity. Some argue that the distal, non-malleable nature of socioeconomic status, and the small effect sizes for socioeconomic status noted in regression analyses, negate its importance as an etiologic factor (Blum et al., 2000). This individualistic line of reasoning does not account for the population-level effects. Socioeconomic status is a root cause of morbidity and mortality that has been shown to continue to create health disparities even in the face of changing patterns of more proximal risk factors, such as diet and physical activity (Link & Phelan, 1995). A focus on such proximal risk factors belies the fundamental nature of the socioeconomic status – health relationship, and fails to incorporate the pervasive, multidimensional nature of the exposure.

Adolescent obesity is a particular focus of this chapter because adolescence may be a critical developmental period for the interaction of social, psychological, and physiologic risks—in particular obesity (De Spiegelaere, Dramaix, & Hennart, 1998). The dramatic increase in adolescent obesity over the past two decades suggests an urgent need to explore these processes among young people. In addition, adolescents are at a developmental stage where they are developing greater autonomy. This means that, while they are becoming more responsible for the obesity problem, they can also actively and independently be involved in the solution. Recent data from NHANES indicate that disparities in adolescent overweight are increasing among poor older adolescents, but not younger youth (Miech et al., 2006). The greater autonomy older adolescents exert over both their diets and levels of physical activity may explain these age-related trends, and suggests the need for developmentally appropriate interventions to reduce overweight disparities. Preventive and treatment interventions aimed at youth can have direct effects that are not dependent on parental behavioral change, as is often the case with preventive and interventions programs aimed at younger children. This is particularly important because recent work suggests that parental behaviors and functioning are not extremely important causes of the social status gradient in adolescent obesity (Mustillo et al., 2003). Adolescence is also a time of profound physiologic change. Puberty is the most obvious manifestation of these physiologic changes, but there are other less obvious changes, as well. For example, all adolescents experience a decrease in insulin sensitivity during puberty (Ball et al., 2006). There are neurotransmitter changes such as dopamine and serotonin that lead to alterations in the functioning of the limbic system, increasing stress responsivity and emotionality. Because lower socioeconomic status can be considered a chronic stressor, this suggests that physiologic pathways involved in weight regulation may be different in lower status youth (Goodman, Daniels, & Dolan, in press; Goodman, McEwen, Huang, Dolan, & Adler, 2005).

This chapter is organized in four sections. The first section gives an overview of the concept of socioeconomic status—defined both objectively and subjectively. The second section discusses the relationship between social status and obesity. The third section synthesizes the preceding sections and discusses how lower socioeconomic status creates risk for development and persistence of obesity. Although low socioeconomic status may create significant risk for obesity through physical environmental variables associated with low socioeconomic status environments—such as lack of access to safe walking routes and high density of fast food restaurants—these factors will be just briefly touched on throughout the chapter (see Chapter 10, the "Obesogenic Environment" for more details). A concluding section will be presented last.

THE CONCEPT OF SOCIAL STATUS

Dual trends of increasing income inequality and rising prevalence of overweight among children and adolescents have led to a greater focus on social inequalities in pediatric obesity. As noted in Chapter 1, obesity has been increasing in all age and ethnic groups and within both genders. Thirty-one percent of adolescents 12–19 years of age are now considered overweight, and 16 percent are considered obese (Hedley et al., 2004). In parallel to these increasing trends in pediatric overweight and obesity, there has been growth in income inequality in the United States. Despite economic prosperity, the gap between the rich and the poor in this country has widened. Since 1980, family income for those in the two upper-fifths of household incomes in the U.S. population has increased while family income for those in the lower three-fifths has, in fact, decreased (Auerbach, Krimgold, & Lefkowitz, 2000). The temporal association between increasing socioeconomic inequality and the rise in pediatric obesity suggests that these phenomena may be linked and highlights the need to understand the relationship between socioeconomic status and obesity for all age groups.

To understand the relationship between socioeconomic status and obesity, socioeconomic status itself must be understood. This concept, although familiar to all, is actually quite difficult to define and is often misused. In the United States, minority race/ethnicity is correlated with lower socioeconomic status, and race/ethnicity has been used as a proxy for socioeconomic status. These are vastly different concepts, however, and while they are both related to social disadvantage, race/ethnicity is not synonymous with socioeconomic status and should not be considered as a measure of socioeconomic status in clinical work or in research (Braveman et al., 2005). Socioeconomic status itself is a multifaceted, dense, and highly complex social construct. This section briefly reviews major theorists who developed the context for understanding social status, and describes the current conceptualization of socioeconomic status.

Objective Social Status

In 1927, Pitirim Sorokin defined social stratification as "the differentiation of a given population into hierarchically superposed classes. It is manifested in the very existence of upper and lower social layers. Its basis and very existence consist of unequal distribution of rights and privileges, duties and responsibilities, social values and privations, social power and influence among members of a society" (Sorokin, 1927, p. 11). Despite dramatic changes in industrialization and global societal development, this definition lays out many of the factors theorists associate with the concept of social position 80 years hence.

Karl Marx and Max Weber are the two of the most prominent theorists in this area. Their conceptualizations of social stratification have been widely applied in many disciplines ranging from history to sociology to public health and medicine. Marx saw social class as a fundamental characteristic that determined a person's complete existence from his cultural and community experiences, to his financial and environmental resources, to health-related behaviors (Johnson & Hall, 1995). For Marx, class was made up of distinct, bounded social groups that were categorical in nature (Vanneman & Pampel, 1968). In contrast, Weber's theories of a social status continuum, characterized by differential access to social resources and/or prestige, gave rise to the concept of socioeconomic status commonly used in the scientific literature (Nam & Powers, 1983).

Socioeconomic status, which is based in a Weberian tradition, is the predominant concept applied to the study of social status' impact on obesity. Socioeconomic status is a multidimensional construct that is most often measured by some combination of income, education, and occupation. In the past, these factors were conglomerated to derive indices of socioeconomic status, such as the Hollingshead index (Hollingshead, 1975). However, research suggests these factors act through differing pathways and may not be comparable across cultural and ethnic groups. Income can influence the ability to purchase expensive fresh fruits and vegetables, rather than cheaper, energy dense foods that have high palatability due to increased sugar and fat content (Drewnowski & Specter, 2004). Poor families who spend less on food may be drawn to such inexpensive, concentrated sources of energy, leading to poorer diet quality (Drewnowski & Specter). This economic pathway between socioeconomic status and obesity suggests that consumer food choices and the availability of energy-dense, low-cost, high-sugar and high-fat content foods partially mediate the relationship between low income and obesity. Income also influences neighborhood context, which varies in safety, availability of parks and recreational space, fast food developments, and extracurricular activities. Education may enable people to utilize knowledge and resources more efficiently and effectively to prevent or reduce obesity. Education may also be associated with beliefs and behaviors related to diet and physical activity, and may influence how individuals cope with the stress of living in a lower status environment. Occupation—such as shift work—may influence the ability of a parent to provide home-prepared meals. All of these interconnected factors—environmental, behavioral, physiological, and psychological—can influence obesity risk in children and youth and work through varying mechanisms. In addition, the different domains of socioeconomic status are not necessarily correlated. For example, shift work can be highly lucrative, and some occupations that require a high degree of education and training are not well-compensated. Therefore, current research recommendations include using these measures of social status separately—not as composite indices. The conceptualization of socioeconomic status is gaining in complexity, too. Wealth and assets are growing areas of interest. There has been increasing recognition of the importance of the intergenerational transfer of wealth to morbidity and mortality (Oliver & Shapiro, 1995). These new areas of inquiry reflect the burgeoning interest in capital, be that human capital (education), financial capital (wealth and assets), or social capital (social networks, reciprocity) (Coleman, 1990). Each of these types of capital influence social position, and may affect access to resources and their utilization, and ultimately health and well-being.

Subjective Social Status

The pathway from an objective social force to the creation of health differentials has been termed "the sociobiologic translation" (Tarlov, 1996). This process has also been termed "embodiment" (Krieger, 2001). One example of this process is the association between traditional measures of socioeconomic status and obesity (Figure 9.1). In this example, the objective social force of socioeconomic status measured by income, education, or occupation somehow gets *under the skin* to determine the creation of differential prevalence of obesity in lower socioeconomic status groups. Subjective social status is identified in Figure 9.1 as the mechanism partially mediating the sociobiologic translation between socioeconomic status and obesity. The concept of subjective social status grew from the recognition that, although the traditional variables used to measure socioeconomic status (income, education, and occupation) are only moderately correlated with each other, all are associated with health in a similar fashion. This suggests that all three individually reflect an underlying common component of social status. However, little is known about peoples' perceptions of their placement in the social hierarchy, or what determines these perceptions.

Early work on perceived social status relied on measures of social class identification and focused on political attitudes and behavior (Centers, 1949). Use of such class-based tools that rely on assessing class membership, rather than perceptions of stratification, had two major problems. The categorical nature of measures of social class identification did not adequately tap the full spectrum of socioeconomic stratification. In addition, the socially charged nature of the language used to describe the discrete classes may have affected how people responded to these measures. In 2001, Goodman et al. reported on the development of a youth-specific measure of the subjective social status that circumvented these problems (Goodman et al., 2001). Early work with this youth-specific measure indicated that there are developmental

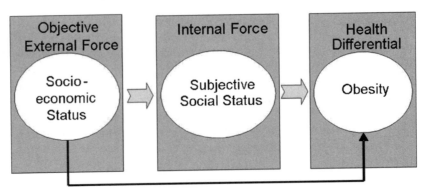

Figure 9.1. The sociobiologic translation.

trajectories in perceptions of social stratification that may influence obesity risk (Goodman et al.). In analyses that looked at mother-child dyads, the adolescents tended toward higher perceived social status compared to their mothers, and perceptions of subjective social status between mothers and their adolescent children were more strongly correlated among older teens.

These findings suggest a convergence of beliefs between parent and child as an adolescent matures, which may reflect a broader understanding of social positioning that accompanies the growth in cognitive ability and experience during the adolescent years. Changing conceptualization of social status may influence stress levels, health-related behaviors, and physiological process—all of which are relevant to childhood and adolescent obesity. Thus, it is important to consider both objective indicators of socioeconomic position, and subjective perceptions of socioeconomic status, to fully understand the relationship between social stratification and health.

RELATIONSHIPS BETWEEN SOCIAL STATUS AND OBESITY

The Influence of Socioeconomic Status on Obesity

Socioeconomic status gradients in obesity have been clearly demonstrated in adults, children, and adolescents (Ball & Crawford, 2005; Goodman, 1999; Gordon-Larsen, Adair, & Popkin, 2003; Greenlund et al., 1996; Kaplan & Keil, 1993; Pamuk, Makuc, Heck, Reuben, & Lochner, 1998; Sobal & Strunkard, 1989; Troiano & Flegal, 1998; Whitaker, Wright, Pepe, Seidel, & Dietz, 1997). Sobal & Strunkard's (1989) earlier review showed that a strong inverse relationship exists in developed societies between socioeconomic status and obesity among women, but no consistent relationship was found among men—although, more recent data suggests the socioeconomic status – obesity relationship is more complex (Ball &

Crawford). For nonblack adults (both men and women), there appears to be a consistent relationship between occupation and obesity. This relationship is less robust when education is used as the measure of socioeconomic status, and is quite inconsistent when income is assessed (Ball & Crawford). Among adolescents, the findings are mixed. In the National Health and Examination Survey (NHANES), socioeconomic status was a significant predictor of body mass index among adolescent girls but not boys, (Winkleby, Robinson, Sundquist, & Kraemer, 1999). However, Goodman found that obesity defined as BMI greater than or equal to the 95th percentile for age and gender was associated with lower household income and less parental education, after adjusting for gender and race/ethnicity using data from the National Longitudinal Study of Adolescent Health (Goodman). Other studies have found inconsistent associations between socioeconomic status and BMI in race/ethnicity-stratified analyses (Gordon-Larsen et al.; Kimm et al., 1996). Although the relationship between socioeconomic status and obesity in childhood and adolescence is inconsistent, the relationship appears strongest for nonHispanic white girls (Goodman et al., 2003; Gordon-Larsen et al.; Kimm et al.). Longitudinal studies have shown that as girls mature, the strong inverse relationship between socioeconomic status and obesity seen among adult women emerges (Braddon, Rodgers, Wadsworth, & Davies, 1986; Power, Lake, & Cole, 1997).

It is interesting to note that both Type 2 diabetes in adolescence, and the socioeconomic status gradient in obesity, show a female predominance. It may be that girls are more vulnerable to the detrimental effects of lower social status. This may reflect, for example, the stronger association of socioeconomic status with sedentary lifestyle for girls than for boys (Pamuk et al., 1998). It appears that boys from all socioeconomic status levels are active, but that low socioeconomic status girls may have relatively less access to resources that support exercise, or may be more restricted in their outside activities because of fears about safety than are boys of low socioeconomic status. This could explain both the female predominance of Type 2 diabetes in adolescence and the socioeconomic status gradient for female, but not male, obesity.

Many of the studies noted above show relatively modest effect sizes for socioeconomic status factors in regression models. Because they are weak, distal predictors of health, some investigators have concluded that the focus should be placed on more proximal risks, like diet and physical activity, and that socioeconomic factors should be discarded as useful mechanisms for understanding adolescent obesity. This perspective is based on studies that demonstrate the weak influence of socioeconomic status on the risk for obesity at the individual level. However, despite the weak-to-modest effects of socioeconomic status on obesity at the individual level, socioeconomic status has a broad and important influence on obesity across the population level. Population-attributable risk is a concept that determines the population-level, or public-health, impact of an exposure to an outcome by representing the proportion of cases of a disease that would be prevented if the risk factor or exposure were removed from the population (Levin, 1953).

Using population-attributable risks, Goodman, Slap, & Huang (2003) have shown that lower household income and parental education were each associated with approximately one-third of obesity in a nationally representative sample of youth. Parent education accounted for more of the proportion of adolescent obesity than household income. Why education should have a stronger effect than income is not clear. Education's effect may relate more to coping styles and other interpersonal skills, such as communication, while income's effect may be more strongly associated with material goods and services. When the focus was shifted from looking at the population-level effects across the entire socioeconomic status gradient to looking at the most vulnerable (the poor for income or those without a high school degree for education), the effects were also striking (Goodman, Slap, & Huang). Low household income accounts for 27.0 percent of obesity among teens from poor families. Low parent education accounts for 25.0 percent of obesity in teens from families where the highest level of parent education was high school or less. This suggests that policies that focus on eliminating poverty or ensuring a high school education for all can have important effects amongst the most vulnerable. However, the overall population-attributable risks decreased significantly in these analyses. The overall population-attributable risk for income—when it was defined as poor versus nonpoor—was 4.8 percent. Likewise, the overall population-attributable risk for parent education, when education was defined as *lack of a high school diploma* versus *high school diploma or better* was 3.2 percent. These differences suggest that, for the population as a whole, antipoverty policies will not change the adverse effects of socioeconomic status for most individuals in the population. Realistic policy options that could apply throughout the socioeconomic status spectrum are likely to have a broader effect.

Subjective Social Status and Obesity

Subjective social status has been associated with obesity among both adults and adolescents. Adler, Epel, Castellazzo, and Ickovics (2000) showed that higher society ladder rank was associated with lower waist/hip ratio. Subjective social status has been used in two separate cohort studies among adolescents with similar findings. In a largely nonHispanic white, advantaged cohort, lower subjective social status was associated with greater risk for obesity (Goodman et al., 2001). Similar findings emerged when subjective social status was assessed in a racially and socioeconomically diverse cohort of nonHispanic black and white students from the Princeton School District (PSD) Study (Goodman et al., 2003). This study indicated that subjective social status in the more immediate, local setting of the school community has a stronger impact on obesity than societal subjective social status, which was not associated with obesity here. Race and gender were important effect moderators. School subjective social status was significantly associated with obesity in all groups but black girls. The association was strongest among white girls, and intermediate for white and black boys.

When the data regarding the associations of obesity to both socioeconomic status and subjective social status are looked at as a whole, an interesting pattern becomes apparent. Despite the fact that black girls demonstrate the lowest subjective social status, have low socioeconomic status, and have the highest BMI and highest prevalence of overweight, they are the only group for whom no measure of social status appears related to obesity. In contrast, the associations between social status indicators and obesity were strongest for white girls. Cultural norms regarding weight and perceptions of beauty may help explain these differences. Evidence suggests that young black women see obesity as less stigmatizing than similar-aged white peers, or young men of either racial group (Latner, Stunkard, & Wilson, 2005).

It should also be noted that the race-based differences in the social status-obesity relationships seen among girls are not present among adolescent boys (Goodman et al., 2003). Because the socioeconomic status – obesity association has been inconsistent or nonexistent for black girls, some have postulated that genetic factors may underlie racial disparities in obesity prevalence (Gordon-Larsen et al., 2003; Kimm et al., 1996). The lack of effect among boys of either race/ethnicity in the PSD Study data argues against racial distribution of genetic susceptibility as the cause of socioeconomic status gradient in obesity, and points to social and cultural factors as the driving forcers behind disparities in obesity among young people.

The fact that subjective socioeconomic status was not associated with obesity in a more diverse cohort of youth—and that the associations of parent education and household income to obesity were weaker than that of school subjective social status—are also intriguing. For a teenager, understanding one's place in the social structure within school is likely to be easier and more apparent than one's place in society at large. Adolescents spend a great deal of their time in school and school-related activities, and their worldview is largely framed by their school experience. The presence of vending machines in schools where foods of minimum nutritional value can be easily obtained, and the decreases in physical activity during the school day due to lack of physical education classes may influence obesity risk, although it is not known if these risks are differentially distributed by socioeconomic status.

PATHWAYS BETWEEN SOCIOECONOMIC FACTORS AND OBESITY

The conceptual complexity of socioeconomic status makes the development of specific hypotheses regarding the pathways through which each domain of socioeconomic status influences obesity risk critically important for researchers (Kaplan & Keil, 1993; Libratos, Link, & Kelsey, 1988; Susser, Watson, & Hopper, 1985). Such hypotheses are also important for the clinician to consider, because discussion of risks and potential interventions need to be geared to the specific circumstances of the family and child involved. If both parents are shift workers, and there is little mealtime supervision, discussion about meal planning would be paramount, because it is unlikely that parents will be able to alter their job schedules.

However, if family dinners occur nightly, portion size or nutritional evaluation might be the most effective avenue for discussion. In high violence neighborhoods, strategies to decrease stress and find safe outlets for physical activity may be the most cogent. Given the multidimensional nature of the concept, flexibility in understanding and defining the nature of the risks is key to decreasing social inequalities in childhood and adolescent obesity.

The complexity of the interrelationships between objective and subjective measures of social position and weight status suggest multiple pathways for the development of social inequalities in obesity (Goodman et al., 2003). Three prominent school sof thought in the United States endeavor to explain the pathways through which social status influences health—the materialist/neomaterialist school, the psychosocial-social comparisons school, and the fundamental cause theorists. Materialists believe that social status indicators serve as markers for material advantage over the life course, and that these advantages in education, income occupation, and wealth have direct influence on health and well-being (Raphael, 2003). Material disadvantage leads to experiences with fewer health-enhancing environments and more exposure to health-threatening environments. Deprivation also leads to the development of more health-risk behaviors. Material deprivation may lead children and adolescents to live in neighborhoods with greater availability of energy-dense foods and lower availability of playgrounds and parks for recreation. Eating can be used to self-medicate and sooth the harsh realities of the young person's current environment. In the United Kingdom, greater area deprivation has been associated with an increased likelihood of obesity in children (Kinra, Nelder, & Lewendon, 2000). The neomaterialist interpretation is similar to the materialist theory, but emphasizes how resources are allocated within a society (Kaplan, Pamuk, Lynch, Cohen, & Balfour, 1996). Such a view suggests that higher socioeconomic status individuals are less likely to be overweight or obese because they have greater access to tangible resources such as the healthy foods, services, and amenities that promote development and maintenance of a healthy weight (Lynch & Kaplan, 2000).

Complementary to both the materialist and neomaterialist explanations, the psychosocial interpretation contends that stress caused by being lower in the social hierarchy also has both direct and indirect effects on health. Wilkinson (1999) points to evidence that, as social status hierarchies within societies deepen, the quality of the social relations within the country lessen. He argues that social cohesion—a by-product of strong social relations—is beneficial to health and is eroded when social relations are weakened by a deeply hierarchical society. In Wilkinson's model, social comparisons create evaluative responses that can lead to a sense of relative deprivation, and hence, social anxiety, shame, and depression. These, in turn, influence emotional health as well as physiologic well-being. With respect to obesity, depression (more common in lower SES groups) has been shown to predict development of obesity in children and adolescents (Anderson, Cohen, Naumova, & Must, 2006; Goodman & Whitaker, 2002). Population-level studies of adolescent obesity also support Wilkinson's theory of the causal relationship between inequality obesity (Goodman et al., 2003).

The highest population-attributable risks for socioeconomic factors are demonstrated in race by gender group strata, with the steepest socioeconomic status gradients. Conversely, the lowest population-attributable risks are in strata where no graded relationship was present.

Link and Phelan (1995) argue that lower social status is a fundamental, root cause of health inequalities because increased status brings with it better resources, such as knowledge, money, power, prestige, and beneficial social connections; and that such resources are used to reduce risk regardless of the specific diseases and risk factors that are relevant at any given time. Thus, to effect long-range changes in obesity prevalence, they argue that the focus needs to be on the distal societal factors, not just proximal risks such as specific behaviors like diet and physical activity or healthcare.

Although these differing schools of thought have been portrayed as competing explanations for underlying health inequalities, they are not mutually exclusive and it is difficult to disentangle their effects. For example, lower socioeconomic status could increase risk for obesity, and obesity, in turn, could lead to lower subjective perceptions of subjective social status within the school context. This is a social causation model, which suggests that obesity mediates the association between socioeconomic status and subjective social status, and is most consistent with Wilkinson's psychosocial theory. Although studies of discrimination and stigmatization of obese children in schools have not linked the development of obesity to lower socioeconomic status, a number of studies have documented harassment and discrimination of obese children by schoolmates (Puhl, & Brownell, 2001).

It is also possible that the roles of obesity and subjective social status could be reversed—lower socioeconomic status might lead to lower perceptions of status, which in turn create a stressful psychological environment and increased stress responses in the limbic system (Goodman et al., 2003). Such stressors could affect weight regulation and energy balance through activation of such regulatory pathways as the HPA axis, autonomic nervous system, and the immune system, to name a few (Chrousos, 2000; McEwen, 1998a). In this model, subjective social status mediates the association of socioeconomic status and obesity and provides an avenue through which the external environment becomes internalized.

A third possible pathway is one in which obesity itself influences objective socioeconomic status, because negative social and economic consequences in adulthood have been shown to be related to overweight in adolescence (Gortmaker, Must, Perrin, Sobol, & Dietz, 1993). This model suggests social drift, rather than social causation, is the etiologic mechanism underlying social inequalities in obesity. The social selection process is less relevant to childhood and adolescent obesity, because it is unlikely that a child's weight would influence familial socioeconomic position. Williams (2003, p. 743) noted that the debate pitting social causation theorists against social selection proponents was obscuring the key issue— understanding the "causal chain leading from low socioeconomic status to death and disease" to develop more effective preventive and treatment interventions.

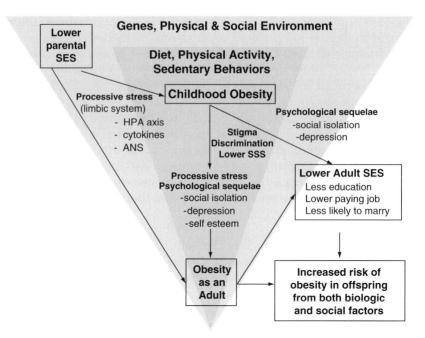

Figure 9.2. Intergenerational transfer of socioeconomic inequalities in obesity.

As an individual progresses through the lifecourse, this third pathway becomes possible—as do the likelihood that these pathways may intersect. When placed in the context of an individual's genetic makeup, and their physical and social environment, these pathways together create the convoluted set of experiences that can lead to an intergenerational transfer of social inequalities in health. Figure 9.2 outlines an example focusing on obesity. Lower parental education can, in addition to effects mediated through diet and physical activity/inactivity, create a environment that the brain processes as stressful. This leads to chronic and/or repeated activation of the HPA axis and autonomic nervous system, as well as cytokine release such as IL-6. These, in turn, influence weight regulation and cause development of obesity in childhood and adolescence. Childhood obesity has psychological sequelae that can influence educational attainment, occupation, wages, and household income, leading to lower socioeconomic status in adulthood. Childhood obesity also increases the likelihood of adult obesity, which can influence these same factors, leading to lower adult socioeconomic status. Lower adult socioeconomic status then restarts the cycle for the next generation.

Stress responses related to corticotrophin-releasing hormone (CRH) secretion in the central nucleus of the amygdala and the hippocampus are one mechanism for how social status can cause HPA axis dysfunction (see Schulkin, Gold, & McEwen, 1998 for review). The hippocampus, which has high levels of steroid receptors, is very important for declarative and contextual memory. The hippocampus can repeatedly process the common stressors found in a lower status environment as stressful, leading to repeated CRH release and HPA axis activation. Hypothalamic CRH neurons in the bed nucleus of the stria terminalis, responsible for the termination of the HPA stress response, are also inhibited by the hippocampus, which can engender chronic activation (Herman & Cullinan, 1997). In addition, long-term stress and persistence of hippocampal release of excitatory amino acids after stress has been shown to cause neuronal loss (Lowy, Wittenberg, & Yamamoto, 1995). This may lead to hippocampal dysfunction that enhances the heightened stress responses through more frequent appraisal of situations as stressful and through failure to terminate the stress response. CRH causes HPA axis stimulation, which, in turn, increases a number of neurohormonal mediators, including cortisol and insulin. The alterations in these hormones then cause secondary effects, such as hyperglycemia, hypertension, central obesity, and dyslipidemia, which promote development and progression of disease, including cardiovascular disease. This chain of events, and the multi-system deregulation and development of disease that follows, has been termed "allostatic load" (McEwen, 1998b).

This framework links the external social, political, historical, and physical environments that socially disadvantaged youth grow up in to the internal processes that allow an individual to adapt to that external reality, and is consistent with Halfon and Hochstein's (2002) life course health development model. The framework suggests that adolescents' experience of social disadvantage affects how their bodies adapt to environmental stressors such as lower social status. The notion of individual differences in the internal experience of the outside world is key to understanding how disparities develop. Differences in the brain's processing of an environment creates variation in how individuals respond to similar, or even shared, environments, which in turn leads to differing levels of physiological and psychological adaptation. This may explain why obesity can be differentially distributed among children and adolescents within a family or other shared environment. If a child perceives the environment as harsh and challenging, increased adaptation is required, which creates cumulative wear and tear of central regulatory processes—some of which may eventually lead to obesity. Data on the relationship between parent education and insulin resistance, which is closely associated with obesity, exemplifies this chain of events. Lower parent education increases the likelihood of obesity and insulin resistance (Goodman et al., 2005), and leads to worsening insulin resistance, especially among obese youth (Goodman et al., 2007).

CONCLUSION

Although the United States is a democracy, the structure of our society is a hierarchical one. Stratification is part of the American experience and the culture in which our children develop. This stratification has health effects that influence pediatric overweight and obesity. The direct link between social structure and health has not been the dominant lens through which obesity disparities among children and adolescents have been approached. Rather, policies, practices, and much research have focused on the need for individual behavioral change or the provision of better healthcare. Children and youth are told to eat better and exercise more. Yet, at the same time, physical education programs are being cut from schools, fast food and foods of minimum nutritional value have invaded school cafeterias, the availability of healthy choices has decreased in disadvantaged neighborhoods, food marketing to young children has increased, portion sizes have sky-rocketed, and opportunities for children to play safely and even walk to school have diminished. These factors may be differentially distributed by socioeconomic status, although there is a marked dearth of literature addressing these influences. In addition, while it is acknowledged by many that growing up today is more *stressful* than it was in the past, and growing up in a socially disadvantaged home is clearly more stressful than growing up surrounded by social advantage, how stress affects the body—including development and persistence of overweight—is often ignored. Socioeconomic factors have a profound influence on pediatric overweight through environmental, psychological, physiological, and behavioral paths. Until all the pathways by which this broader social context influences obesity risk are taken into account in policy and program-planning, and in the provision of healthcare, disparities will continue to accrue and the *epidemic* of childhood obesity is likely to go on unabated.

REFERENCES

Adler, N. E., Boyce, T., Chesney, M. A., Cohen, S., Folkman, S., Kahn, R. L., et al. (1994). Socioeconomic status and health: The challenge of the gradient. *American Psychologist, 49*, 15–24.

Adler, N. E., Epel, E. S., Castellazzo, G., & Ickovics, J. R. (2000). Relationship of subjective and objective social status with psychological and physiological functioning: preliminary data in healthy white women. *Health Psychology, 19*, 586–592.

Anderson, N. B., & Armstead, C. A. (1995). Toward understanding the association of socioeconomic status and health: A new challenge for the biopsychosocial approach. *Psychosomatic Medicine, 57*, 213–225.

Anderson, S. E., Cohen, P., Naumova, E. N., & Must, A. (2006). Association of depression and anxiety disorders with weight change in a prospective community-based study of children followed up into adulthood. *Archives of Pediatric and Adolescent Medicine, 160*, 285–291.

Auerbach, J., Krimgold, B., & Lefkowitz, B. (2000). *Improving Health; It Doesn't Take A Revolution* (No. 298). Washington, DC: National Policy Association.

Ball, K., & Crawford, D. (2005). Socioeconomic status and weight change in adults: A review. *Social Science & Medicine, 60*, 1987–2010.

Ball, G. D. C., Huang, T. T. K., Gower, B. A., Cruz, M. L., Shaibi, G. Q., Weigensberg, M. J., et al. (2006). Longitudinal changes in insulin sensitivity, insulin secretion, and [beta]-cell function during puberty. *The Journal of Pediatrics, 148*, 16.

Blum, R. W., Beuhring, T., Shew, M. L., Bearinger, L. H., Sieving, R. E., & Resnick, M. D. (2000). The effects of race/ethnicity, income, and family structure on adolescent risk behaviors. *American Journal of Public Health, 90*, 1879–1884.

Braddon, F. E., Rodgers, B., Wadsworth, M. E., & Davies, J. M. (1986). Onset of obesity in a 36 year birth cohort study. *British Medical Journal Clinical Research Education, 293*, 299–303.

Bradley, R. H., & Corwyn, R. F. (2002). Socioeconomic status and child development. *Annual Review of Psychology, 53*, 371–399.

Braveman, P. A., Cubbin, C., Egerter, S., Chideya, S., Marchi, K. S., Metzler, M., et al. (2005). Socioeconomic status in health research: One size does not fit all. *Journal of the American Medical Association, 294*, 2879–2888.

Cassel, J. (1976). The contribution of the social environment to host resistance: The fourth Wade Hampton Frost lecture. *American Journal of Epidemiology, 104*, 107–123.

Centers, R. (1949). *The Psychology of Social Classes: A Study of Class Consciousness.* Princeton: Princeton University Press.

Chrousos, G. P. (2000). The role of stress and the hypothalamic-pituitary-adrenal axis in the pathogenesis of the metabolic syndrome: Neuro-endocrine and target tissue-related causes. *International Journal of Obesity Related Metabolic Disorders, 24*, S50–55.

Coleman, J. S. (1990). *Foundations of Social Theory.* Cambridge, MA: Belknap Press.

De Spiegelaere, M., Dramaix, M., & Hennart, P. (1998). The influence of socioeconomic status on the incidence and evolution of obesity during early adolescence. *International Journal of Obesity Related Metabolic Disorders, 22*, 268–274.

Drewnowski, A., & Specter, S. (2004). Poverty and obesity: The role of energy density and energy costs. *American Journal of Clinical Nutrition, 79*, 6–16.

Goodman, E. (1999). The role of socioeconomic status gradients in explaining differences in U.S. adolescents' health. *American Journal of Public Health, 89*, 1522–1528.

Goodman, E., Adler, N. E., Daniels, S. R., Morrison, J. A., Slap, G. B., & Dolan, L. M. (2003). Impact of objective and subjective social status on obesity in a biracial cohort of adolescents. *Obesity Research, 11*, 1018–1026.

Goodman, E., Adler, N. E., Kawachi, I., Frazier, A. L., Huang, B., & Colditz, G. A. (2001). Adolescents' perceptions of social status: Development and evaluation of a new indicator. *Pediatrics, 108*, e31.

Goodman, E., Daniels, S. R., & Dolan, L. M. (2007). Socioeconomic disparities in insulin resistance: Results from the Princeton school district study. *Psychosomatic Medicine, 69*, 61–67.

Goodman, E., McEwen, B. S., Huang, B., Dolan, L. M., & Adler, N. E. (2005). Social inequalities in biomarkers of cardiovascular risk in adolescence. *Psychosomatic Medicine, 67*, 9–15.

Goodman, E., Slap, G. B., & Huang, B. (2003). The public health impact of socioeconomic status on adolescent depression and obesity. *American Journal of Public Health, 93*, 1844–1850.

Goodman, E., & Whitaker, R. C. (2002). A prospective study of the role of depression in the development and persistence of adolescent obesity. *Pediatrics, 110*, 497–504.

Gordon-Larsen, P., Adair, L. S., & Popkin, B. M. (2003). The relationship of ethnicity, socioeconomic factors, and overweight in U.S. adolescents. *Obesity Research, 11*, 121–129.

Gortmaker, S. L., Must, A., Perrin, J. M., Sobol, A. M., & Dietz, W. H. (1993). Social and economic consequences of overweight in adolescence and young adulthood. *New England Journal of Medicine, 329*, 1008–1012.

Greenlund, K. J., Liu, K., Dyer, A. R., Kiefe, C. I., Burke, G. L., & Yunis, C. (1996). Body mass index in young adults: Associations with parental body size and education in the CARDIA Study. *American Journal of Public Health, 86*, 480–485.

Halfon, N., & Hochstein, M. (2002). Life course health development: An integrated framework for developing health, policy, and research. *Milbank Quarterly, 80*, 433–479.

Hedley, A. A., Ogden, C. L., Johnson, C. L., Carroll, M. D., Curtin, L. R., & Flegal, K. M. (2004). Prevalence of overweight and obesity among U.S. children, adolescents, and adults, 1999–2002. *Journal of the American Medical Association, 291*, 2847–2850.

Herman, J. P., & Cullinan, W. E. (1997). Neurocircuitry of stress: Central control of the hypothalamo-pituitary-adrenocortical axis. *Trends in Neurosciences, 20*, 78–84.

Hollingshead, A. B. (1975). *Four Factor Index of Social Status* (Working Paper, Dept of Sociology). New Haven: Yale University Press.

Johnson, J. V., & Hall, E. M. (1995). Class, Work, and Health. In B. J. Amick, S. Levine, A. R. Tarlov, & D. C. Walsh (Eds.), *Society and Health* (pp. 247–271). New York: Oxford University Press.

Kaplan, G. A., & Keil, J. E. (1993). Socioeconomic factors and cardiovascular disease: A review of the literature. *Circulation, 88*, 1973–1988.

Kaplan, G. A., Pamuk, E. R., Lynch, J. W., Cohen, R. D., & Balfour, J. L. (1996). Inequality in income and mortality in the United States: Analysis of mortality and potential pathways [published erratum appears in BMJ 1996 May 18;312(7041):1253]. *British Medical Journal, 312*, 999–1003.

Kimm, S. Y., Obarzanek, E., Barton, B. A., Aston, C. E., Similo, S. L., Morrison, J. A., et al. (1996). Race, socioeconomic status, and obesity in 9- to 10-year-old girls: The NHLBI Growth and Health Study. *Annals of Epidemiology, 6*, 266–275.

Kinra, S., Nelder, R. P., & Lewendon, G. J. (2000). Deprivation and childhood obesity: A cross sectional study of 20,973 children in Plymouth, United Kingdom. *Journal of Epidemiology and Community Health, 54*, 456–460.

Krieger, N. (2001). Theories for social epidemiology in the 21st century: An ecosocial perspective. *International Journal of Epidemiology, 30*, 668–677.

Latner, J. D., Stunkard, A. J., & Wilson, G. T. (2005). Stigmatized students: Age, sex, and ethnicity effects in the stigmatization of obesity. *Obesity Research, 13*, 1226–1231.

Levin, M. (1953). The occurrence of lung cancer in man. *Acta Unio Internationalis Contra Cancrum, 9*, 531–541.

Libratos, P., Link, B. G., & Kelsey, J. L. (1988). The measurement of social class in epidemiology. *Epidemiologic Reviews, 10*, 87–121.

Link, B. G., & Phelan, J. (1995). Social conditions as fundamental causes of disease. *Journal of Health and Social Behavior*, Spec: 80–94.

Lowy, M. T., Wittenberg, L., & Yamamoto, B. K. (1995). Effect of acute stress on hippocampal glutamate levels and spectrin proteolysis in young and aged rats. *Journal of Neurochemistry, 65*, 268–274.

Lynch, J., & Kaplan, G. A. (2000). Socioeconomic Position. In L. Berkman & I. Kawachi (Eds.), *Social Epidemiology*. New York: Oxford University Press.

McEwen, B. S. (1998a). Protective and damaging effects of stress mediators. *New England Journal of Medicine, 338*, 171–179.

McEwen, B. S. (1998b). Stress, adaptation, and disease: Allostasis and allostatic load. *Annals of the New York Academy of Sciences, 840*, 33–44.

Miech, R. A., Kumanyika, S. K., Stettler, N., Link, B. G., Phelan, J. C., & Chang, V. W. (2006). Trends in the association of poverty with overweight among U.S. adolescents, 1971–2004. *Journal of the American Medical Association, 295*, 2385–2393.

Mustillo, S., Worthman, C., Erkanli, A., Keeler, G., Angold, A., & Costello, E. J. (2003). Obesity and psychiatric disorder: Developmental trajectories. *Pediatrics, 111*, 851–859.

Nam, C. B., & Powers, M. G. (1983). *The Socioeconomic Approach to Status Measurement with a Guide to Occupational and Socioeconomic Status Scores*. Houston: Cap and Gown Press.

Oliver, M. L., & Shapiro, T. M. (1995). *Black Wealth/White Wealth: A New Perspective on Racial Inequality*. New York: Routledge.

Pamuk, E., Makuc, D., Heck, K., Reuben, C., & Lochner, K. (1998). *Health, United States, 1998 with Socioeconomic Status and Health Chartbook* (No. DHHS Publication # (PHS) 98-1232). Hyattsville, Maryland: U.S. Department of Health and Human Services, Centers for Disease Control and Prevention, National Center for Health Statistics.

Power, C., Lake, J. K., & Cole, T. J. (1997). Body mass index and height from childhood to adulthood in the 1958 British born cohort. *American Journal of Clinical Nutrition, 66*, 1094–1101.

Puhl, R., & Brownell, K. D. (2001). Bias, discrimination, and obesity. *Obesity Research, 9*, 788–805.

Raphael, D. (2003). A society in decline. In R. Hofrichter (Ed.), *Health and Social Justice: Politics, Ideology, and Inequality in the Distribution of Disease* (pp. 59–88). San Francisco: Jossey-Bass.

Schulkin, J., Gold, P. W., & McEwen, B. S. (1998). Induction of corticotropin-releasing hormone gene expression by glucocorticoids: implication for understanding the states of fear and anxiety and allostatic load. *Psychoneuroendocrinology, 23*, 219–243.

Sobal, J., & Strunkard, A. J. (1989). Socioeconomic status and obesity: A review of the literature. *Psychological Bulletin, 105*, 260–275.

Sorokin, P. (1927). *Social Mobility*. New York: Harper.

Susser, M., Watson, W., & Hopper, K. (1985). *Sociology in Medicine* (3rd ed.). New York: Oxford University Press.

Tarlov, A. R. (1996). Social determinants of health: The sociobiological translation. In D. Blaine, E. J. Brunner, & R. G. Wilkinson (Eds.), *Health and Social Organizations* (pp. 71–93). London: Routledge Publications.

Troiano, R. P., & Flegal, K. M. (1998). Overweight children and adolescents: Description, epidemiology, and demographics. *Pediatrics, 101*, 497–504.

Vanneman, R., & Pampel, F. (1968). The American perception of social class and status. *American Sociological Review, 42*, 422–437.

Whitaker, R. C., Wright, J. A., Pepe, M. S., Seidel, K. D., & Dietz, W. H. (1997). Predicting obesity in young adulthood from childhood and parental obesity. *New England Journal of Medicine, 337*, 869–873.

Wilkinson, R. G. (1999). Health, hierarchy, and social anxiety. *Annals of the New York Academy of Sciences, 896*, 48–63.

Williams, D. R. (1990). Socioeconomic differentials in health: A review and a redirection. *Social Psychology Quarterly, 53*, 81–99.

Williams, R. B. (2003). Invited commentary: Socioeconomic status, hostility, and health behaviors - Does it matter which comes first? *American Journal of Epidemiology, 158*, 743–746.

Winkleby, M. A., Robinson, T. N., Sundquist, J., & Kraemer, H. C. (1999). Ethnic variation in cardiovascular disease risk factors among children and young adults: Findings from the Third National Health and Nutrition Examination Survey, 1988–1994. *Journal of the American Medical Association, 281*, 1006–1013.

10

The Obesogenic Environment

AMY A. GORIN and MELISSA M. CRANE

The rates of childhood obesity continue to rise, with poor dietary habits and sedentary lifestyles as the most proximal causes. Historically, researchers have focused on individual-level variables such as health-related know-ledge, motivation, and self-efficacy to understand eating, exercise, and obesity. This approach is limited in that internal psychological characteristics are often poor predictors of weight-regulating behaviors (Strauss, Rodzilsky, Burack, & Colin, 2001; Timperio et al. 2006) and behavioral weight loss treatment focused on the obese patient alone has struggled to produce long-term weight control (Epstein, Myers, Raynor, & Saelens, 1998). Moreover, this individual-level approach fails to address how the numerous societal trends observed over the past 30 years—such as the proliferation of fast food restaurants and increased access to television—influence the weight of children. Researchers have recently begun to approach obesity from an ecological perspective, revealing several environmental correlations between unhealthy eating, sedentary lifestyles, and obesity (French, Story, & Jeffery, 2001; Hill & Peters, 1998; Nestle & Jacobson, 2000), leading many to conclude that for obesity, "genetics loads the gun, [but] the environment pulls the trigger" (Bray, 1996).

AN ECOLOGICAL MODEL OF OBESITY

American society has been described as a *toxic environment* that promotes passive overeating and inactivity (Brownell & Horgen, 2003). In fact, a dose-response relationship between exposure to U.S. culture and risk

AMY A. GORIN • University of Connecticut, Storrs, CT 06269.
MELISSA M. CRANE • The Miriam Hospital, Providence, RI 02903.

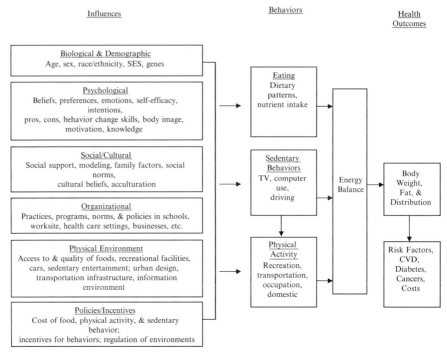

Developed for the NHLBI Workshop on Predictors of Obesity, Weight Gain, Diet, and Physical Activity; August 4-5, 2004, Bethesda MD

Figure 10.1. An ecological model of diet, physical activity, and obesity.

for obesity has been reported. Kaplan, Huguet, Newsom, & McFarland, (2004) found that Hispanic immigrants living in the United States for more than 15 years had a four-fold higher risk of obesity than immigrants living in the United States for less than five years, and that U.S.-born Hispanic individuals had the highest rates of obesity. To understand how the environment impacts body weight, an ecological model of obesity has been proposed (see Figure 10.1). This framework identifies several micro- and macrolevels of influence on weight regulation, including social and cultural factors (e.g., acculturation), organizational structures (e.g., school programs), the physical environment (e.g., proximity of restaurants), and larger policies and incentives (e.g., food pricing). Starting with the home and moving outward to schools, neighborhoods, and beyond, this chapter reviews some of the key environmental factors contributing to the increase in childhood obesity rates and describes some initial attempts to prevent and treat obesity from an ecological—rather than an individual—perspective.

HOME ENVIRONMENT

The home environment is the behavioral setting for many eating and exercise choices and can certainly be obesogenic. Parents and children tend to be similar in their weight status (Lake, Power, & Cole, 1997; Whitaker, Deeks, Baughcum, & Specker, 2000) and in dietary and physical activity habits (Freedman & Evenson, 1991; Salmon, Timperio, Telford, Carver, & Crawford, 2005), likely reflecting both genetic and environmental vulnerabilities to obesity. The weights of marital partners are also correlated, with some evidence that these weights change in a similar fashion over time (Jeffery & Rick, 2002; Katzmarzyk, Perusse, Rao, & Bouchard, 1999), underscoring the influence that the shared home environment can have on obesity. Household factors associated with eating and exercise behaviors include food availability, access to exercise equipment and televisions, and the level of cognitive stimulation in the home.

Food in the Home: Availability, Portion Sizes, and Presentation

By an early age, children's eating habits are influenced by their surrounding environments. Children tend to eat the foods that are available in amounts proportional to what they are served (Patrick & Nicklas, 2005). For example, having fruits and vegetables available in the home is associated with increased consumption of these foods in adolescents (Befort et al. 2006; Hanson, Neumark-Sztainer, Eisenberg, Story, & Wall, 2005). In a study of almost 4,000 adolescents, availability of fruits and vegetables in the home was the strongest predictor of fruit and vegetable intake, even when taste preferences for these foods were low (Neumark-Sztainer, Wall, Perry, & Story, 2003). Likewise, the amount of food children eat is influenced by environmental cues. While supersizing is often discussed in the context of fast food restaurants (Young & Nestle, 2002), corresponding increases in the portion sizes of foods served at home have been observed over the past 20 years (Nielsen & Popkin, 2003). This is problematic because it is well established that children, particularly those with greater body fat stores, eat significantly more when given portions larger than the appropriate size (Johnson & Birch, 1994; Orlet Fisher, Rolls, & Birch, 2003).

How food is served and stored can also alter consumption. A series of studies by Wansink and colleagues (2003, 2006) suggests that intake is dependent in part on visual cues, some of which can be misleading. Children and adults pour more juice when using short, wide glasses than when using tall, slender glasses, but perceive themselves as having less (Wansink & Van Ittersum, 2003). Proximity and visibility of food also influence eating behaviors. Wansink recently reported that adults underestimate how much candy they have eaten if the candy is kept on their work desk, yet overestimate consumption when candy is stored a few feet away (Wansink, Painter, & Lee, 2006). On the positive side, proximity and visibility can be manipulated to increase consumption of healthy foods. Fruit and vegetable intake at home is higher when these foods are stored in accessible locations and in child-friendly sizes (Baranowski, Cullen, & Baranowski, 1999), and when parents eat these foods themselves (Hanson et al., 2005). Thus, reflecting the basic behavioral principle of stimulus control, it appears important to structure the home environment to have healthy, accessible snacks in visible locations and to keep less healthy items out of reach and out of the sight of children.

Physical Activity in the Home: Availability of Exercise Equipment and Models for Physical Activity

The number of homes with exercise equipment has been steadily increasing (Jeffery & Utter, 2003) and home access to this equipment is associated with higher overall activity levels (Atkinson, Sallis, Saelens, Cain, & Black, 2005; Jakicic, Wing, Butler, & Jeffery, 1997). Living in a home where parents provide support and encouragement for physical activity is also associated with higher activity levels in children and adolescents (Heitzler, Martin, Duke, & Huhman 2006; McGuire, Hannan, Neumark-Sztainer, Cossrow, & Story, 2002). In a nationwide representative survey of 9–13 year olds, activity levels were higher in children who perceived strong support from their parents and in children whose parents engaged in physical activity with them (Heitzler et al.).

Sedentary Activity in the Home: Television Access

Television sets are found in over 98 percent of U.S. households, and 75 percent of households have multiple sets (Nielsen Media Research, 2000). Having multiple TVs in the home, and/or having a TV in the bedroom, significantly increases viewing hours in children (Dennison, Erb, & Jenkins, 2002). Having a TV in the bedroom is surprisingly common—approximately 20 percent of children under the age of one have a TV in their bedroom, increasing to 43 percent in four- to six-year old children (Kaiser Family Foundation, 2006). Over 30 percent of children age six and younger live in homes where the TV is on most or all of the time (Kaiser Family Foundation). These trends are disturbing in light of evidence that obesity rates rise as children watch more than the recommended amount (Giammattei, Blix, Marshak, Wollitzer, & Pettitt, 2003; Saelens et al., 2002). In a recent prospective study, weight status over three years was associated with the amount of TV viewing and physical activity in preschool-age children, and these relationships became stronger over time (Jago, Baranowski, Baranowski, Thompson, & Greaves, 2005). Prolonged TV viewing, when paired with either a low-level activity or a high-fat diet, was also prospectively linked to increases in excessive body fat from preschool to early adolescence in the Framingham Children's Study (Proctor et al., 2003).

Television viewing appears to increase obesity risk primarily by increasing energy intake. For each hour adolescents increase their TV viewing on a daily basis, their daily dietary intake increases by over 160 calories (Wiecha et al., 2006). Watching TV while having immediate access to food may be particularly harmful to children. Eating meals in front of the TV increases screen time (Saelens et al., 2002) and research suggests that children who eat dinner while watching TV are heavier (Matheson, Killen, Wang, Varady, & Robinson, 2004).

Cognitive Stimulation

More broadly, lack of cognitive stimulation in the home may put children at risk for overeating, inactivity, and ultimately weight gain. In a prospective study of nearly 3,000 children under the age of nine, children whose homes were characterized by low or average cognitive stimulation (e.g., limited access to toys, books, musical instruments, and safe playing environments) were much more likely to become obese over a six-year period than children living in homes with the highest level of cognitive stimulation—even after controlling for socioeconomic status (SES; Strauss & Knight, 1999). Interestingly, the emotional home environment (e.g., how often the child was kissed, hugged, spanked) was not related to obesity development for these same children, Others have also reported significant relationships between cognitive stimulation in the home and childhood BMI (Lumeng, Gannon, Appugliese, Cabral, & Zuckerman, 2005), indicating this may be a potential target for obesity prevention and treatment.

Taken together, the empirical evidence suggests that factors within the home may contribute to food choices, activity patterns, and weight status in children and adolescents. To promote healthy food choices at home, plenty of fruits and vegetables should be offered in appropriate portion sizes, and less desirable foods should be stored in less visible containers (Ritchie, Welk, Styne, Gerstein, & Crawford, 2005). Access to TVs, particularly in the bedroom, should be limited, and opportunities to exercise with parental support and involvement should be encouraged.

SCHOOL ENVIRONMENT

During the academic year, more than 7 hours each day are spent in school, making this environment an important behavioral setting for weight regulation in children and adolescents. In recent years, several concerns have been voiced about the obesogenic nature of the school environment, including the increased availability of both competitive foods and soft drinks, and the decreased opportunity for physical activity during the school day.

Food Choice in Schools

The National School Lunch Program federally regulates the types of foods that can be served in public school cafeterias. The nutritional quality of these lunches are debatable (Kant & Graubard, 2003), the perceived quality is low (Bauer, Yang, & Austin, 2004), and participation rates hover just below 60 percent (Gleason, 1995). Many more desirable options for beverage and food consumption (i.e., *competitive foods*) are offered outside of the federal lunch program. Nearly all schools have vending and beverage machines, as well as *a la carte* programs (Kubik, Lytle, Hannan, Perry, & Story, 2003) and students are drawn to these options for many reasons, including feeling like they are not given enough time to eat a sit-down meal (Bauer et al.) and a general distrust of school foods (Gleason). Approximately one-third of foods offered in *a la carte* programs and vending machines are low in fat (French, Story, Fulkerson, & Gerlach, 2003), but the majority of foods purchased from these sources are overwhelmingly high in sugar and/or fat and are consumed at the expense of healthier choices (Kubik et al.). Students at schools with vending machines eat less fruit than students at schools without vending machines, and students in schools with *al la carte* programs eat less fruit and vegetables and consume more fat than students in other schools (Kubik et al.). The number of snack machines in schools is also positively correlated with the amount of snack purchases (Neumark-Sztainer, French, Hannan, Story, & Fulkerson, 2005).

Soft drinks and sweetened beverages—a mainstay of vending machines—are also of concern. The consumption of high fructose corn syrup (the sweetener used in soft drinks) increased by more than 1000 percent from 1970 to 1990, and some have argued that this increase is responsible for the rise in obesity rates (e.g., Bray, Nielsen, & Popkin, 2004). Upwards of 40 percent of total caloric intake in 2 to 19-year olds comes from sweetened beverages (Troiano, Briefel, Carroll & Bialostosky, 2000) and each additional daily serving of sweetened beverages is associated with a .24 unit increase in BMI (Ludwig, Peterson, & Gortmaker, 2001). Over 30 percent of elementary schools offer sport or fruit drinks and another 9–12 percent offer soft drinks (Parasad & Lewis, 2006). Limiting access to soda machines during lunch periods is associated with lower rates of soda purchases in high school students (Neumark-Sztainer et al., 2005), and many states are now adopting legislation to limit access to soft drinks and sweetened beverages in schools (Nestle, 2003).

Opportunities for Physical Activity

Opportunities for physical activity as part of the school day include active commuting, physical education (PE) classes, and recess. Unfortunately, the numbers of students participating in all of these activities are declining. Active commuting is associated with higher physical activity levels and lower BMIs than other forms of school transportation (Cooper, Andersen, Wedderkopp, Page, & Froberg, 2005; Heelan et al., 2005), but only 10–30 percent of students currently walk or bike to school (Gordon-Larsen, Nelson, & Beam, 2005)—a decrease of 60 percent since 1977 (Center for Disease Control and Prevention [CDC], 2002). Common barriers to active commuting include living too far from school, and having a route with busy roads, steep inclines, and/or inadequate street crossings (Merom, Tudor-Locke, Bauman, & Rissel, 2006; Timperio et al., 2006). However, even in students living within one mile of school, rates have decreased from 90 percent in 1969 to 31 percent today (CDC), suggesting that more than just proximity to school is a factor in commuting decisions.

During the school day, physical education (PE) classes provide a structured, supervised opportunity for exercise. Students who engage in daily PE are more likely to engage in high levels of moderate to vigorous physical activity than students who do not (Gordon-Larsen, McMurray, & Popkin, 2000) and there is some evidence to suggest that exposure to PE at school fosters an overall increase in physical activity interest (Chen & Zhu 2005). The number of students engaging in at least 20 minutes of daily PE in high school has dropped from 34 percent in 1991 to 22 percent in 1997 (Lowry, Wechsler, Kann, & Collins, 2001). Students in urban settings and in lower socioeconomic areas, who are already at increased risk for obesity, are offered significantly fewer PE classes (Parasad & Lewis, 2006), impacting their immediate energy expenditure and perhaps also their lifelong enjoyment of physical activity.

Unstructured recess or free periods provide another opportunity for physical activity, however many schools do not offer recess and in those that do, many students do not use the time to exercise (Sallis et al., 2001). Approximately 10 percent of public elementary schools do not offer recess, and similar to PE, schools with large minority populations and high rates of poverty are less likely to provide this opportunity to their students (Parasad & Lewis, 2006). Sallis and colleagues found that while less than 5 percent of middle school students engage in physical activity on school grounds during free periods, significantly higher levels of physical activity were found in students at schools where supervision was provided and where simple physical improvements had been made on school grounds—such as the installation of basketball hoops or volleyball nets.

In sum, children and adolescents spend a significant part of their day at school—an environment that offers many unhealthy food options and limited opportunities for physical activity. More research is needed to inform policies for improving access to physical activity—particularly in urban and low SES schools—and to identify effective strategies for modifying the school food environment.

NEIGHBORHOOD AND COMMUNITY ENVIRONMENT

The built environment and larger communities in which we live may also influence the health behaviors and weight of children and adolescents (Booth, Pinkston, & Poston, 2005). Researchers from diverse fields have revealed some consistent findings regarding how the temporal trends concerning the availability of food and exercise facilities, food pricing, urban sprawl, and neighborhood safety coincide with the rise in childhood obesity rates.

Food Availability and Pricing

From 1970 to 1995, the per capita per day availability of food energy increased by 15 percent (Harnack, Jeffery, & Boutelle, 2000). Access to food in the community differs by SES and may be related to dietary habits and obesity (Popkin, Duffey, & Gordon-Larsen, 2005). In lower SES neighborhoods, where residents rely on smaller grocery stores, access to whole-grain breads and low-fat meats and cheeses is reduced (Jetter & Cassady, 2006), while in higher SES neighborhoods, more supermarkets are available that provide greater access to low-cost, healthy food options (Popkin et al.). Availability of low-cost healthy foods at local stores may translate into a decrease in obesity risk. Smaller gains were observed in children's BMI over a three-year period in neighborhoods with easy access to lower-priced fruits and vegetables than in neighborhoods with higher prices (Sturm & Datar, 2005).

Almost 40 percent of the U.S. food dollar is spent on food eaten away from home, and the number of ready-to-eat food locations has nearly doubled over the past 30 years (Jeffery & Utter, 2003). Fast food is often identified as a causal contributor to the obesity epidemic (Brownell & Horgen, 2003). A representative, nationwide survey revealed that 30 percent of children ages 4–19 years eat fast food daily, and that children who frequent these restaurants consume more calories and fat and fewer fruits than children who do not eat fast food (Bowman, Gortmaker, Ebbeling, Pereira, & Ludwig, 2003). Many children live and go to school in close proximity to fast food outlets. In Chicago, 80 percent of primary and secondary schools are located with a half mile of a fast food establishment, with a significant clustering of these types of restaurants within one mile of most schools (Austin et al., 2005). Fast food restaurants are also more common in predominately black neighborhoods than predominately white neighborhoods (Block, Scribner, & DeSalvo, 2004).

There is conflicting data about whether proximity to fast food restaurants impacts consumption and obesity rates. At the statewide and regional levels, the number of fast food chains is associated with obesity (Maddock, 2004) as well as acute coronary syndrome and mortality rates (Alter & Eny, 2005). Two recent studies, however, report that there is no relationship between proximity to fast food and consumption or weight status at the individual level (i.e., identifying the exact proximity and availability of fast food restaurants with individualized geocoded maps). While frequent fast food consumption is clearly undesirable, more research is needed to understand how proximity to fast food establishments impacts eating behavior and weight in children.

Urban Sprawl, Automobile Use, and Walkability

Urban sprawl is characterized by low-density residential development and single-use zoning (i.e., separate zones for residential, commercial, and industrial development)—a pattern that has flourished due to increased personal wealth, a rejection of traditional city living, and an increased interest in larger house sizes and lots (Lopez, 2004). Living in urban sprawl areas is associated with an increased risk of overweight and obesity in adults (Ewing, Schmid, Killingsworth, Zlot, & Raudenbush, 2003). This link has yet to be established in children; however, urban sprawl is associated with a greater reliance on automobiles and less walkable neighborhoods—two factors that may decrease physical activity in children.

Americans now take 90 percent of their trips in private vehicles, and 75 percent of trips of less than one mile are made by car (CDC, 2003). Increased time spent in a car is associated with an increased risk of obesity. Counties with the highest vehicle miles of travel have the highest rates of obesity (Lopez-Zetina, Lee, & Friis, 2006) and each additional hour per day spent in a car is associated with a 6 percent increase in obesity risk (Frank, Andresen, & Schmid, 2004). The impact automobile use can have on body weight has been demonstrated in Chinese adults. Acquisition of a motorized vehicle was prospectively associated with weight gain and a greater risk of obesity over an eight-year period, with Chinese adults owning a motorized vehicle showing a 2:1 risk of developing obesity compared to those who did not own a vehicle (Bell, Ge, & Popkin, 2002).

Urban sprawl is also associated with a decrease in neighborhood walkability (e.g., land-use mix of an area, residential density, intersection density, sidewalk conditions, neighborhood tidiness). This is unfortunate, because neighborhood walkability is related to rates of physical activity. Frank, Schmid, Sallis, Chapman, & Saelens (2005) found that 37 percent of individuals living in the most walkable areas of Seattle walked 30 minutes or more each day compared to only 18 percent in the least walkable areas. Similar trends have been observed in adolescents. Jago, Baranowski, Zakeri, & Harris (2005) found that sidewalk characteristics, such as the location of the sidewalk and the presence of street lights and trees, were associated with activity levels in adolescent boys. Other environmental variables, such as walking/cycling ease, tidiness, and street access and condition, however, were not associated with activity levels in these adolescents. Further research is needed to understand which physical characteristics of a neighborhood have the most influence on children and adolescents' exercise choices.

Safety

Whether parents and children perceive their neighborhoods to be safe is a major determinant of outdoor activity. Children and adolescents are less likely to use walking as a form of transportation and are more likely to be overweight when their parents are concerned about road safety and/or perceive their local streets as heavy with traffic (Carver et al., 2005; Timperio, Salmon, Telford, & Crawford, 2005). Higher rates of serious and violent crimes and neighborhood disorder are also associated with lower levels of physical activity (Gomez, Johnson, Selva, & Sallis, 2004; Molnar, Gortmaker, Bull, & Buka, 2004; Popkin et al., 2005) and increased TV time (Burdette & Whitaker, 2004). In inner-city adolescents, greater amounts of violent crimes within a half mile of the child's home are associated with decreased physical activity in girls (Gomez et al.). One study (Lumeng, Appugliese, Cabral, Bradley, & Zuckerman, 2006) found that parents' perceptions of neighborhood safety (e.g., satisfaction with police protection, amount of drug activity) are related to children's weight status in 7–10 year olds. In the least safe neighborhoods, 17 percent of children were overweight, in comparison to four percent in the safest neighborhoods, and this was not accounted for by SES or by the child's weight status three years earlier.

Neighborhood Access to Exercise Facilities

Another important determinant of physical activity is whether children have access to appropriate exercise facilities. Having access to open play space, afterschool programs, and a neighborhood community recreation center, are all associated with higher activity levels in children and adolescents (Gomez et al., 2004; Heitzler et al., 2006; Mota, Almeida, Santos, & Ribeiro, 2005; Popkin et al., 2005; Romero, 2005). Proximity to these facilities may exert a strong influence on physical activity choices—having to walk just five minutes to an exercise facility decreased adolescents' physical activity by more than 50 percent compared to adolescents who had immediate access to similar facilities (Raynor, Coleman, & Epstein, 1998). However, there are disparities in access to exercise facilities, with high SES neighborhoods having many more options than low SES neighborhoods (Popkin et al.). In a large study of the built environment, having at least one exercise facility decreased adolescents' odds of being overweight by five percent, yet high-minority, low-educated neighborhoods were much less likely to have at least one physical activity facility than other neighborhoods (Gordon-Larsen, Nelson, Page, & Popkin, 2006). Lack of appropriate adult supervision (Romero, 2005) and the cost of using neighborhood exercise facilities are additional barriers cited by adolescents (Allison et al., 2005).

As is evident, the literature on the relationship between the built environment and obesity is growing rapidly, and most studies to date have focused on adults. Neighborhood factors, such as safety and access to exercise facilities, appear to be related to weight-regulating behaviors in children and adolescents, posing a significant challenge for communities to address.

MODIFYING OBESOGENIC ENVIRONMENTS

In light of the mounting evidence of an association between the environment and obesity, efforts are being made to broaden the focus of obesity prevention and treatment to the home, school, and neighborhood/community settings in which eating and exercise choices are made (e.g., U.S. Department of Health and Human Services, 2001). Several ecological approaches to obesity are discussed below as models of how environmental factors can be modified to change weight-regulating behaviors.

Interventions Targeting the Home Environment

Many studies have examined ways to structure the physical home environment to promote positive weight-related changes. In a recent study, household TV time was reduced by approximately 50 percent by having families use behavioral techniques (e.g., goal setting, reinforcement) in combination with electronic devices that limited TV access (Gorin, Raynor, Chula-Maguire, & Wing, 2006). Another strategy that has proven effective in decreasing TV time is requiring children to ride a stationary bike to activate their TV set. This strategy reduced TV viewing to a mere 1.6 hours per week compared to 21 hours per week in a control group (Faith et al., 2001). Provision of food and exercise equipment also decreases the obesogenic nature of the home environment. In adults, providing a treadmill for home use is one of the few strategies known to be effective in changing long-term exercise behaviors (Jakicic, Winters, Lang, & Wing, 1999). Similarly, changing the home food environment by providing food, prepared meals, and/or detailed meals plans and grocery lists improves weight loss outcomes in overweight adults for up to 18 months (Jeffery et al., 1993; Wing et al., 1996).

Interventions Targeting the School Environment

Interventions in schools have targeted both the foods available and the opportunities for physical activity. Studies on vending machine purchases indicate that lowering the price of healthier options can alter consumption without impacting total purchases or overall profits (French, Jeffery, Story, Hannan, & Snyder, 1997; French et al., 2001). Increasing the number of low-fat food items available in *a la carte* areas and encouraging student purchase of low-fat items through peer-based promotions (e.g., taste tests, media campaigns) has also been shown to increase students' low-fat food purchases (French, Story, Fulkerson, & Hannan, 2004).

A model program that has demonstrated some initial success in increasing students' physical activity through active commuting is Marin County's Safe Routes to School program (www.saferoutestoschool.org). The program involves identifying and creating safe routes for active commuting, organizing parent-led *walking school buses* and *bike trains*, and community advertising. Children also participate in classroom discussions of pedestrian and bicycling safety and receive small incentives for active commuting (Staunton, Hubsmith, & Kallins, 2003). During the first two years of the program, walking and biking to school increased by 64 percent and 114 percent, respectively (Boarnet, Anderson, Day, McMillan, & Alfonzo, 2005). Other researchers have found that basic environmental strategies, such as providing balls and inexpensive equipment for recess, are also effective in increasing activity levels at school (Verstraete, Cardon, De Clercq & De Bourdeaudhuij, 2006).

Interventions Targeting the Neighborhood/Community Environment

Specific strategies that have shown success in modifying the built environment include encouraging stair use at public places through visual prompts, structuring communities to increase physical activity, and using media campaigns to increase daily walking. Simple interventions, such as placing signs in public places that emphasize the health or weight benefits of exercise significantly increases stair use in adults (Anderson, Franckowiak, Synder, Bartlett, & Fontaine, 1998; Brownell, Stunkard, & Albaum, 1980). Using motivational signs to promote the use of stairs, in combination with environmental changes designed to enhance the sensory appeal of the stairs (e.g., new carpeting, paint, art work, and stereo system), can result in even greater increases in stair use (Kerr, Yore, Ham, & Dietz, 2004). More recently, a national campaign has been initiated (www.americaonthemove.org), encouraging people to walk 2000 more steps and eat 100 fewer calories each day. Ongoing research studies are examining the impact of this type of environmental manipulation on physical activity and weight.

OBESOGENIC ENVIRONMENTS: WHERE DO WE GO FROM HERE?

As the importance of the environment as both a contributing factor and a potential prevention/treatment context for obesity is increasingly recognized, it is necessary to note some limitations of the existing empirical evidence. Most of the studies pertaining to the environment and obesity are cross sectional in nature, limiting the certainty with which causal conclusions can be drawn (Jeffery & Utter, 2003). Moreover, much of the literature has focused on adults, requiring caution when applying these findings to child and adolescent populations. It is also important to consider that not all studies support an environment-obesity connection (Burdette & Whitaker, 2005; Jeffery, Baxter, McGuire & Linde, 2006; Norman et al., 2006). Methodological differences are common in this emerging literature (Booth et al., 2005) and may account for some discrepant findings. Despite these limitations, the pattern of results across a growing number of studies supports an association between the environment and obesity. Modifiable factors within the home, school, neighborhood, and larger community have been identified as related to eating and exercise behaviors and, in some cases, weight status. In general, interventions targeting these environmental influences have shown promise in changing weight-regulating behaviors, leading to calls for more policy-wide changes in areas such as food pricing and urban planning (Hill, Wyatt, Reed, & Peters, 2003; Nestle & Jacobson, 2000). Continued research is needed to understand the long-term impact of environmental factors on obesity development in children and adolescents, and innovative strategies are needed to conceptualize, prevent, and treat obesity from an ecological perspective.

REFERENCES

Allison, K. R., Dwyer, J. J., Goldenberg, E., Fein, A., Yoshida, K. K., & Boutilier, M. (2005). Male adolescents' reasons for participating in physical activity, barriers to participation, and suggestions for increasing participation. *Adolescence, 40,* 155–70.

Alter, D. A. & Eny, K. (2005). The relationship between the supply of fast-food chains and cardiovascular outcomes. *Canadian Journal of Public Health, 96,* 173–177.

Anderson, R. E., Franckowiak, S. C., Synder, J., Bartlett, S. J., & Fontaine, K. R. (1998). Can inexpensive signs encourage the use of stairs? Results from a community intervention. *Annals of Internal Medicine, 129,* 363–369.

Atkinson, J. L., Sallis, J. F., Saelens, B. E., Cain, K. L., & Black, J. B. (2005). The association of neighborhood design and recreational environments with physical activity. *American Journal of Health Promotion, 19,* 304–309.

Austin, S. B., Melly, S. J., Sanchez, B. N., Patel, A., Buka, S., & Gortmaker, S. L. (2005). Clustering of fast-food restaurants around schools: A novel application of spatial statistics to the study of food environments. *American Journal of Public Health, 95,* 1575–1581.

Baranowski, T., Cullen, K. W., & Baranowski, J. (1999). Psychosocial correlates of dietary intake: Advancing dietary intervention. *Annual Review of Nutrition, 19,* 17–40.

Bauer, K. W., Yang, Y. W., & Austin, S. B. (2004). "How can we stay healthy when you're throwing all this in front of us?" Findings from focus groups and interviews in middle schools on environmental influences on nutrition and physical activity. *Health Education and Behavior, 31,* 34–46.

Befort, C., Kaur, H., Nollen, N., Sullivan, D., Nazir, N., Choi, W. S., et al. (2006). Fruit, vegetable, and fat intake among non-Hispanic black and non-Hispanic white adolescents: Associations with home availability and food consumption. *Journal of the American Dietetic Association, 106*, 367–373.

Bell, A. C., Ge, K., & Popkin, B. M. (2002). The road to obesity or the path to prevention: Motorized transportation and obesity in china. *Obesity Research, 10*, 277–283.

Block, J. P., Scribner, R. A., & DeSalvo, K. B. (2004). Fast food, race/ethnicity, and income: A geographic analysis. *American Journal of Preventive Medicine, 27*, 211–217.

Boarnet, M. G., Anderson, C. L., Day, K., McMillan, T., & Alfonzo, M. (2005). Evaluation of the California Safe Routes to School legislation: Urban form changes and children's active transportation to school. *American Journal of Preventive Medicine, 28*, 134–140.

Booth, K. M., Pinkston, M. M., & Poston, W. S. (2005). Obesity and the built environment. *Journal of the American Dietetic Association, 105*, S110–S117.

Bowman, S. A., Gortmaker, S. L., Ebbeling, C. B., Pereira, M. A., & Ludwig, D. S. (2003). Effects of fast-food consumption on energy intake and diet quality among children in a national household survey. *Pediatrics, 113*, 112–118.

Bray, G. A., (1996). Eat slowly – from laboratory to clinic: Behavioral control of eating. *Obesity Research, 4*, 397–400.

Bray, G. A., Nielsen, S. J., & Popkin, B. M. (2004). Consumption of high-fructose corn syrup in beverages may play a role in the epidemic of obesity. *American Journal of Clinical Nutrition, 79*, 537–543.

Brownell, K. D., & Horgen, K. B. (2003). *Food Fight : The Inside Story of the Food Industry, America's Obesity Crisis, and What We Can Do About It.* New York: McGraw-Hill.

Brownell, K. D., Stunkard, A. J., & Albaum, J. M. (1980). Evaluation and modification of exercise patterns in the natural environment. *American Journal of Psychiatry, 137*, 1540–1545.

Burdette, H. L., & Whitaker, R. C. (2004). Neighborhood playgrounds, fast food restaurants, and crime: Relationships to overweight in low-income preschool children. *Preventive Medicine, 38*, 57–63.

Burdette, H. L., & Whitaker, R. C. (2005). A national study of neighborhood safety, outdoor play, television viewing, and obesity in preschool children. *Pediatrics, 116*, 657–62.

Carver, A., Salmon, J., Campbell K., Baur L., Garnett S., & Crawford, D. (2005). How do perceptions of local neighborhood relate to adolescents' walking and cycling? *American Journal Of Health Promotion, 20*, 139–147.

Centers for Disease Control and Prevention. (2002). Barriers to children walking and bicycling to school United States, 1999. *Morbidity and Mortality Weekly Report, 51*, 701–704.

Centers for Disease Control and Prevention. (2003). Physical activity levels among children aged 9–13 years United States, 2002. *Morbidity and Mortality Weekly Report, 52*, 785–788.

Chen, A., & Zhu, W. (2005). Young children's intuitive interest in physical activity: Personal, school, and home factors. *Journal of Physical Activity and Health, 2*, 1–15.

Cooper, A. R., Andersen, L. B., Wedderkopp, N., Page, A. S., & Froberg, K. (2005). Physical activity levels of children who walk, cycle, or are driven to school. *American Journal of Preventive Medicine, 29*, 179–184.

Dennison, B. A., Erb, T. A., & Jenkins, P. L. (2002). Television viewing and television in bedroom associated with overweight risk among low-income preschool children. *Pediatrics, 109*, 1028–1035.

Epstein, L. H., Myers, M. D., Raynor, H. A., & Saelens, B. E. (1998). Treatment of pediatric obesity. *Pediatrics, 101*, 554–570.

Ewing, R., Schmid, T., Killingsworth, R., Zlot, A., & Raudenbush, S. (2003). Relationship between urban sprawl and physical activity, obesity, and morbidity. *American Journal of Health Promotion, 18*, 47–57.

Faith, M. S., Berman, N., Heo, M., Pietrobelli, A., Gallagher, D., Epstein, L. H., et al. (2001). Effects of contingent television on physical activity and television viewing in obese children. *Pediatrics, 107*, 1043–1048.

Frank, L. D., Andresen, M. A., & Schmid, T. L. (2004). Obesity relationship with community design, physical activity, and time spent in cars. *American Journal of Preventive Medicine, 27*, 87–96.

Frank, L. D, Schmid, T. L, Sallis, J. F., Chapman, J., & Saelens, B. E. (2005). Linking objectively measured physical activity with objectively measured urban form: Findings from SMARTRAQ. *American Journal of Preventive Medicine, 28,* 117–125.

Freedman, P. S., & Evenson, S. (1991). Familial aggregation in physical activity. *Research Quarterly on Exercise and Sport, 62,* 384–389.

French, S. A., Jeffery, R. W., Story, M., Hannan, P. & Snyder, M. P. (1997). A pricing strategy to promote low-fat snack choices through vending machines. *American Journal of Public Health, 87,* 849–851.

French, S. A., Jeffery, R. W., Story, M., Breitlow, K. K., Baxter, J. S., Hannan, P., et al. (2001). Pricing and promotion effect on low-fat vending snack purchases: The CHIPS study. *American Journal of Public Health, 91,* 112–117.

French, S. A., Story, M., Fulkerson, J. A., & Gerlach, A. F. (2003). Food environment in secondary schools: A la carte, vending machines, and food policies and practices. *American Journal of Public Health, 93,* 1161–1167.

French, S. A., Story, M., Fulkerson, J. A., & Hannan, P. (2004). An environmental intervention to promote lower-fat food choices in secondary schools: Outcomes of the TACOS study. *American Journal of Public Health, 94,* 1507–1512.

French, S. A., Story, M., & Jeffrey, R. W. (2001). Environmental influences on eating and physical activity. *Annual Review of Public Health, 22,* 309–335.

Giammattei, J., Blix, G., Marshak, H. H., Wollitzer, A. O., & Pettitt, D. J. (2003). Television watching and soft-drink consumption: Associations with obesity in 11 to 13-year-old schoolchildren. *Archives of Pediatric and Adolescent Medicine, 157,* 882–886.

Gleason, P. M. (1995). Participation in the National School Lunch Program and the School Breakfast Program. *American Journal of Clinical Nutrition, 61,* 213S–220S.

Gomez, J. E., Johnson, B. A., Selva, M., & Sallis, J. F. (2004). Violent crime and outdoor physical activity among inner-city youth. *Preventive Medicine, 39,* 876–881.

Gordon-Larsen P., McMurray, R. G., & Popkin, B. M. (2000). Determinants of adolescent physical activity and inactivity patterns. *Pediatrics, 105,* E83.

Gordon-Larsen, P., Nelson, M.C., & Beam, K. (2005). Associations among active transportation, physical activity, and weight status in young adults. *Obesity Research, 13,* 868–75.

Gordon-Larsen, P., Nelson, M. C., Page, P., & Popkin, B. M. (2006). Inequality in the built environment underlies key health disparities in physical activity and obesity. *Pediatrics, 117,* 417–424.

Gorin, A., Raynor, H., Chula-Maguire, K., & Wing, R. R. (2006). Decreasing household television time: A pilot study of a combined environmental/behavioral intervention. *Behavioral Interventions, 21,* 273–280.

Hanson, N. I., Neumark-Sztainer, D., Eisenberg, M. E., Story, M., & Wall, M. (2005). Associations between parental report of the home food environment and adolescent intake of fruits, vegetables, and dairy foods. *Public Health Nutrition, 8,* 77–85.

Harnack, L. J., Jeffery, R. W., & Boutelle, K. N. (2000). Temporal trends in energy intake in the United States: An ecologic perspective. *American Journal of Clinical Nutrition, 71,* 1478–1484.

Heelan, K. A., Donnelly, J. E., Jacobsen, D. J., Mayo, M. S., Washburn, R., & Greene, L. (2005). Active commuting to and from school and BMI in elementary school children-preliminary data. *Child Care Health Development, 31,* 341–349.

Heitzler, C. D., Martin, S. L., Duke, J., & Huhman, M. (2006). Correlates of physical activity in a national sample of children aged 9–13 years. *Preventive Medicine, 42,* 254–260.

Hill, J. O., & Peters, J. C. (1998). Environmental contributions to the obesity epidemic. *Science, 280,* 1371–1374.

Hill, J.O., Wyatt, H.R., Reed, G.W., & Peters, J.C. (2003). Obesity and the environment: Where do we go from here? *Science, 299,* 853–855.

Jago, R., Baranowski, T., Baranowski, J. C., Thompson, D., & Greaves, K. A. (2005). BMI from 3–6 years of age is predicted by TV viewing and physical activity, not diet. *International Journal of Obesity, 29,* 557–564.

Jago, R., T., Baranowski, T., Zakeri, I., & Harris, M. (2005). Observed environmental features and the physical activity of adolescent males. *American Journal of Preventive Medicine, 29,* 98–104.

Jakicic, J. M., Wing, R. R., Butler, B. A., & Jeffery, R. W. (1997). The relationship between presence of exercise equipment in the home and physical activity level. *American Journal of Health Promotion, 11*, 363–365.

Jakicic, J. M., Winters, C., Lang, W., & Wing, R. R. (1999). Effects of intermittent exercise and use of home exercise equipment on adherence, weight loss, and fitness in overweight women: A randomized trial. *Journal of the American Medical Association, 282*, 1554–1560.

Jeffery, R. W., Baxter, J., McGuire, M., & Linde, J. (2006). Are fast food restaurants an environmental risk factor for obesity? *International Journal of Behavioral Nutrition and Physical Activity, 3*, 2.

Jeffery, R. W., & Rick, A. M. (2002). Cross-sectional and longitudinal associations between body mass index and marriage related factors. *Obesity Research, 10*, 809–815.

Jeffery, R. W., & Utter, J. (2003). The changing environment and population obesity in the United States. *Obesity Research, 11*, 12S–22S.

Jeffery, R. W., Wing, R. R., Thorson, C., Burton, L. R., Raether, C., Harvey, J., et al. (1993). Strengthening behavioral interventions for weight loss: A randomized trial of food provision and monetary incentives. *Journal of Consulting and Clinical Psychology, 61*, 1038–1045.

Jetter, K. M., & Cassady, D. L. (2006). The availability of healthier food alternatives. *American Journal of Preventive Medicine, 30*, 38–44.

Johnson, S. L., & Birch, L. L. (1994). Parents' and children's adiposity and eating style. *Pediatrics, 94*, 653–661.

Kaiser Family Foundation. (2006). The media family: Electronic media in the lives of infants, toddlers, preschoolers, and their parents. CA: Menlo Park.

Kant, A. K. & Graubard, B. I. (2003). Predictors of reported consumption of low-nutrient-density foods in a 24-h recall by 8–16 year old US children and adolescents. *Appetite, 41*, 175–180.

Kaplan, M. S., Huguet, N., Newsom, J. T., & McFarland, B. H. (2004). The association between length of residence and obesity among Hispanic immigrants. *American Journal of Preventive Medicine, 27*, 323–326.

Katzmarzyk, P. T., Perusse, L., Rao, D. C., & Bouchard, C. (1999). Spousal resemblance and risk of 7-year increases in obesity and central adiposity in the Canadian population. *Obesity Research, 7*, 545–551.

Kerr, N. A., Yore, M. M., Ham, S. A., & Dietz, W. H. (2004). Increasing stair use in a worksite through environmental changes. *American Journal of Health Promotion, 18*, 312–315.

Kubik, M. Y., Lytle, L. A., Hannan, P. J., Perry, C. L., & Story, M. (2003). The association of the school food environment with dietary behaviors of young adolescents. *American Journal of Public Health, 93*, 1168–1173.

Lake, J. K., Power, C., & Cole, T. J. (1997). Child to adult body mass index in the 1958 British birth cohort: Associations with parental obesity. *Archives of Diseases of Childhood, 77*, 376–381.

Lopez, R. (2004). Urban sprawl and risk for being overweight or obese. *American Journal of Public Health, 94*, 1574–1579.

Lopez-Zetina, J., Lee, H., & Friis, R. (2006). The link between obesity and the built environment. Evidence from an ecological analysis of obesity and vehicle miles of travel in California. *Health and Place, 12*, 656–664.

Lowry, R., Wechsler, H., Kann, L., & Collins, J. L. (2001). Recent trends in participation in physical education among U. S. high school students. *Journal of School Health, 71*, 145–152.

Ludwig, D. S., Peterson, K. E., & Gortmaker, S. L. (2001). Relation between consumption of sugar sweetened drinks and childhood obesity: A prospective analysis. *Lancet, 357*, 505–508.

Lumeng, J. C., Appugliese, D., Cabral, H. J., Bradley, R. H., & Zuckerman, B. (2006). Neighborhood safety and overweight status in children. *Archives of Pediatric and Adolescent Medicine, 160*, 25–31.

Lumeng, J. C., Gannon, K., Appugliese, D., Cabral, H. J., & Zuckerman, B. (2005). Preschool child care and risk of overweight in 6- to 12-year-old children. *International Journal of Obesity, 29*, 60–66.

Maddock, J. (2004). The relationship between obesity and the prevalence of fast food restaurants: State-level analysis. *American Journal of Health Promotion, 19,* 137–143.

Matheson, D. M., Killen, J. D., Wang, Y., Varady, A., & Robinson, T. N. (2004). Children's food consumption during television viewing. *American Journal of Clinical Nutrition, 79,* 1088–1094.

McGuire, M. T., Hannan, P. J., Neumark-Sztainer, D., Cossrow, N. H., & Story, M. (2002). Parental correlates of physical activity in a racially/ethnically diverse adolescent sample. *Journal of Adolescent Health, 30,* 253–261.

Merom, D., Tudor-Locke, C., Bauman, A., & Rissel, C. (2006). Active commuting to school among NSW primary school children: Implications for public health. *Health and Place, 12,* 678–687.

Molnar, B. E., Gortmaker, S. L., Bull, F. C, & Buka, S. L. (2004). Unsafe to play? Neighborhood disorder and lack of safety predict reduced physical activity among urban children and adolescents. *American Journal of Health Promotion, 18,* 378–86.

Mota, J., Almeida, M., Santos, P., & Ribeiro, J. C. (2005). Perceived neighborhood environments and physical activity in adolescents. *Preventive Medicine, 41,* 834–6.

Nestle, M. (2003). *Food Politics: How the Food Industry Influences Nutrition and Health.* Berkeley, CA: University of California Press.

Nestle, M., & Jacobson, M. F. (2000). Halting the obesity epidemic: A public health policy approach. *Public Health Reports, 115,* 12–24.

Neumark-Sztainer, D., French, S. A., Hannan, P. J., Story, M., & Fulkerson, J. A. (2005). School lunch and snacking patterns among high school students: Associations with school food environment and policies. *International Journal of Behavioral Nutrition and Physical Activity, 6,* 14.

Neumark-Sztainer, D., Wall, M., Perry, C., & Story, M. (2003). Correlates of fruit and vegetable intake among adolescents. Findings from Project EAT. *Preventive Medicine, 37,* 198–208.

Nielsen, S. J., & Popkin, B. M. (2003). Patterns and trends in food portion sizes, 1977–1998. *Journal of the American Medical Association, 289,* 450–453.

Nielsen Media Research. (2000). *2000 Report on Television: The First 50 Years.* New York: AC Nielsen.

Norman, G. J., Nutter, S. K., Ryan, S., Sallis, J. F., Calfas, K. J., & Patrick, K. (2006). Community design and access to recreational facilities as correlates of adolescent physical activity and body mass index. *Journal of Physical Activity and Health, 3,* S118–S128.

Orlet Fisher, J., Rolls, B. J., & Birch, L. L. (2003). Children's bite size and intake of an entree are greater with large portions than with age-appropriate or self-selected portions. *American Journal of Clinical Nutrition, 77,* 1164–1170.

Parasad, B. & Lewis, L. (2006). *Calories in, Calories out: Food and exercise in public elementary schools, 2005* (NCES 2006–057). U.S. Department of Education. Washington, DC: National Center for Education Statistics.

Patrick, H. & Nicklas, T. A. (2005). A review of family and social determinants of children's eating patterns and diet quality. *Journal of the American College of Nutrition, 24,* 83–92.

Popkin, B. M., Duffey, K., & Gordon-Larsen, P. (2005). Environmental influences on food choice, physical activity, and energy balance. *Physiology and Behavior, 86,* 603–613.

Proctor, M. H., Moore, L. L., Gao, D., Cupples, L. A., Bradlee, M. L., Hood, M. Y., et al. (2003). Television viewing and change in body fat from preschool to early adolescence: The Framingham Children's Study. *International Journal of Obesity, 27,* 828–833.

Raynor, D. A., Coleman, K.J., & Epstein, L. H. (1998). Effects of proximity on the choice to be physically active or sedentary. *Research Quarterly on Exercise and Sport, 69,* 99–103.

Ritchie, L. D., Welk, G. Styne D., Gersetin, D. E., & Crawford, P. B. (2005). Family environment and pediatric overweight: What is a parent to do? *Journal of the American Dietetic Association, 105,* S70–S79.

Romero, A. J. (2005). Low-income neighborhood barriers and resources for adolescents' physical activity. *Journal Of Adolescent Health, 36,* 253–259.

Saelens, B. E., Sallis, J. F., Nader, P. R., Broyles, S. L., Berry, C. C., & Taras, H. L. (2002). Home environmental influences on children's television watching from early to middle childhood. *Journal of Developmental and Behavioral Pediatrics, 23*, 127–132.

Sallis, J. F., Conway, T. L., Prochaska, J. J., McKenzie, T. L., Marshall, S. J., & Brown, M. (2001). The association of school environments with youth physical activity. *American Journal of Public Health, 91*, 618–620.

Salmon, J., Timperio, A., Telford, A., Carver, A., & Crawford, D. (2005). Association of family environment with children's television viewing and with low level of physical activity. *Obesity Research, 13*, 1939–1951.

Staunton, C. E., Hubsmith, D., & Kallins, W. (2003). Promoting safe walking and biking to school: The Marin County success story. *American Journal of Public Health, 93*, 1431–1434.

Strauss, R. S. & Knight, J. (1999). Influence of the home environment on the development of obesity in children. *Pediatrics, 103*, 1–8.

Strauss, R. S., Rodzilsky, D., Burack, G., & Colin, M. (2001). Psychosocial correlates of physical activity in healthy children. *Archive of Pediatric and Adolescent Medicine, 155*, 897–902.

Sturm, R., & Datar, A. (2005). Body mass index in elementary school children, metropolitan area food prices and food outlet density. *Public Health, 119*, 1059–1068.

Timperio, A., Salmon, J., Telford, A., & Crawford, D. (2005). Perceptions of local neighborhood environments and their relationship to childhood overweight and obesity. *International Journal of Obesity, 29*, 170–175.

Timperio, A., Ball, K., Salmon, J., Roberts, R., Giles-Corti, B., Simmons, D., et al. (2006). Personal, family, social, and environmental correlates of active commuting to school. *American Journal of Preventive Medicine, 30*, 45–51.

Troiano, R. P., Briefel, R. R., Carroll, M. D., & Bialostosky, K. (2000). Energy and fat intakes of children and adolescents in the United States: Data from the national health and nutrition examination surveys. *American Journal of Clinical Nutrition, 72*, 1343S–1353S.

U.S. Department of Health and Human Services. (2001). *The Surgeon General's call to action to prevent and decrease overweight and obesity.* Rockville, MD: Author.

Verstraete, S. J., Cardon, G. M., De Clercq, D. L., & De Bourdeaudhuij, I. M. (2006). Increasing children's physical activity levels during recess periods in elementary schools: The effects of providing game equipment. *European Journal of Public Health, 16*, 415–419.

Wansink, B., Painter, J. E., & Lee, Y. K. (2006). The office candy dish: Promixity's influence on estimated and actual consumption. *International Journal of Obesity, 30*, 871–875.

Wansink, B. & Van Ittersum, K. (2003). Bottoms up! The influence of elongation on pouring and consumption volume. *Journal of Consumer Research, 20*, 455–463.

Whitaker, R. C., Deeks, C. M., Baughcum, A. E., & Specker, B. L. (2000). The relationship of childhood adiposity to parent body mass index and eating behavior. *Obesity Research, 8*, 234–240.

Wiecha, J. L., Peterson, K. E., Ludwig, D. S., Kim, J., Sobol, A., & Gortmaker, S. L. (2006). When children eat what they watch: Impact of television viewing on dietary intake in youth. *Archives of Pediatric and Adolescent Medicine, 160*, 436–442.

Wing, R. R., Jeffery, R. W., Burton, L. R., Thorson, C., Sperber Nissinoff, K., & Baxter, J. E. (1996). Food provision vs structured meal plans in the behavioral treatment of obesity. *International Journal of Obesity, 20*, 56–62.

Young, L. R., & Nestle, M. (2002). The contribution of expanding portion sizes to the US obesity epidemic. *American Journal of Public Health, 92*, 246–249.

11

Application of Genetic Epidemiology to Understanding Pediatric Obesity

ROBERT MAIR and STEPHEN T. McGARVEY

The prevalence of overweight in children and adolescents has increased significantly over the last two decades in the United States, especially in families of lower social status and ethnic minorities (Ogden, Flegal, Carroll, & Johnson, 2002). Childhood obesity has also been increasing globally due to rapid changes in diet and physical activity with economic development, generally referred to as the *nutrition transition* (Popkin & Gordon-Larsen, 2004). While the temporal increases in childhood overweight are ultimately attributable to macrolevel changes in childhood energy budgets—such as family socioeconomic factors, food quality and pricing, the built environment, and organized and unstructured activity patterns—genetic variation very likely plays an important role in increasing susceptibility to childhood obesity. Because of the rise in childhood obesity in the United States and throughout the world, there is a clear need for genetic studies of pediatric obesity among representative families and the detection of more subtle genetic influences that operate in interaction with the modern obesogenic childhood environment.

The purpose of this chapter is to provide a concise review of genetic epidemiology studies of body size, weight, and obesity among children and adolescents. Although most of the published studies in this age group focus on uncommon monogenic obesity syndromes, we emphasize the concept of genetic susceptibility and the multifactorial determination of pediatric obesity, and thus are somewhat selective in the papers we describe. The review suggests that research is just beginning to assess the complex

ROBERT MAIR and STEPHEN T. McGARVEY • Brown University, Providence, RI 02903.

nature of genetic predispositions to childhood obesity, and that future pediatric obesity studies will detect increasingly subtle genetic influences, gene and environment interactions, and gene-gene interactions.

When reading the literature, one must keep in mind that certain polymorphisms confer small risks that may only be detectable when measuring specific obesity related phenotypes—in particular, environments or populations. Because adiposity and obesity are complex phenotypes, there are many known and unknown physiologic mechanisms and molecular biology pathways contributing to them. Thus, we are just starting to unravel the complex combinations and interactions among the different genetic influences on childhood obesity.

The following sections describe the chromosomal regions identified in linkage studies, or the common polymorphisms identified in candidate gene association studies. We identified these candidate genes through the 2005 update of the Human Obesity Gene Map (Rankinen et al., 2006) and searches on the PubMed database involving word combinations such as childhood, adolescence, obesity, and genetics.

Human Obesity Gene Map

A review of the 2005 Human Obesity Gene Map update demonstrates that only 12/127 obesity candidate genes and 16/580 positive genotype-phenotype linkages are attributed to child study samples. Similarly, 10/317 candidate genome loci are listed as verified or identified in child populations (Rankinen et al., 2006). The tables and charts from the 2005 Human Obesity Gene Map only notate associations observed exclusively in children and these figures, therefore, do not account for studies identifying both child and adult linkages. Thus, the preponderance of genetic studies of obesity pertains to adults, and there is an absolute and relative paucity of genetic information about obesity in children and adolescents.

Genome Scans

Studies using genome scan methods attempt to identify genomic regions harboring susceptibility loci or quantitative trait loci (QTL) by estimating linkage (Blangero & Almasy, 1997). Linkage is generally quantified with logarithm of odds (LOD) scores. Higher LOD scores indicate a higher likelihood of linkage, and a score of 3 or above has traditionally been considered significant evidence (Teare & Barrett, 2005). One influential paper suggests that an LOD score ≥ 3.3 should be taken as evidence of significant linkage, which is equivalent to a p-value of .0001 or less (Lander & Kruglyak, 1995). The same authors suggest that LOD scores ≥ 1.175 and ≥ 1.9 show potential linkage and evidence of suggestive linkage, respectively

Despite the fact that the significance of inheritance in early onset obesity is well established, there are few genome scan studies among pediatric samples relative to adults (Meyre et al., 2004). The studies described in this section demonstrate the approaches that have been taken to identifying pediatric obesity susceptibility genes, and determining whether such influence persists into adulthood. The success of the few existing studies suggests that childhood obesity genome scans are an important technique for identifying the chromosomal regions containing such genes.

One such pediatric obesity genome scan examined 369 German children from 89 families with at least two obese children (Saar et al., 2003). An initial whole genome scan identified three genomic regions with LOD scores above 1.5 on chromosome 10, 10p11.23, LOD = 2.24, chromosome 11, 11q11-11q13.1, LOD = 1.65, and chromosome 19, 19q12, LOD = 1.97. Researchers then carried out more detailed fine-mapping in these identified chromosomal regions, and detected weaker LOD peaks in two locations—10p, LOD = 0.68, and 11q, LOD = 0.71. The 10p locus has been identified in several genome scans for adult obesity and contains the candidate gene glutamic acid decarboxylase 2 (GAD-2) (Meyre, Boutin, et al., 2005). The obesity candidate's genes' uncoupling protein (UCP) 2 and UCP 3 are located in the 11q region (Yanovski et al., 2000).

Another whole genome scan for childhood obesity examined 506 French subjects of European ancestry from 115 families with one or more obese children (Meyre et al., 2004). Subjects were grouped according to percentiles of BMI (95th, 97th, and 99th percentile, or PCT) and age of adiposity rebound (less than 2 years, 2–3 years, 3–5 years, more than 5 years). *Adiposity rebound* is defined as the beginning of the second rise in childhood adiposity following stabilization at one year of age. In the initial whole genome scan, significant linkages were detected with all three BMI groups: 2q33.2-q36.3 was linked to PCT 97, LOD = 2.08, and PCT99, LOD = 2.73; 6q22.31-q23.2 with PCT95, LOD = 3.13, and PCT97, LOD = 3.27; and 17p13 with PCT95, LOD = 2.25. The chromosome 6 QTL with PCT97 was the only association to meet a genome-wide significance test ($p = .01$). This locus overlaps with one identified in an obesity scan of adult and child subjects from the Framingham Heart study (Atwood et al., 2002). Several candidate genes exist in this region, including PC-1 (plasma cell membrane glycoprotein, also known as ENPP-1). The relationship of PC-1 polymorphisms to childhood obesity is discussed below in the candidate gene section (Meyre, Bouatia-Naji, et al., 2005).

All 62 children with an adiposity rebound under the age of two, or lacking such a rebound, became obese, and none of the 38 lean children underwent such a low age of rebound. Linkages with age of adiposity rebound were found for three QTL: 15q12-q15.1, LOD = 2.53; 16q22.1-q24.1, LOD = 2.54; and 19p13.3-p13.11, LOD = 2.31. These findings suggest that age of adiposity rebound is an important obesity-related phenotype to consider in future childhood genetic studies because it captures important nutritional and growth changes (Meyre et al., 2004).

The Bogalusa Heart Study used whole-genome scans to detect linkage with BMI trends from childhood to young adulthood (Chen et al., 2004). The average age of BMI measurement in the 782 Louisiana siblings of European ancestry was 17.3 years old and BMI was recorded once every three years for an average span of 20 years. Researchers looked for QTLs with both long-term obesity burden (total area under the BMI growth curve, area under the curve (AUC)) and long-term trend (total AUC minus baseline AUC). QTL for long-term burden were detected in three genomic locations: 5q23.1; 7p12.3; and 7p15.3. QTL for long-term trend were identified in eight locations: 1p12; 1p31.1; 5q21.1; 7q11.1; 12p12.2; 12q21.1; 13q11.2; and 18p11.3. The locus 12q24.1 was the only region linked with both phenotypes (LOD = 3.0 for total AUC and 2.3 for incremental AUC). Candidate genes in this region of chromosome 12 include insulin-like growth factor-1 (IGF-1) and scavenger receptor class B, type 1 (SR-B1). This study demonstrates that combining linkage methods with longitudinal phenotypes allows researchers to identify candidate genes for childhood obesity whose influence persists into young adulthood (Chen et al.).

A recent genome-wide association (GWA) study provides evidence that certain candidate genes may contribute to both child and adult obesity (Herbert et al., 2006). GWA studies take advantage of large numbers of single nucleotide polymorphisms (SNPs) to identify—in finer-grained detail—the genetic variants associated with phenotypes. GWA studies in one population are most often followed by replication in other study samples of the association between the phenotype and specific genetic variants that were detected in the first sample. Over 86,600 SNPs were genotyped in 694 participants from the Framingham Heart Study, who were not selected for obesity. After a screening and testing step, researchers identified one SNP—rs7566605 in the 2q14.1 region, which was significantly associated with BMI. The C polymorphism in this location was found to have a frequency of 0.37, and CC homozygotes had 1 kg/m^2 greater BMI and were more likely to be obese. In the replication analyses, this genotype was also associated with increased BMI and likelihood of obesity in several other populations: 3,996 Germans of Western European ancestry; 1,775 obese and 926 lean individuals of European ancestry; and 1,268 African-American individuals selected for extreme high and low BMI distribution. No association was found between BMI and the rs7566605 polymorphism in 2,726 individuals of European ancestry from the Nurses Health Study Cohort.

The positive associations identified in the GWA study of adults were replicated in a study of children involving 368 parent-obese child trios, in which the C allele was overtransmitted to the overweight children ($p = .0017$). The polymorphism is located upstream of the INSIG2 gene, which is known to inhibit fatty acid synthesis. This study demonstrates that a SNP consistently linked to obesity in adults carries the same association in a cohort of children. The result suggests that the large number of obesity genome screens that have examined adult subjects provide a reasonable basis for identifying candidate genes for childhood obesity (Herbert et al., 2006).

The four genome scan studies among children described here were able to detect linkage at several sites in the genome. There was close correspondence of the childhood adiposity QTLs and those identified in studies of adults. Of course, a cursory review of the 2005 Human Obesity Gene Map (Rankinen et al., 2006), indicates that QTLs for adult body weight or obesity are found virtually everywhere in the human genome! Thus, further research is needed using linkage and genome scan techniques. Advances in high-throughput and low-cost SNP genotyping and bioinformatics are leading to testing large numbers of SNPs using GWA study designs. This promises to give more specific evidence of genetic variants and replication across different study populations.

Candidate Genes

Another type of genetic epidemiology design explores the relationship between known polymorphisms in candidate genes and the development of human obesity. Many of these candidate genes are identified in nonhuman animal studies where breeding experiments, environmental control, and genetic knock-out methods are possible. Candidate gene studies start with a pre-existing biological hypothesis based on plausible molecular biological and physiological mechanisms. This contrasts with genome scan and GWA studies that rely on statistical evidence of greater sharing of genetic variants among those with similar phenotypic values or the same disease or condition. The complex relationship between genetic and environmental factors has made it difficult to identify such common candidate genes for childhood obesity. No meta-analysis has drawn a clear connection between a common polymorphism and risk for obesity (Bell, Walley, & Froguel 2005a). Replication generally results in mixed findings and negative evidence exists for nearly all the candidate genes. Outcomes often depend on the specific study design, ancestry of subjects, the obesity phenotype chosen, and the diet and activity patterns of the study environment. This concise review does not attempt to summarize all candidate genes. Emphasis is given to studies and candidate genes that present important insights into the complexity of demonstrating genetic predisposition to childhood obesity.

Melanocortin Receptors (MCRs). Researchers have identified many rare monogenic obesity disorders (Farooqi, 2005). Mutations in the melanocortin-4 receptor (MC4R) are the most common identified forms of autosomal-dominant obesity. These receptors are expressed on effector neurons downstream of anorectic POMC/CART neurons of the hypothalamic arcuate nucleus, and MC4R activation is known to limit food consumption. A study examining the MC4R gene sequences in 500 severely obese children provides strong evidence that common mutations in the gene contribute to childhood obesity (Farooqi et al. 2003). MC4R sequences were screened and the function of mutant MC4R alleles was examined by transfecting wild type and mutant MC4R sequences into an *in vitro* cell line. Almost 6 percent of the subjects carried mutations that impaired MC4R function. Individuals heterozygous for nonfunctional mutants had higher BMI than those with partially functional alleles ($p = .005$). BMI, height, bone mineral density, energy intake, and plasma insulin were higher in individuals with inactive MC4Rs in comparison to partially functional variants. These findings suggest that there is a link between the number of functional MC4Rs and adiposity.

Although the study by Farooqi et al. (2003) provides solid evidence for the physiological significance of common MC4R mutations, the prevalence of such variants is not clear. Other studies examining cohorts of obese children have observed rates of potentially pathogenic MC4R mutations of 6.3 percent in 63 obese French children (Dubern et al., 2001), 3.9 percent in 306 obese German children (Hinney et al., 1999) and 3.3 percent in 243 obese U.K. children (Farooqi et al., 2000). Ancestry and the precise cutoff used to define obesity are potential explanations for this variation. One study involving 208 Mediterranean children reports a mutation rate of only

0.5 percent, but this could be explained by the fact that this figure only reflects genes that cosegregated with the phenotype in all familial carriers (Miraglia del Giudice et al., 2002). This is clearly a complex system, and as demonstrated in the Farooqi et al., (2003) study, putatively significant MC4R mutations do not necessarily correspond with obesity phenotypes in all carriers. Nonetheless, the MC4R literature does show that common polymorphisms in this form of autosomal-dominant obesity contribute to subtle variations in BMI.

Other melanocortin receptors also revealed associations with childhood obesity. Feng et al. (2003) report that children doubly homozygous for the MC3R missense mutations Thr6Lys and Val8Ile are significantly heavier than individuals lacking this genotype. The project examined 190 overweight and 165 nonoverweight African-American and European-American 5–18 year olds recruited from a community in Bethesda, Maryland. Approximately 8 percent carried the double homozygous genotype, and this group had a significantly higher BMI, body fat mass, and percentage fat mass ($p < .001$). Because15.8 percent (24/152) of African-Americans and 1.7 percent (3/176) of Americans of European ancestry carried the risk haplotype, the authors suggest it could contribute to the higher rate of overweight and insulin resistance in African-Americans (Feng et al.).

Insulin-like Growth Factor (IGF-1). Insulin-like growth factor (IGF-1) has been shown to influence body composition and metabolism. Polymorphisms in the length of a cytosine-adenosine (CA) repeat microsatellite upstream of the IGF-1 coding region affect both birthweight and adult IGF-I serum levels (Voorhoeve et al., 2006). To determine its influence on obesity, Voorhoeve et al. examined the longitudinal relationship between body composition and the IGF-1 promoter polymorphism in 359 Dutch subjects of European ancestry born between 1961 and 1965, and 258 children from the same background born in the 1980s (Voorhoeve et al.). Anthropometric measurements were taken from the older generation four times from ages 12 to 16 years and at 39 years, and from the younger generation four times from ages 10 to 14 years. The authors defined the variant IGF carriers as all individuals possessing a non-192 or-194 base pair allele (19 and 20 CA repeats, respectively). Such a variable polymorphism was detected in approximately 28 percent of subjects, and was associated with significantly higher body weight, BMI, fat mass, and waist circumference in females than the younger generation. These trends were present but not statistically significant in male carriers of this generation but were not observed in the older, leaner generation. This finding suggests a potential gene-environment interaction between the IGF-1 promoter polymorphism and contemporary nutritional exposures, as well as developmental age-related influences.

Insulin-related Candidate Genes. Several of the childhood obesity candidate genes affect insulin secretion and signal transduction. Insulin has a complex set of regulatory functions, acting as a satiety signal in the brain but enhancing the storage of fatty acids through its signaling in adipose tissues. The fact that the mechanism underlying the association between obesity and type II diabetes is not understood makes the link between fat deposition and changes in insulin sensitivity particularly interesting.

INS-related Candidate Genes: Plasma Cell Membrane Glycoprotein (PC-1 or ENPP-1). The Meyre et al. (2004) pediatric obesity scan identified plasma cell membrane glycoprotein (PC-1 or ENPP-1) as a positional candidate. A follow-up case-control study examined the gene sequence in 6,147 individuals and found an association between a three-allele risk haplotype and childhood obesity and type II diabetes (Meyre, Bouatia-Naji et al., 2005). The wild type haplotype was observed in 60.3 percent of obese children and 64 percent of controls, whereas the risk haplotype was present in 11.2 percent of severely obese children and 7.2 percent of controls. Although the molecular effects of the haplotype are not clear, functional evidence suggests it might enhance the genes' function of inhibiting insulin receptor activation, therefore potentially blocking insulin's anorectic effects on the brain and skeletal muscles and causing excess energy intake. This model presents a molecular mechanism through which a common polymorphism could place children at risk for both insulin resistance and obesity. The mechanism remains unclear, however, and it is uncertain why the ENPP-1 variant would inhibit insulin's anorectic effect but not its fatty acid storage enhancing signaling in adipose tissue.

INS-related Candidate Genes: Variable Number of Tandem Repeats (VNTR) in Insulin Promoter. Another polymorphism potentially linking insulin and obesity is the variable number of tandem repeats (VNTR) located in the promoter region upstream of the insulin gene. The number of such repeats varies greatly throughout populations, and studies generally classify individuals with fewer repeats as Class I and those with higher numbers of repeats as Class III. One study of 1,207 randomly selected U.K. births reports that at age seven the III/III genotype is associated with higher BMI and waste circumference (Ong et al., 2004). However, when researchers examined the 25 percent of children who experienced a weight catch-up pattern during their first three years of life, seven- year old I/I children had significantly higher BMI and waist circumference than III/ III children of the same age. The risk associated with the polymorphism therefore appears to depend on the tempo and timing of growth patterns. The INS VNTR III/III genotype was also associated with higher concentrations of cord blood's Insulin Growth Factor II (IGF-II)—also downstream of the polymorphism—and with higher fasting insulin levels in girls, implying that INS VNTR's influence on obesity could involve changes in the regulation of these hormones.

To further examine the relationship between INS VNTR polymorphism, catch-up growth patterns, and BMI, the research group collected data from 947 of the same children at age nine (Heude, Petry, Pembrey, Dunger, & Ong, 2006). III/III children again had higher BMI and were also found to have a higher fat mass index, but no significant difference in fat-free mass. The rate of weight gain between birth and three years of age was associated with higher BMI and fat mass index at nine years of age in children carrying a type I gene, but not in the III/III children. The study also observed no association between genotype and total insulin secretion in nine-year old children, but did report that Class I carriers displayed a stronger positive correlation between BMI and insulin secretion. Children with this genotype appear to secrete greater amounts of insulin in association with rapid weight gain. This could lead to increases in the deposition of fat in adipose tissue, and contribute to the Class I allele-associated risk of obesity through the early growth pathway.

Because the type I INS VNTR variant is associated with higher BMI in children who experience rapid weight gain in infancy, its influence on obesity is likely to appear greater in a cohort with extreme early onset obesity than a randomly selected population. Indeed, an examination of 201 obese Mediterranean children and 257 obese Central European children revealed that I/I children had higher BMI than I/III or III/III children, gained weight more rapidly during adolescence, and secreted higher levels of insulin (Le Stunff et al., 2000a). Another study of 238 obese European children found that paternal transmission of class I VNTR was associated with obesity (Le Stunff, Fallin, & Bougneres, 2001). Similarly, an examination of 431 French children with a mean age of 13.5 found that III/III alleles are under-transmitted to overweight offspring (Heude et al., 2004). On the other hand, a study of 256 nonobese children reported that III/III females have significantly higher fat mass (Thorsby, Berg, & Birkeland, 2005).

These findings imply that Class I genotypes confer a risk of obesity through a rapid infancy weight gain associated pathway, and that Class III genotypes confer risk through a pathway independent of this early growth. It appears as though the VNTR Class I polymorphism tends to be associated with obesity risk in case-control studies of overweight children and with some protection from obesity in randomly selected child study samples. This pattern of findings indicates that both lifespan developmental stage and study design must be carefully considered when examining genes with pathway-specific influence.

INS-related Candidate Genes: Adiponectin. Low levels of adiponectin—a hormone secreted by adipose tissue—have been associated with obesity in adults and children. A recent case-control study examined adiponectin gene polymorphisms in 534 obese French Caucasian children, and a comparable number of normal-weight control adults (Bouatia-Naji et al., 2006). Severe obesity was associated with the −11,377C and +276G polymorphisms in the promoter region. The same percentage of −11,377C carriers were observed in obese children as were in a cohort of morbidly obese adults, implying the possibility of a genetic influence that persists from youth through adulthood. Although obesity has been associated with lower adiponectin in past studies, evidence from this and other studies suggests that the −11,377C variant is associated with a higher likelihood of obesity, higher adiponectin levels, and protection from type II diabetes (Bouatia-Naji et al; Petrone et al., 2006). These complex results likely reflect adiponectin's function of sensitizing insulin's fat storage signals in adipose tissue. Such a mechanism could explain the counterintuitive association between increased adiponectin and both obesity and protection from type II diabetes.

Glutamic Acid Decarboxylase (GAD2). The Saar et al. (2003) genome scan identified glutamic acid decarboxylase (GAD2) as a positional candidate for childhood obesity, and studies involving adult subjects have inconsistently observed protective SNPs in the GAD2 promoter region (Bell, Walley, & Froguel, 2005a). A case-control study examining 635 severely obese French children of European ancestry and 421 unrelated nonobese controls observed that the GAD2 risk polymorphism is associated with obesity in children (Meyre, Boutin, et al., 2005). At GAD2-243, 63.7 percent of obese children and 68.8 percent of controls were AA, whereas 5.8 percent of obese children and 3.3 percent of controls were GG. This association between the G polymorphism and obesity was modest but significant (OR = 1.25, p = .04). The GAD2-243 GG carriers also had a 270 g lower birth weight than AA carriers (p = .009), 25 percent lower insulin secretion in response to glucose load (not significant), and higher self-reported binge eating (18 vs. 5.7 percent, p = .04). The GAD2 gene encodes an enzyme involved in the production of the neurotransmitter GABA, and the 243G variant is known to display enhanced promoter activity, suggesting that individuals with the mutation may produce more GABA, which has an orexigenic effect in the hypothalamus (GABA inhibits the anorectic POMC/CART neurons of the arcuate nucleus). Therefore, the GAD2 polymorphism appears to both reduce birth weight (possibly by inhibiting insulin secretion) and then—as the orexigenic GABA-ergic neurons of the hypothalamus develop—cause an increase in feeding behavior. This proposed mechanism could contribute to the counterintuitive association that has been observed between low birth weight and childhood overweight (Meyre, Boutin, et al.).

β3 Adrenergic Receptors. β3 adrenergic receptors are expressed in adipose tissue, and their activation influences the regulation of fatty acid metabolism and thermogenesis. The receptor is therefore a plausible candidate gene, and studies in adults have inconsistently identified relationships between Trp/Arg substitution in β3-adrenergic receptor codon 64 and type II diabetes and overweight (Arashiro, Katsuren, Fukuyama, & Ohta, 2003). Several studies involving German and Danish children of European ancestry report no association between the β3-adrenergic receptor Trp64Arg polymorphism and BMI (Hinney et al., 1997; Tafel et al., 2004; Urhammer, Hansen, Borch-Johnsen, & Pedersen, 2000).

A few projects examining Asian subjects have observed a positive association between adrenergic receptor polymorphisms and obesity. One screening of 329 Korean teenagers identified a positive relationship between BMI and the 1053G/C variant in the β2-adrenergic receptor (p < .05) and Trp64Arg in β3-adrenergic receptor (p < .01), explaining 4.3 and 10.1 percent of variation in BMI, respectively (Park, Kim, & Lee, 2005). The Trp64Arg substitution was also associated with a higher percentage of body fat (p < .01). Further analysis showed a significant interaction between these two polymorphisms and—taking this effect into account—they were calculated to explain 18.3 percent of the obesity variation. Arashiro et al., (2003) screened 105 obese Japanese children and found that boys with the Trp64Arg version of the β3-adrenergic receptor gene had a higher obesity index and BMI. No significant effect was found in females (n = 48). The authors concluded that the polymorphism might affect obesity.

The fact that the prevalence of Trp64Arg polymorphism in Japan and in China (0.20) is higher than reported in children of European ancestry (0.12–0.18) suggests that geographic differences in prevalence could partially explain discrepancies with previous studies conducted in European populations. There are, of course, conflicting findings even in Asian populations—for instance, a screening of 311 randomly selected Chinese children uncovered no association between BMI and the Trp64Arg polymorphism, but did report that obese children without the mutation lost significantly more weight in response to a dietary intervention than children with the mutation (Xinli, Xiaomei, Meihua, & Song, 2001).

Peroxisome Proliferator-activated Receptor Υ2 (PPARΥ2) and its Interactions with β3-Adrenergic Receptors. Peroxisome proliferator-activated receptor Υ2 (PPARΥ2) is a nuclear receptor activated by fatty acids and is thought to be involved in the specialization of adipocyte cells. The PPARΥ2 Pro12Ala polymorphism, detected in .08 to .25 of population samples, has been associated with both obesity and lower BMI in adults, but a meta-analysis reports no clear relationship with adult BMI (Hamann et al., 1999; Masud, ye, & SAS Group, 2003; Ochoa et al., 2004). The association between PPARΥ2 polymorphism and pediatric obesity is similarly inconsistent and inconclusive. A study involving 311 randomly selected Finnish children reports that the Ponderal Index (kg/m^3) at birth and weight at seven years of age were higher in children with Pro12Ala than Pro12Pro genotypes (Pihlajamaki, Vanhala, Vanhala, & Laakso, 2004). However, research examining 554 obese French children of European ancestry and 374 lean controls observed no association between BMI and the Pro12Ala polymorphism (Ghoussaini et al., 2005). Likewise, a case-control study examining 296 obese German children and 130 lean controls identified the Pro12Ala in 13 percent of obese and 14 percent of lean children (Hamann et al.).

Evidence suggests that the relationship between the PPARλ2 Pro12Ala substitution and obesity phenotypes may depend on an interaction with other polymorphisms. Because previous adult-subject research observed a genetic interaction between the β3-adrenergic receptor Trp64Arg and the PPARλ2 Pro12Ala polymorphisms, Ochoa et al. (2004) examined the relationship between this interaction and body composition in children. This research team screened β3 adrenergic receptors and PPARλ2 genotypes in 185 obese and 185 control children from Navarra, Spain (Ochoa et al.). The PPARλ2 12Ala variant was associated with a higher risk for obesity after adjustment for sex, age, and physical activity (OR = 2.18; 95 percent confidence intervals [CI] = 1.09–4.36). Five percent of overweight subjects and three percent of controls carried both substitutions, and these double carriers were significantly more likely to be obese (OR = 5.3; 95 percent CI = 1.08–26). The association between double carriers and obesity rose to OR = 19.5, 95 percent CI = 2.4–146.8. When researchers adjusted for a family history of obesity, an attempt to control for other genetic factors may be an overadjustment. Although the mechanism of the interaction is unclear, previous *in vitro* functional data suggests that activation of β3 adrenergic receptors could upregulate PPARλ2 expression. This study demonstrates the importance of considering interactions between candidate genes, and suggests that the influence of a substitution may only be detectible in combination with other polymorphisms.

Ghrelin. Ghrelin is a ligand thought to be involved in meal initiation. Studies in adults have implied an association between the Leu72Met polymorphism upstream of the ghrelin and preparoghrelin genes, and BMI and fat mass (Ukkola et al., 2002). A case-control screen of the ghrelin gene in 300 obese Italian children (BMI 97th percentile, 10.5 years old), and in 200 lean controls, observed the same Leu72Met polymorphism frequency in both groups (10.3 percent Met heterozygotes, 1.3 percent homozygotes). However, the Leu72Met polymorphism was associated with the age of obesity onset within the obese group (5.3 for Leu 72 vs. 3.3 for Met 72, $p = .003$). Another examination of the ghrelin gene in 81 obese Italian children of European ancestry, and 168 healthy-weight control subjects, also reports an association between Met72 and an earlier age of obesity onset, and with higher neonatal weight for age. In normal-weight children, the 72Met variant was significantly associated with lower BMI, so it could influence a complex set of mechanisms (Vivenza et al., 2004). The fact that several studies have identified an association between common ghrelin variants and age of obesity onset suggests that this is an important obesity-related phenotype to consider in future candidate gene studies.

Propiomelanocortin (POMC). POMC is a precursor to proteins such as adrenocotricotropin hormone (ACTH) that signal hypothalamic melanocortin receptors. Rare POMC mutations have been associated with severe child obesity (Farooqi, 2005). A case-control study of 242 African-American children reports that certain POMC sequences were more common in this cohort than in children of European ancestry, but found no association between sequence and obesity (Feng et al., 2003). Another study looked at the POMC coding region sequence in 262 Caucasian children, and identified the missense mutation R236G in two subjects. Combining these numbers with previous research, the authors estimate that 0.88 percent of individuals with early-onset obesity carry this POMC mutation, and that the number is 0.22 percent for normal-weight persons. Functional studies suggest that this mutation leads to the creation of a fusion protein that interferes with normal MC4R satiety signaling (Challis et al., 2002).

Uncoupling Protein (UCP). UCP 2—another candidate gene identified in the Saar et al. genome scan of German children—reverses the proton gradient across the mitochondrial matrix and therefore affects ATP synthesis. The UCP-866 G/A polymorphism has been linked to increased expression of the gene and adult obesity. Researchers examined UCP2 sequences in 105 African-, Asian-, and European-American six to 10-year old children in Montgomery Country, Maryland who were either overweight or normal weight with overweight relatives (Yanovski et al., 2000). Of the 89 genotyped at exon 8, 50 had del/ins genotypes and 6 ins/ins. BMI and body fat mass were higher in del/ins than del/del ($p < .001$, $p < .005$). A case-control study examining 296 obese Mediterranean and Central European children, and 568 young adult controls, observed no difference between UCP-2 genotypes of obese children and controls (Le Fur, Le Stunff, Dos Santos, & Bougneres, 2004). This study also detected no association between BMI and genotype within the obese group. However, children homozygous for −866A (15/129) had a greater glucose oxidation rate (plus 34 percent, $p = .03$) and a lower lipid oxidation rate (minus 23 percent, $p = .03$) than G/A or G/G obese children. Thus, the A/A children demonstrated a carbohydrate-to-lipid calorie ratio of 3.6, and others showed a ratio of 1.4—suggesting that the polymorphism affects metabolic balance.

Leptin. Leptin levels vary with fat mass, and mutations have been associated with severe childhood obesity (Farooqi, 2005). A review reports no consistent association between any of the commonly identified leptin polymorphisms and adult obesity (Heo et al., 2002). An examination of 233 obese French girls of European ancestry observed that those carrying the −2549 −/− transcription initiation start site polymorphism demonstrated a more positive relationship between fat mass and serum leptin concentrations than +/+ homozygotes (Le Stunff, Le Bihan, Schork, & Bougneres, 2000b). This indicates that the mutation could potentially influence set point regulation, although no effect on BMI was observed within the cohort. Similarly, case control study comparing 55 obese and 48 non-obese Mexican adolescents detected no association between BMI and leptin polymorphisms, but does report a significant relationship between the Gln223Arg polymorphism and insulin, body fat, and leptin levels (Guizar-Mendoza et al., 2005). Although there does not appear to be a clear link between leptin polymorphisms and obesity, common variants have physiological influences that could affect obesity in certain environments or populations.

The previous descriptions of positional and functional candidate genes do not address all alleles associated with childhood obesity, and reflect our selection. The 2005 update of the Human Obesity Gene Map reports that markers in the candidate genes acid phosphatase (ACP1), melanocortin receptor 1 (MCR1 or GPR 24), dehydroxysteroid dehydrogenase type 1 (HSD 11), the serotonin Class 2C receptor (HTR2C), and glucocorticoid receptor NR3C4 have also been linked to obesity-related phenotypes in studies of children, and provides relevant references (Rankinen et al., 2006).

CONCLUSION

Our descriptions of the heterogeneous findings on genetic influences on childhood obesity are intended to convey the limitations of current understanding and the promises of future research. In summary, the few whole-genome scans that have tested for links with child obesity have identified several important candidate genes, such as ENPP-1, GAD-2, and UCP-2. The Bogalusa Heart Study demonstrated that combining genome scans with long-term measurement allows researchers to identify candidate genes for childhood obesity whose influence persists into young adulthood (Chen et al., 2004). Literature concerning MC4R receptors shows how combining functional assays with anthropometric measures can reveal the significance of partial-loss-of-function mutations. The complicated influence of insulin promoter repeats emphasizes the fact that a single allele variant may not have the same effect on all pathways to childhood obesity, and demonstrates how study design affects outcome. Work on GAD2 and ENPP-1 polymorphisms has suggested potential molecular mechanisms to explain the connections between childhood obesity, low birth weight, and insulin resistance. The fact that the influence of β3-adrenergic receptors varies by populations emphasizes the importance of careful description of study population ancestry and its apparent interaction with PPARγ2 polymorphisms. This demonstrates the importance of considering such haplotypes. Screens of ghrelin and UCP-2 suggest that traits such as age of obesity onset and carbohydrate-to-lipid calorie ratios may be important obesity-related phenotypes to consider, in addition to the more commonly measured phenotypes of BMI, waste circumference, and body fat mass. A cross-generational study of an IGF promoter polymorphism makes a strong case that certain allele variants influence body composition only in obesity-promoting environments. Leptin and UCP-2 are examples of genes with physiologic effects, whose influence on common obesity-associated phenotypes may depend on pathway, environment, and interactions between polymorphisms. Such insights demonstrate that research is just beginning to capture the complex nature of genetic predisposition to childhood obesity, and that future pediatric obesity studies will detect increasingly subtle genetic influences.

This brief review suggests that the future yield from genetic studies of pediatric obesity depends on at least three important factors:

1) Careful selection—and highly accurate measurement—of the adiposity phenotypes of interest, with longitudinal phenotypes being the most informative, yet practically difficult to measure. The use of both whole-body phenotypes, such as BMI and percent body fat, is encouraged, but measurement of regional adiposity and adiposity endophenotypes such as leptin and adiponectin will be important, as well as obesity-related cardiovascular disease risk factors.
2) Use of the increasing amount and inexpensively measured genomic information through genotyping of many thousands of SNPs. In combination with longitudinal designs, this will provide more accurate understanding of the complex system of regulation of gene expression of adiposity phenotypes at different ages and developmental periods.
3) Use of replication samples to determine, across multiple human groups, how consistently certain genetic factors are associated with pediatric obesity. Our reading of this literature indicates that almost all of the identified polymorphisms confer only small risks for obesity in unselected study populations.

It appears that we have a long way to go to understand the genetic architecture of childhood obesity in the general population. This suggests the need to share data, and—more importantly, moving into the future—the urgent need for commonly agreed upon study designs and statistical approaches, genotyping techniques, environmental measures, and explicit phenotypic outcomes. These common and/or shared studies must be done while also considering the heterogeneous human histories of global study populations, and the likely crucial role that evolutionary and adaptive forces play in determining variations in energy acquisition, storage, and use throughout the lifecycle (Wells, 2006).

Finally, what are the clinical implications for childhood obesity of this review? First, individual childhood risk of obesity aggregates with general family risk. This suggests that pediatricians should inquire vigilantly about family history of overweight, obesity, and severe obesity in siblings, parents, and other extended family members. Second, personalized medicine in the form of individual genetic tests for obesity risk in children are likely many years away from standard pediatric practice. In the absence of genetic tests indicating pharmaceutical interventions on childhood obesity along specific biological pathways, clinicians must be prepared for behavioral interventions after identifying children and families at risk for obesity. The intertwined nature of family genetic transmission and the family's nutritional environment suggests that pediatricians should be educated about, and prepared for, informal discussions and advice, formal structured education, and referrals about diet, exercise, and health risks of obesity. Such behavioral interventions are available and effective, though not easy. Third, human evolutionary reconstructions and recent historical data conclusively indicate that the contemporary levels of child adiposity in the developed world are due to recent alterations in the nutritional environment. Although genetic factors certainly play a role in the response to the current nutritional exposures, scientists, clinicians, and citizens need not wait for advancements in genetic studies to advocate for preventive interventions at all societal levels to combat pediatric obesity.

REFERENCES

Arashiro, R., Katsuren, K., Fukuyama, S., & Ohta, T. (2003). Effect of Trp64Arg mutation of the beta3-adrenergic receptor gene and C161T substitution of the peroxisome proliferator activated receptor gamma gene on obesity in Japanese children. *Pediatrics International, 45*, 135–141.

Atwood, L. D., Heard-Costa, N. L., Cupples, L. A., Jaquish, C. E., Wilson, P. W., & D'Agostino, R. B. (2002). Genomewide linkage analysis of body mass index across 28 years of the Framingham heart study. *American Journal of Human Genetics 71*, 1044–1050.

Bell, C. G., Walley, A. J., & Froguel, P. (2005a). The genetics of human obesity. *Nature Reviews of Genetics, 6*, 221–234.

Bell, C. G., Meyre, D., Samson, C., Boyle, C., Lecoeur, C., Tauber, M., et al. (2005b). Association of melanin-concentrating hormone receptor 1 5′ polymorphism with early-onset extreme obesity. *Diabetes, 54*, 3049–3055.

Blangero, J., & Almasy, L. (1997). Multipoint oligogenic linkage analysis of quantitative traits. *Genetic Epidemiology, 14*, 959–964.

Bouatia-Naji, N., Meyre, D., Lobbens, S., Seron, K., Fumeron, F., Balkau, B., et al. (2006). ACDC/adiponectin polymorphisms are associated with severe childhood and adult obesity. *Diabetes, 55*, 545–550.

Challis, B. G., Pritchard, L. E., Creemers, J. W., Delplanque, J., Keogh, J. M., Luan, J., et al. (2002). A missense mutation disrupting a dibasic prohormone processing site in pro-opiomelanocortin (POMC) increases susceptibility to early-onset obesity through a novel molecular mechanism. *Human Molecular Genetics, 15*, 1997–2004.

Chen, W., Li, S., Cook, N. R., Rosner, B. A., Srinivasan, S. R., Boerwinkle, E., et al. (2004). An autosomal genome scan for loci influencing longitudinal burden of body mass index from childhood to young adulthood in white sibships: The Bogalusa heart study. *International Journal of Obesity and Related Metabolic Disorders, 28*, 462–469.

Dubern, B., Clement, K., Pelloux, V., Froguel, P., Girardet, J. P., Guy-Grand, B., et al. (2001). Mutational analysis of melanocortin-4 receptor, agouti-related protein, and alpha-melanocyte-stimulating hormone genes in severely obese children. *Journal of Pediatrics, 139*, 204–209.

Farooqi, I. S. (2005). Genetic and hereditary aspects of childhood obesity. *Best practice & Research Clinical Endocrinology & Metabolism, 19*, 359–374.

Farooqi, I. S., Keogh, J. M., Yeo, G. S., Lank, E. J., Cheetham, T., & O'Rahilly, S. (2003). Clinical spectrum of obesity and mutations in the melanocortin 4 receptor gene. *The New England Journal of Medicine, 348,* 1085–1095.

Farooqi, I. S., Yeo, G. S., Keogh, J. M., Aminian, S., Jebb, S. A., Butler, G., et al. (2000). Dominant and recessive inheritance of morbid obesity associated with melanocortin 4 receptor deficiency. *The Journal of Clinical Investigation, 106,* 271–279.

Feng, N., Adler-Wailes, D., Elberg, J., Chin, J. Y., Fallon, E., Carr, A., et al. (2003). Sequence variants of the POMC gene and their associations with body composition in children. *Obesity Research, 11,* 619–624.

Ghoussaini, M., Meyre, D., Lobbens, S., Charpentier, G., Clement, K., Charles, M. A., et al. (2005). Implication of the Pro12Ala polymorphism of the PPAR-gamma 2 gene in type 2 diabetes and obesity in the French population. *BioMed central Medical Genetics, 22,* 11–15.

Guizar-Mendoza, J. M., Amador-Licona, N., Flores-Martinez, S. E., Lopez-Cardona, M. G., Ahuatzin-Tremary, & R., Sanchez-Corona, J. (2005). Association analysis of the Gln223Arg polymorphism in the human leptin receptor gene, and traits related to obesity in Mexican adolescents. *Journal of Human Hypertension, 19,* 341–346.

Hamann, A., Munzberg, H., Buttron, P., Busing, B., Hinney, A., Mayer, H., et al. (1999). Missense variants in the human peroxisome proliferator-activated receptor-gamma2 gene in lean and obese subjects. *European Journal of Endocrinology, 141,* 90–92.

Heo, M, Leibel, R. L., Fontaine, K. R., Boyer, B. B., Chung, W. K., Koulu, M., et al. (2002). A meta-analytic investigation of linkage and association of common leptin receptor (LEPR) polymorphisms with body mass index and waist circumference. *International Journal of Obesity and Related Metabolic Disorders, 26,* 640–646.

Herbert, A., Gerry, N. P., McQueen, M. B., Heid, I. M., Pfeufer, A., Illig, T., et al. (2006). A common genetic variant is associated with adult and childhood obesity. *Science, 312,* 279–283.

Heude, B., Dubois, S., Charles, M. A., Deweirder, M., Dina, C., Borys, J. M., et al. (2004). VNTR polymorphism of the insulin gene and childhood overweight in a general population. *Obesity Research 12,* 499–504.

Heude, B., Petry, C. J., Pembrey, M., Dunger, D. B., & Ong, K. (2006). The insulin gene VNTR: associations and interactions with childhood body fat mass and insulin secretion in normal children. *Journal of Clinical Endocrinology Metabolism, 91,* 11–15.

Hinney, A., Lentes, K. U., Rosenkranz, K., Barth, N., Roth, H., Ziegler, A., et al. (1997). Beta 3-adrenergic-receptor allele distributions in children, adolescents and young adults with obesity, underweight or anorexia nervosa. *Intetnational Journal of Obesity and Related Metabolic Disorders, 21,* 224–230.

Hinney, A., Schmidt, A., Nottebom, K., Heibult, O., Becker, I., Ziegler, A., et al. (1999). Several mutations in the melanocortin-4 receptor gene including a nonsense and a frameshift mutation associated with dominantly inherited obesity in humans. *Journal of Clinical Endocrinology & Metabolism, 84,* 1483–1486.

Lander, E., & Kruglyak, L. (1995). Genetic dissection of complex traits: Guidelines for interpreting and reporting linkage results. *Nature Genetics, 11,* 241–247.

Le Fur, S., Le Stunff, C., Dos Santos, C., & Bougneres, P. (2004). The common -866 G/A polymorphism in the promotor of uncoupling protein 2 is associated with increased carbohydrate and decreased lipid oxidation in juvenile obesity. *Diabetes, 53,* 235–239.

Le Stunff, C., Fallin, D., & Bougneres, P. (2001). Paternal transmission of the very common class I INS VNTR alleles predisposes to childhood obesity. *Nature Genetics, 29,* 96–99.

Le Stunff, C., Fallin, D., Schork, N. J., & Bougneres, P. (2000a). The insulin gene VNTR is associated with fasting insulin levels and development of juvenile obesity. *Nature Genetics, 26,* 444–446.

Le Stunff, C., Le Bihan, C., Schork, N. J., & Bougneres, P. (2000b). A common promotor variant of the leptin gene is associated with changes in the relationship between serum leptin and fat mass in obese girls. *Diabetes, 49,* 2196–2200.

Masud, S., Ye, S., & SAS Group. (2003). Effect of the peroxisome proliferator activated receptor-gamma gene Pro12Ala variant on body mass index: A meta-analysis. *Journal of Medical Genetics, 40,* 773–780.

Meyre, D., Boutin, P., Tounian, A., Deweirder, M., Aout, M., Jouret, B., et al. (2005). Is glutamate decarboxylase 2 (GAD2) a genetic link between low birth weight and subsequent development of obesity in children? *Journal of Clinical Endocrinology & Metabolism, 90,* 2384–2390.

Meyre, D., Bouatia-Naji, N., Tounian, A., Samson, C., Lecoeur, C., Vatin, V., et al. (2005). Variants of ENPP1 are associated with childhood and adult obesity and increase the risk of glucose intolerance and type 2 diabetes. *Nature Genetics, 37,* 863–867.

Meyre, D., Lecoeur, C., Delplanque, J., Francke, S., Vatin, V., Durand, E., et al. (2004). A genome-wide scan for childhood obesity-associated traits in French families shows significant linkage on chromosome 6q22.31–q23.2. *Diabetes, 53,* 803–811.

Miraglia Del Giudice, E., Cirillo, G., Nigro, V., Santoro, N., D'Urso, L., Raimondo, P., et al. (2002). Low frequency of melanocortin-4 receptor (MC4R) mutations in a Mediterranean population with early-onset obesity. *International Journal of Obesity and Related Metabolic Disorders, 26,* 647–651.

Ochoa, M. C., Marti, A., Azcona, C., Chueca, M., Oyarzabal, M., Pelach, R., et al. (2004). Gene-gene interaction between PPAR gamma 2 and ADR beta 3 increases obesity risk in children and adolescents. *International Journal of Obesity and Related Metabolic Disorders, 28* (Suppl 3): S37–S41.

Ogden, C. L., Flegal, K. M., Carroll. M. D., & Johnson, C. L. (2002). Prevalence and trends in overweight among US children and adolescents, 1999–2000. *The Journal of American Medical Association, 288,* 1728–32.

Ong, K. K., Petry, C. J., Barratt, B. J., Ring, S., Cordell, H. J., Wingate, D. L., Avon Longitudinal Study of Pregnancy and Childhood Study Team. (2004). Maternal-fetal interactions and birth order influence insulin variable number of tandem repeats allele class associations with head size at birth and childhood weight gain. *Diabetes, 53,* 1128–1133.

Park, H. S., Kim, Y., & Lee, C. (2005). Single nucleotide variants in the beta2-adrenergic and beta3-adrenergic receptor genes explained 18.3% of adolescent obesity variation. *Journal of Human Genetics, 50,* 365–369.

Petrone, A., Zavarella, S., Caiazzo, A., Leto, G., Spoletini, M., Potenziani, S., et al. (2006). The promoter region of the adiponectin gene is a determinant in modulating insulin sensitivity in childhood obesity. *Obesity, 14,* 1498–1504.

Pihlajamaki, J., Vanhala, M., Vanhala, P., & Laakso, M. (2004). The Pro12Ala polymorphism of the PPAR gamma 2 gene regulates weight from birth to adulthood. *Obesity Research, 12,* 187–190.

Popkin, B. M., & Gordon-Larsen, P. (2004). The nutrition transition: worldwide obesity dynamics and their determinants. *International Journal of Obesity and Related Metabolic Disorders, 28* (Suppl 3): S2–9.

Rankinen, T., Zuberi, A., Chagnon, Y. C., Weisnagel, S. J., Argyropoulos, G., Walts, B., et al. (2006). The human obesity gene map: The 2005 update. *Obesity Research, 14,* 529–644.

Saar, K., Geller, F., Ruschendorf, F., Reis, A., Friedel, S., Schauble, N., et al. (2003). Genome scan for childhood and adolescent obesity in German families. *Pediatrics, 111,* 321–327.

Tafel, J., Branscheid, I., Skwarna, B., Schlimme, M., Morcos, M., Algenstaedt, P., et al. (2004). Variants in the human beta 1-, beta 2-, and beta 3-adrenergic receptor genes are not associated with morbid obesity in children and adolescents. *Diabetes, Obesity and Metabolism, 6,* 452–455.

Teare, M., & Barrett, J. H. (2005). Genetic linkage studies. *Lancet, 366,* 1036–44.

Thorsby, P. M., Berg, J. P., Birkeland, K. I. (2005). Insulin gene variable number of tandem repeats is associated with increased fat mass during adolescence in non-obese girls. *Scandinavian Journal of Clinical & Laboratory Investigation, 65,* 163–168.

Ukkola, O., Ravussin, E., Jacobson, P., Perusse, L., Rankinen, T., Tschop, M., et al. (2002). Role of ghrelin polymorphisms in obesity based on three different studies. *Obesity Research, 10,* 782–791.

Urhammer, S. A., Hansen, T., Borch-Johnsen, K., & Pedersen, O. (2000). Studies of the synergistic effect of the Trp/Arg64 polymorphism of the beta3-adrenergic receptor gene and the -3826 A-->G variant of the uncoupling protein-1 gene on features of obesity and insulin resistance in a population-based sample of 379 young Danish subjects. *Journal of Clinical Endocrinology & Metabolism, 85*, 3151–3154.

Vivenza, D., Rapa, A., Castellino, N., Bellone, S., Petri, A., Vacca, G., et al. (2004). Ghrelin gene polymorphisms and ghrelin, insulin, IGF-I, leptin and anthropometric data in children and adolescents. *European Journal of Endocrinology, 151*, 127–133.

Voorhoeve, P. G., van Rossum, E. F., Te Velde, S. J., Koper, J. W., Kemper, H. C., Lamberts, S. W., et al. (2006). Association between an IGF-I gene polymorphism and body fatness: Differences between generations. *European Journal of Endocrinology, 154*, 379–388.

Xinli, W., Xiaomei, T., Meihua, P., & Song, L. (2001). Association of a mutation in the beta3-adrenergic receptor gene with obesity and response to dietary intervention in Chinese children. *Acta Paediatrica, 90*, 1233–1237.

Wells, J. C. (2006). The evolution of human fatness and susceptibility to obesity: An ethological approach. *Biological Reviews of the Cambridge Philosophical Society, 81*, 183–205.

Yanovski, J. A., Diament, A. L., Sovik, K. N., Nguyen, T. T., Li, H., Sebring, N. G., et al. (2000). Associations between uncoupling protein 2, body composition, and resting energy expenditure in lean and obese African American, white, and Asian children. *American Journal of Clinical Nutrition, 71*, 1405–1420.

Section IV

Interventions

12

Developmental Considerations in the Prevention of Pediatric Obesity

MELISSA XANTHOPOULOS, CHANTELLE HART, and ELISSA JELALIAN

The number of children and adolescents who are overweight or at risk of obesity in the United States has increased dramatically in the last two decades (Ogden et al., 2006), leading to a public health epidemic (Wang & Dietz, 2004). Prevalence of overweight has increased significantly in children of all age groups. Particularly noteworthy is the increase in overweight in young children two to seven-years old (Ogden et al.). Overweight in childhood increases the risk of adult overweight (Whitaker et al., 1997, Whitaker, Pepe, Wright, Seidel, & Dietz, 1998; Freedman et al., 2004; Guo et al., 2002), highlighting the importance of addressing weight concerns in pediatric populations. Paralleling age-related trends in weight are developmental progressions in nutritional needs, and physical activity patterns and capacities. The objective of this chapter is to provide a developmental context for considering growth, dietary intake, and physical activity patterns with the goal of highlighting potential key periods and strategies for pediatric weight control interventions across childhood and adolescence.

MELISSA XANTHOPOULOS • The Children's Hospital of Philadelphia, Philadelphia, PA 19104. **CHANTELLE HART** • Warren Alpert Medical School of Brown University, Providence, RI 02903. **ELISSA JELALIAN** • Warren Alpert Medical School of Brown University, Providence, RI 02903.

NATURAL GROWTH TRAJECTORY

An individual's growth is influenced by heredity, nutrition, and environmental factors, as well as a myriad of other physical and psychological factors. Normal growth, including both height and weight, is one of the best indicators of good health and nutrition. However, there is wide variation in the height and weight of normal children, which is why placing a child's growth in a normative context is valuable. In general, children's length increases very rapidly during the first two years of life, with the average child reaching about 50 percent of adult stature by age two (Wilmore & Costill, 1994). After two years of age, growth continues but at a slower and steady rate of about 6 cm per year until about the age of 11–12 years in girls and 13–14 years in boys (Tanner & Davies, 1985; Abbassi, 1998). During puberty, and for approximately two years thereafter, another growth spurt begins, and peak velocity of height growth occurs. For girls, growth velocity during puberty is approximately 6–11 cm per year, and for boys during puberty, the rate is 7–13 cm per year (Tanner & Davies; Abbassi). Normal growth stops when the growing ends of the bones fuse—usually between the ages of 13 and 15 for girls, and 14 and 17 for boys (Tanner & Davies; Abbassi). Thus, peak times for growth occur during the first two years of life and then again during adolescence.

The natural trajectory of normal weight gain is more complex because it is based on age, gender, and height. Therefore, weight cannot be considered in and of itself, but BMI for age and gender is used to indicate a child's weight in relation to his or her height. For each individual, it is necessary to obtain a series of BMI plots to determine the growth trend and whether or not the individual's growth chart pattern deviates from normal growth patterns. In general, by one year of age, a child's birth weight has usually tripled, and he or she will gain about a half to two pounds per month (Insel, Turner, & Ross, 2007, p. 668). Children grow at a slower rate than infants, and will gain about five pounds per year (Insel et al., p. 692). During adolescence, boys typically gain about 45 pounds, and girls gain about 35 pounds; however, if a child gains slightly more weight per year during this period, then he or she will quickly become overweight (Insel et al., p. 700).

In addition to the parameters of height and weight, more specific developmental changes in muscle mass and fat deposition occur. Muscle mass increases steadily as weight is gained from birth through adolescence. The rate of muscle mass increase peaks at puberty between the ages of 18–25 in males, and between the ages of 16–20 in females, although females do not experience as dramatic an increase in muscle mass as males (Wilmore & Costill, 1994). The amount of fat accumulation depends on diet, habits, and heredity. Further, fat cells can increase in number and size throughout life. Body fatness normally declines starting between nine and 12 months up to the age of five to six years, when it reaches a minimum, and gradually increases through adolescence and most of adulthood (Dietz, 1994; Whitaker et al., 1998). The point of maximal leanness is known as adiposity rebound (Rolland-Cachera et al., 1984). Early adiposity rebound is associated with higher BMI in adolescence and adulthood (Rolland-Cachera et al.; Siervogel, Roche, Guo, Mukherjee, & Chumlea, 1991; Whitaker et al., 1998). At physical maturity, normal male body fat averages about 15 percent of total body weight, and females average about 23 percent (Spear, 2002).

Considerable attention has been given to the construct of adiposity rebound defined as the point during childhood at which BMI is lowest, and also thought to be associated with the point of least body fat (Rolland-Cachera et al., 1984). While not all researchers agree on the clinical utility of adiposity rebound (Cole, 2004), there are some data to suggest that early adiposity or BMI rebound may be related to increased risk of overweight in adulthood (Taylor, Grant, Goulding, & Williams, 2005). Early adiposity rebound defined as less than 4.8 years was associated with increased risk of adult obesity in a retrospective cohort study (Whitaker et al., 1998). Both early BMI rebound and childhood BMI were related to greater adult weight in a sample followed through the Bogalusa Heart study (Freedman et al., 2001). In a review of the topic, Taylor and colleagues (Taylor et al., 2005) concluded that earlier adiposity rebound is a clear risk factor and that the utility of the construct lies in the potential to identify children who may become overweight prior to actual onset of obesity.

Several aspects of physical fitness ability improve due to physiological maturation of children's nervous, cardiovascular, and respiratory systems during the first 18 years of life. For example, motor ability gradually increases during this period, but girls tend to plateau around puberty— potentially due to increased estrogen levels and possibly the onset of a more sedentary lifestyle at that time (Wilmore & Costill, 1994). Strength increases as muscle mass increases and neuromuscular control is complete—usually around sexual maturity. Pulmonary function improves as lung volumes increase until physically mature. Cardiovascular fitness naturally improves as cardiac output increases with the maturation of the child through late adolescence due to increases in heart size and blood volume, but can be improved even more in physically active children and adolescents (Wilmore & Costill). Similarly, aerobic capacity improves as pulmonary and cardiovascular function improves through development and physical fitness. Anaerobic capacity is limited in childhood, but becomes comparable to adults in late adolescence.

GUIDELINES AND RECOMMENDATIONS

These developmental variations in growth, muscle mass, and fat deposition are paralleled by variations in caloric and micro/macronutrient needs and abilities related to physical activity, and provide a framework for prevention and intervention strategies.

Caloric and Micronutrient Consumption Needs

Caloric requirements of children vary over time based upon the body's growth and development. During infancy and toddlerhood (1–3 years), children require 900–1000 calories/day (American Heart Association [AHA], 2006).

By four years of age, there are separate caloric guidelines for girls and boys. Calorie needs increase over time for both genders, with young girls (4–8 years old) needing to consume approximately 1200 calories/day and adolescent girls (14–18 years) needing approximately 1800 calories/day. Young boys need approximately 1400 calories/day and adolescent boys need approximately 2200 calories/day (AHA). In addition to developmental variability in caloric needs, there is also variability in the macronutrients that children should consume to attain the appropriate energy intake.

Throughout childhood and adolescence, it is recommended that 45–65 percent of calories consumed come from carbohydrates (ADA, 2004). However, added sugars should not exceed a maximum of 25 percent of calories consumed. Fat intake should decrease over time, with toddlers (1–3 years) consuming 30–40 percent of calories from fat and children 4–18 years of age consuming 25–35 percent of calories from fat—similar to the lower fat intake that is recommended for adults. Protein consumption should, conversely, increase over time with younger children consuming 5–20 percent of calories from protein and older children consuming 10–30 percent (ADA). Finally, fiber consumption should increase over time as well, with 1 to 3-year old children consuming 19 grams/day of fiber and 4 to 8-year old children consuming approximately 25 grams of dietary fiber (ADA; AHA et al., 2006). During adolescence, it is recommended that boys continue to increase their fiber consumption to 31 grams/day, while girls essentially maintain their fiber intake at 26 grams/day (ADA; AHA et al.). It is recommended that sources of the above micronutrients consist of lean meats, poultry, fish, legumes, low-fat dairy, fruits, vegetables, and whole grains (AHA et al.).

Physical Activity

Ideally, physical activity should be enjoyable for each individual at any age, and should involve a variety of lifelong leisure-time activities. Developmental level will dictate the kind, intensity, and duration of physical activity best suited to an individual. Recent recommendations from the U.S. Department of Health and Human Services suggest that children and adolescents should engage in at least 30–60 minutes of physical activity on most, and preferably all, days of the week (Strong et al., 2005; USD-HHS and USDA, 2005). It has also been determined that activity may be broken into smaller segments of 10 or 15 minutes throughout the day and still provide significant health benefits (Strong et al.). Breaking physical activity up into multiple bouts of shorter duration may improve motivation for youth—especially preadolescent children—given their relatively shorter attention span compared to adults. To accomplish this goal, parents are encouraged to incorporate regular physical activity into their family's everyday lives, which does not necessarily mean joining an expensive gym or committing to a rigorous exercise or training routine. It is sufficient to choose lifestyle activities that fit into the daily routine that speed heart rate and breathing, or increase strength and flexibility (Strong et al.). Examples include walking or riding a bike to school or work, getting off a bus at an earlier stop and walking the remainder of the way to the destination, taking the stairs whenever possible, stretching or doing resistance exercises such as sit-up or push-ups while watching television, or taking vacations that emphasize activity.

In terms of guidelines for specific age groups, the American College of Sports Medicine recommends that the primary goal of activity for preadolescence is to maintain a schedule of activity that children enjoy to establish a foundation for lifelong activity habits (Zwerin & Manos, 1998). To accomplish this goal, it is recommended that the child be allowed to be naturally active and in control of the intensity and duration of the activity, and that the activity should be enjoyable to the child. Play should be encouraged outside away from the television and computer, with motor and sport skill acquisition being increasingly emphasized as children become adolescents.

The International Consensus Conference on Physical Activity developed two guidelines for physical activity in adolescence (Sallis & Patrick, 1994). The first guideline states that all adolescents should be physically active daily—or nearly every day—as part of play, games, sports, work, transportation, recreation, physical education, or planned exercise, in the context of family, school, and community activities. The second guideline emphasizes more specific recommendations for activity, such as engaging in three or more sessions per week of activities that last 20 minutes or more, and that require moderate to vigorous levels of exertion. Moderate to vigorous activities are those that require at least as much effort as brisk or fast walking and burn 3–7 kcal/min (Sallis & Patrick). Further, a diverse variety of activities that use large muscles groups are recommended as part of sports, recreation, chores, transportation, work, school, physical education, or planned exercise.

One dimension that is less often considered in encouraging physical activity in both children and adolescents is resistance training. Strength gains achieved from resistance training in preadolescents result primarily from improved motor skill coordination, increased motor unit activation, and neurological adaptation. The risk of injury from resistance training in young children is relatively low provided maturation is considered. Specific benefits associated with resistance training include reduction of activity-related injury (American College of Sports Medicine, 1993) and potential improvement in motor tasks (Lillegard, Brown, Wilson, Henderson, & Lewis, 1997). There are also some data to suggest that resistance training may serve to positively impact muscular strength and endurance in school age children (Faigenbaum, Westcott, LaRosa Loud, & Long, 1999). The reader is referred to Kraemer and Fleck (1992) for a more detailed discussion of recommended resistance exercise programs based on age.

With this general developmental context regarding nutrition and physical activity, we will consider the trajectory of nutrition and physical activity habits across childhood and adolescence as these relate to opportunities for weight control and prevention efforts.

LONGITUDINAL STUDIES RELATED TO EATING HABITS AND PHYSICAL ACTIVITY

Eating Habits

Longitudinal studies of eating habits across childhood, adolescence, and young adulthood suggest that while overall macronutrient intake tracks over time (i.e., individuals maintain their relative position for intake over time) (Singer Moore, Garrahie, & Ellison, 1995; Mannino, Lee, Mitchell, Smickilas-Wright, & Birch, 2004), trends in diet quality and consumption of specific foods and micronutrients vary (Demory-Luce et al., 2004; Kelder, Perry, Klepp, & Lytle, 1994; Singer et al.). For example, Mannino and colleagues found that while the intake of vitamins C and D, calcium, phosphorous, magnesium and zinc tracked from five to nine years of age in girls, there were significant decreases in the nutrient densities of these micronutrients in nine-year olds' diets (as compared to five-year olds). Furthermore, although consumption of fruits, vegetables, and dairy were related across time, total energy intake increased over time. Thus, although nine-year olds consumed the same number of fruits, vegetables, and dairy, their overall diet quality decreased over time (Mannino et al.).

Additional studies in childhood have reported similar findings. Results from a sample of children in the Framingham Children's Study suggest that nutrient density intakes are consistent throughout early childhood (i.e., 3–8 years old) (Singer et al., 1995). Furthermore, Fiorito, Mitchell, Smiciklas-Wright, and Birch (2006) found that dairy intake remains stable in girls from five to 11 years old. However, milk consumption declines over time and, while total dairy consumption remains stable, this results in girls not having enough calcium and phosphorous in their diets by the time they are nine and 11 years old (Fiorito et al.).

Results from the Bogalusa Heart study show that consumption of fruits and vegetables (Demory-Luce et al., 2004) and total calcium (Rajeshwari Nicklas, Yang, & Berenson 2004) remains relatively stable from childhood (i.e., 10 years) through early adulthood (i.e., 19–28 years)(Demory-Luce et al.). However, the nutrient quality of foods consumed decreases from childhood to early adulthood. Furthermore, mean consumption of meats and sweets increases over time, while consumption of dairy products decreases in young adulthood. When looking more specifically at individual foods, increased variability in consumption patterns can be found with fruits/fruit juices, candy, desserts, milk, and mixed meats being consumed more in childhood than adulthood, and sweetened beverages, salty snacks, beef, poultry, and seafood being consumed more in early adulthood than in childhood (Demory-Luce et al.). Thus, although many eating patterns track over time, overall diet quality frequently decreases both due to the addition of less healthy options into the diet as well as the inability of individuals to *keep up* with increasing nutritional needs over time.

Physical Activity

Research regarding the tracking of physical activity across the lifespan has revealed significant but modest relationships over time. Overall, it has been reported that physical activity tracks at low to moderate levels in the transition from early to middle childhood, and from late childhood through adolescence (Janz, Burns, & Levy, 2005; Janz, Dawson, & Mahoney, 2000; Kemper, Snel, Verschuur, & Storm-van Essen, 1990; Malina, 1996; Raitakari et al., 1994; Sallis, Berry, Broyles, McKenzie, & Nader, 1995). Similarly, low to moderate relationships between childhood and adolescent physical activity and adult physical activity have been documented (Malina, 2001). However, sedentary behaviors tend to be more predictable and stable over time (Janz et al., 2000, 2005).

A number of studies have documented age-related declines in activity in both boys and girls, with girls demonstrating a predictable decrease in physical activity during preadolescence (Livingstone, Robson, Wallis, & McKinley, 2003). A 26 percent decrease was observed during a four-year longitudinal study of adolescents, with analysis suggesting a decrease in the number of activities in which adolescents participate rather than the time spent in activities (Aaron, Storti, Robertson, Kriska, & LaPorte, 2002). Vigorous physical activity declined significantly in girls between the 8th and 12th grades, and participating in activities during 8th grade was a strong predictor of participation in 12th grade (Pate, Dowda, O'Neill, & Ward, 2007).

A recent study offers an interesting perspective with regard to further understanding such gender differences. Researchers found an overall decrease in activity and increase in sedentary behavior over a three-year period in children entering middle childhood (Janz et al., 2005). However, while the rate of change was similar for boys and girls in morning and afternoon activities, evening activity levels decreased at greater rates in girls than boys (Janz et al.). In addition, boys transitioning from middle childhood to adolescence report increases in their vigorous activity levels, whereas girls remain the same (Centers for Disease Control and Prevention, 1997; Janz et al., 2000). The overall decrease in physical activity in boys and girls during this period may be the result of school-related requirements and routines. This suggests that targeting sedentary behavior after school and on weekends may be a useful focus of individual and family-based interventions. Alternatively, increasing opportunities for physical activity within the context of the school setting provides another option for addressing this concern.

Research has also documented the consistency of some sedentary behaviors. Boys who watched the most television, and the girls and boys who played the most video games in childhood, continued to do so during adolescence, indicating that certain sedentary behavior patterns may be established early and persist through sexual maturation (Janz et al., 2000, 2005). In a longitudinal study assessing changes in physical activity and sedentary behavior from early to mid-adolescence, and mid-adolescence to late adolescence, time spent in moderate to vigorous physical activity decreased significantly in girls from early to mid-adolescence, and again from mid- to late adolescence (Nelson, Neumark-Sztainer, Hannan, Sirard, & Story, 2006). Boys showed similar declines from mid- to late adolescence. These changes were paralleled by increases in leisure-time computer use from mid- to late adolescence in girls, and during both time periods for boys.

Although there has been less focus on examining physical activity patterns from late adolescence into adulthood, evidence suggests a modest relationship. Gordon-Larsen, Nelson, and Popkin (2004) evaluated changes in physical activity and sedentary behavior during the transition from adolescence to adulthood in a multiethnic sample. A significant decrease was observed in the number of youth who achieved five sessions or more of moderate to vigorous physical activity from adolescence to young adulthood—particularly for girls. There was also a tendency for screen time to increase into adulthood.

Several factors have been identified as important targets in adolescence that impact adult activity participation. Adult exercise habits have been positively related to preteen and teen skill in physical activity, as well as preteen participation in a team sport (Taylor, Blair, Cummings, Wun, & Malina, 1999). Further, being more physically fit during childhood and adolescence may be predictive of increased adult physical activity (Malina 2001). Not surprisingly, being forced to exercise during the preteen and teen years is negatively related to adult exercise habits (Taylor et al.). These results suggest that a significant challenge for interventions is development of physical activity opportunities that are nonthreatening and foster skill development in children of all physical abilities. For a detailed review of the effectiveness of interventions for increasing physical activity, including school, family, primary care, community, and internet-based settings, the reader is referred to Kahn et al. (2002) and Salmon, Booth, Phongsavan, Murphy, and Timperio (2007).

THE UTILITY OF DEVELOPMENTAL PERIODS IN TREATMENT AND PREVENTION OF OVERWEIGHT

This section considers the impact of development on opportunities for establishing or changing eating and activity habits related to the prevention and treatment of overweight. Examples of effective intervention strategies at different ages will be highlighted.

Key Periods for Prevention and Intervention

Weight maintenance has been recommended as the first step in weight control for all children two years of age and older (Dietz & Robinson, 2005). Historically, weight maintenance has been recommended for school-age children and adolescents whose BMI for age and gender places them between the 85th and 95th percentiles, and gradual weight loss is the goal when BMI for age and gender is above the 95th percentile (Barlow & Dietz, 1998). Recent expert committee recommendations suggest the appropriateness of weight loss for children two years old and above whose height and weight places them at higher BMI percentiles for their age and gender, with clear guidelines regarding appropriate rates of weight loss depending upon the child's age and BMI status (Barlow and the Expert Committee, 2007). The overall goal for children across the age continuum is to achieve a weight percentile that is less than the 85th percentile for age and sex.

These guidelines provide a context for reviewing developmental considerations in the onset and treatment of obesity. It has been proposed that there may be *critical periods* during childhood for the onset of obesity, including the prenatal period, the timing of adiposity rebound, and adolescence (Dietz, 1994). Furthermore, basic eating research shows that the preschool period may be an additional critical time during which environmental cues for eating begin to play a greater role. As such, a better understanding of the significant variables associated within these timeframes for later obesity risk may provide key opportunities for the prevention of obesity (Dietz & Gortmaker, 2001). Given that recommendations for evaluation and treatment begin in early childhood (Barlow & Dietz, 1998), and the chapter's focus on developmental considerations for assessment and treatment, the present review will focus on the preschool period and beyond.

Preschool. The preschool period may be a particularly critical time for the development of healthy eating habits for a number of reasons. First, lifelong eating and activity habits are being developed within this timeframe (Brent & Weitzman, 2004). Interventions that capitalize on the development of food preferences by promoting healthier eating habits could serve to decrease the likelihood of children engaging in eating behaviors associated with obesity (e.g., drinking sweetened beverages, eating snack foods). Attempting to influence food preferences during this period may be particularly important because food neophobia is less of a concern for younger children than older children. For example, while food preferences are relatively stable from toddlerhood (2–3 years) through early childhood (8 years), younger children are more receptive to trying new foods than older children (Skinner, Carruth, Bounds, & Ziegler, 2002). Finally, younger children are less influenced by environmental cues for eating than are older children, and therefore are better able to self-regulate based on internal hunger and satiety cues rather than on environmental influences such as portion size. For example, for five-year-old children, amount of food presented is correlated with amount of food eaten, with larger portion sizes being associated with larger amounts of food consumed (Rolls, Engell, & Birch, 2000). The relationship between amount of food presented and consumed is not significant in three-year-old children. Moreover, between five and seven years of age, eating in the absence of hunger is a stable trait for girls and is significantly associated with being overweight (Fisher & Birch, 2002). Thus, the preschool period may be particularly important for the development of prevention or early intervention approaches for obesity and associated disease. Given current research on children's dietary habits, studies that capitalize on increased food acceptability during this age through increasing the variety of healthy foods in children's diets may help to promote greater preferences for a larger variety of healthy foods and thus prevent the development of obesity later in life.

Preschool is also an opportunity to encourage involvement with play and enjoyment of physical activity. Prior to four years of age, physical activity should be encouraged in the form of play and leisure activities because children younger than four years of age are not ready for organized team play. Parents are also especially important role models for lifestyle activity during this time, and should be encouraged to incorporate physical activity into their own lives. Given the dependence of children in this age group on their parents, physical activities, games, and play that include the whole family should be emphasized.

Also of relevance to the end of the preschool period is the timing of the adiposity rebound. Given that earlier adiposity rebound has been identified as a risk factor for onset of obesity (Taylor et al., 2005), identification and close surveillance of children with early adiposity rebound provides a potential opportunity for early intervention efforts. Parental weight status has also been identified as a risk factor for overweight in children (Safer, Agras, Bryson, & Hammer, 2001), and has been associated with early adiposity rebound (Dorosty et al., 2000), suggesting its utility as another marker for early intervention and prevention efforts. At least one study targeted modification of dietary habits in nonoverweight school age children of overweight parents (Epstein et al., 2001).

School Age. Given that the nutrient quality of foods consumed decreases from childhood to early adulthood, one opportunity for obesity prevention efforts is to maintain the quality of diet through school-age years. Primary targets with regard to dietary intake include limited consumption of sugar-sweetened beverages and increased consumption of fruits and vegetables (Barlow and the Expert Committee, 2007).

A second area for prevention efforts in school-age children relates to eating habits. It has been suggested that encouraging daily consumption of breakfast may be an effective strategy in the prevention of pediatric obesity (Expert Committee on the Assessment, Prevention and Treatment of Child and Adolescent Overweight and Obesity, 2007; O'Dea & Wilson, 2006). Another recommendation relates to the encouragement of family meals (Expert Committee on the Assessment, Prevention and Treatment of Child and Adolescent Overweight and Obesity). Eating fewer family meals and watching more TV was associated with an increased probability of overweight in a longitudinal study of young school-age children—suggesting the potential benefits of increasing frequency of family meals for prevention efforts (Gable, Chang, & Krull, 2007).

Encouragement of physical activity, and a reduction in sedentary behaviors, are also key targets for prevention efforts. When children reach age four years and older, they are able to participate in more structured activities and team sports (e.g., pee wee soccer). As children's nervous systems mature, myelination of nerve fibers finishes—therefore, fast reactions and skilled movements can fully develop, resulting in improvements in balance, agility, coordination, and ability to participate in a structured sport (Wilmore & Costill, 1994). An estimated 45 million children in the United States participate in youth sports (Weinberg & Gould, 2007, p 514). However, participation peaks at a critical developmental period in the child's life (between the ages of 10 and 13 years), and slowly continues to decline to the age of 18 years (Weinberg and Gould, p 514). Most of the motives children have to participate in nonschool and school sports are intrinsic (e.g., to have fun, learn skills) (Weinberg and Gould, p 515). A positive approach to coaching during this time leads to fewer dropouts (5%) compared to untrained coaching (26%)—therefore, special attention should be paid to the kind and quality of coaching, especially during this period (Weinberg and Gould, p 525).

Preadolescence is an especially sensitive time for encouraging participation in physical activity, given the documented drop-off—especially for girls. Parental or coaching strategies to increase physical activity participation during this period include: 1) giving praise sincerely and immediately; 2) developing realistic expectations; 3) rewarding effort as much as outcome; 4) focusing on teaching and practicing skills; and 5) focusing on limiting screen time and increasing outdoor time (Weinberg & Gould, 2007, p 526). Limiting television viewing and other screen time to one or two hours daily and removing televisions from children's sleeping areas has been explicitly recommended as a strategy to prevent the onset of obesity in children (Expert Committee on the Assessment, Prevention and Treatment of Child and Adolescent Overweight and Obesity, 2007).

Other potential strategies for increasing physical activity in school-age children include encouraging those variables that have been associated with involvement in physical activity. For example, motor proficiency was positively related to time spent in physical activity as measured by accelerometer, and negatively related to sedentary behavior in a sample of school-age children—suggesting the potential utility of proficiency as an appropriate target to support increased physical activity (Wrotniak, Epstein, Dorn, Jones, & Kondilis, 2006). Similarly, self-efficacy and parental involvement have been identified as other potential targets for intervention. Low self-efficacy related to physical activity was related to decline in physical activity participation for girls and boys over a one-year period (Barnett, O'Loughlin, & Paradis, 2002). Other important variables included lack of participation in team sports and the amount of time spent watching TV—suggesting the potential utility of these dimensions as targets for interventions to prevent declines in physical activity in this age group. Investigators have also noted the importance of increasing self-efficacy related to physical activity, and parent modeling of physical activity, and providing access to outlets as strategies for promoting physical activity in overweight school-age children (Trost, Kerr, Ward, & Pate, 2001). Finally, in a sample of African-American school-age girls, parental self-efficacy related to girls' activity was related to girls' participation in physical activity—suggesting a potential role for increasing parental self-efficacy (Adkins, Sherwood, Story, & Davis, 2004).

Adolescence. Given the significant tracking of weight status from adolescence through adulthood (Guo et al., 2002), adolescence may offer a critical period for prevention of adult overweight. Ideally, prevention efforts and establishment of healthy eating and physical activity habits begin well before adolescence. With that in mind, we briefly review potential key targets for this age group. A key consideration in prevention strategies with adolescents relates to the development of increasing autonomy, necessitating an ongoing negotiation of responsibility related to both diet and physical activity. While fostering adolescent independence is important, parents continue to play a key role in supporting health behaviors in this age group (DeVore & Ginsburg, 2005).

A key variable related to dietary intake in adolescence is the consumption of sugar-sweetened beverages, which has been positively related to weight status in a number of studies (Malik, Schulze, & Hu, 2006; Sanigorski, Bell, & Swinburn, 2007). As noted above, limiting consumption of sugar-sweetened beverages has been identified as an important strategy in obesity prevention efforts (Barlow and the Expert Committee, 2007). An environmental intervention to replace sugar-sweetened beverages with noncaloric alternatives was effective in significantly reducing sweetened beverage consumption, and showed promise in decreasing BMI in the heaviest adolescents (Ebbeling et al., 2006). Frequency of family meals constitutes a second key dietary target with adolescents. The frequency of family meals has been associated with increased consumption of fruits, vegetables, and dairy (Videon & Manning, 2003) and making family meals a priority was protective against disordered eating in a large sample of adolescents (Neumark-Sztainer, Wall, Story, & Fulkerson, 2004). The current data do not yet provide an understanding of the mechanisms through which family meals are beneficial; however, it is possible that family meals provide an opportunity to model healthful choices (Neumark-Sztainer, Story, Perry, & Casey, 1999) or reflect a more general pattern of family connectedness (Neumark-Sztainer, et al., 2004).

Encouraging participation in physical activity during the younger years is important to the ability of girls to maintain involvement through adolescence (Pate et al., 2007). Also of importance is the identification of variables related to physical activity involvement during adolescence. In a longitudinal study of adolescent girls, time constraints were negatively related to time spent in physical activity, and social support from family, peers, and teachers. To a lesser extent, self-perception was positively related to involvement in physical activity (Neumark-Sztainer, Story, Hannan, Tharp, & Rex, 2003). The authors noted the potential benefit of targeting these dimensions in interventions to promote physical activity in adolescent girls. Similarly, support from family and friends, higher self-efficacy, and more enjoyment in physical activity were found to correlate with physical activity involvement in both overweight and nonoverweight adolescents—suggesting these as key factors in engaging adolescents in physical activity (DeBourdeaudjuij et al., 2005). Several studies have documented relationships between parental support and involvement and adolescent participation in physical activity (Sallis, Prochaska, & Taylor, 2000). Higher levels of physical activity were reported by young adolescents who perceived strong parent support for physical activity, and whose parents engaged in physical activity with them (Heitzler, Martin, Duke, & Huhman, 2006). Parental support for physical activity was directly related to adolescent participation in physical activity (Trost et al., 2003) and parent transportation for physical activity was significantly related to adolescent participation in physical activity outside of school (Hoefer, McKenzie, Sallis, Marshall, & Conway, 2001). Finally, adolescent perception of parental encouragement of physical activity was related to time spent in physical activity (McGuire et al., 2002).

Engaging adolescents in physical activity may require novel approaches. As an example, a resistance-training intervention specifically targeted at overweight adolescents was effective in increasing insulin sensitivity in teens at risk for developing type II diabetes (Shaibi et al., 2006). While involvement with video and computer games is typically counter-intuitive with regard to increasing physical activity, there may be a role for computer activities such as Dance Dance Revolution to captivate adolescent involvement in physical activity (Brown, 2006). Such programs need to be evaluated empirically, as novelty does not necessarily increase efficacy. In a brief intervention delivered through print material or the Web to increase physical activity self-efficacy and intentions, comparable increases were seen in physical activity self-efficacy, but the print group demonstrated greater increases in physical activity intentions (Marks et al., 2006).

Recent guidelines from the American Heart Association Council on nutrition, physical activity, and metabolism regarding increasing physical activity for school-age children and adolescents center on an expanded role for schools, including children and teens receiving a minimum of 30 minutes of moderate to vigorous physical activity during the school day; expanded opportunities for intramurals; clubs, etc.; encouragement of physical activity to get to school; and linkages to community agencies that offer physical activity (Pate et al., 2006). Opportunities for alternatives to *traditional organized sports* such as afterschool fitness classes, intramural sports, open gymnasium time, and playing fields not dedicated to varsity sports, as well as afterschool and community-based programs, would also support adolescent involvement in physical activity. Improvements in physical activity and fitness have been reported as a result of such noncurricular and community-based programs (Colchico, Zybert, & Basch, 2000; Resnicow et al., 2005); however, city-wide assessment and access to these programs needs to be performed to determine the implications of such programs on a larger scale (Hannon et al., 2006; Pate et al., 2000). Multiple community settings outside of school should emphasize physical activity, including public and private organizations, worksites, government agencies, and businesses (Baranowski et al., 2000; Pate et al.).

CONCLUSIONS

In summary, consideration of developmental status provides important direction regarding normative growth, energy demands, and capacity to engage in physical activity. While there is considerable continuity in these dimensions over time, there is also opportunity for change and intervention. Of critical importance to the prevention of pediatric obesity is establishment of healthy eating and activity habits during the preschool years, which need to be supported through anticipated declines in physical activity and quality of dietary intake through preadolescence and adolescence.

REFERENCES

Aaron, D. J., Storti, I. L., Robertson, R. J., Kriska, A. M., & LaPorte, R. E. (2002). Longitudinal study of the number of choice of leisure time physical activities from mid to late adolescents: Implications for school curricula and community recreation programs. *Archives of Pediatrics & Adolescent Medicine, 156*(11), 1075–1080.

Abbassi, V. (1998). Growth and normal puberty. *Pediatrics, 102*(2, Pt. 3), 507–511.

Adkins, S., Sherwood, N. E., Story, M., & Davis, M. (2004). Physical activity among African-American girls: The role of parents and the home environment. *Obesity Research, 12*(Suppl.), 38S–45S.

American College of Sports Medicine. (1993). The prevention of sports injuries of children and adolescents. *Medicine and Science in Sports and Exercise, 25*(Suppl. 8), 1–7.

American Dietetic Association (2004). Position of the American Dietetic Association: Dietary guidance for healthy children ages 2 to 11 years. *Journal of the American Dietetic Association, 104*, 660–677.

American Heart Association, Gidding, S. S., Dennison, B. A., Birch, L. L., Daniels, S. R., Gilman, M. W., et al. (2006). Dietary recommendations for children and adolescents: A guide for practitioners. *Pediatrics, 117*, 544–559.

Baranowski, T., Mendlein, J., Resnicow, K., Frank, E., Cullen, K. W., & Baranowski, J. (2000). Physical activity and nutrition in children and youth: An overview of obesity prevention. *Preventative Medicine, 31*, S1–S10.

Barlow, S. E., & Dietz, W. H. (1998). Obesity evaluation and treatment: Expert committee recommendations. *Pediatrics, 102*, e29. Retrieved from http://www.pediatrics.org/ cgi/content/full/102/3/e29.

Barlow, S. E., & the Expert Committee (2007). Expert committee recommendations regarding the prevention, assessment, and treatment of child and adolescent overweight and obesity: Summary report. *Pediatrics*, S164–S192.

Barnett, T. A., O'Loughlin, J., & Paradis, G. (2002). One- and two-year predictors of decline in physical activity among inner-city schoolchildren. *American Journal of Preventive Medicine, 23*(2), 121–128.

Brent, R. L. & Weitzman, M. (2004). The pediatricians' role and responsibility in educating parents about environmental risk. *Pediatrics, 113*, 1167–1172.

Brown, D. (2006). Playing to win: Video games and the fight against obesity. *Journal of the American Dietetic Association, 106*(2), 188–189.

Centers for Disease Control and Prevention (1997). Youth risk behavior surveillance: United States. *MMWR, 47*(1), 89.

Colchico, K., Zybert, P., & Basch, C. E. (2000). Effects of after-school physical activity on fitness, fatness and cognitive self-perceptions: A pilot study among urban, minority adolescent girls. *American Journal of Public Health, 90*(6), 977–978.

De Bourdeaudhuij, I., Lefevre, J., Deforche, B., Wijndaele, K., Matton, L., & Philippaerts, R. (2005). Physical activity and psychosocial correlates in normal weight and overweight 11 to 19 year olds. *Obesity Research, 13*(6), 1097–1105.

Demory-Luce, D., Morales, M., Nicklas, T., Baranowski, T., Zakeri, I., & Berenson, G. (2004). Changes in food group consumption patterns from childhood to young adulthood: The Bogalusa Heart Study. *Journal of the American Dietetic Association, 104*, 1684–1691.

DeVore, E. R. & Ginsburg, K. R. (2005). The protective effects of good parenting on adolescents. *Current Opinions in Pediatrics, 17*, 460–465.

Dietz, W. H. (1994). Critical periods in childhood for the development of obesity. *American Journal of Clinical Nutrition, 59*, 955–959.

Dietz, W. H., & Gortmaker, S. L. (2001). Preventing obesity in children and adolescents. *Annual Review in Public Health, 22*, 337–353.

Dietz, W. H., & Robinson, T. N. (2005). Overweight children and adolescents. *New England Journal of Medicine, 352*, 2100–2109.

Dorosty, A. R., Emmett, P. M., Cowin, S., & Reilly, J. J. (2000). Factors associated with early adiposity rebound. ALSPAC study team. *Pediatrics, 105*, 1115–1118.

Ebbeling, C. B., Feldman, H. A., Osganian, S. K., Chomitz, V. R., Ellenbogen, S. J. & Ludwig, D. S. (2006). Effects of decreasing sugar-sweetened beverage consumption on body weight in adolescents: A randomized, controlled pilot study. *Pediatrics, 117*, 673–80.

Epstein, L. H., Gordy, C. C., Raynor, H. A., Beddome, M., Kilanowski, C. K., & Paluch, R. (2001). Increasing fruit and vegetable intake and decreasing fat and sugar intake in families at risk for childhood obesity. *Obesity Research, 9*, 171–178.

Faigenbaum, A. D., Westcott, W. L., LaRosa L., R., & Long, C. (1999). The effects of resistance training protocols on muscular strength and endurance development in children. *Pediatrics, 104*, e5–e11.

Fiorito, L. M., Mitchell, D. C., Smiciklas-Wright, H., & Birch, L. L. (2006). Dairy and dairy- related nutrient intake during middle childhood. *Journal of the American Dietetic Association, 106*, 534–542.

Fisher, J. O., & Birch, L. L. (2002). Eating in the absence of hunger and overweight in girls from 5 to 7y of age. *American Journal of Clinical Nutrition, 76*, 226–231.

Gable, S., Chang, Y., & Krull, J. L. (2007). Television watching and frequency of family meals are predictive of overweight onset and persistence in a national sample of school-aged children. *Journal of the American Dietetic Association, 107*(1), 53–61.

Gordon-Larsen, P., Nelson, M. C., & Popkin, B. M. (2004). Longitudinal physical activity and sedentary behavior trends: Adolescence to adulthood. *American Journal of Preventative Medicine, 27*(4), 277–283.

Guo, S. S., Wu, W., Chumlea, W. C., & Roche, A. F. (2002). Predicting overweight and obesity in adulthood from body mass index values in childhood and adolescene. *American Journal of Clinical Nutrition, 76*, 653–658.

Hannon, C., Cradock, A., Gortmaker, S. L., Wiecha, J., El Ayandi, A., Keefe, L., et al. (2006). Play across Boston: A community initiative to reduce disparities in access to after-school physical activity programs for inner-city youths. *Preventing Chronic Disease* [serial online] 2006 Jul [June 25, 2007]. Retrieved from: URL: http//www.cdc.gov/pcd/issues/2006/jul/05_0125.htm.

Heitzler, C. D., Martin, S. L., Duke, J., & Huhman, M. (2006). Correlates of physical activity in a national sample of children aged 9–13 years. *Preventive Medicine, 42*, 254–260.

Hoefer, W. R., McKenzie, T. L., Sallis, J. F., Marshall, S. J., & Conway, T. L. (2001). Parental provision of transportation for adolescent physical activity. *American Journal of Preventive Medicine, 21*, 48–51.

Insel, P. Turner, R. E., & Ross, D. (2007). Nutrition. In P. Insel, R. E. Turner, & D. Ross (Eds.). Sudbury, MA: Jones and Bartlett.

Janz, K. F., Burns, T. L., & Levy, S. M. (2005). Tracking of activity and sedentary behaviors in childhood: The Iowa Bone Development Study. *American Journal of Preventative Medicine, 29*(3), 171–178.

Janz, K. F., Dawson, J. D., & Mahoney, L. T. (2000). Tracking physical fitness and physical activity from childhood to adolescence: The muscatine study. *Medicine & Science in Sports & Exercise, 32*(7), 1250–1257.

Kahn, E. B., Ramsey, L. T., Brownson, R. C., Heath, G. W., Howze, E. H., Powell, K. E., et al. (2002). The effectiveness of interventions to increase physical activity. A systematic review. *American Journal of Preventative Medicine, 22*(Suppl. 4), 73–107.

Kelder, S. H., Perry, C. L., Klepp. K. I., & Lytle, L. L. (1994). Longitudinal tracking of adolescent smoking, physical activity, and food choice behaviors. *American Journal of Public Health, 84*, 1121–1126.

Kemper, H. C., Snel, J., Verschuur, R., & Storm-van Essen, L. (1990). Tracking of health and risk indicators of cardiovascular diseases from teenager to adult: Amsterdam Growth and Health Study. *Preventative Medicine, 19*(6), 642–655.

Lillegard, W., Brown, E., Wilson, D., Henderson, R., & Lewis, E. (1997). Efficacy of strength training in prepubescent to early postpubescent males and females: Effects of gender and maturity. *Pediatric Rehabilitation, 1*, 147–157.

Livingstone, M. B., Robson, P. J., Wallace, J. M., & McKinley, M. C. (2003). How active are we? Levels of routine physical activity in children and adults. *Proceedings of the Nutrition Society, 62*(3), 681–701.

Malik, V. S., Schulze, M. B., & Hu, F. B. (2006). Intake of sugar-sweetened beverages and weight gain: A systemic review. *American Journal of Clinical Nutrition, 84*, 274–288.

Malina, R. M. (1996). Tracking of physical activity and physical fitness across the lifespan. *Research Quarterly for Exercise and Sport, 67*(Suppl. 3), S48–57.

Malina, R. M. (2001). Physical activity and fitness: pathways from childhood to adulthood. *American Journal of Human Biology, 13*(2), 162–172.

Mannino, M. L., Lee, Y., Mitchell, D. C., Smiciklas-Wright, H., & Birch, L. L. (2004). The quality of girls' diets declines and tracks across middle childhood. *International Journal of Behavioral Nutrition and Physical Activity, 1*, 5–15.

Marks, J. T., Campbell, M. K., Ward, D. S., Ribisl, K. M., Wildemuth, B. M., & Symons, M. J. (2006). A comparison of web and print media for physical activity promotion among adolescent girls. *Journal of Adolescent Health, 39*(1), 96–104.

McGuire, M. T., Hannan, P. J., Neumark-Sztainer, D., Cossrow, N. H., & Story, M. (2002). Parental correlates of physical activity in a racially/ethnically diverse adolescent sample. *Journal of Adolescent Health, 30*(4), 253–261.

Nelson, M. C., Neumark-Sztainer, D., Hannan, P. J., Sirard, J. R., & Story, M. (2006). Longitudinal and secular trends in physical activity and sedentary behavior during adolescence. *Pediatrics, 118*(6), 1627–1634.

Neumark-Sztainer, D., Story, M., Hannan, P. J., Tharp, T., & Rex, J. (2003). Factors associated with changes in physical activity: A cohort study of inactive adolescent girls. *Archives of Pediatric and Adolescent Medicine, 157*, 803–810.

Neumark-Sztainer, D., Story, M., Perry, C. & Casey, M.A. (1999). Factors influencing food choices of adolescents: Findings from focus-group discussions with adolescents. *Journal of the American Dietetic Association, 99*, 929–937.

Neumark-Sztainer, D., Wall, M., Story M., Fulkerson, J. A. (2004). Are family meal patterns associated with disordered eating behaviors among adolescents? *Journal of Adolescent Health, 35*(5), 350–359.

O'Dea, J. A. & Wilson, R. (2006). Socio-cognitive and nutritional factors associated with body mass index in children and adolescents: Possibilities for childhood obesity prevention. *Health education research, 21*(6), 796–805.

Ogden, C. L., Carroll, M. D., Curtin, L. R., McDowell, M. A., Tabak, C. J., & Flegal, K. M. (2006). Prevalence of overweight and obesity in the United States, 1999–2004. *Journal of the American Medical Association, 295*(13), 1549–1555.

Pate, R. R., Davis, M. G., Robinson, T. N., Stone, E. J., McKenzie, T. L., & Young, J. C. (2006). Promoting physical activity in children and youth: A leadership role for schools: a scientific statement from the American Heart Association Council on Nutrition, Physical Activity, and Metabolism (Physical Activity Committee) in collaboration with the Councils on Cardiovascular Disease in the Young and Cardiovascular Nursing. *Circulation, 114*(11), 1214–1224.

Pate, R. R., Dowda, M., O'Neill, J. R., & Ward, D. S. (2007). Change in physical activity participation among adolescent girls from 8th to 12th grade. *Journal of Physical Activity and Health, 4*(1), 3–16.

Pate, R. R., Trost, S. G., Mullis, R., Sallis, J. F., Wechsler, H., & Brown, D. R. (2000). Community interventions to promote proper nutrition and physical activity among youth. *Preventative Medicine 31*, S138–S149.

Resnicow, K., Jackson, A., Blissett, D., Want, T., McCarty, F., Rahotep, S., & Periasamy, S. (2005). Results of the Healthy Body Healthy Spirit Trial. *Health Psychology, 24*(4), 339–348.

Raitakari, O. T., Porkka, K. V., Taimela, S., Telama, R., Rasanen, L., & Viikari, J. S. (1994). Effects of persistent physical activity and inactivity on coronary risk factors in children and young adults. The Cardiovascular Risk in Young Finns Study. *American Journal of Epidemiology, 140*(3), 195–205.

Rajeshwari, R., Nicklas, T.A., Yang, S.J., Berenson, G.S. (2004). Longitudinal changes in intake and food sources of calcium from childhood to young adulthood: The Bogalusa heart study. *Journal of the American College of Nutrition, 23*, 341–350.

Rolland-Cachera, M. F., Deheeger, M., Bellisle, F., Sempe, M., Guilloud-Bataille, M., & Patois, E. (1984). Adiposity rebound in children: A simple indicator for predicting obesity. *American Journal of Clinical Nutrition, 39*(1), 129–135.

Rolls, B. J., Engell, D., & Birch, L. L. (2000). Serving portion size influences 5-year-old children's food intakes. *Journal of the American Dietetic Association, 100*, 232–234.

Safer, D. L., Agras, W. S., Bryson, S., & Hammer, L. D. (2001) Early body mass index and other anthropometric relationships between parents and children. *International Journal of Obesity, 25*, 1532–1536.

Sallis, J. F., & Patrick, K. (1994). Physical activity guidelines for adolescents: consensus statement. *Pediatric Exercise Science, 6*, 302–314.

Sallis, J. F., Prochaska, J. J., Taylor, W. C. (2000). A review of correlates of physical activity of children and adolescents. *Medicine and Science in Sports and Exercise, 32*(5), 963–975.

Sallis, J. F., Berry, C. C., Broyles, S. L., McKenzie, T. L., & Nader, P. R. (1995). Variability and tracking of physical activity over 2 yr in young children. *Medicine & Science in Sports & Exercise, 27*(7), 1042–1049.

Salmon, J., Booth, M. L., Phongsavan, P., Murphy, N., & Timperio, A. (2007). Promoting physical activity participation among children and adolescents. *Epidemiology Reviews, 29*, 144–159.

Sanigorski, A. M., Bell, A. C., & Swinburn, B. A. (2007). Association of key foods and beverages with obesity in Australian school children. *Public Health Nutrition, 10*, 152–157.

Shaibi, C. Q., Cruz, M. L., Ball, G. D., Weigensberg, M. J., Salem, G. J., Crespo, N. C., et al. (2006). Effects of resistance training on insulin sensitivity in overweight Latino adolescent males. *Medicine & Science in Sports & Exercise, 38*, 1208–15.

Siervogel, R. M., Roche, A. F., Guo, S. M., Mukherjee, D., & Chumlea, W. C. (1991). Patterns of change in weight/stature2 from 2 to 18 years: findings from long-term serial data for children in the Fels longitudinal growth study. *International Journal of Obesity, 15*(7), 479–485.

Singer, M. R., Moore, L. L., Garrahie, E. J., & Ellison, R. C. (1995). The tracking of nutrient intake in young children: The Framingham children's study. *American Journal of Public Health, 85*, 1673–1677.

Skinner, J. D., Carruth, B. R., Bounds, W., & Ziegler, P. J. (2002). Children's food preferences: A longitudinal analysis. *Journal of the American Dietetic Association, 102*, 1638–1647.

Spear, B. A. (2002). Adolescent growth and development. *Journal of the American Dietetics Association, 102*(Suppl. 3), S23–29.

Strong, W. B., Malina, R. M., Blimkie, C. J., Daniels, S. R., Dishman, R. K., Gutin, B., et al. (2005). Evidence based physical activity for school-age youth. *Journal of Pediatrics, 146*(6), 732–737.

Tanner, J. M., & Davies, P. S. (1985). Clinical longitudinal standards for height and height velocity for North American children. *Journal of Pediatrics, 107*(3), 317–329.

Taylor, R. W., Grant, A. M., Goulding, A., & Williams, S. M. (2005). Early adiposity rebound: Review of papers linking this to subsequent obesity in children and adults. *Current Opinion in Clinical Nutrition and Metabolic Care, 8*(6), 607–661.

Taylor, R. W., Grant, A. M., Goulding, A., & Williams, S. M. (2005). Early adiposity rebound. Review of papers linking this to subsequent obesity in children and adults. *Current Opinions in Clinical Nutrition & Metabolic Care, 8*, 607–612.

Taylor, W. C., Blair, S. N., Cummings, S. S., Wun, C. C., & Malina, R. M. (1999). Childhood and adolescent physical activity patterns and adult physical activity. *Medicine & Science in Sports & Exercise, 31*(1), 118–123.

Trost, S. G., Kerr, L. M., Ward, D. S., & Pate, R. R. (2001). Physical activity and determinants of physical activity in obese and non-obese children. *International Journal of Obesity and Related Metabolic Disorders, 25*(6), 822–829.

Trost, S. G., Sallis, J. F., Pate, R. R., Freedson, P. S., Taylor, W. C., & Dowda, M. (2003). Evaluating a model of parental influence on youth physical activity. *American Journal of Preventive Medicine, 25*, 277–282.

U.S. Department of Human Services, & U.S. Department of Agriculture (2005). *Dietary Guidelines for Americans, 2005.* Washington D.C.: US Department of Health and Human Services/US Department of Agriculture.

Videon, T. M. & Manning C. K. (2003). Influences on adolescent eating patterns: the importance of family meals. *Journal of Adolescent Health, 32*(5), 365–373.

Wang, G., & Dietz, W. H. (2002). Economic burden of obesity in youths aged 6 to 17 years: 1979–1999. *Pediatrics, 109*, E81.

Whitaker, R. C., Pepe, M. S., Wright, J. A., Seidel, K. D., & Dietz, W. H. (1998). Early adiposity rebound and the risk of adult obesity. *Pediatrics, 101*(3), E5.

Weinberg, R. S. & Gould, D. (2007). Children and sport Psychology. In R. S. Weinberg & D. Gould (Eds.), *Foundations of Sport and Exercise Ppsychology* (pp. 514–532). Champaign, IL: Human Kinetics.

Wilmore, J. H. & Costill, D. L. (1994). Physiology of sport and exercise. In J. H. Wilmore & D. L. Costill (Eds.), *Growth, Development, and the Young Athlete* (pg. 400–421). Champaign, IL: Human Kinetics.

Wrotniak, B. H., Epstein, L. H., Dorn, J. M., Jones, K. E., & Kondilis, V. A. (2006). The relationship between motor proficiency and physical activity in children. *Pediatrics, 118*(6), 1758–1765.

Zwerin, L. D. & Manos, T. M. (1998). ACSM's Resource manual for guidelines for exercise testing and prescription. In J. L. Roitman, M. Kelsey, T. P. LaFontaine, D. R. Southard, M. A. Williams, & T. York (Eds.). *Exercise Testing and Prescription Considerations throughout Childhood* (pp. 507–515). Philadelphia, PA: Williams & Wilkins.

13

Evidence-Based Treatments for Childhood Obesity

HOLLIE A. RAYNOR

The prevalence of obesity in all age groups has increased dramatically over the past 30 years, such that overweight and obesity are considered to be a major public health concern in the United States (Baskin, Aard, Franklin, & Allison, 2005). Currently, 1.3 out of every 10 children aged 2 to 11 years is overweight ($\geq 95^{th}$ percentile body mass index [BMI]) (Hedley et al., 2004). The adverse medical and psychosocial effects of overweight in children have been well-established (Dietz, 1998). Childhood obesity is also associated with the development of several risk factors for heart disease, including hyperlipidemia, hyperinsulemia, and hypertension, and other chronic diseases in adulthood (Berenson et al., 1998; Janssen et al., 2005). Finally, being overweight as a child increases the likelihood of being overweight as an adult (Janssen et al.; Whitaker, Wright, Pepe, Seidel, & Dietz, 1997).

Due to the negative and potentially lifelong consequences of childhood obesity, treatment of overweight is necessary at its earliest detection in childhood (Yin, Wu, Liu, & Yu, 2005). Treatment of overweight during childhood is believed to have behavioral and biological advantages over treatment in adulthood (Epstein, Myers, Raynor, & Saelens, 1998) that may aid in better long-term weight loss maintenance. Changing eating and activity behaviors may be easier in childhood; problematic behaviors have not been in place as long for children as they have usually been for adults. Moreover, research indicates that preferences, particularly for food, are learned. Thus, in children, food experiences can be encouraged to shape patterns of food preference that are consistent with healthier diets starting at a young age—thereby assisting with better long-term dietary adherence

HOLLIE A. RAYNOR • University of Tennessee, Knoxville, TN 37996.

This paper was supported by Grant 7-05-HFC-27 from the American Diabetes Association, and by Grant DK074919 from the National Institute of Diabetes and Digestive and Kidney Diseases.

(Birch, 1999; Birch & Fisher, 1998). Family support for behavior change may also be easier to establish for children than for adults (Epstein et al.). Treatment of obesity in childhood has the added benefit of taking advantage of linear growth, and increases in lean muscle mass, as well as reductions in weight, that are not possible in the treatment of adults (Epstein, Valoski, & McCurley, 1993). The advantage of growth may mean that smaller and/or fewer changes in the diet and/or leisure-time activity may produce a healthier weight status in children, as compared to adults, and these smaller changes may be easier to successfully maintain. Finally, while obesity treatment in adults causes shrinkage but not loss of excess adipose cells, treatment of obesity in children may prevent the development of excess adipose cells, again helping with long-term weight loss maintenance (Epstein et al.).

Indeed, findings from childhood obesity research interventions provide evidence that treatment during childhood may produce better long-term outcomes than treatment during adulthood. Two research groups have shown successful long-term weight loss maintenance in children, during follow-up periods of five (Knip & Nuutinen, 1993) and 10 years (Epstein, Valoski, Kalarchian, & McCurley, 1995; Epstein, Valoski, Wing, & McCurley, 1990, 1994), in which almost one-third of treated preadolescent children were nonobese after 10 years. These outcomes are better than what is found with obesity treatment in adults (Wing, 2002). While long-term weight loss outcomes in children appear to be better, there is still a considerable amount of relapse in treated children (Epstein, Valoski, Kalarchian, et al.), thus research is still needed to improve long-term success in childhood obesity treatments.

Ideally, pediatric obesity treatment should regulate body weight through providing adequate nutrition for growth and development, so that loss of lean muscle mass is minimized and linear growth is not compromised (Rees, 1990). Treatment should also change eating and activity behaviors, and variables that regulate these behaviors, in such a way that the new behaviors are sustainable throughout the lifetime (Epstein et al., 1998). Finally, treatment should be associated with improvements in physiological and psychological consequences of obesity, and not produce new negative outcomes (i.e., the development of an eating disorder). The purpose of this chapter is to review evidence-based pediatric obesity interventions that involve modifications to the diet and/or leisure-time activity that are conducted within a clinical research setting. Evidence-based interventions were defined in accordance with criteria outlined in the Consolidated Standard for Reporting Trials (CONSORT) (Altman et al., 2001; Davidson et al., 2003). The goal of the CONSORT guidelines is to facilitate the design, reporting, and review of research to identify evidence-based treatments (EBTs). This review is organized by the major treatment components of childhood obesity, including diet, leisure-time activity, behavioral strategies, and structure of treatment. While these components are described separately, it is important to note that outcomes are best when dietary, leisure-time activities, and behavior modification components are integrated (Epstein et al.). Also, because the interventions provide components from several arenas (i.e., diet, leisure-time activities, and behavior modification) with differing doses or prescription within the different components, extracting the contribution of each treatment component is not possible.

STUDY SELECTION

Relevant studies for this review were found using two methods. The first involved reviewing the references of two reviews of pediatric obesity treatment (Epstein et al., 1998; Jelalian & Saelens, 1999). The second involved searches through computerized databases (i.e., Medline and PsychInfo) using the following keywords: childhood, pediatric, juvenile, obese, obesity, overweight, treatment, and intervention. Only randomized trials were included in this review (if studies did not provide detail about how groups were selected, these studies were not considered to be random). Included studies also investigated participants ≤ 13 years of age (adolescent obesity interventions are reviewed in a separate chapter), targeted weight loss as a primary objective, and delivered the intervention in an outpatient setting. Exclusionary criteria included: 1) intervention delivered within a school, camp, or residential housing setting; 2) intervention conducted with special populations (i.e., children with chronic illness/developmental disability); and 3) interventions using medication, dietary supplements, or surgery. Based upon these criteria, 29 studies were identified.

The CONSORT guidelines include 22 items to include in publications to help determine EBTs (Davidson et al., 2003). None of the 29 studies identified included all 22 items. Therefore, 10 key items were identified. These key items included: 1) scientific background and explanation of rationale; 2) eligibility criteria for participants; 3) precise details of the intervention intended for each group; 4) specific hypotheses or objectives; 5) clearly defined primary outcome measures; 6) a separate statistical methods section that described statistical methods used to compare groups for primary outcomes; 7) baseline demographics and clinical characteristics of participants; 8) a summary of results for primary outcomes; 9) interpretation of results; and 10) general interpretation of results in context of current evidence. Based upon these criteria, 13 of the previously identified 29 studies were included in this review. For reviews that do not use the CONSORT guidelines, and thereby include more pediatric obesity intervention studies, please see Epstein et al. (1998) and Jelalian and Saelens (1999).

Details of the randomized studies that were included in this review are presented in Tables 13.1 and 13.2. Table 13.1 includes a description of the studies, which includes age, group assignment, randomized sample size, gender distribution, dietary components, leisure-time activity components, and behavior modification components. Table 13.2 contains the primary anthropometric outcomes of the investigations. There were several dependent measures used across the studies, but the most common ones that have been included in the table are percent overweight, BMI, standardized BMI (z-BMI), and body weight. In Table 13.2, the baseline values are provided, along with change during treatment and change during follow-up from baseline.

Table 13.1. Characteristics of randomized trials of childhood obesity treatment in outpatient settings

Source	Age (y)	Group assignment	Between-group variable	N	% Girls	Diet	Leisure-time	B Mod
Becque, Katch, Rocchini, Marks, and Moorehead (1988)	12–13	R	1. PA 2. No PA 3. No treatment control	36	58.3	ADA exchange for ↓ 1–2lb/wk (1,2)	50 min, 3x/wk supervised aerobic activity (1); no SI (1,2)	PR,SC, SM (1,2)
Epstein, Wing, Koeske, Andrasik, and Ossip (1981) and Epstein et al. (1994)	6–12	RS	1. Mother and child targeted 2. Child targeted 3. Nonspecific target	76	69.6[a]	Traffic-light diet 1200 or 1500 kcals (1,2,3)	EI (1,2,3); no SI (1,2,3)	M,PR,SC, SM (1,2,3)
Epstein, Paluch, Kilanowski, and Raynor (2004)	8–12	R	1. Reinforced ↓ SB (15 hrs/wk) 2. Stimulus control ↓ SB (15 hrs/wk)	63	61.9	Traffic-light diet 800–1200 kcals (1,2)	EI (1,2); ↓ SB 15 hrs/wk (1,2)	M,PP,PR, PS,SC, SM (1,2)
Epstein, Paluch, Gordy, and Dorn (2000)	8–12	RS	1. ↓ SB high 2. ↓ SB low 3. ↑ PA high 4. ↑ PA low	90	68.4[a]	Traffic-light diet 1000–1200 kcals (1,2,3,4)	↓ SB 20 hrs/wk (1); ↓ SB 10 hrs/wk (2); ↑ PA 20 miles/wk (3); ↑ PA 10 miles/wk (4)	M,PP,PR, PS,SC.SM (1,2,3,4)
Epstein, Paluch, Gordy, Saelens, and Ernst (2000)	8–12	RS	1. Problem solving with parent and child 2. Problem solving with child 3. Standard family-based treatment	67	57.9[a]	Traffic-light diet 1200 kcals (1,2,3)	Lifestyle PA (1,2,3); no SI (1,2,3)	M,PP,PR, SC, SM (1,2,3); PS (1,2)
Epstein, Paluch, and Raynor (2001)	8–12	R	1. ↑ PA 2. ↑ PA + ↓ SB	67	50.7	Traffic-light diet 1200–1500 kcals (1,2)	↑ PA 180 min/wk (1,2); ↓ SB 15 hrs/wk (2)	M,PP,PR, PS, SC,SM (1,2)
Epstein, Valoski, Vara, et al. (1995)	8–12	R	1. ↑ PA 2. ↓ SB 3. ↑ PA + ↓ SB	61	73[a]	Traffic-light diet 1000–1200 kcals (1,2,3)	↑ PA 1500 kcal/wk (1); ↓ SB 15 hrs/wk (2); ↑ PA and ↓ SB (3)	M,PR,SC SM (1,2,3)
Epstein, Wing, Koeske, and Valeski (1985) and Epstein et al. (1994)	8–12	R	1. Programmed aerobic activity 2. Lifestyle activity 3. Calisthenics	41	60[a]	Traffic-light diet 1200 kcals (1,2,3)	Aerobic 3x/wk (1); lifestyle (2); calisthenics 3x/wk (3) activity; isocaloric across groups; no SI (1,2,3)	M,PR,SM (1,2,3)

Study	Age		Conditions	N	%	Diet	Physical Activity	Behavioral Techniques
Epstein, Wing, Penner, and Kress (1985)	8–12	RS	1. PA 2. No PA	23	100	Traffic-light diet 900–1200kcals (1,2)	Supervised exercise, 3-mile walk, 3x/wk (1); no SI (1,2)	M,PR,SC SM (1,2)
Golan, Wiezman, Apter, and Fainaru (1998)	6–11	RM	1. Parent as change agent 2. Child as change agent	60	61.7	NI, lower fat content of family diet (1); 1500kcals (2)	EI (1,2); no SI (1,2)	M,PS,SC (1);PS,SC, SM (2)
Goldfield Epstein. Kilanowski, Paluch & Kogut-Bossler, 2001	8–12	R	1. Group and individual treatment 2. Group treatment	31	70.8a	Traffic-light diet 1000–1200 kcals (1,2)	↑ PA 180 min/wk (1,2); no SI (1,2)	M, PP, PR, PS, SC, SM (1,2)
Graves, Meyers, and Clark (1988)	6–12	RS	1. Parent problem-solving 2. No parent problem-solving 3. Education only	40	NR	NI (1,2,3)	EI (1,2,3); no SI (1,2,3)	PR,SC,SM (1,2); PS (1)
Senediak and Spence (1985)	6–13	R	1. Rapid schedule behavior modification 2. Gradual schedule behavior modification 3. Attention control 4. Wait-list control	45	–33.3	Traffic-light diet, food exchange (1,2)	30min, 4x/wk aerobic activity, lifestyle activity (1,2); no SI (1,2)	M, PR,SC SM (1,2)

a. Percentage based upon children that finished treatment.

Notes. N = number of participants randomized to conditions; B Mod = behavior modification techniques; R= participants were randomly assigned to conditions; PA = physical activity; ADA = American Diabetes Association; SI = sedentary information; PR = positive reinforcement; SC = stimulus control; SM = self-monitoring; RS = participants were stratified on key variables and then randomly assigned to conditions; EI = exercise information; M = Modeling; SB = sedentary behaviors; PP = pre-planning; PS = problem-solving; RM = participants were randomized to conditions matched on key variables; NI = Nutrition information; NR = not reported.

Table 13.2. Outcomes of randomized trials of childhood obesity treatment in outpatient settings

Source	OW %*	BMI*	z-BMI*	BW, lb*	Rx, mos	OW, %*	BMI*	z-BMI*	BW, lb*	FU, mos	OW, %*	BMI*	z-BMI*	BW, lb*	Results
Becque et al. (1988)					0–5					None					BW, Rx: 1=2=3
				149.4	1				↓ 3.5						
				169.8	2				↓ 0.9						
				151.1	3				↑ 7.0						
Epstein et al. (1981, 1994)					0–8					0–120					OW, Rx: 1=2=3
	39.0	24.1			1	↓ 16.0‡				1	↓ 15.3				OW, FU: 1>3
	41.2	25.0			2	↓ 17.0‡				2	↓ 3.0				
	45.4	25.1			3	↓ 19.0‡				3	↑ 7.6				
Epstein et al. (2004)					0–6					0–12					z-BMI, Rx, FU: 1=2
	64.9		3.2		1			↓ 1.0‡		1			↓ 0.6‡		
	65.0		3.3		2			↓ 1.0‡		2			↓ 0.9‡		
Epstein et al. (2000)					0–6					0–24					OW, BW, Rx, FU: 1=2=3=4
	66.6			139.7	1	↓ 27.4‡			↓ 14.7‡	1	↓ 14.3‡			↑ 19.8‡	
	55.8			126.3	2	↓ 22.4‡			↓ 10.1‡	2	↓ 11.6‡			↑ 20.0‡	
	62.3			130.2	3	↓ 26.4‡			↓ 13.9‡	3	↓ 13.2‡			↑ 19.8‡	
	62.7			135.7	4	↓ 25.6‡			↓ 14.1‡	4	↓ 12.4‡			↑ 19.6‡	
Epstein, Paluch, Gordy, Saelens, et al. (2000)					0–6					0–24					z-BMI, BW, Rx: 1=2=3; z-BMI, BW, FU: 3>1, 2=1, 2=3
			2.8	141.2	1			↓ 1.3	↓ 15.0	1			↓ 0.5	↑ 26.2	
			2.6	128.0	2			↓ 1.4	↓ 15.4	2			↓ 0.9	↑ 15.8	
			2.7	125.4	3			↓ 1.5	↓ 13.6	3			↓ 1.1	↑ 15.8	
Epstein, Paluch, and Raynor (2001)					0–6					0–12					OW, Rx, FU: 2 boys> 1 girls, 2 girls; 2 boys=1 boys BMI, FU: 2 boys> 1 girls, 2 girls; 2 boys=1 boys
	58.4	27.3		134.5	1-boys	↓ 11.0				1-boys	↓ 9.0‡	↓ 0.65			
	56.8	26.9		127.8	1-girls	↓ 7.0				1-girls	↓ 6.5‡	↓ 0.27			
	61.9	27.5		132.8	2-boys	↓ 17.0				2-boys	↓ 15.5‡	↓ 1.76			
	64.1	27.9		134.7	2-girls	↓ 6.0				2-girls	↓ 0.5‡	↑ 1.00			
Epstein, Valoski, Vara, et al. (1995)					0–4					0–12					OW, Rx: 2>1
	51.8 Total				1	↓ 13.0				1	↓ 9.0				OW, FU: 2>1,3
					2	↓ 20.0				2	↓ 18.0				
					3	↓ 17.0				3	↓ 10.0				

Study	Baseline*	Rx (mos)	Change†	Change†	FU (mos)	Change†	Change†	Significant effects
Epstein, Wing, Koeske et al. (1985) and Epstein et al. (1994)	47.8	0–12 1	↓ 16.3‡	↑ 2.4	0–120 1	↓ 10.9		OW, BW, Rx: 1=2=3
	48.3	2	↓ 16.1‡	↓ 2.3	2	↓ 19.7		OW, FU: 1,2>3
	48.0	3	↓ 17.5‡	↓ 2.3	3	↑ 12.2		
Epstein, Wing, Penner, et al. (1985)	48.0	0–12 1	↓ 25.4‡	↓ 8.5‡	None			OW, BW, Rx: 1=2
	48.1	2	↓ 18.7‡	↓ 3.0				
Golan et al. (1998)	39.6	0–12 1	↓ 14.6‡		0–18 1	↓ 12.4		OW, Rx, FU: 1>2
	39.1	2	↓ 8.1‡		2	↓ 3.2		
Goldfield, et al. (2001)	60.4 3.0	0–6	↓ 10.0‡ Total	↓ 0.6‡ Total	0–12	↓ 8.0‡ Total	↓ 0.6‡ Total	OW, z-BMI, Rx, FU: 1=2
	56.4 2.7							
Graves et al. (1988)	53.0	0–2 1	↓ 13.5‡	↓ 8.3‡	0–8 1	↓ 24.5	↓ 9.1	OW, BW, Rx, FU: 1>2.3
	56.3	2	↓ 8.6‡	↓ 4.7‡	2	↓ 10.2	↓ 0.5	
	51.8	3	↓ 4.7	↓ 3.2	3	↓ 9.5	↑ 2.5	
Senediak and Spence (1985)	34.6	Varied 1 0–1	↓ 5.3	↓ 3.7	0–7 1	↓ 13.0	↓ 2.4	OW, BW, Rx: 2>1>3,4
	34.9	2 0–4	↓ 13.6	↓ 7.9	2	↓ 19.2	↓ 6.1	OW, BW, FU: 1,2>3
	41.7	3 0–1	↓ 1.4	↓ 0.7	3	↓ 5.9	↑ 0.6	
	37.6	4 0–1	↑ 2.3	↑ 1.7				

* Baseline

† Change from baseline values

‡ Value significantly different from baseline value

Notes. OW = indicates overweight; BMI = body mass index; z-BMI = standardized body mass index; BW = body weight; Rx = treatment period; FU = follow – up; lb = pounds; mos = months.

DIET

Diet interventions for obesity treatment predominantly focus on reducing energy intake and/or restructuring dietary intake to follow current dietary recommendations. There are several methods in which caloric reduction and/or improvements in nutrient quality of the diet can occur. One method is to provide nutrition guidelines that encourage dietary choices to be lower in fat and or more nutrient dense (i.e., fruits and vegetables over energy-dense, low-nutrient quality foods [chips and candy]) by using a food classification system without prescribing a daily energy goal (Golan et al., 1998; Graves et al., 1988; Senediak & Spence, 1985). Another method would involve solely prescribing a daily energy goal (Golan et al.). Finally, a combination of the previous two methods can occur (Becque et al., 1988; Epstein, Paluch, Gordy, & Dorn, 2000; Epstein, Paluch, Gordy, Saelens et al., 2000; Epstein et al. 2004; Epstein, Paluch, & Raynor, 2001; Epstein, Valoski, Vara, et al., 1995; Epstein, Wing, Koeske, Andrasik and Ossip, 1981; Epstein, Wing, Koeske, et al., 1985; Epstein, Wing, Penner, et al., 1985; Goldfield et al., 2001).

Of these dietary interventions, the combination of a hypocaloric diet combined with recommended intakes from specific food groups has been used most commonly in the reviewed interventions—predominantly by Epstein and colleagues—and is called the "Traffic-Light Diet." The Traffic-Light Diet uses a caloric prescription of 800 to 1,500 kcals/day, and foods in the food groups of the Food Guide Pyramid (United States Department of Agriculture; USDA, 1996) are broken down into three color categories— green foods (go) are low in fat and added sugars, are of high nutrient quality for the foods within their food group, and may be consumed in unlimited quantities; yellow foods (caution) have moderate levels of fat and/or added sugars, are of average nutrient quality for the foods within their food group, and should be eaten in moderation; and red foods (stop) are high in fat and/or added sugars, are of poor nutrient quality for the foods within their food group, and usually have a prescribed limit on number of servings consumed per week.

Interventions that have used the Traffic Light Diet within the context of a comprehensive, family-based program have shown significant reductions in obesity in children, predominantly between the ages of 8 to 12 years (Becque et al., 1988; Epstein et al., 1981, 2004; Epstein, Paluch, Gordy, & Dorn, 2000; Epstein, Paluch, Gordy, Saelens, et al., 2000; Epstein, Paluch, & Raynor, 2001; Epstein, Valoski, Vara, et al., 1995; Epstein, Wing, Koeske, et al., 1985; Epstein, Wing, Penner, et al., 1985; Goldfield et al., 2001). There is some evidence that the use of this diet in overweight children improves the nutrient quality of the diet (Valoski & Epstein, 1990) and helps shape food preferences that may assist in the consumption of a healthy diet long-term (Epstein et al., 1989). Indeed, when implemented in a comprehensive, family-based intervention, this diet has shown long-term obesity reductions, extending from five to 10 years after the initiation of treatment (Epstein et al., 1990, 1994; Epstein, Valoski, Kalarchian, et al., 1995).

Unfortunately, within the reviewed studies there were no comparative studies in which all aspects of treatment, except for the diet, were held constant so that the effects of different diets on weight loss in children could be studied. While a low-calorie, low-fat diet has traditionally been prescribed in childhood obesity treatments, many questions still remain about the optimum dietary prescription for weight loss in children. Recently, randomized trials with adults and adolescents examined the effects of a low-carbohydrate diet on weight loss, and results indicated that weight loss with a low-carbohydrate diet as compared to a low-fat diet may be greater in the short term (6 months) with no detrimental effect on blood lipids or renal functioning (Foster et al., 2003; Sondike, Copperman, & Jacobson, 2003). Due to the high protein content of the low-carbohydrate diet, it may be appropriate to prescribe during periods of growth; however, the effect of this diet on weight loss and other physiological outcomes in children has not been examined. Questions have also arisen about how a weight-loss diet could be formulated to improve satiation and satiety—aiding in long-term adherence. Diets that have been hypothesized to improve satiation include a low glycemic load and a low-energy-dense diet.

The types of diets described above encourage children to make large changes in the diet, and most likely would require children and their parents to monitor several aspects of the diet (i.e., calories and specific types of foods consumed), which may be difficult—especially with younger children who developmentally may be less able to engage in extensive monitoring. Another approach may be to target a few specific foods that have been associated with overweight status in children, rather than changing most of the diet. Recent epidemiological research shows that intake of sweetened drinks is positively related to weight status in children (Ludwig, Peterson, & Gortmaker, 2001). Perhaps targeting a reduction of these specific foods in overweight children who regularly consume these foods may be a successful strategy. Targeting a few foods may be more ideal for interventions with young children—monitoring a few behaviors may be easier for parents and young children to do, and by changing only a few foods in the diet, smaller changes in energy balance will most likely occur. This small change in energy balance may have little affect on larger, older children, but may be enough for smaller, younger children who still have a decade or more of linear growth.

There are several other dietary questions that need to be investigated in pediatric obesity treatment. One area that has not been examined is the role of *snacking*. It has been proposed that snacking could be very helpful in reducing overall energy intake by warding off excessive hunger that may cause overeating, but snacking also increases the number of eating opportunities occurring during the day, which may promote over consumption. Due to differences in growth and development, snacking may be more appropriate for younger children, but not for older children. Another target area that needs further examination in childhood obesity is the premise that with young children—as eating patterns and food preferences are being established (Birch, 1999; Birch & Fisher, 1998)—weight loss diets should not only focus on reducing energy intake, but should also concentrate on developing preferences for healthy foods. If that concept is valid, it is not clear what the consequences of including modified foods (i.e., diet soda, reduced-fat ice cream) in children's diets are on the development of food preferences and weight loss. Also, increasing the structure in the diet during weight loss interventions has improved weight loss in adults (Wing & Jeffery, 2001). Perhaps this strategy would also improve weight outcomes in children. An easy way to increase dietary structure is through the use of portion-controlled foods. Because the variety of portion-controlled foods has increased in the marketplace (i.e., oatmeal, yogurt, crackers, cereal), parents could be encouraged to use portion-controlled foods with their children, which may be incredibly helpful for reducing energy intake.

Finally, questions remain about the overall dietary message that should be provided to children. This message could be positive (focusing on healthy foods to eat) or restrictive (focusing on non-nutrient-dense foods to reduce in the diet) (Epstein, Gordy, et al., 2001). While it is theorized that a positive focus will increase long-term adherence, and that a prescription that encourages increased intake of fruits and vegetables and skim milk will push other non-nutrient-dense foods and sweetened drinks out of the diet, thereby reducing energy intake, this has not currently been examined in a randomized trial for childhood obesity treatment.

LEISURE-TIME ACTIVITY

In childhood obesity treatment, leisure-time activity has been broken into two components: physical activity and sedentary behaviors (TV watching, video and computer games). Both behaviors affect energy balance, with increases in physical activity directly increasing energy expenditure, and decreases in sedentary behaviors—particularly TV watching—are hypothesized to increase energy expenditure (time is reallocated from sedentary behaviors to physical activity) and decrease energy intake (reducing eating prompted by TV watching). While physical activity interventions on their own do not usually impact energy balance enough to produce significant changes in weight (Epstein et al., 1998), interventions for TV watching in which only TV watching is reduced have been found to positively affect weight status in children (Robinson, 1999). This may be because reducing sedentary behaviors may influence both sides of the energy balance equation.

Physical Activity

The addition of regular physical activity to the Traffic Light Diet in eight- to 12-year old children results in greater reductions in overweight percentage at six months as compared to the Traffic Light Diet alone (Epstein, Wing, Penner, et al., 1985). Moreover, combining changes in the diet with increased physical activity also improved fitness in the children. Pediatric obesity research interventions currently incorporate some way of increasing physical activity, along with making changes in the diet, to produce optimum weight loss outcomes (Becque et al., 1988; Epstein, Paluch, Gordy, & Dorn, 2000; Epstein, Paluch, Gordy, Saelens, et al., 2000; Epstein, Paluch,

& Raynor, 2001; Epstein, Valoski, Vara, et al., 1995; Epstein, Wing, Koeske, et al., 1985; Goldfield et al., 2001; Senediak & Spence, 1985).

Questions about physical activity during treatment tested in randomized trials in children include what type of physical activity produces the greatest weight loss, and does a greater amount of physical activity produce more weight loss? Epstein and colleagues (Epstein, Wing, Koeske, et al., 1985) examined the Traffic Light Diet combined with lifestyle activity, programmed aerobic activity, or calisthenics on weight loss in eight- to 12-year old children. All groups showed significant reductions in overweight percentage through one year, with no significant differences between the groups. However, at a two-year follow-up, only the lifestyle group maintained a reduction in overweight percentage from baseline, while the other two groups returned to baseline levels. At a 10-year follow-up, however, the lifestyle intervention group still had greater overweight percentage reductions than the other two conditions, but only the lifestyle and calisthenics conditions were significantly different (Epstein et al., 1994). This demonstrates that lifestyle activity, which is less structured and a more flexible type of physical activity, may be easier for young children to maintain, producing better maintenance of weight improvements.

In regard to whether or not prescribing more physical activity helps achieve more weight loss, one investigation (Epstein, Paluch, Gordy, & Dorn, 2000) randomized eight- to 12-year old children to one of four conditions—of which two of the conditions increased physical activity to a low (10 mile/week) or a high (20 mile/week) level. At six months, there was a significant reduction in overweight percentage from baseline, but no difference was found in overweight percentage reduction between the two conditions (−25.6 % overweight vs. −26.4% overweight in the low- and high-level physical activity, respectively). At a two-year follow-up, again both conditions showed significant reductions in percent overweight from baseline, with no difference between the two conditions (−12.4% overweight vs. −13.2% overweight in the low- and high-level physical activity conditions, respectively). This suggests that greater prescriptions of physical activity of up to 20 miles of activity per week do not improve weight loss outcomes in children.

A number of areas still remain to be tested about physical activity in childhood obesity treatment. For example, it is unknown what affect the current guidelines for children of 60 minutes of moderately-intense physical activity most days of the week (USDA, 2005) have on weight loss, or what the best principles are to help children increase physical activity—such as encouraging team or group activities (i.e., soccer, dance), individual activities (i.e., walking, biking), or a combination of the two. Also, to help increase physical activity, the focus of an intervention could be on developing a skill and achieving a sense of accomplishment or on having fun with physical activity. To help children find physical activities they like, encouraging a variety of activities—in which children are introduced to many activities, including activities that they have not engaged in previously—may help to increase physical activity. Perhaps focusing on fun and new activities is not the best approach to increase physical activity in children, and the focus should be on increasing only those activities that they normally do, and develop a routine of physical activity with these activities. Most importantly, activity recommendations are not usually based upon age and/or developmental level of children (i.e., based upon play and family activities for younger children and skill-based, peer activities for older children). As children's days become more organized by school schedules and activities, a transition to encourage older children to plan for fairly structured activity (i.e., get up in the morning and go for a 30-minute walk)—in a similar way that adults are encouraged to get physical activity in during the day instead of engaging in *play*—may also be key.

Sedentary Behaviors

In the 1980s, epidemiological research showed a positive relationship between TV watching and obesity in children (Dietz & Gortmaker, 1985). TV watching may influence weight status by reducing physical activity (Epstein, Paluch, Gordy, & Dorn, 2000; Epstein, Valoski, Vara, et al., 1995). While a one-to-one inverse relationship between physical activity and TV watching has not been found, several studies have documented an inverse relationship between these two leisure-time activities in children (Dietz and Gortmaker; Gortmaker et al., 1996). TV watching may also influence weight status by increasing energy intake (Epstein, Roemmich, Paluch, & Raynor, 2005). TV watching may become a conditioned stimulus for eating through repeated occasions of eating in front of the TV, and food commercials may also serve as prompts for eating (Epstein, Valoski, Vara, et al., 1995). Indeed, an investigation found that when sedentary behaviors were decreased by 50 percent from baseline levels, energy and percent of energy from fat intake decreased (Epstein et al., 2005).

Four of the reviewed studies targeted reductions in sedentary behaviors as part of a comprehensive, family-based childhood obesity intervention (Epstein et al. 2004; Epstein, Paluch, Gordy, & Dorn, 2000; Epstein, Paluch, & Raynor, 2001; Epstein, Valoski, Vara, et al., 1995). Two studies provided comparisons between conditions that either decreased sedentary behaviors or increased physical activity in children aged eight to 12 years of age (Epstein, Paluch, Gordy, & Dorn; Epstein, Valoski, Vara, et al.). Both studies found significant improvements in weight status when sedentary behaviors were decreased. Most interestingly, while one study found no difference in weight outcomes between conditions that targeted physical activity or sedentary behavior (Epstein, Paluch, Gordy, & Dorn), the other study found that decreasing sedentary behavior produced greater reductions in overweight percentage at one year than increasing physical activity (–18% overweight vs. –9% overweight), and that both conditions had comparable improvements in fitness (Epstein, Valoski, Vara, et al.).

These outcomes suggest that perhaps an intervention that targets decreasing sedentary behaviors along with increasing physical activity may be the best way to intervene in children's leisure time for obesity treatment. Interestingly, when eight- to 12-year old children were randomized to decrease sedentary behaviors, increase physical activity, or increase physical activity and decrease sedentary behaviors at the same time, the decreased sedentary condition still produced the greatest reductions in overweight percentage at one year (Epstein, Valoski, Vara, et al., 1995). In another study that compared outcomes in males and females who had been randomized to conditions that either increased physical activity only or combined increased physical activity with decreased sedentary behaviors, males from the combined group had significantly better weight status outcomes than females from either of the two conditions—with no difference in outcomes for males from the two conditions (Epstein, Paluch, & Raynor, 2001). These results, along with those from another intervention that targeted reduction in sedentary behavior during childhood obesity treatment (Epstein et al., 2004), suggest that there may be differences in responses to reductions in sedentary behavior such that some children may be better at reallocating time from sedentary behavior to physical activity (substitutors), while others may reallocate their time from one sedentary activity to another and thus show little change in physical activity (nonsubstitutors). Both studies indicate that male children are more inclined to substitute physical activity for reductions in sedentary behaviors, indicating that interventions that reduce sedentary behavior during obesity treatment may be more helpful for male children.

Incorporating reductions in sedentary behaviors during childhood obesity treatment appears to be a promising approach to improving weight-loss outcomes. More research is needed to identify which method produces the best weight-loss outcome—decreasing sedentary behavior or a combination of decreasing sedentary behavior and increasing physical activity. Furthermore, developing an intervention for decreasing sedentary behaviors that is better at influencing all children to substitute active for sedentary behaviors would be helpful. Finally, it is not clear which sedentary behaviors should be targeted in obesity interventions—TV watching, computer/video game use (eating may be unaffected by changes in these sedentary behaviors), or both.

BEHAVIORAL STRATEGIES

The reviewed studies all incorporated behavior modification techniques in the active intervention conditions. These techniques included self-monitoring of targeted behaviors, positive reinforcement, stimulus control, preplanning, and modeling, if parents were involved in treatment. Three of the reviewed studies specifically examined behavioral techniques on weight control outcomes in children. The first study investigated the effect of rapid (eight sessions in four weeks) or gradual (eight sessions over 15 weeks) behavioral treatment in children aged six to 13 years (Senediak & Spence, 1985). The different schedules of treatment caused several differences other than scheduling to occur between the two conditions, including shaping versus nonshaping of targeted behaviors, and fading versus nonfading of therapist contact during treatment. This investigation found that the gradual condition produced better weight outcomes at the end of treatment than the rapid condition, but at seven months follow-up, there was no difference in weight outcomes between the two conditions, with both conditions producing better weight outcomes than a nonspecific control. Currently, the schedule of treatment over six months is usually weekly for the initial phase of treatment, with a decline in the frequency of meetings as treatment comes to a close (i.e., initially weekly, then biweekly, followed by monthly meetings).

Two studies examined the effectiveness of problem-solving on weight-loss outcomes in children aged six to 12 years (Epstein, Paluch, Gordy, Saelens, et al., 2000; Graves et al., 1988). In one investigation (Graves et al.), families in the parent problem-solving condition spent time at each session using problem-solving techniques for those areas of difficulty associated with children's weight control. In comparison to a family-based, behavioral intervention and an education-only condition, the parent problem-solving condition produced better weight outcomes at the end of two months of treatment and an 8-month follow-up visit. In the second study, the technique of problem-solving was taught either to the parent and child, or the child only, and these conditions were compared to a standard family-based treatment (Epstein, Paluch, Gordy, Saelens, et al.). At the end of treatment, there were no significant differences between the conditions in weight outcomes, and at a 2-year follow-up, the standard intervention had better weight outcomes than the parent and child problem-solving condition, with no other differences in conditions. Problem-solving is now viewed as a standard component of childhood obesity treatment.

Given the recent emphasis on environmental factors greatly influencing the prevalence of obesity (Hill, Wyatt, Reed, & Peters, 2003; Lowe, 2003), methods that assist in controlling the home environment to promote healthy eating and leisure-time activity behaviors may be even more important in present-day treatment than in treatment 30 years ago. On the other hand, stimulus control—in which participants are encouraged to alter the home environment to help reduce energy intake and increase physical activity—was a behavioral technique included in the majority of the reviewed studies. It is unclear how well participants actually use stimulus control. One of the reviewed studies did investigate the effects of using stimulus control or positive reinforcement for reducing sedentary behaviors, and no differences were found in reductions in sedentary behaviors between the groups (Epstein et al., 2004). However, it was unclear how well stimulus control was implemented for reducing sedentary behaviors. Perhaps implementation of stimulus control should be monitored during treatment (i.e., monthly recording of the number of high-energy-dense foods, the pieces of activity equipment that are visible and in working condition, the number of TVs/computers in the house or bedroom, the number of channels available in the home, etc.). Because basic eating studies are finding more evidence that factors such as portion size (Rolls, Roe, Meengs, & Wall, 2004) and the size of plates/cups influence intake (Wansink & Cheney, 2005; Wansink & Van Ittersum, 2003), encouraging participants to focus more on stimulus control of these elements could help with influencing consumption.

STRUCTURE OF TREATMENT

The role of the parent in treatment has also been closely examined in several studies (Epstein et al., 1981; Epstein, Paluch, Gordy, Saelens, et al., 2000; Golan et al., 1998). Specifically, these investigations addressed the question of who is the better target for treatment—the parent, the child, or both? Two studies investigated conditions in which the child (or the combination of the parent and child) were targeted for different components of treatment, and found no differences in weight outcomes in children aged six to 12 years at the end of treatment (Epstein et al., Epstein, Paluch, Gordy, Saelens, et al.), but a 10-year follow-up found that the parent and child combination produced the best reduction in overweight percentage (Epstein et al., 1994). Golan and colleagues (Golan et al.) targeted either the parent or child only in the treatment of six- to 11-year old children and found that percent reductions in overweight were greater in the parent-only group at the end of 12 months of treatment and an 18-month follow-up. Adding evidence to the importance of parental involvement during treatment, analyses of changes in weight status in family-based programs in which parents and children participate in treatment find that parental weight change during treatment is a significant predictor of child weight change during treatment (Epstein et al.; Wrotniak, Epstein, Paluch, & Roemmich, 2004). This is hypothesized to be a consequence of parental modeling (Wrotniak, Epstein, Paluch, & Roemmich, 2005). This suggests that in children under the age of 13, an intervention that involves the parent produces the best outcomes. However, it is unclear if an intervention that targets the parent only for childhood obesity treatment is the optimum strategy. While Golan and colleagues' (Golan et al.) outcomes indicate this is the most appropriate way to treat childhood obesity, the sample in that investigation consisted of children between the ages of six and 11 years. Potentially, for younger children—in which self-monitoring may be very difficult due to developmentally appropriate difficulties with reading, writing, and math—targeting the parents only, and emphasizing stimulus control, positive reinforcement, and modeling, may be the best approach in treatment. In older children, cognitive development is such that self-monitoring is more feasible, thus allowing older children to take a more active role in treatment. For these children, an intervention that involves both the parent and the child might produce the best outcomes.

A final area that has been investigated regarding treatment structure is the effect of providing behavioral family-based treatment in a group versus a group-plus-individual format. Goldfield and colleagues (Goldfield et al., 2001) studied changes in z-BMI in eight- to 12-year olds receiving a family-based, six-month intervention solely in a group or in a group combined with brief individual sessions with an interventionist. Total treatment contact time was equal between the two conditions. Both conditions showed significant reductions in z-BMI from baseline to six and 12 months, but there were no differences between the two conditions. This outcome demonstrates that effective treatment can be delivered using a group format only.

One area of treatment structure that has not been examined in obesity treatment for children is the length of treatment needed to optimize maintenance outcomes. Treatment in children has most commonly been provided over an approximately six-month period, with no contact during follow-up (Becque et al., 1988; Epstein et al., 2004; Epstein, Paluch, Gordy, & Dorn, 2000; Epstein, Paluch, Gordy, Saelens, et al., 2000; Epstein, Paluch, & Raynor, 2001; Goldfield et al., 2001). Treatment in adults has found that lengthening the initial phase of treatment (Perri, Nezu, Patti, & McCann, 1989), and/or biweekly contact during maintenance (Perri et al., 2001), produces better long-term weight loss. It is unknown if either of these strategies would improve long-term weight outcomes in children.

THEORIZED NEGATIVE CONSEQUENCES OF CHILDHOOD OBESITY TREATMENT

Besides improvements in weight status, numerous studies have also documented improvements in blood pressure (Figueroa-Colon, von Almen, Franklin, Schuftan, & Suskind, 1993), serum lipids (Knip & Nuutinen, 1993), insulin sensitivity (Hoffman, Stumbo, Janz, & Nielson, 1995), and psychosocial status (Braet, Tanghe, Bode, Franckx, & Winckel, 2003; Myers, Raynor, & Epstein, 1998) in children receiving obesity treatment. Due to the reduction of energy intake during treatment, one hypothesized negative consequence is the impairment of linear growth. Sothern and colleagues (Sothern, Udall, Suskind, Vargas, & Blecker, 2000) investigated the influence of a very low-calorie diet on growth in overweight children aged seven to 17 years, and reported that 80 percent of the children sustained growth velocities appropriate for chronological and/or height age over a year of follow-up. Moreover, 17 percent of the children who did not sustain appropriate growth velocities during treatment were taller than other children at the same age at the start of treatment, and at the one-year follow-up mark they were at or above an appropriate height for age. These results coincide with previous outcomes (Epstein et al., 1990).

Another area of concern in pediatric obesity treatment is the potential increased risk of developing an eating disorder (Butryn & Wadden, 2005). Decreased energy intake is the primary dietary treatment for childhood obesity, yet dieting, which is believed to be an important contributor to the pathogenesis of eating disorders (Schmidt, 2002), is theorized to increase the risk of developing eating pathologies—particularly in females (Garner & Wooley, 1991). However, several studies have examined the effect of obesity treatment on eating behaviors in children and have found either a decrease (Braet et al.; Braet & Van Winckel, 2000; Levine, Ringham, Kalarchian, Wisniewski, & Marcus, 2001) or no change (Epstein, Paluch, Saelens, Ernst, & Wilfley, 2001) in eating pathology. Moreover, a 10-year follow-up of children receiving obesity treatment found that 4 percent of participants reported receiving treatment for bulimia nervosa, and none reported treatment for anorexia nervosa (Epstein et al., 1994). These rates of treatment are similar to those reported in community samples (Butryn & Wadden, 2005). The outcomes of these studies suggest that professionally administered childhood obesity treatments pose minimal risk for the development of an eating disorder.

FUTURE DIRECTIONS

This review provides support for the success of evidence-based pediatric obesity treatment. The reviewed studies demonstrate that an intervention that incorporates dietary and leisure-time activity pre-scriptions, provides behavior modification techniques, and includes a parental involvement in the treatment plan, produces improvements in weight status in children. Aside from addressing the previously identi-fied areas that need to be investigated, three large areas in the treat-ment of childhood obesity need to be examined. The first two areas are a consequence of the obesity epidemic. As the prevalence of obesity has increased in children, the number of overweight young children (ages two to seven years) has also increased. Most interventions have targeted children between the ages of eight and 12 years, thus it is not known how effective treatment is, or what treatment should be like, for younger children. Another area that needs further investigation is treatment for severely overweight children (> 100% overweight). Again, as the number of overweight children has increased, so has the number of severely over-weight children. Many of the reviewed investigations deemed severely overweight children (> 100% overweight) ineligible, thus it is not clear if the reviewed programs are effective for these children. Finally, there is very little research on preventing childhood overweight (Johnson, Ger-stein, Evans, & Woodward-Lopez, 2006). This approach may be the best for addressing the obesity epidemic. However, while there are hypoth-esized behaviors to target in prevention (i.e., breast feeding, TV watching, sweetened drink intake), none have been investigated. Thus, although progress has been made in the area of pediatric obesity treatment, con-tinued research is needed to improve long-term outcomes and address these new areas of need.

REFERENCES

Altman, D. G., Schulz, K. F., Moher, D., Egger, M., Davidoff, F., Elbourne, D., et al. (2001). The revised CONSORT statement for reporting randomzied trails: Explana-tion and elaboration. *Annals of Internal Medicine, 134,* 663–694.

Baskin, M. L., Aard, J., Franklin, F. A., & Allison, D. B. (2005). Prevalence of obesity in the United States. *Obesity Reviews, 6,* 5–7.

Becque, M. D., Katch, V. L., Rocchini, A. P., Marks, C. R., & Moorehead, C. (1988). Coronary risk incidence of obese adolescents: Reduction by exercise plus diet inter-vention. *Pediatrics, 81,* 605–612.

Berenson, G. S., Srinivasan, S. R., Bao, W., Newman, W. P., Tracy, R. E., & Wattingney, W. A. (1998). Association between multiple cardiovascular risk factors and arthero-sclerosis in children and young adults: The Bogalusa heart study. *New England Journal of Medicine, 338,* 1650–1656.

Birch, L. L. (1999). Development of food preferences. *Annual Review of Nutrition, 19,* 41–62.

Birch, L. L., & Fisher, J. O. (1998). Development of eating behaviors among children and adolescents. *Pediatrics, 101,* 539–548.

Braet, C., Tanghe, A., Bode, P. D., Franckx, H., & Winckel, M. V. (2003). Inpatient treatment of obese children: A multicomponent program without stringent calorie restriction. *European Journal of Pediatrics, 162,* 391–396.

Braet, C., & Van Winckel, M. (2000). Long-term follow-up of a cognitive behavioral treatment program for obese children. *Behavior Therapy, 31,* 55–74.

Butryn, M. L., & Wadden, T. A. (2005). Treatment of overweight in children and adolescents: Does dieting increase the risk of eating disorders? *International Journal of Eating Disorders, 37,* 285–293.

Davidson, K. W., Goldstein, M., Kaplan, R. M., Kaufmann, P. G., Knatterud, G. L., Orleans, C. T., et al. (2003). Evidence-based behavioral medicine: What is it and how do we acheive it? *Annals of Behavioral Medicine, 26,* 161–171.

Dietz, W. H. (1998). Health consequences of obesity in youth: Childhood predictors of adult onset. *Pediatrics, 101,* 518–525.

Dietz, W. H., & Gortmaker, S. L. (1985). Do we fatten our children at the television set? Obesity and television viewing in children and adolescents. *Pediatrics, 75,* 807–812.

Epstein, L. H., Gordy, C. C., Raynor, H. A., Beddome, M., Kilanowski, C. K., & Paluch, R. (2001). Increasing fruit and vegetable intake and decreasing fat and sugar intake in families at risk for childhood obesity. *Obesity Research, 9,* 171–178.

Epstein, L. H., Myers, M. D., Raynor, H. A., & Saelens, B. E. (1998). Treatment of pediatric obesity. *Pediatrics, 10,* 554–569.

Epstein, L. H., Paluch, R. A., Gordy, C. C., & Dorn, J. (2000). Decreasing sedentary behaviors in treating pediatric obesity. *Archives of Pediatrics & Adolescent Medicine, 154,* 220–226.

Epstein, L. H., Paluch, R. A., Gordy, C. C., Saelens, B. E., & Ernst, M. M. (2000). Problem solving in the treatment of childhood obesity. *Journal of Consulting and Clinical Psychology, 68,* 717–721.

Epstein, L. H., Paluch, R. A., Kilanowski, C. K., & Raynor, H. A. (2004). The effect of reinforcement or stimulus control to reduce sedentary behavior in the treatment of pediatric obesity. *Health Psychology, 23,* 371–380.

Epstein, L. H., Paluch, R. A., & Raynor, H. A. (2001). Sex differences in obese children and siblings in family-based obesity treatment. *Obesity Research, 9,* 746–753.

Epstein, L. H., Paluch, R. A., Saelens, B. E., Ernst, M. M., & Wilfley, D. E. (2001). Changes in eating disorder symptoms with pediatric obesity treatment. *Journal of Pediatrics, 139,* 58–65.

Epstein, L. H., Roemmich, R. A., Paluch, R. A., & Raynor, H. A. (2005). Influence of changes in sedentary behavior on energy and macronutrient intake in youth. *American Journal of Clinical Nutrition, 81,* 361–366.

Epstein, L. H., Valoski, A. M., Kalarchian, M. A., & McCurley, J. (1995). Do children lose and maintain weight easier than adults: A comparison of child and parent weight changes from six months to ten years. *Obesity Research, 3,* 411–417.

Epstein, L. H., Valoski, A., & McCurley, J. (1993). Effect of weight loss by obese children on long-term growth. *American Journal of Diseases in Children, 147,* 1076–1080.

Epstein, L. H., Valoski, A. M., Vara, L. S., McCurley, J., Wisniewski, L., Kalarchian, M. A., et al. (1995). Effects of decreasing sedentary behavior and increasing activity on weight change in obese children. *Health Psychology, 14,* 109–115.

Epstein, L. H., Valoski, A., Wing, R. R., & McCurley, J. (1990). Ten-year follow-up of behavioral, family-based treatment for obese children. *Journal of the American Medical Association, 264,* 2519–2523.

Epstein, L. H., Valoski, A., Wing, R. R., & McCurley, J. (1994). Ten year outcomes of behavioral family based treatment for childhood obesity. *Health Psychology, 13,* 373–383.

Epstein, L. H., Valoski, A., Wing, R. R., Perkins, K. A., Fernstrom, M. D., Marks, B. L., et al. (1989). Perception of eating and exercise in children as a function of child and parent weight status. *Appetite, 12,* 105–118.

Epstein, L. H., Wing, R. R., Koeske, R., Andrasik, F., & Ossip, D. (1981). Child and parent weight loss in family-based behavior modification programs. *Journal of Consulting and Clinical Psychology, 49,* 674–685.

Epstein, L. H., Wing, R. R., Koeske, R., & Valoski, A. (1985). A comparison of lifestyle exercise, aerobic exercise, and calisthenics on weight loss in obese children. *Behavior Therapy, 16,* 345–356.

Epstein, L. H., Wing, R. R., Penner, B. C., & Kress, M. J. (1985). Effect of diet and controlled exercise on weight loss in obese children. *Journal of Pediatrics, 107,* 358–361.

Figueroa-Colon, R., von Almen, T. K., Franklin, F. A., Schuftan, C., & Suskind, R. M. (1993). Comparison of two hypocaloric diets in obese children. *American Journal of Diseases in Children, 140,* 160–166.

Foster, G., Wyatt, H. R., Hill, J. O., McGuckin, B. G., Brill, C., Mohammed, B. S., et al. (2003). A randomized trial of a low-carbohydrate diet for obesity. *The New England Journal of Medicine, 348,* 2082–2090.

Garner, D. M., & Wooley, S. C. (1991). Confronting the failure of behavioral and dietary treatments for obesity. *Clinical Psychology Review, 11,* 729–780.

Golan, M., Wiezman, A., Apter, A., & Fainaru, M. (1998). Parents as the exclusive agents of change in the treatment of childhood obesity. *American Journal of Clinical Nutrition, 67,* 1130–1135.

Goldfield, G. S., Epstein, L. H., Kilanowski, C. K., Paluch, R. A., & Kogut-Bossler, B. (2001). Cost-effectiveness of group and mixed family-based treatment for childhood obesity. *International Journal of Obesity, 25,* 1843–1849.

Gortmaker, S. L., Must, A., Sobol, A. M., Peterson, K., Colditz, G. A., & Dietz, W. H. (1996). Television viewing as a cause of increasing obesity among children in the United States, 1986–1990. *Archives of Pediatrics and Adolescent Medicine, 150,* 356–362.

Graves, T., Meyers, A. W., & Clark, L. A. (1988). An evaluation of parental problem-solving training in the behavioral treatmenmt of childhood obesity. *Journal of Consulting and Clinical Psychology, 56,* 246–250.

Hedley, A. A., Ogden, C. L., Johnson, C. L., Carroll, M. D., Curtin, L. R., & Flegal, K. M. (2004). Prevalence of overweight and obesity among US children, adolescents, and adults, 1999–2002. *Journal of the American Medical Association, 291,* 2847–2850.

Hill, J. O., Wyatt, H. R., Reed, G. W., & Peters, J. C. (2003). Obesity and the environment: Where do we go from here? *Science, 299,* 853–855.

Hoffman, R. P., Stumbo, P. J. E., Janz, K. F., & Nielson, D. H. (1995). Altered insulin resistance is associated with increased dietary weight loss in obese children. *Hormone Research, 44,* 17–22.

Janssen, I., Katzmarzyk, P. T., Srinivasan, S. R., Chen, W., Malina, R. M., Bouchard, C. et al. (2005). Utility of childhood BMI in the prediction of adult disease: Comparison of national and international references. *Obesity Research, 13,* 1106–1115.

Jelalian, E., & Saelens, B. E. (1999). Empirically-supported treatments in pediatric psychology: Pediatric obesity. *Journal of Pediatric Psychology, 24,* 223–248.

Johnson, D. B., Gerstein, D. E., Evans, A. E., & Woodward-Lopez, G. (2006). Preventing obesity: A lifecycle perspective. *Journal of the American Dietetic Association, 106,* 97–102.

Knip, M., & Nuutinen, O. (1993). Long-term effects of weight reduction on serum lipids and plasma insulin in obese children. *American Journal of Clinical Nutrition, 54,* 490–493.

Levine, M. D., Ringham, R. M., Kalarchian, M. A., Wisniewski, L., & Marcus, M. D. (2001). Is family-based behavioral weight control appropriate for severe pediatric obesity? *International Journal of Eating Disorders, 30,* 318–328.

Lowe, M. R. (2003). Self-regulation of energy intake in the prevention and treatment of obesity: Is it feasible? *Obesity Research, 11,* 44S–59S.

Ludwig, D. S., Peterson, K. E., & Gortmaker, S. L. (2001). Relation between consumption of sugar-sweetened drinks and childhood obesity: A prospective, observational analysis. *Lancet, 357,* 505–508.

Myers, M. D., Raynor, H. A., & Epstein, L. H. (1998). Predictors of child psychological changes during family-based treatment for obesity. *Archives of Pediatric and Adolescent Medicine, 152,* 855–861.

Perri, M. G., Mckelvey, W. F., Renjilian, D. A., Nezu, A. M., Shermer, R. L., & Viegener, B. J. (2001). Relapse prevention training and problem-solving therapy in the long-term managment of obesity. *Journal of Consulting and Clinical Psychology, 69*, 722–726.

Perri, M. G., Nezu, A. M., Patti, E. T., & McCann, K. L. (1989). Effect of length of treatment on weight loss. *Journal of Consulting and Clinical Psychology, 57*, 450–452.

Rees, J. M. (1990). Management of obesity in adolescence. *Medical Clinics of North America, 74*, 1275–1292.

Robinson, T. (1999). Reducing children's television viewing to prevent obesity. *Journal of the American Medical Association, 282*, 1561–1567.

Rolls, B. J., Roe, L. S., Meengs, J. S., & Wall, D. E. (2004). Increasing the portion size of a sandwich increases energy intake. *Journal of the American Dietetic Association, 104*, 367–372.

Schmidt, U. (Ed.). (2002). *Risk Factors for Eating Disorders* (2nd ed.). New York: Guilford Press.

Senediak, C., & Spence, S. H. (1985). Rapid versus gradual scheduling of therapuetic contact in a family based behavioral weight control programme for children. *Behavioural Psychotherapy, 13*, 265–287.

Sondike, S. B., Copperman, N., & Jacobson, M. S. (2003). Effects of a low-carbohydrtae diet on weight loss and cardiovascular risk factors in overweight adolescents. *Journal of Pediatrics, 142*, 253–258.

Sothern, M. S., Udall, J. N., Suskind, R. M., Vargas, A., & Blecker, U. (2000). Weight loss and growth velocity in obese children after very low calorie diet, exercise, and behavior modification. *Acta Paediatric, 89*, 1036–1043.

United States Department of Agriculture. (2005). *Dietary Guidelines for Americans, 2005* (6th ed.). Washington, DC: U.S. Government Printing Office.

United States Department of Agriculture. (1996). The food guide pyramid. *Home and Garden Bulletin, 252*. Washington, DC: Author.

Valoski, A., & Epstein, L. H. (1990). Nutrient intake of obese children in a family-based behavioral weight control program. *International Journal of Obesity, 14*, 667–677.

Wansink, B., & Cheney, M. M. (2005). Super bowls: Serving bowl size and food consumption. *Journal of the American Medical Association, 293*, 1727–1728.

Wansink, B., & Van Ittersum, K. (2003). Bottoms up! The influence of elongation on pouring and consumption volume. *Journal of Consumer Research, 30*, 455–463.

Whitaker, R. C., Wright, J. A., Pepe, M. S., Seidel, K. D., & Dietz, W. H. (1997). Predicting obesity in young adulthood from childhood and parental obesity. *The New England Journal of Medicine, 25*, 869–873.

Wing, R. R. (2002). Behavioral weight control. In T. A. Wadden & A. J. Stunkard (Eds.), *Handbook of Obesity Treatment* (pp. 301–316). New York: Guilford Press.

Wing, R. R., & Jeffery, R. W. (2001). Food provision as a strategy to promote weight loss. *Obesity Research, 9*(Suppl.), 271–275.

Wrotniak, B. H., Epstein, L. H., Paluch, R. A., & Roemmich, J. N. (2004). Parent weight change as a predictor of child weight change in family-based behavioral obsity treatment. *Archives of Pediatrics and Adolescent Medicine, 158*, 342–347.

Wrotniak, B. H., Epstein, L. H., Paluch, R. A., & Roemmich, J. N. (2005). The relationship between parent and child self-reported adherence and weight loss. *Obesity Research, 13*, 1089–1096.

Yin, T. J. C., Wu, F. L., Liu, Y. L., & Yu, S. (2005). Effects of a weight-loss program for obese children: A "mix of attributes" approach. *Journal of Nursing Research, 13*, 21–29.

14

Empirically Supported Treatment of Overweight Adolescents

ALAN M. DELAMATER, JASON F. JENT, CORTNEY T. MOINE, and JESSICA RIOS

In this chapter, we address empirically supported treatment approaches for overweight adolescents. We consider various approaches to treatment for overweight adolescents, including dietary and physical activity interventions, outpatient multicomponent interventions, camp and residential programs, primary care interventions, and medical approaches including pharmacological interventions and bariatric surgery. We conclude with a discussion of implications for clinical practice and future research in this area.

While the literature on the treatment efficacy of childhood overweight is promising (Baur & O'Connor, 2004; Epstein, Valoski, Wing, & McCurley, 1994; Jelalian & Mehlenbeck, 2003), relatively less attention has been placed on the efficacy of treatment for adolescent overweight. Interventions for adolescent overweight vary across treatment approaches (e.g., dietary intervention, physical activity intervention, multicomponent behavioral therapy, medication management, and surgery), treatment settings (e.g., specialty outpatient clinic, hospital inpatient, primary care, school, residential camp, church, and community center), and treatment formats (e.g., individual, group, classroom, peer, dyadic, and family). However, even with the development of several different treatment approaches, there are few well-controlled studies examining the efficacy of adolescent overweight interventions.

ALAN M. DELAMATER, JASON F. JENT, CORTNEY T. MOINE and JESSICA RIOS • University of Miami, Miami, FL 33101.

DIETARY AND PHYSICAL ACTIVITY INTERVENTIONS

Relatively few studies have compared the effects of different dietary interventions with overweight adolescents; preliminary findings suggest that the type of nutritional intake affects weight loss, but varies by the setting of treatment. In a 12-week randomized controlled trial (RCT) comparing the effects of a low-carbohydrate diet with those of a low-fat diet on weight loss and serum lipids in overweight adolescents, those in the low-carbohydrate group (n = 12) displayed significantly greater reductions in their body mass index (BMI) and improvements in nonHDL cholesterol levels relative to adolescents in the low-fat group (n = 14; Sondike, Copperman, & Jacobsen, 2003). Adolescents in the low-fat group displayed improvements in LDL cholesterol level, but not in the low-carbohydrate group. Less than half of treatment participants returned for a one-year follow-up assessment, but none of them returned to their baseline BMI. In another overweight adolescent RCT (n = 14) comparing reduced-carbohydrate and fat diets, the reduced-carbohydrate treatment group displayed greater reductions in BMI and fat mass at six and 12 month follow-ups (Ebbeling, Leidig, Sinclair, Hangen, & Ludwig, 2003).

With regard to other comparative studies of dietary restrictions, a residential nine-month intervention randomized extremely overweight adolescents (n = 121) into either an increased protein dietary intake or decreased carbohydrate intake group. Participants significantly reduced their weight, but there were no differences between dietary groups in weight loss (Rolland-Cachera et al., 2004). At their two-year follow-up, adolescents regained a significant portion of their weight due to increased energy intake (particularly snacking) and sedentary behaviors after returning home.

In a standalone dietary intervention where overweight adolescents (n = 17) were admitted into a hospital for one month and then followed in an outpatient setting for a total of 12 months to implement a protein-sparing modified fast diet (a high-protein, low-calorie diet), 47 percent displayed significant decreases in body weight after one year (Stallings, Archibald, Pencharz, Harrison, & Bell, 1988).

Despite preliminary support for the use of reduced carbohydrate and increased protein dietary interventions to reduce adolescent obesity, these studies generally had small sample sizes and unclear follow-up data. Larger-scale RCTs are needed to gain a better understanding of the differences between high-protein and low-carbohydrate dietary interventions, and the long-term effectiveness of these interventions with adolescents.

Similar to dietary interventions, only a few studies have examined the independent effect of physical activity on overweight adolescents (Epstein & Goldfield, 1999). In a study of the independent effects of exercise on overweight children and adolescent girls, participants (n = 19) engaged in aerobic activity for 40 minutes a session, three times a week for a period of 12 weeks. Girls displayed significant improvement in cardiorespiratory fitness and insulin sensitivity, but no changes in BMI (Nassis et al., 2005). While physical activity interventions alone do not appear to impact weight reduction in adolescents, they do appear to confer benefits to adolescents beyond weight loss—including increased physical activity and insulin sensitivity.

MULTI-COMPONENT INTERVENTIONS: PHYSICAL ACTIVITY, NUTRITION, AND BEHAVIORAL THERAPY

Given that overall energy expenditure must exceed energy intake to lose weight, several interventions have been designed to increase energy expenditure (increasing exercise and decreasing sedentary activities) and to decrease energy intake (diet) simultaneously. Further, the presence of behavioral treatment components within overweight interventions has also been found to be an important factor in the treatment of childhood overweight (Epstein et al., 1994). That is, research has consistently demonstrated the importance of including behavioral strategies (e.g., self-monitoring of caloric intake and weight, goal-setting, positive reinforcement, stimulus control, and behavioral contracting) in treatment programs for childhood overweight. However, relatively few well-controlled RCTs have demonstrated the efficacy of multicomponent interventions that include physical activity, nutrition, and behavioral treatment components for overweight adolescents. Studies of this type have been conducted in various treatment settings, including outpatient specialty clinics, community centers, schools, churches, primary care practices, and in patients' homes via the Internet.

Several RCTs have examined the effects of multicomponent treatments on overweight adolescents. In one of the most promising, well-controlled studies of adolescent overweight interventions, the efficacy of adding a peer-based *adventure therapy* to a cognitive behavioral weight-control program was evaluated (Jelalian, Mehlenbeck, Lloyd-Richardson, Birmaher, & Wing, 2006). Adolescents were randomly assigned to a cognitive behavioral weight-loss program plus a peer-enhanced adventure therapy group ($n = 37$), a standard cognitive behavioral weight-loss program plus exercise group ($n = 39$), or a standard care group ($n = 13$). Both cognitive-behavioral therapy (CBT) group interventions included 16 weekly sessions with parents and adolescents attending separate simultaneous meetings. Adolescents were prescribed a balanced deficit diet and physical activity 30 minutes daily/five days a week. Both CBT group interventions learned about self-monitoring, motivation for weight loss, goal-setting, the importance of physical activity, stimulus control strategies, parent-teen contracts, social influences on dietary intake, stress, and relapse prevention. In addition, the peer-enhanced group attended an additional weekly session where the group engaged in a physical and challenging group activity together (e.g., mazes, rope courses) to develop social skills, problem-solving abilities, and self confidence. The standard CBT group received an additional weekly aerobic exercise session.

Results indicated that the two cognitive-behavioral treatment groups had significant weight loss over time, but the peer-enhanced adventure therapy group had more success with *maintenance* of weight loss. In addition, findings indicated that, not only did the average weight loss in this intervention group exceed that of prior controlled trials with youth in this age range, but they also suggested that the adventure-therapy component was particularly effective for the older adolescents.

In an RCT of a family-based intervention conducted in Israel for the treatment of child and adolescent overweight (6–16 years of age), participants were randomly assigned to a multicomponent three-month treatment group (n = 24) or a control group (n = 22; Nemet et al., 2005). Youth were first invited to a session with their parents and a dietitian, and then youth meetings alternated with parent meetings for a total of six meetings in the three-month program. Participants were placed on a balanced hypocaloric diet, with a deficit of 30 percent from reported intake or intake that was 15 percent less than the daily required intake. Youths participated in an hour-long physical training program twice a week, and were also encouraged to complete 30–45 minutes of walking or weight-bearing sport activities at least once per week. At post-treatment, youths in the multicomponent intervention group achieved significant decreases in body weight, BMI, and body fat percentage, and significant increases in physical activity and endurance relative to the control group. Long-term effects of the intervention were also very positive, with maintenance of body weight and a reduction in BMI and body fat percentages in the intervention group. The maintenance effects of the intervention are encouraging, but the treatment needs to be replicated in the other settings with an entirely adolescent population to gain a better understanding of whether or not the findings can be generalized.

In another multicomponent intervention, families were randomly assigned to either a "mother and adolescent (ages 13–17) seen separately" condition or an "adolescent seen alone" condition (Coates, Killen, & Slinkard, 1982). Treatment included 14 weekly, 90-minute group sessions, two parent sessions, onsite exercise, and leader-facilitated interactions about weight control behaviors. At post-treatment, the "adolescent and mother seen separately" condition and the "adolescent seen alone" condition both displayed decreases in overweight percentage (8.6% and 5.1%, respectively). At an 18-month follow-up, both groups continued to display decreases in overweight percentage from baseline (8.4% adolescent-mother; 8.2% child alone).

In a study with a predominately Caucasian sample of adolescents (ages 12–16) that were randomly assigned to treatment format (i.e., mothers and adolescents seen separately; mothers and adolescents seen together; adolescents seen alone), treatment type affected outcomes (Brownell, Kelman, & Stunkard, 1983). Treatment included 45- to 60-minute group sessions for one year (16 weekly sessions, then one session every two months) and participants were provided with nutrition and exercise education, rewards for attendance and weight loss, stimulus control, and behavior modification. At post-treatment, the mothers and adolescents that were seen separately displayed better outcomes (17.1% decrease in percent overweight) than when mothers and adolescents were seen together (7.0% decrease in percent overweight) or when adolescents were seen alone (6.8% decrease in percent overweight). However, a study that sought to replicate these findings in a predominately African-American adolescent sample was unsuccessful (Wadden et al., 1990). That is, treating the adolescent and the mother separately did not have a differential impact on treatment outcomes, although weight loss was positively correlated to the number of sessions attended by the parent.

Other multicomponent interventions that utilized RCT methodology did not result in reductions in BMI, but several improved health markers and psychological outcomes were found. In an RCT designed to explore the effects of exercise intensity on cardiovascular fitness and insulin resistance in overweight adolescents over an eight-month treatment program, participants ($n = 80$) were randomly assigned to one of three groups: lifestyle education (LSE), LSE and moderate intensity physical training, or LSE and high intensity physical training (Gutin et al., 2002; Kang et al., 2002). The majority of participants (69%) were African-American and were provided transportation to the community-based program after school. During LSE, adolescents received information about nutrition, physical activity, psychosocial factors associated with obesity, coping skills, and behavior modification. While no groups displayed changes in BMI, the combined physical training (high-intensity and moderate- intensity groups) and LSE group displayed significant improvements in cardiovascular fitness, and the high intensity group displayed improvements in insulin resistance compared to the LSE-alone group. However, the maintenance effects of this program were not reported. A similar RCT examined differences between 1) a diet and behavioral treatment; 2) an exercise, diet, and behavioral treatment; and 3) a control group. Results indicated that the exercise, diet, and behavioral treatment group achieved significant improvements in high density lipoprotein cholesterol levels, systolic blood pressure, and diastolic blood pressure relative to other groups over a five-month treatment period (Becque, Katch, Rocchini, Marks, & Moorehead, 1988). Similar to the previous reports (Gutin et al.; Kang et al.), the intervention did not result in reduced BMIs and there was no follow-up data.

Another RCT evaluated the effectiveness of an exercise program on BMI and psychological outcomes in overweight adolescents (Daley, Copeland, Wright, Roalfe, & Wales, 2006). Overweight youth (ages 11–16 years) were randomly assigned to receive exercise therapy ($n = 28$), an equal contact exercise placebo ($n = 23$), or usual care ($n = 30$). The exercise therapy group engaged in aerobic exercise activities for 30 minutes three times weekly for eight weeks (24 sessions). During the first 12 sessions, participants were also introduced to cognitive behavioral strategies consistent with the transtheoretical model, including cognitive reappraisal and consciousness-raising. During the last 12 sessions, behavioral interventions including goal setting, self-monitoring, and increasing social support were introduced to participants. While the intervention did not result in significant reductions in BMI, the exercise therapy group and exercise contact group displayed significant improvements in physical self-worth compared to the usual care group at post-treatment and physical and global self-worth effects were found for the exercise therapy group at 14- and 28-week follow-ups.

In an innovative treatment approach, a recent RCT evaluated the efficacy of an Internet-based lifestyle behavior modification program that included interactive Internet behavioral weight-loss counseling for overweight African-American adolescent girls and their overweight parents over a two-year period of intervention (Williamson et al., 2006). The Internet behavioral group lost more mean body fat, and parents in the behavioral program lost significantly more mean body weight during the first six months. However, differences between groups disappeared after two years, which was attributed to reduced utilization of the Internet program after the initial six months of treatment.

The findings from several nonrandomized multicomponent interventions suggest positive effects in reducing adolescents' weight. One promising short-term intervention for adolescent overweight is the SHAPEDOWN program (Mellin, Slunkard, & Irwin, 1987). In this program, adolescents (ages 12–18) attended 14 weekly, 90-minute group sessions. Sessions included nutrition education, onsite exercise, two parent sessions, and discussions about weight-control behaviors. At post-treatment, adolescents who participated in the program demonstrated a significant decrease in their overweight percentage (5.9 percent), and at a 15-month follow-up, program participants displayed further decreases in the overweight percentage (9.9 percent).

Sothern Udall, Suskind, Vargas, and Blecker (2000) developed a phased outpatient intervention that included an acute very low calorie diet (VLCD), followed by a hypocaloric diet, exercise, and behavior modification. All participants were billed $750 for enrolling in the program. Fifty-two overweight children and adolescents (ages 7–17) completed the VLCD phase, with 35 youth completing the one-year program. Mildly overweight (130–149% Ideal Body Weight [IBW]) adolescents followed the VLCD for 10 weeks, whereas moderately (150–199% IBW) and severely overweight adolescents (≥ 200% IBW) maintained the diet for 20 weeks. The second phase of treatment included following a less-restrictive balanced hypocaloric diet, a moderate-intensity exercise program at the clinic, a prescribed exercise regimen for home, and family-based behavioral modification. The acute VLCD resulted in a significant average weight loss of 9.4 kg and a reduction in body fat percentage. Participants who completed the entire one-year program maintained significant weight loss from pretreatment, but did not reduce their BMI during the second phase of treatment. Only the extremely overweight adolescents continued to display reductions in BMI during the multidisciplinary phase. This study provides preliminary support for VLCD, but the expense of the program and age disparity makes it difficult to determine for whom this diet would be effective. Furthermore, the dynamic involvement of parents in the behavior modification component makes it difficult to evaluate the unique effects of parent participation and diet on treatment outcome. More controlled work using this approach is needed.

Other recent adolescent overweight interventions have built upon empirically-based interventions by utilizing additional behavioral strategies, such as daily reminders, motivational interviewing, and conducting the interventions in novel settings—however, these studies have had limited success. In a multicomponent intervention for overweight African-American girls ages 12 to 16, a total of 10 churches were randomly assigned to either a high-intensity or moderate-intensity intervention (Resnicow, Taylor, Baskin, & McCarty, 2005). The high intensity intervention included 24 to 26 sessions, and girls participated in every session with parents attending every other session. Each session included information about dietary intervention and 30 minutes of physical exercise. In addition, girls were provided two-way paging devices so that they could receive messages throughout the day about dietary intake and physical exercise. Participants also received four to six motivational interviewing telephone calls over the course of treatment. The moderate-intensity intervention included six sessions and the topics addressed included fat, fad diets, barriers to physical activity, and benefits of physical activity. The results showed no significant differences in BMI over time or between groups over the six-month intervention period. However, girls who attended greater than 75 percent of sessions showed a small decrease in BMI (.8 units). This suggests that actual attendance to treatment may have an impact on adolescent treatment outcomes.

CAMP-BASED AND RESIDENTIAL INTERVENTIONS

The effectiveness of nontraditional treatment approaches for adolescent overweight, such as residential inpatient and camp programs, have also been examined. In camp or residential settings, adolescents' daily regimen, including physical activity, dietary intake, and participation in behavioral interventions, can be controlled—increasing the likelihood that participants can experience more immediate success.

The effectiveness of a short-term residential weight-loss camp based in Britain has been examined in a series of studies (Barton, Walker, Lambert, Gately & Hill, 2004; Gately et al., 2005; Walker, Gately, Bewick, & Hill, 2003). Overweight campers (n = 185; mean age 13.9 years) who attended a month-long weight-loss camp were compared to a nonrandomized control group of overweight and average weight children of similar ages (n = 94). It should be noted that all children who attended the camp normally resided in boarding schools. Campers participated in six hours of fun-based physical activities per day, and daily nutrition was structured based on each participant's estimated basal metabolic rate. Campers also attended weekly nutrition, lifestyle, and group sessions to promote awareness of behavioral patterns related to eating and physical activity. Group sessions included didactics and discussions related to self-monitoring, goal-setting, problem-solving, cognitive restructuring, stimulus control, and enhancing natural sources of social support. Significant group-by-time interactions showed that campers reduced their BMI, systolic blood pressure, diastolic blood pressure, and body fat percentage, and increased aerobic fitness in comparison to the control group. Further, longer durations at the camp resulted in greater improvements on these measures (Gately et al.). In addition, the camp had a generally positive impact on campers' psychological well-being. That is, campers displayed increases in self-esteem, global self-worth, athletic competence, and physical appearance esteem, and decreases in body shape dissatisfaction and negative automatic thoughts (Barton et al.; Walker et al.). However, no follow-up was conducted and, therefore, the long-term impact of this camp program on youths' weight and psychological functioning remains unknown.

The effects of long-term inpatient/residential interventions in Europe was examined in 122 children and adolescents (ages 7 to 17) who were admitted to a 10-month inpatient treatment program for overweight in Belgium (Braet, Tanghe, Decaluwe, Moens, & Rosseel, 2004). All were referred by medical doctors after outpatient treatments had failed. The youths stayed in a treatment center with an attached school, and were allowed to visit home two weekends a month. Meals were regulated by the center. During the first four months of treatment, all children received CBT in small groups (4–6 per group). Children were taught self-regulation skills, self-observation, self-instruction, self-evaluation, and self-reward. Children were also invited to develop personal eating plans for the weekend with therapist assistance. Parents were provided with information to assist their child in adopting a new lifestyle.

Significant effects were found over time for decreased percent overweight, BMI, and weight, as well as parent reports of decreases in internalizing behavior and increases in children's global psychological well-being. With regard to eating pathology, significant improvements over time were found in drive for thinness, bulimia, body dissatisfaction, external eating, eating concern, weight concern, and shape concern. Gender differences in outcome were also found because boys achieved greater weight loss, demonstrated improved self-reported physical appearance, and showed less eating pathology than girls. Average maintained weight loss at 14 months from pretreatment was 31.7 percent. In addition, 82 percent of children reached the goal of a 10 percent weight reduction. Psychological well-being gains were also maintained by participants at a 14-month follow-up.

A separate study of the same inpatient treatment program examined specific changes in physical activity and psychosocial determinants of physical activity in 30 youth enrolled in the inpatient program that did not exhibit any other significant psychological or medical problems other than overweight (Deforche, De Bourdeaudhuij, Tanghe, Hills, & De Bode, 2004). During treatment, adolescents displayed significant increases in high-intensity exercise and reductions in the amount of television watched. However, at a six-month follow-up in a less-controlled natural environment, youths' moderat-e to high-intensity physical activity levels and hours of television viewed relapsed to baseline levels. This suggests that while inpatient treatment can provide significant short-term outcomes in the treatment of overweight, changes made during treatment are unlikely to be maintained without ongoing support for behavioral changes from family members.

In a 10-month inpatient multidisciplinary weight-reduction program in France for extremely overweight adolescents (n = 26), participants were provided with prescribed diets, physical training, psychological follow-up, and nutrition education (Lazzer et al., 2005). At the end of the program, adolescents achieved significant decreases in BMI and time spent in sedentary activities. However, no follow-up data was collected once the adolescents returned home. Therefore, it is unknown if participants maintained their weight once they completed the program. Overall, this study appeared somewhat successful for reducing weight in very overweight adolescents, but the expense of inpatient programs likely limits its accessibility.

PRIMARY CARE INTERVENTIONS

Besides the outpatient specialty clinic setting and residential treatment facilities, interventions for overweight adolescents have been attempted in the primary care setting. Pediatricians have an excellent opportunity to screen adolescents for overweight at regular office visits. However, a national survey of pediatrician's practices indicated that adolescent overweight is diagnosed significantly less by pediatricians than the national prevalence of adolescent overweight (Cook, Weitzman, Auinger, & Barlow, 2005). This suggests that a large number of overweight children and adolescents go undiagnosed and untreated. Despite this, innovative attempts are being made to develop feasible overweight interventions that can be conducted in primary care settings.

For example, a multicomponent treatment called Patient-centered Assessment and Counseling for Exercise plus Nutrition (PACE+) was developed for use in a primary care setting (Patrick et al., 2001). Participants (n = 117) ages 11–18 years (n = 117) completed an interactive computer program designed to increase their moderate physical activity, vigorous physical activity, reduce fat intake, and increase fruit and vegetable intake. PACE+ components were based on the trans-theoretical model and guided participants to set specific change plans for one nutrition and one physical activity behavior they were most ready to change. After completing the computer program, participants received physical activity and nutrition counseling from a healthcare provider. Participants were then randomly assigned to a no-contact control group, frequent mail group, infrequent mail and telephone group, or frequent mail and telephone group to evaluate a low-cost follow-up strategy over a four-month trial. All groups displayed significant improvements in healthy dietary intake, and in moderate physical activity, and adolescents who targeted a specific behavior improved more than those who did not target a behavior—unless that behavior was vigorous physical activity.

In a multicomponent behavioral weight-control intervention implemented in a primary care office, overweight adolescents were randomly assigned to the Healthy Habits program group (n = 23), or a traditional single session of physician-moderated weight counseling group (n = 21; Saelens, et al., 2002). The Healthy Habits group completed a computer program adapted from the PACE+ specifically designed for overweight adolescents who developed an individualized action plan. The action plan was subsequently discussed with their physicians, who tailored their counseling to the specific action plans. Treatment participants then received weekly follow-up phone counseling calls for eight weeks, and then bi-weekly calls for an additional six to eight weeks. Phone counseling included teaching adolescents about the association between weight change and nutritional and physical activity behaviors, goals, self-monitoring, and the use of behavioral skills related to goal achievement. Adolescents were also provided with manuals to assist them in acquiring behavioral skills related to weight change, and parents were sent information sheets highlighting how to reinforce their child and assist their child with structuring the environment to promote healthy lifestyle habits. The primary care behavioral intervention resulted in modest decreases in BMI and the intervention group did not return to their baseline weight at follow-up, but the control group's BMI increased at post-treatment and follow-up. This suggests that the Healthy Habits program at least helps overweight adolescents maintain their BMI, whereas those who did not receive the intervention continued to gain weight.

CORRELATES OF TREATMENT OUTCOME

Given the mixed evidence for the efficacy of various types of adolescent overweight interventions, research has been conducted to gain a better understanding of what treatment and patient characteristics may be associated with better treatment outcomes. Several predictors of treatment outcomes in overweight adolescents have emerged. Specifically, daily monetary reinforcement (Coates, Jeffrey, Slinkard, Killen, & Danaher, 1982), increased self-monitoring (Kirschenbaum, Germann, & Rich, 2005), higher BMI at pretreatment (Braet, 2006), initial weight loss (Braet), higher treatment attendance (Germann, Kirschenbaum, Rich, & O'Koon, 2006; Resnicow et al., 2005), and peer involvement (Jelalian et al., 2006), have all been linked to greater weight reduction while participating in a multidisciplinary treatment program. However, there is no consistent evidence to help determine whether adolescents and parents should attend treatment separately or if they should be seen together (Brownell et al., 1983; Coates et al.; Wadden et al., 1990). Parent and family participation in treatment is nevertheless an important factor in treating pediatric overweight (Golan & Crow, 2004; Goldfield, Raynor, & Epstein, 2002).

MEDICAL INTERVENTIONS

Although multicomponent interventions continue to be the most widely used approach to weight loss for overweight adolescents, recent advances in medical approaches, such as pharmacological and surgical treatments, are generating increased options for the treatment of overweight adolescents. However, relatively few medical intervention studies have been reported in the literature for children and adolescents. Nevertheless, initial findings suggest the potential for effectively integrating medical interventions into existing empirically-based multicomponent interventions to better address adolescent overweight.

Pharmacological Therapies

Three of the most commonly discussed anti-obesity drugs in current research include sibutramine, orlistat, and metformin. Recent studies suggest the potential for the use of these relatively safe and well-tolerated pharmacological treatments for adolescent overweight. In two RCTs, the efficacy of combined sibutramine and behavior treatment on reducing weight in overweight adolescents was evaluated (Berkowitz, Wadden, Tershakovec,

& Cronquist, 2003; Berkowitz et al., 2006). A previous RCT ($n = 82$) demonstrated the short-term efficacy of the addition of sibutramine to a six-month family-based behavioral weight-loss program in reducing weight compared to the behavioral therapy and placebo control group (Berkowitz et al., 2003). However, the medication dose had to be reduced ($n = 23$) or discontinued ($n = 10$) to manage the increases in blood pressure, heart rate, and other symptoms.

In a larger multicenter double blind RCT (3:1 randomization ratio) of the efficacy of a one-year sibutramine and behavior intervention, the behavior therapy plus sibutramine treatment group ($n = 368$) showed significantly greater improvements in overweight adolescents' (ages 12–16) BMI, body weight, triglyceride levels, high-density lipoprotein cholesterol levels, insulin levels, and insulin sensitivity relative to the behavior therapy plus placebo group ($n = 130$; Berkowitz et al., 2006). Overall, adverse events led to the removal of 23 sibutramine participants (6.3%) from the medication. In much smaller RCTs, significant reductions in BMI were also found when examining the efficacy of sibutramine on Brazilian and Mexican overweight adolescents (Garcia-Morales et al., 2006; Godoy-Matos et al., 2005).

In a study that employed similar multicenter RCT (2:1 randomization ratio) methodology, the efficacy of a one-year trial of an orlistat, plus diet, exercise, and family-based behavioral intervention, was evaluated with overweight adolescents ages 12–16 (Chanoine, Hampl, Jensen, Boldrin, & Hauptman, 2005). There was a significant decrease in BMI in both treatment groups until Week 12. The orlistat treatment group's BMIs ($n = 232$) stabilized from 12 weeks to one year, whereas the control group's BMIs ($n = 117$) slightly increased. A much smaller RCT also supported the use of orlistat in reducing overweight adolescents' weight, BMI, total cholesterol, low-density lipoprotein-cholesterol, fasting insulin, and fasting glucose (Ozkan, Bereket, Turan, & Keskin, 2004).

Metformin has also been evaluated for the treatment of adolescent overweight. However, the trials specific to overweight treatment have been much smaller relative to orlistat and sibutramine. Three RCTs (n ranges from 24 to 29 overweight) provided preliminary support for the use of metformin in treating adolescent overweight. Specifically, metformin treatment (from eight weeks to six months in length) resulted in greater weight loss, reductions in BMI, and fasting insulin, in comparison to control groups (Freemark & Bursey, 2001; Kay et al., 2001; Srinivasan et al., 2006). However, the long-term effect of metformin on adolescent overweight is unknown. Larger multisite RCTs of all three drugs are needed to gain a better understanding of their relative long-term effectiveness for weight control in adolescents, as well as their potential side effects.

Bariatric Surgery

Drawing further attention, interest, and controversy is the issue of adolescent bariatric surgery. The continuing development of effective weight management surgery is leading to a decrease in possible post-operative complications (e.g., mortality, nutrition, physical development, pregnancy) associated with surgery (Inge et al., 2004). Decreased complications and increased safety of surgery are providing adolescents who have a significant history of failing (≥ six months) in other organized weight-loss interventions an alternative intervention for managing their weight.

Several studies suggest that bariatric gastric bypass surgery is efficacious for treating overweight adolescents and related comorbidities (Garcia, Langford, & Inge, 2003). Research has shown that bariatric surgery has demonstrated larger improvements in short-term and long-term follow-up BMIs relative to other weight interventions (Inge, Xanthakos, & Zeller, 2007; Rand & MacGregor, 1994). However, the effectiveness of bariatric surgery in reducing weight should be viewed with caution because most adolescents that receive the surgery have a BMI ≥ 40. As a result, these individuals have more weight to lose than moderately or mildly overweight adolescents. Other positive surgery results discussed in a study with 34 adolescents interviewed six years post-surgery included excellent psychosocial adjustment (i.e., improved self-esteem, social relationships, and appearance) as reported by the patients (Rand & MacGregor).

The recently approved (for adults) adjustable banding is gaining more interest, particularly for adolescent patients where the adjustability in the gastric band can better accommodate the needs of a physically developing individual. The adjustability of the device can permit for a progression of weight loss and degree of restriction most appropriate over time, avoiding the problem with nutritional deficiencies (Garcia et al., 2003). Also, if complications persist, the gastric band can be surgically removed. Preliminary studies have demonstrated that laparoscopic adjustable gastric banding in severely overweight adolescents results in significant reductions in weight at short-term follow-up (as early as six months) and at long-term follow-up (up to six years post-operative) (Angrisani et al., 2005; Fielding & Duncombe, 2005; Nadler, Youn, Ginsburg, Ren, & Fielding, 2007). However, more well-controlled larger studies of adolescent bariatric surgery are needed to further explore the potential benefits and risks associated with bariatric surgery before surgery is integrated as a standard treatment for extreme adolescent overweight. In addition, more studies concerning the psychosocial outcomes for adolescents after bariatic surgery are needed.

COMMENTARY

A number of studies addressing various treatments for overweight adolescents have been reported in recent years, including over two dozen randomized controlled trials. Most of the studies reported in the literature focus on multicomponent outpatient treatment programs. The results of these studies provide some evidence supporting the efficacy of behavioral interventions that target lifestyle changes in dietary intake and physical activity (Brownell et al., 1983; Coates et al., 1982; Jelalian et al., 2006; Nemet et al., 2005; Wadden et al., 1990). While multicomponent intervention studies that emphasize increased physical activity have not consistently showed significant weight loss—they have demonstrated improvements in physical fitness and reductions in cardiovascular and metabolic risks (Becque et al., 1988; Gutin et al., 2002; Kang et al., 2002), as well as improved self-worth (Daley et al., 2006).

It is worth noting that the few reported studies that intervened separately on the side of either dietary intake or physical activity did not produce very significant reductions in body weight or improvements in BMI over time, suggesting that addressing both of these components may be essential for successful treatment outcomes. However, there is some evidence supporting the idea that reduced-carbohydrate diets produce better weight loss than reduced-fat diets (Ebbeling et al., 2003; Sondike et al., 2003). Nevertheless, reductions in total caloric intake are clearly needed for successful weight loss, whether by reductions in fat or carbohydrate intake. More research is needed with larger study samples to determine which types of dietary caloric restriction are more appealing and feasible with overweight adolescents. Few studies have considered the use of very low calorie diets for the treatment of extremely overweight youth. While there is some support for this approach in a clinical study (Sothern et al., 2000), more controlled research with larger study samples is needed to determine the efficacy in the short- and long-term, and whether this approach is feasible and acceptable for overweight adolescents.

Findings regarding the role of parents in adolescent weight-loss treatment suggest that equal outcomes were obtained when the adolescent was treated with a parent or with the parent seen separately, although only a few studies have specifically addressed this issue (Brownell et al., 1983; Coates et al., 1982; Wadden et al., 1990). The key point for clinical practice is that parents must be involved to some extent for adolescent weight loss to be successful. Not only are parents an important source of support for adolescents' weight-loss efforts, but they obviously play a major role in the types of foods provided for adolescents in the home setting, as well as providing a role model for their children in terms of lifestyle habits.

Because peer groups are so important to adolescents, it is reasonable to involve them to some degree in adolescent weight-loss programs. Most programs are conducted in a group setting with overweight peers. A recent study by Jelalian et al. (2006) showed that overweight adolescents who received an enhanced peer group intervention focusing on recreational outdoor physical activity and skill-building had better maintenance of weight loss during the follow-up period—suggesting the important role of peer support for overweight adolescents. However, little is known about the effects of normal-weight peers on the overweight adolescent's efforts to make effective health behavior changes, and there are no intervention studies specifically addressing the potential positive effects of their involvement on overweight youths' weight loss.

It is important to consider the settings in which weight-loss interventions are conducted. While most reported studies were traditional clinic-based interventions, there is a clear need to reach more of the overweight population than may be possible using clinics as the site of intervention. Research shows that several settings hold considerable promise for adolescent weight-loss intervention. For example, the primary care setting has particular advantages at least for the identification of overweight status, as well as initiating some type of weight-loss program. Initial research in this area indicates that overweight adolescents can be provided brief interventions in the primary care setting targeting specific health behavior changes, and that—when followed up with over time with mail and telephone support—they can achieve improvements in dietary intake and physical activity (Patrick et al., 2001; Saelens et al., 2002). Again, more controlled work with larger study samples are needed, with effects on weight loss demonstrated over time.

An innovative study was reported by Resnicow et al. (2005) that provided behavioral intervention for overweight African-American girls in the church setting. This study added unique treatment components, including motivational interviewing and daily electronic reminders. The results indicated that better weight loss occurred for those girls who attended more treatment sessions. More research is needed to evaluate the use of motivational interviewing, as well as technology that can provide daily interaction and feedback with youth regarding their health behaviors. More work is also needed in exploring the use of church and other community settings to conduct weight-loss interventions.

As more of the population has access to the Internet, there is a tremendous potential to reach more of the overweight adolescent population. Initial work in this area is promising (Williamson et al., 2006), and indicates positive short-term effects but a lack of maintenance over time. More work in this area should focus on ways to engage adolescents over time with informative, fun, and interactive methods so that they continue to utilize the weight loss program.

There are many summer camp programs for overweight youth, yet few have been empirically evaluated. The studies reviewed in this chapter suggest the potential of the summer camp approach for achieving significant reductions in body weight, improvements in cardiovascular fitness, and improved psychosocial functioning (Barton et al., 2004; Gately et al., 2005; Walker et al., 2003). However, it is important to note that these reports were nonrandomized studies, and the effects were not evaluated through follow-up after the camp program ended.

Extremely overweight youth have also been treated in the inpatient residential setting. Several nonrandomized studies were recently reported from Europe indicating that significant reductions in weight can be achieved (Braet et al., 2004; Deforche et al., 2004; Lazzer et al., 2005). However, it is important to consider the tremendous expense of these residential programs that often last up to 10 months, and the lack of follow-up. In the one study reporting outcomes six months after residential treatment (Deforche et al., 2004), there was a return to baseline functioning in terms of reduced levels of physical activity and increases in sedentary behavior.

Medical interventions have also been recently examined, including both pharmacological and surgical approaches. Two randomized controlled trials with sibutramine indicate it can promote better weight loss than that achieved by family behavioral intervention alone (Berkowitz et al., 2003, 2006). However, side effects requiring either reductions or discontinuation of the medication were noted for significant numbers of patients. Similarly, two RCTs demonstrated that orlistat helped to achieve reduced weight in adolescents, as well as improved cardiovascular risk profiles (Chanoine et al., 2005; Ozkan et al., 2004), but the gastrointestinal side effects of this medication may make this an unattractive treatment option for adolescents. The results of three RCTs provide some evidence that metformin may be a reasonable medication to promote weight loss in adolescents, as well as reduce cardiovascular and metabolic risk (Freemark & Bursey, 2001; Kay et al., 2001; Srinivasan et al., 2006). More controlled research with these medications, as well as other medications, is needed to determine the efficacy and safety of pharmacological interventions for overweight adolescents. It is unlikely that pharmacologic approaches would be effective in the absence of behavioral interventions to promote healthier lifestyles behaviors.

When all else fails for the extremely overweight adolescent, surgical approaches are a treatment option that has been increasingly used in recent years. While the outcome data support the efficacy of bariatric surgery for overweight adolescents (Garcia et al., 2003), there are significant complications that can result from these procedures, and the long-term safety and efficacy of this approach has not been demonstrated.

Overall, these initial medical intervention studies demonstrate that pharmacological therapy and surgical procedures, in addition to the behavioral intervention targeting healthy dietary intake and increased physical activity, may have a greater positive effect for weight loss in adolescents than standard multicomponent treatments alone. Regardless of which medical treatment may be used, it is generally accepted that an interdisciplinary team approach consisting of medical specialists, psychologists, dietitians, and exercise physiologists, is needed to effectively work with overweight adolescent patients. More research is required to address various issues such as ethnic differences, side effects of medications, surgical complications, and both physical and psychosocial development using larger-sample, randomized trials before drugs and surgeries can be safely integrated with current multicomponent treatment options.

CONCLUSIONS

Overweight in adolescents has reached epidemic proportions in the United States, with approximately 17 percent categorized as overweight, and 34 percent categorized as at-risk for overweight (Ogden et al., 2006). Obese adolescents are at increased risk for various health-related and psychosocial comorbidities. The likelihood is very high that overweight adolescents will remain overweight as adults, increasing their risk of developing various health problems, including cardiovascular disease and type II diabetes. Identifying and implementing effective treatments for overweight adolescents is therefore an urgent issue of great public health significance.

Review of research studies provide some support for the efficacy of multicomponent interventions that address weight loss through modification of dietary and physical activity lifestyle behaviors. Such interventions that include parental involvement and support, as well as the involvement of peers, appear to hold promise for sustained weight loss. Given the numbers of overweight adolescents needing treatment, researchers must focus on ways to reach and deliver efficacious interventions, considering the fact that most families will likely not seek out specialty outpatient programs located in medical centers. More research is needed to evaluate the efficacy and costs of interventions delivered in community settings such as schools, churches, and primary care clinics—as well as over the Internet—to provide treatment to more adolescents. More work is also needed on methods to motivate, engage, and sustain adolescents and their families in treatment, as research indicates better outcomes with increased program participation and longer duration of treatment. While camp and residential programs are another treatment option, there are currently no controlled studies with long-term follow-up to support their use. Medical interventions including both pharmacological and surgical approaches have shown some efficacy, but more research is needed to demonstrate their safety and acceptability, as well as their long-term effects.

REFERENCES

Angrisani, L., Favretti, F., Furbetta, F., Paganelli, M., Basso, N., Soldi, S. B., et al., (2005). Obese teenagers treated by lap-band system: The Italian experience. *Surgery, 138,* 877–881.

Barton, S. B., Walker, L. L., Lambert, G., Gately, P. J., & Hill, A. J. (2004). Cognitive change in obese adolescents losing weight. *Obesity Research, 12,* 313–319.

Baur, L. A., & O'Connor, J. (2004). Special considerations in childhood and adolescent obesity. *Clinics in Dermatology, 22* (4), 338–344.

Becque, M. D., Katch, V. L., Rocchini, A. P., marks, C. R., & Moorehead, C. (1988). Coronary risk of obese adolescents: Reduction by exercise plus diet intervention. *Pediatrics, 81,* 605–612.

Berkowitz, R. I., Fujioka, K., Daniels, S. R., Hoppin, A. G., Owen, S., Perry, A. C., et al., (2006). Effects of sibutramine treatment in obese adolescents: A randomized trial. *Annals of Internal Medicine, 145,* 81–90.

Berkowitz, R. I., Wadden, T. A., Tershakovec, A. M., & Cronquist, J. L. (2003). Behavior therapy and sibutramine for the treatment of adolescent obesity. *Journal of the American Medical Association, 289,* 1805–1812.

Braet, C. (2006). Patient characteristics as predictors of weight loss after an obesity treatment for children. *Obesity, 14,* 148–155.

Braet, C., Tanghe, A., Decaluwe, V., Moens, E., & Rosseel, Y. (2004). Inpatient treatment for children with obesity: Weight loss, psychological well-being, and eating behavior. *Journal of Pediatric Psychology, 29,* 519–529.

Brownell, K. D., Kelman, S. H., & Stunkard, A. J. (1983). Treatment of obese children with and without their mothers: Changes in weight and blood pressure. *Pediatrics, 71,* 515–523.

Chanoine, J., Hampl, S., Jensen, C., Boldrin, M., & Hauptman, J. (2005). Effect of orlistat on weight and body composition in obese adolescents. *Journal of American Medical Association, 293,* 2873– 1491

Coates, T. J., Jeffrey, R. W., Slinkard, L. A., Killen, J. D., & Danaher, B. G. (1982). Frequency of contact and monetary reward in weight loss, lipid change, and blood pressure reduction with adolescents. *Behavior Therapy, 13,* 175–185.

Coates, T. J., Killen, J. D., & Slinkard, L. A. (1982). Parent participation in a treatment program for overweight adolescents. *International Journal of Eating Disorders, 1,* 37–48.

Cook, S., Weitzman, M., Auinger, P., & Barlow, S. (2005). Screening and counseling associated with obesity diagnosis in a national survey of ambulatory pediatric visits. *Pediatrics, 116,* 112–116.

Daley, A. J., Copeland, R. J., Wright, N. P., Roalfe, A., & Wales, J. K. (2006). Exercise therapy as a treatment for psychopathologic conditions in obese and morbidly obese adolescents: A randomized controlled trial. *Pediatrics, 118*, 2126–2134.

Deforche, B., De Bourdeaudhuij, I., Tanghe, A., Hills, A. P., & De Bode, P. (2004). Changes in physical activity and psychosocial determinants of physical activity in children and adolescents treated for obesity. *Patient Education and Counseling, 55*, 407–415.

Ebbeling, C. B., Leidig, M. M., Sinclair, K. B., Hangen, J. P., & Ludwig, D. S. (2003). A reduced-glycemic load diet in the treatment of adolescent obesity. *Archives of Pediatric Adolescent Medicine, 157*, 773–779.

Epstein, L., & Goldfield, G. (1999). Physical activity in the treatment of childhood overweight and obesity: Current evidence and research issues. *Medicine & Science in Sports & Exercise, 31*, S553–S559.

Epstein, L. H., Valoski, A. M., Wing, R. R., & McCurley, J. (1994). Ten year outcomes of behavioral family-based treatment for childhood obesity. *Health Psychology, 13*, 373–383.

Fielding, G. A., & Duncombe, J. E. (2005). Laparoscopic adjustable banding in severely obese adolescents. *Surgery for Obesity and Related Diseases, 1*, 399–407.

Freemark, M., & Bursey, D. (2001). The effects of metformin on body mass index and glucose tolerance in obese adolescents with fasting hyperinsulinemia and a family history of type 2 diabetes. *Pediatrics, 107*, E55.

Garcia, V. F., Langford, L., & Inge, T. H. (2003). Application of laparoscopy for bariatric surgery in adolescents. *Current Opinion in Pediatrics, 15*, 248–255.

Garcia-Morales, L. M., Berber, A., Macias-Lara, C. C., Lucio-Ortiz, C., Del Rio-Navarro, B. E., & Dorantes-Alvarez, L. M. (2006). Use of sibutramine in obese Mexican adolescents: A 6-month, randomized, double-blind, placebo-controlled, parallel-group trial. *Clinical Therapeutics, 28*, 770–782.

Gately, P. J., Cooke, C. B., Barth, J. H., Bewick, B. M., Radley, D., & Hill, A. J. (2005). Children's residential weight-loss programs can work: A prospective cohort study of short-term outcomes for overweight and obese children. *Pediatrics, 116*, 73–77.

Germann, J. N., Kirschenbaum, D. S., Rich, B. H., & O'Koon, J. C. (2006). Long-term evaluation of multi-disciplinary treatment of morbid obesity in low-income minority adolescents: LaRabida Children's Hospital Fitmatters Program. *Journal of Adolescent Health, 39*, 553–561.

Godoy-Matos, A., Carraro, L., Vieira, A., Oliveira, J., Guedas, E. P., Mattos, L., et al., (2005). Treatment of obese adolescents with sibutramine: A randomized, double-blind, controlled study. *The Journal of Clinical Endocrinology & Metabolism, 90*, 1460–1465.

Golan, M., & Crow, S. (2004). Targeting parents exclusively in the treatment of childhood obesity: Long-term results. *Obesity Research, 12*(2), 357–361.

Goldfield, G. S., Raynor, H. A., & Epstein, L.H. (2002). Treatment of pediatric obesity. In A. J. Stunkard & T. A. Wadden (Eds.), *Obesity: Theory and Therapy.* (2nd ed., pp. 137–149). New York: Raven Press.

Gutin, B., Barbeau, P., Owens, S., Lemmon, C.R., Bauman, M., Allison, J., et al., (2002). Effects of exercise intensity on cardiovascular fitness, total body composition, and the visceral adiposity of obese adolescents. *American Journal of Clinical Nutrition, 75*, 818–826.

Inge, T. H., Krebs, N. F., Garcia, V. F., Skelton, J. A., Guice, K. S., Strauss, R. S. et al., (2004) Bariatric surgery for severely overweight adolescents: Concerns and recommendations. *Pediatrics, 114*, 217–223.

Inge, T. H., Xanthakos, S. A., & Zeller, M. H. (2007). Bariatric surgery for pediatric obesity: Now or later? *International Journal of Obesity, 31*, 1–14.

Jelalian, E. and Mehlenback, R. (2003). Pediatric Obesity. In M. Roberts (Ed.,) *Handbook of Pediatric Psychology*, (3rd ed., pp. 529–543). New York, NY: Guilford Press.

Jelalian, E., Mehlenbeck, R., Lloyd-Richardson, E. E., Birmaher, V., & Wing, R. R., (2006). 'Adventure therapy' combined with cognitive-behavioral treatment for overweight adolescents. *International Journal of Obesity, 30*, 31–39.

Kang, H. S., Gutin, B., Barbeau, P., Owens, S., Lemmon, C. R., Allison, J. et al., (2002). Physical training improves insulin resistance syndrome markers in obese adolescents. *Medicine and Science in Sports and Exercise, 34,* 1920–1927.

Kay, J. P., Alemzadeh, R., Langley, G., D'Angelo, L., Smith, P., & Holshouser, S. (2001). Beneficial effects of metformin in normoglycemic morbidly obese adolescents. *Metabolism, 50,* 1457–1461.

Kirschenbaum, D. S., Germann, J. N., & Rich, B. H. (2005). Treatment of morbid obesity in low-income adolescents: Effects of parental self-monitoring. *Obesity Research, 13,* 1527–1529.

Lazzer, S., Boirie, Y., Poissonnier, C., Petit, I., Duche, P., Taillardat, M., et al., (2005). Longitudinal changes in activity patterns, physical capacities, energy expenditure, and body composition in severely obese adolescents during a multidisciplinary weight-reduction program. *International Journal of Obesity, 29,* 37–46.

Mellin, L. M., Slunkard, L. A. & Irwin, C. E. (1987). Adolescent obesity intervention: Validation of the SHAPEDOWN program. *Journal of the American Dietetic Association, 87,* 333–338.

Nadler, E. P., Youn, H. A., Ginsburg, H. B., Ren, C. J., & Fielding, G. A. (2007). Short-term results in 53 US obese pediatric patients with laparoscopic adjustable gastric banding. *Journal of Pediatric Surgery, 42,* 137–142.

Nassis, G. P., Papatakou, K., Skenderi, K., Triandafillopoulou, M., Kavouras, S. A., Yannakoulia, M., et al., (2005). Aerobic exercise training improves insulin sensitivity without changes in body weight, body fat, adiponectin, and inflammatory markers in overweight and obese girls. *Metabolism: Clinical and Experimental, 54,* 1472–1479.

Nemet, D., Barkan, S., Epstein, Y., Friedland, O., Kowen, G., & Eliakim, A. (2005). Short- and long-term beneficial effects of a combined dietary-behavioral-physical activity intervention for the treatment of childhood obesity. *Pediatrics, 115,* 443–449.

Ogden, C. L., Carroll, M. D., Curtin, L. R., McDowell, M. A., Tabak, C. J., & Flegal, K. M. (2006). Prevalence of overweight and overweight in the United States, 1999–2004. *Journal of the American Medical Association, 295,* 1549–1555.

Ozkan, B., Bereket,A., Turan, S., & Keskin, S. (2004). Addition of orlistat to conventional treatment in adolescents with severe obesity. *European Journal of Pediatrics, 163,* 738–741.

Pate, R. R., et al. (2005). Promotion of Physical Activity Among High-School Girls: A Randomized Controlled Trial. *American Journal of Public Health, 95,* 1582–1600.

Patrick, K., Sallis, J. F., Prochaska, J. J., Lydston, D. D., Calfas, K. J., Zabinski, M. F., et al., (2001). A multicomponent program for nutrition and physical activity change in primary care. *Pediatric and Adolescent Medicine, 155,* 940–946.

Rand, C. S. & MacGregor, A. M. (1994). Adolescents having obesity surgery: A six year follow-up. *Southern Medical Journal, 87,* 1208–1213.

Reinehr, T., Brylak, K., Alexy, U., Kersting, M., & Andler, W. (2003). Predictors to success in outpatient training in obese children and adolescents. *International Journal of Obesity & Related Metabolic Disorders, 27,* 1087–1092.

Resnicow, K., Taylor, R., Baskin, M., & McCarty, F. (2005). Results of Go Girls: A weight control program for overweight African-American adolescent females. *Obesity Research, 13,* 1739–1748.

Rolland-Cachera, M. F. et al. (2004). Massive obesity in adolescents: Dietary interventions and behaviours associated with weight regain at 2 year follow-up. *International Journal of Obesity, 28,* 514–519.

Saelens, B. E., Sallis, J. F., Wilfey, D. E., Patrick, K., Cella, J. A., & Butcha, R. (2002). Behavioral weight control for overweight adolescents initiated in primary care. *Obesity Research, 10,* 22–32.

Sondike, S. B., Copperman, N., & Jacobson, M. S. (2003). Effects of a low-carbohydrate diet on weight loss and cardiovascular risk factors in overweight adolescents. *Journal of Pediatric Psychology, 142,* 253–258.

Sothern, M., Udall, J. N., Jr., Suskind, R. M., Vargas, A., & Blecker, U. (2000). Weight loss and growth velocity in obese children after very low calorie diet, exercise and behavior modification. *Acta paediatrica, 89,* 1036–1043.

Srinivasan, S., Ambler, G. R., Baur, L. A., Garnett, S. P., Tepsa, M., Yap, F. et al., (2006). Randomized, controlled trial of metformin for obesity and insulin resistance in children and adolescents: Improvement in body composition and fasting insulin. *The Journal of Clinical Endocrinology & Metabolism, 91,* 2074–2080.

Stallings, V. A., Archibald, E. H., Pencharz, P. B., Harrison, J. E., & Bell, L. E. (1988). One-year follow-up of weight, total body potassium, and total body nitrogen in overweight adolescents treated with the protein-sparing modified fast. *The American Journal of Clinical Nutrition, 48,* 91–94.

Wadden, T. A., Stunkard, A. J., Rich, L., Rubin, C. J., Sweidel, G., & McKinney, S. (1990). Obesity in black adolescent girls: A controlled clinical trial of treatment by diet, behavior modification, and parent support. *Pediatrics, 85,* 345–352.

Walker, L. L. M., Gately, P. J., Bewick, B. M., & Hill, A. J. (2003). Children's weight-loss camps: Psychological benefit or jeopardy? *International Journal of Obesity, 27,* 748–754.

Williamson, D. A., Walden, H. M., White, M. A., York-Crowe, E., Newton, Jr., R. L., Alfonso, A., et al., (2006). Two-year internet-based randomized controlled trial for weight loss in African-American girls. *Obesity Research, 14,* 1231–1243.

15

Intensive Therapies for the Treatment of Pediatric Obesity

JOAN C. HAN and JACK A. YANOVSKI

For children and adolescents with abnormally high body adiposity, therapies for minimizing future weight gain and inducing weight loss may play important roles in the prevention and treatment of the comorbid conditions associated with obesity. While the initial approach to the management of obesity in children and adolescents should be moderate caloric restriction in combination with behavior modification, increased physical activity, and decreased time spent in sedentary behaviors (Barlow & Dietz, 1998; Speiser et al., 2005), these conservative measures are not always successful in producing long-term weight control (Epstein, Valoski, Wing, & McCurley, 1990, 1994). Therefore, more aggressive approaches—such as restriction of energy intake below 1000 kcal/d, pharmacotherapy, and bariatric surgery—have been suggested as treatment options for severe pediatric obesity. In this chapter, we will review the limited available data for the safety and efficacy of these intensive therapies in children and adolescents.

JOAN C. HAN and JACK A. YANOVSKI • National Institute of Child Health and Human Development National Institutes of Health, Bethesda, MD 20892.

Supported by the Intramural Research Program of the NIH, Grant ZO1-HD-00641 (NICHD, NIH) to Dr. Yanovski.

INDICATIONS AND CONSIDERATIONS FOR INTENSIVE THERAPY

Regardless of the severity of obesity, the first-line approach should always be moderate caloric restriction and increased activity. Should these measures fail to achieve satisfactory weight control, the aggressiveness of therapy should be commensurate with the degree of obesity. In general, only those children and adolescents who have a body mass index (BMI) greater than the 95th percentile for age and sex (as defined by the Center for Disease Control; Kuczmarski et al., 2000), who have also developed a demonstrable medical complication that may be remediable through weight reduction should be considered for intensive treatment regimens (Yanovski, 2001). In many older studies, the severity of obesity was gauged not by the subject's BMI percentile, but by the subject's weight expressed as a percentage of his/her ideal body weight (IBW), defined as the 50th percentile weight-for-height for a child of the same age and sex. Pharmacotherapy has generally been considered appropriate as an adjunct to standard therapy for children and adolescents with BMI ≥ 95th percentile (or who are ≥120 percent IBW) who also have an obesity-related comorbidity, such as dyslipidemia, hypertension, insulin resistance, steatohepatitis, obstructive sleep apnea, or orthopedic complications. Very low energy diets have generally been reserved for those ≥140 percent IBW. Recent recommendations for adolescent bariatric surgery suggest it should be offered only to those who are very severely obese (defined as BMI ≥40 kg/m²), who have largely completed skeletal growth (age ≥13 years for girls and ≥15 years for boys), and who have obesity-related comorbidities that might be remedied by long-lasting weight loss (Inge, Krebs, et al., 2004).

Each of these intensive therapies for pediatric obesity should be administered in conjunction with behavioral modification programs, designed to improve diet, increase physical activity, and decrease inactivity. Comprehensive family-based programs managed by multidisciplinary teams tend to yield better results, and therefore, whenever possible, patients with severe obesity should be referred to specialized centers with expertise in these regimens (Whitlock, Williams, Gold, Smith, & Shipman, 2005).

Finally, many intensive therapies are still considered investigational when used in children. Thus, obtaining written informed consent from parents before initiating such therapies may be advisable.

VERY LOW ENERGY DIETS

The standard pediatric dietary prescription for weight loss aims to reduce intake by approximately 500–700 kcal/day (to induce a 0.5 kg weight loss each week), and except for the youngest children, generally results in a total intake greater than 1000 kcal/day. More restrictive diet prescriptions are termed very low energy diets. Very low energy diets are often prescribed in the form of a protein-sparing modified fast (PSMF), intended to maximize fat loss while minimizing loss of lean body mass. PSMF regimens generally supply a daily intake of 600–800 kcal/day and 1.5–2.5 g high quality protein per kg of ideal body weight, while restricting carbohydrate intake to 20–40 g/day. Such formulations do not cause cardiac dysrhythmias or sudden death, as was observed in the 1970s when liquid protein diets containing only hydrolyzed collagen as a protein source were used (Anon., 1979; Michiel, Sneider, Dickstein, Hayman, & Eich, 1978). Many PSMF programs use readily available lean meats, poultry, and fish as protein sources (Sothern, von Almen, Schumacher, Suskind, & Blecker, 1999), although there are also commercially available liquid diet formulations. It is recommended that patients using a PSMF take a daily vitamin and mineral supplement and consume >1500 mL free water/day. In most programs, a PSMF is prescribed for no longer than 12 weeks, and is conducted under medical supervision.

In one study (Figueroa-Colon, Franklin, Lee, von Almen, & Suskind, 1996), 12 third to fifth graders weighing more than 140 percent IBW, who were enrolled in a comprehensive six-month school-based program that included a nine-week PSMF, lost 5.6 ± 7.1 kg vs. a weight gain of 2.8 ± 3.1 kg in seven untreated control children. In another study (Stallings, Archibald, Pencharz, Harrison, & Bell, 1988), 17 obese adolescents were treated with a PSMF for three months along with diet and activity counseling. At follow-up one year later, 48 percent had maintained at least some weight loss with a mean change in percent IBW of 29 percentage points. In a larger study (Sothern et al., 1999) of 87 children who weighed more than 120 percent IBW and remained enrolled in a one-year multidisciplinary weight-reduction program that included 10 weeks of PSMF, an exercise program, and behavior modification sessions, weight was 8.4 kg less after one year of treatment compared to baseline. However, no information about those who left the program was presented, and no control groups using a higher energy diet were studied.

Some investigators have employed PSMFs for longer periods of time. One study (Suskind et al., 1993) enrolled 50 obese children (aged 7 to 17-years old) in a 10-week nutrition, activity, and behavior modification education program plus a PSMF, and allowed those who were still more than 150 percent of IBW to continue taking the PSMF for as long as 30 weeks. When they stopped the PSMF, all subjects were offered a 1,200 kcal/d balanced diet maintenance program consisting of weekly exercise sessions and bimonthly educational programs. Fifteen subjects (30%) took the PSMF for more than 15 weeks. While 80 percent completed the 10-week program, only 60 percent were reported to have entered the weight maintenance program, and only 40 percent were reported as having 26-week follow-up. However, those subjects with 26-week follow-up reduced their body weight by approximately 9 kg, and had improvements in plasma lipids. Whether these results are better than those achievable with conventional dietary interventions has not been proven. In another study (Figueroa-Colon, von Almen, Franklin, Schuftan, & Suskind, 1993), 19 obese children aged 7 to 17 years in age were randomized to participate in a PSMF (600–800 kcal/d) or a hypocaloric balanced diet (800–1000 kcal/d) plus a behavior modification program for 10 weeks, and subsequently, both groups were then placed on a 1,000–1,200 kcal/d balanced diet. At the 10-week point, the PSMF group had greater weight loss (-11.2 ± 4.4 kg vs. -5.1 ± 4.1 kg, $p < 0.01$), but at one-year follow-up, both groups had similar weights, suggesting no long-lasting benefit of the PSMF relative to a balanced hypocaloric diet.

The potential risks of PSMF regimens include cholelithiasis, hyperuricemia (Mathew & Lifshitz, 1974), decreases in serum proteins including transferrin, retinol-binding protein, and complement β1c (Merritt, Blackburn, Bistrian, Palombo, & Suskind, 1981), orthostatic hypotension, halitosis, and diarrhea (Brown, Klish, Hollander, Campbell, & Forbes, 1983). Serious complications in patients treated with modern PSMFs appear to be rare. In summary, PSMF programs appear to be reasonably safe when carried out under medical supervision, and produce more rapid weight loss in the short term than conventional diets, but have not been shown to offer significant improvements in long-term outcome compared to less restrictive diets offered in the context of a comprehensive program. While there may be selected patients who will benefit from a PSMF, particularly when rapid short-term weight loss is desirable (for example, those who must lose weight before a surgical procedure can be performed, or who have life-threatening complications of obesity), it remains unclear whether programs employing a PSMF are superior at inducing the long-lasting significant weight changes desired for treatment of pediatric obesity than long-term programs using moderate caloric restriction.

PHARMACOTHERAPY

Because obesity is considered to be a chronic disease best treated using a long-term medical therapy model (Anon., 1996), there is great interest in identifying medications that may be safely prescribed over extended periods to treat pediatric obesity. Compared with the body of literature on medications to treat obesity in adults, there are relatively few data from pediatric-age patients. In this section, we will review the medications that have been studied in children, with a focus on randomized, double-blind, controlled trials.

Appetite Suppressants

Appetite suppressants act within the central nervous system to alter the release and reuptake of neurotransmitters involved in appetite—primarily norepinephrine, serotonin, and dopamine (Samanin & Garattini, 1993). Phentermine, diethylpropion, mazindol, ephedrine, racemic amphetamine, and dextroamphetamine are sympathomimetic drugs that increase the synaptic release of norepinephrine and/or dopamine and inhibit their reuptake. Racemic fenfluramine, dexfenfluramine, and chlorphentermine are halogenated amphetamine-like drugs that increase the release of serotonin and dopamine and inhibit their reuptake. Sibutramine is a cyclobutane-methanamine that inhibits the reuptake of norepinephrine, serotonin, and dopamine. Concomitant use of monoamine oxidase inhibitors is contraindicated for all these medications. In addition, it is recommended that patients taking medications affecting serotonin concentrations (such as sibutramine) avoid taking selective serotonin reuptake inhibitors.

Sibutramine is currently the only available appetite suppressant approved by the FDA for long-term use in adults—and, therefore, for adolescents aged ≥16y. There are also limited data studying its use in younger adolescents. In one RCT funded by the manufacturer (Berkowitz, Wadden, Tershakovec, & Cronquist, 2003), 82 obese adolescents (aged 13–17 years) received sibutramine 15mg/day or placebo—both in conjunction with an intensive, family-based, behavior therapy program, a 1200–1500 kcal/day diet, and a prescription for 120 minutes/week of exercise. Those treated with sibutramine lost significantly more weight in the first six months than those who received placebo (–7.8 vs. –3.2 kg, $p < 0.01$). During the second phase of the study, the sibutramine group was offered an additional six months of sibutramine, and on average regained 0.8 kg, while the placebo group was switched to sibutramine at the same dose, and lost an additional 1.3 kg. At 12 months, there was no statistical difference in total weight loss between those who had received 12 months vs. six months of sibutramine. Adverse effects included elevated blood pressure, elevated pulse, premature ventricular contractions, and cholelithiasis, and in 40 percent of subjects, the medication dose was lowered or discontinued due to side effects. In another RCT (Godoy-Matos et al., 2005), 60 obese adolescents (aged 14–17 years) were treated with sibutramine 10mg/day or placebo for six months, both in conjunction with counseling for a 500 kcal/day dietary deficit and 30min/day of physical activity. Those treated with sibutramine had significantly greater weight loss (–10.3 kg vs. –2.4 kg, $p < 0.001$) and decrease in BMI (–3.6 kg/m^2 vs. –0.9 kg/m^2, $p < 0.001$) than those given placebo. Constipation occurred in 40 percent of subjects receiving sibutramine, but no other adverse effects were reported. A 12-month, multicenter RCT of sibutramine plus behavior therapy in 498 obese adolescents, (Berkowitz et al., 2006) also funded by the manufacturer, found that BMI decreased significantly (–2.9 kg/m^2) in the sibutramine-treated group, but changed little (–0.3 kg/m^2) in the placebo-treated group. Taken together, these studies suggest that sibutramine may be useful for improving short-term weight loss in adolescents when used in conjunction with diet and exercise, but long-term efficacy is uncertain and sibutramine's use may be limited by cardiovascular side effects. Trials in younger children have not been reported.

Only short-term data (4–12 weeks of follow-up) are available for the use of phentermine (Spranger, 1965), chlorphentermine (Rauh & Lipp, 1968), mazindol (Golebiowska, Chlebna-Sokol, Kobierska, et al., 1981; Golebiowska, Chlebna-Sokol, Mastalska, & Zwaigzne-Raczynska, 1981; Komorowski, Zwaigzne-Raczynska, Owczarczyk, Golebiowska, & Zarzycki, 1982), amphetamine (Lorber, 1966) or diethylpropion (Andelman, Jones, & Nathan, 1967; Stewart, Bailey, & Patell, 1970) in children. Taken together, all of these studies suggest that these medications induce 2–5 kg greater weight loss compared with placebo. However, none of these studies included comprehensive behavior modification programs or longer-term follow-up. Adverse effects commonly reported with these medications included insomnia, jitteriness, palpitations, and dry mouth.

Coadministration of ephedrine and caffeine not only suppresses appetite, but has also been reported to increase energy expenditure in adult studies (Greenway, De Jonge, Blanchard, Frisard, & Smith, 2004).

One RCT study (Molnar, Torok, Erhardt, & Jeges, 2000) in 32 adolescents examined the use of 100–200 mg caffeine and 10–20 mg ephedrine given three times daily versus placebo. Both groups received nutritional counseling and were prescribed a 500 kcal deficit diet. After 20 weeks, the caffeine/ephedrine treated group had significantly greater decreases in body weight, BMI, and body fat compared with the placebo group (–7.9 kg vs. –0.5 kg weight loss). Reported side effects included nausea, insomnia, tremor, dizziness, and palpitations, but the side effects were reported as not different between the groups. Longer-term data have not been reported. In 2004, as a result of deaths due to hypertensive crises and arrhythmias, the FDA banned the sale of herbal products containing ephedrine, as well as the use of synthetic ephedrine for weight loss.

Both short-term and longer-term data are available for the effects of fenfluramine on body weight in overweight children. In short-term studies ranging from 4–9 weeks, use of fenfluramine or dexfenfluramine coupled with caloric restriction did not result in greater weight loss compared with placebo plus diet (Bacon & Lowrey, 1967; Grugni, Guzzaloni, Ardizzi, Moro, & Morabito, 1997; Malecka-Tendera, Koehler, Muchacka, Wazowski, & Trzciakowska, 1996). In a longer-term study (Pedrinola, Cavaliere, Lima, & Medeiros-Neto, 1994) of fenfluramine versus placebo for 12 months in 68 obese children (aged 10–17 years), the fenfluramine-treated children who remained in the study decreased BMI by 5.1 kg/m^2, while placebo-treated children decreased their BMI by 1.3 kg/m^2 ($p < 0.05$). Because this study was not reported as randomized or double-blind, did not provide results from a substantial portion of enrolled subjects, and did not include a significant behavioral modification, diet, or exercise program, it is not possible to interpret these results as indicating an advantage of fenfluramine treatment over conventional programs. Common side effects reported in these trials on fenfluramine in children included dry mouth, sleep disturbance, and drowsiness. In 1998, the FDA withdrew permission for the use of fenfluramine when cardiac valvulopathies—similar to those seen in the carcinoid syndrome—were found to be associated with fenfluramine use (Anon., 1997; Connolly et al., 1997).

Inhibitors of Nutrient Absorption

Orlistat is a gastric and pancreatic lipase inhibitor that prevents the hydrolysis of triglycerides into absorbable free fatty acids and monoglycerides, thereby reducing the absorption of dietary fat and cholesterol from the gastrointestinal tract (Mittendorfer, Ostlund, Patterson and Klein 2001). At a dose of 120 mg three times daily (TID), orlistat inhibits dietary fat absorption in adolescents and adults by approximately 30 percent (McDuffie, Calis, Uwaifo, et al., 2002; Zhi et al., 1994; Zhi, Moore, & Kanitra, 2003). Orlistat has minimal systemic absorption, and therefore its side effects occur by virtue of its mechanism of action—increased fat in the stool, particularly in subjects who continue to consume high-fat diets. Commonly reported side effects include oily stools, oily spotting of clothing, increased flatulence, and increased defecation. Also, because orlistat has been shown to reduce the absorption of some fat-soluble vitamins (McDuffie, Calis, Booth, Uwaifo, & Yanovski, 2002), it is recommended that all subjects receiving orlistat also be placed on a daily multivitamin taken at least two hours before or after orlistat is given.

There have been three open-label studies on the use of orlistat in obese children and adolescents (McDuffie et al., 2004; McDuffie, Calis, Uwaifo et al., 2002; Norgren, Danielsson, Jurold, Lotborn, & Marcus, 2003; Ozkan, Bereket, Turan, & Keskin, 2004). Follow-up in these studies ranged from 3–15 months, and the number of subjects studied were less than 25 in each group. In sum, these studies showed that orlistat (120 mg TID) combined with behavior modification resulted in 4–6 kg of weight loss. Gastrointestinal side effects were common, but no serious adverse events were reported.

The only published RCT (Chanoine, Hampl, Jensen, Boldrin, & Hauptman, 2005) on the use of orlistat in adolescents was funded by the manufacturer and conducted at 32 institutions with pediatric obesity treatment programs in the United States and Canada. The trial enrolled 539 adolescents, aged 12–16 years, with BMI ≥ two units above the 95th percentile, who were randomized in a 2-to-1 ratio to receive orlistat at 120 mg TID or placebo TID for 52 weeks. Subjects were also prescribed a daily multivitamin and were offered a behavior modification program, a calorie-restricted diet, and prescriptions to increase physical activity. Two-thirds of the subjects completed the study, and the reasons for discontinuation were similar between the two groups. After 52 weeks, those who had received orlistat had significantly less weight gain compared with those who had received placebo (+0.53 kg vs. +3.14 kg, $p < 0.001$), and had decreased BMI by 0.55 kg/m^2 while the placebo group increased BMI by 0.31 kg/m^2 ($p = 0.001$). There were no significant differences between the two groups in lipid levels or glucose and insulin in response to oral glucose challenge. Adverse effects reported with orlistat use included fatty/oily stool (50%), oily spotting (29%), oily evacuation (23%), abdominal pain (22%), fecal urgency (21%), and new development of cholelithiasis (2%). In general, gastrointestinal symptoms were mild, and only 2 percent of the subjects in the orlistat group discontinued the study because of drug-related adverse effects. Fat-soluble vitamin levels remained normal and increased in both groups during treatment, although the orlistat group had statistically smaller increases in beta carotene compared with the control group ($p < 0.001$).

Taken together, these studies suggest that orlistat—when combined with behavior modification, diet, and exercise—may provide short-term improvement in weight management. Whether these findings will translate into improved health outcomes remains to be determined, and further data are needed to better understand the long-term impact of orlistat treatment. Although only 2 percent of subjects in the 52-week RCT (Chanoine et al., 2005) dropped out because of gastrointestinal complaints, the fact that 50–100 percent of subjects in all of these trials had some unpleasant side effects raises concern about the wider applicability of orlistat in pediatric patients. Especially given that orlistat is a medication taken thrice daily, adherence—particularly during school hours—for both logistical and social reasons, may be difficult for children. Overall, however, orlistat appears to be a relatively safe medication with potential benefits when used as adjunctive therapy for weight management in children.

Modulation of Peripheral Insulin Concentrations

Because peripheral insulin stimulates the synthesis and storage of triglycerides in adipose tissue, pharmacotherapy aimed at reducing serum insulin levels has been proposed as a method to promote fat mobilization and weight loss. Two agents modulating insulin concentrations—metformin and octreotide—have been studied in clinical trials of obesity treatment in children. Metformin will be discussed in this section, and octreotide subsequently, when treatment of hypothalamic obesity is discussed.

Metformin is an antihyperglycemic biguanide that inhibits hepatic glucose production, and is presently approved for use in children ≥ 10 years of age with type II diabetes. Metformin is generally safe and well-tolerated, and by itself, does not induce hypoglycemia. However, many patients experience abdominal discomfort, which may be ameliorated by taking the medication with food. Vitamin B12 deficiency has also been reported in as many as 9 percent of patients using metformin. Therefore, a daily multivitamin is recommended with metformin use (Yanovski, 2001). The most feared complication of metformin is lactic acidosis, which is estimated to occur at a rate of three per 100,000 patient-exposure years—primarily in patients with contraindications to the use of metformin (Yanovski). Metformin is contraindicated in children with underlying renal, cardiac, or hepatic disease, although use is permissible with mild elevations in liver enzymes (< 3-fold above normal). Metformin does not undergo hepatic metabolism and its clearance is purely renal; however, the presence of hepatic impairment increases the risk of lactic acidosis, and liver function should be monitored if metformin is used in conjunction with medications that may affect the liver. Metformin should also be withheld when patients become hospitalized with any severe illnesses, with any condition that may cause decreased systemic perfusion, and when use of imaging contrast agents is anticipated.

In adult studies, metformin not only improves hyperglycemic indices, but also decreases food intake and promotes weight loss or weight stabilization in adults (DeFronzo & Goodman, 1995; Lee & Morley, 1998; Stumvoll, Nurjhan, Perriello, Dailey, & Gerich, 1995). Studies are limited, however, regarding the efficacy of metformin for weight control in children with only a handful of open-label studies and small RCTs reported in the literature. One open label study (Lutjens & Smit, 1977) of metformin 500 mg TID in nine obese children (aged 8–14 years) with normal oral glucose tolerance, who were maintained on a constant caloric prescription (1,600–1,900 kcal/d) during hospital admission, showed impressive weight reduction (−10.9 ± 4.1 kg, range −4.0 to −15.0 kg, $p < 0.001$) over a three-month period. Less dramatic results were seen in a six-month open-label study (Schwimmer, Middleton, Deutsch, & Lavine, 2005) of metformin 500 mg twice daily (BID) in obese children (age 8–17 years) with steatohepatitis, in which subjects did not have statistically significant weight loss but did decrease BMI by 1.5kg/m^2

compared with baseline ($p<0.05$), and many had improvement in liver function tests (50% of subjects) and liver fat content (90% of subjects).

In an eight-week RCT (Kay et al., 2001) of 24 obese, normoglycemic adolescents who received metformin 850mg BID or placebo in conjunction with a 1,500–1,800 kcal/d diet, those who received metformin had significantly greater weight loss than the placebo group (–6.1 vs. –3.2 kg, $p<0.01$). Side effects were mild and transient, including nausea (42%), dizziness (17%), and loose stools (17%). In a six-month RCT (Freemark & Bursey, 2001) of 32 obese adolescents with elevated fasting insulin, but normal fasting glucose, who received metformin 500 mg BID or placebo, those who received metformin had a decline in BMI while those who received the placebo increased in BMI (–0.5 kg/m^2 vs. +0.9 kg/m^2, $p<0.05$). Again, side effects were mild gastrointestinal complaints in 40 percent of the subjects. However, because this study did not examine subjects in conjunction with a comprehensive weight management program, it is unclear whether metformin would provide additional benefit when combined with such a program. Also of note, the metformin group in this study had a higher baseline BMI than that the placebo group (41.5 vs. 38.7 kg/m^2, $p<0.05$). Because the reported improvement in BMI seen in the metformin group was quite small (a difference of only 1.4 kg/m^2), it cannot be determined whether the difference in baseline BMI may have accounted for some of the difference in response to treatment.

In sum, the limited data on metformin in the treatment of pediatric obesity (consisting of studies all $\leq$ six months in duration, primarily in adolescents, and mostly without diet, exercise, or behavioral modification programs) suggest that metformin is relatively safe when administered to children. However, the limited data available are insufficient to recommend metformin for weight management. Metformin is approved by the FDA only for the treatment of type II diabetes in children aged $\geq$10 years, and not for insulin resistance or obesity. Longer-term studies are needed, and RCTs in younger prepubertal patients with insulin resistance are currently underway (Anon., 2005).

PHARMACOTHERAPY FOR SPECIFIC PATIENT POPULATIONS

Obesity Associated with Neuropsychiatric Medication Administration

Many neuropsychiatric medications—particularly antipsychotics and mood stabilizers—are associated with weight gain (Schwartz, Nihalani, Virk, Jindal, & Chilton, 2004). Trials of pharmacotherapy for psychotropic medication-related obesity have been limited to case reports and small, open label studies using metformin (Morrison, Cottingham, & Barton, 2002), topiramate (Canitano, 2005; Lessig, Shapira, & Murphy, 2001; Pavuluri, Janicak, & Carbray, 2002) or amantadine (Gracious, Krysiak, & Youngstrom, 2002). Large, long-term RCTs are needed to determine the safety and efficacy of these drugs for treatment of weight gain associated with neuropsychiatric medications.

Hypothalamic Obesity

The ventromedial hypothalamus (VMH) plays an important role in energy homeostasis, and patients who have had hypothalamic damage due to irradiation and/or intracranial surgery frequently exhibit hyperphagia and intractable weight gain. Damage to the VMH may impair appetite regulation, but may also result in loss of inhibitory inputs to the vagus nerve, whose action normally stimulates pancreatic insulin secretion. Unregulated vagal stimulation in patients with hypothalamic damage has therefore been proposed to cause excessive release of insulin, which then promotes weight gain by stimulating adipose tissue accumulation (Lustig et al., 2003). Therefore, pharmacotherapy to reduce insulin secretion has been proposed as a specific therapy for the treatment of hypothalamic obesity. Octreotide is a somatostatin analogue that inhibits the β-cell's voltage-dependent calcium channel, leading to reduction of glucose-dependent insulin secretion. In an RCT (Lustig et al.) of 20 children (ages 8–18 years) with hypothalamic obesity who received octreotide 5–15 μg/kg/day ÷ TID or placebo by subcutaneous injections for six months, those receiving octreotide had significantly less weight gain in comparison to those who received placebo (+1.6 vs. +9.2 kg, $p < 0.001$), and had a stable BMI while the placebo group had increased BMI (−0.2 vs. +2.2 kg/m^2, $p < 0.001$). Adverse effects reported with octreotide use were abdominal discomfort and loose stools (100%), development of cholelithiasis or biliary sludging (44%), and mild glucose intolerance (22%). Because somatostatin has manifold actions, it is uncertain if the weight control observed can be attributed to the effects of octreotide solely on the pancreas. With its many known complications—including cholelithiasis, steatorrhea, abdominal discomfort, suppression of growth hormone secretion, glucose intolerance, and abnormalities in cardiac function—octreotide must be used with great caution. Longer-term RCTs are needed to establish the safety and efficacy of this novel approach in treating hypothalamic obesity.

Leptin Deficiency

Leptin, a hormone secreted by adipocytes, decreases in response to fasting and appears to function as a peripheral signal to the hypothalamus of inadequate food intake. Congenital leptin deficiency is a very rare genetic disorder that leads to hyperphagia and severe, early onset of obesity. Although leptin administration appears remarkably effective in treating the handful of children who have congenital leptin deficiency (Farooqi et al. 1999, 2002; Gibson et al., 2004), it remains unknown whether leptin treatment of obese children or adolescents who do not have leptin deficiency will be of benefit. Studies in leptin-sufficient adults treated with differing regimens of recombinant leptin have show little to no effect on weight loss (Fogteloo, Pijl, Frolich, McCamish, & Meinders, 2003; Hukshorn, Westerterp-Plantenga, & Saris, 2003; Zelissen et al., 2005), but there are recent data in adults that suggest leptin, as an adjunct to caloric restriction, may improve weight control by counteracting neuroendocrine adaptations that tend to favor weight regain (Rosenbaum et al., 2005).

BARIATRIC SURGERY

Weight-loss surgery has been extensively studied in adults, with over 20,000 patients reported in the literature, and has been shown to improve weight loss as well as type II diabetes, hyperlipidemia, hypertension, and obstructive apnea (Buchwald et al., 2004). The National Institutes of Health Consensus guidelines suggest that weight-loss surgery is appropriate for consideration in patients ≥ 18 years of age with BMI ≥ 40 kg/m², or ≥ 35 kg/m² with an obesity-related comorbidity, who have failed with nonsurgical approaches (Anon., 1991). Data in adolescents are very limited, and the use of more stringent eligibility criteria for adolescents has been recommended: BMI ≥ 40 kg/m² (generally ≥ 200% IBW) with comorbidity (Inge, Zeller, Garcia, & Daniels, 2004). In addition, adolescents who have not attained Tanner stage IV and 95 percent of adult height based on bone age have been proposed to be excluded because of concern that post-operative nutrient deficiencies could adversely affect growth and development (Apovian et al., 2005). Options for weight-loss surgery include procedures that restrict food intake, reduce absorption of nutrients, or do both. In this section, we will only discuss procedures that are currently still in use, and for which there are some published data on adolescents—these include gastric bypass, gastroplasty, and gastric banding (Figure. 15.1). Regardless of the procedure, a multidisciplinary team approach is necessary for the management of bariatric surgery patients, who must receive intensive preoperative evaluation and education, as well as extensive post-operative follow-up. Any surgeries involving a reduction in nutrient absorption also require special monitoring to ensure adequate protein, water, vitamin, and mineral intake, as well as prophylaxis against gallstone formation and peptic ulcer development. Finally, as with all therapies for obesity, exercise and calorie control must be continued lifelong.

Gastric Bypass

Roux en Y gastric bypass (RYGB) involves the creation of a small stomach pouch by stapling or banding just beyond the gastroeophageal junction

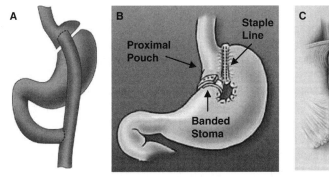

Figure 15.1. Surgical procedures for weight loss: (A) Roux-en-Y gastric bypass, (B) vertical-banded gastroplasty, (C) adjustable gastric band. Adapted from Inge, Zeller, Lawson, and Daniels (2005). Used with permission from Elsevier.

(a procedure which, when performed by itself, is termed gastroplasty), and bypassing the rest of the stomach, duodenum, and proximal jejunum by attaching the distal jejunum to the stomach pouch and reanastomosing the bypassed segment below the gastrojejunostomy. This causes reduced calorie and nutrient absorption, as well as continued low secretion of the stomach-derived orexigen, ghrelin, during weight loss (Cummings et al., 2002). The point at which the stomach pouch attaches to the jejunum defines whether the RYGB is considered proximal (the standard) or distal (used in more severe obesity). Distal procedures result in greater weight loss, but at the risk of greater nutritional deficiencies. Even with proximal RYGB, chewable vitamins and calcium supplementation are necessary, because patients are susceptible to deficiencies in calcium, vitamin D, vitamin E, iron, folate, B12, and thiamine.

In a case series (Anderson, Soper, & Scott, 1980; Soper, Mason, Printen, & Zellweger, 1975), of 30 karyotypically normal adolescents and 11 adolescents with Prader-Willi Syndrome (PWS) who underwent bariatric surgery (80% RYGB, 20% gastroplasty), peri-operative complications included atelectasis (7%), pneumonia (5%), wound infection (10%), stomal obstruction (5%), abscess (2%), and peri-operative death (2%). Both the genetically normal and PWS patients achieved and maintained weight loss of approximately 40 percent of excess body weight loss after five years; however, 27 percent of patients required some type of surgical revision due to failure to lose weight and 12 percent required incisional hernia repair. In a telephone interview study (Rand & Macgregor, 1994), 34 adolescents (mean age at surgery, 17 ± 2 years) 6 ± 3 years after bariatric surgery (88% RYGB, 12% gastroplasty) had average weight decreases from 131 ± 26 kg pre-operatively to 89 ± 24 kg by self-report. Twenty-three patients (67%) weighed within 9 kg of their lowest post-operative weight, but weight regain averaged 23 ± 28 kg (range 0–50 kg). Five patients (15%) had revisional surgery due to inadequate weight loss, and four had cholecystectomies (12%). Of the patients who underwent RYGB, only four patients (13%) reported taking vitamin B12, multivitamins, and calcium as instructed, although 21 (70%) took the supplements with *some* regularity. Such a lack of compliance with vitamin supplementation can have serious consequences. Vitamin B1 (thiamine) deficiency, presenting as dry beriberi (bilateral symmetric lower extremity paresthesia, dysethesia, and allodynia), has been recently reported (Towbin et al., 2004) in three females (ages 14–17 years) two to six months after laparoscopic RYGB. All three patients had been prescribed vitamin supplements, but compliance had been poor or there had been protracted vomiting preceding onset of symptoms.

In a case series (Strauss, Bradley, & Brolin, 2001) of 10 obese adolescents (ages 15–17 years) who underwent RYGB (80% standard, 20% distal) and were followed 8–144 months (*M* = 69 mo), 90 percent had weight losses >30 kg (*M* = −53.6 ± 25.6 kg), comprising 62 percent of their excess body weight. Complications included iron deficiency anemia (50%), transient folate deficiency (30%), need for cholecystectomy (20%), small bowel obstruction (10%), incisional hernia (10%), and protein-calorie malnutrition (10%). In another series (Sugerman et al., 2003) of 33 adolescents, ranging in age from 12–17 years (*M* =16 ± 1), who had undergone weight loss surgery (85% RYGB with open laparotomy, 6% RYGB with laparo-scopic technique, 10% gastroplasty), there were no operative deaths or anastomotic leaks. Early complications included pulmonary embolism (3%), major wound infection (3%), minor wound infections (12%), stomal stenoses (9%), and marginal ulcers (12%). Late complications included small bowel obstruction (3%), incisional hernias (18%), the need for revision from distal-RYGB to standard-RYGB for malnutrition (3%), and the need for revision from standard-RYGB to distal-RYGB for inadequate weight loss (3%). Percentage excess weight loss (EWL) was 58 percent at one year, 63 percent at 5 years, 56 percent at 10 years, and 33 percent at 14 years. Regain of most or all of weight lost at 5–10 years post-procedure occurred in five subjects (15%), and at 15 years in one subject (3%). Of the six patients who regained weight, three had undergone RYGB, one had gastroplasty, and two were not described. Similar results were reported (Stanford et al., 2003) for four adolescents (aged 17–19 years) who under-went uncomplicated laparoscopic RYGB and had an average excess weight loss of 87 percent.

The only study (Lawson et al., 2006) in adolescents comparing surgi-cal patients with a cohort of nonsurgical patients was recently conducted in 39 adolescents (aged 13–21 years) who had undergone RYGB (13% open, 87% laparoscopic), with Roux limb length 75 cm if BMI $<50\,kg/m^2$ and 150 cm if BMI $\geq 50\,kg/m^2$, and gastric pouch size 30–45 ml. In 36 sub-jects, complications reported in the first 12 months included 11 percent with ≥ 1 complication lasting more than seven days, 6 percent with severe complications having long-term consequences of >30 days duration, and death in one patient who developed *C. difficile* colitis at three months. In a subset of 24 subjects studied, metabolic markers at 12 months showed significant decreases in triglycerides ($-65.1 \pm 70.6\,mg/dl$, $p <0.01$), total cholesterol ($-29.7 \pm 30.6\,mg/dl$, $p <0.001$), fasting glucose ($-12\,mg/dl$, no SD reported, $p <0.05$), and fasting insulin ($-21.3\,\mu U/ml$, no SD reported, $p <0.001$). A comparison of 31 subjects treated with RYGB and 13 control subjects who participated for at least 10–14 months in a comprehensive pediatric weight management program, showed that the surgical subjects had significantly greater decreases in BMI compared with the control group (-20.7 vs. $-1.2\,kg/m^2$, $p <0.001$).

Vertical Banded Gastroplasty

In vertical banded gastroplasty (VBG), a small gastric pouch is created using a vertical staple line just below the gastroesophageal junction. A small outlet, reinforced with synthetic material to prevent expansion over time, is produced at the inferior aspect of the pouch, which empties into the distal stomach. VBG induces weight loss by physically restricting food intake, and because it does not involve malabsorption of nutrients, it is somewhat safer, but also appears less effective than RYGB in adult studies (Brolin, Robertson, Kenler, & Cody, 1994; Fobi, 1993; Hell, Miller, Moorehead, & Norman, 2000; Howard et al., 1995). The only major morbidity associated with vertical banded gastroplasty in a case series (Greenstein, 1993) of 260 adult patients was the development of recurrent gastric ulcerations in two patients (<1 percent). Long-term effects of VBG have been reported (Greenstein & Rabner, 1995) in 14 patients aged 13–21 years, interviewed an average of 5.1 years after VBG surgery. All but one subject had a significant decrease in BMI (on average by 14.6 kg/m²). As a group, these patients lost 55 percent of their excess body weight, and 79 percent lost more than 25 percent of their excess body weight.

Laparoscopic Adjustable Gastric Banding

Laparoscopic adjustable gastric banding (LAGB) has been widely used worldwide since the early 1990s, but was not approved for use in the United States until 2001. A synthetic band with an adjustable inner diameter is laparoscopically placed around the proximal stomach. The device is connected to a subcutaneous port, which can be accessed with a needle to inject saline to adjust the tightness of the band, and hence the degree of restriction to food entry. LAGB has essentially replaced VBG because it offers the same restrictive mechanism but is a more reversible procedure, and the degree of restriction can be adjusted gradually to allow for more controlled weight loss.

In one report (Abu-Abeid, Gavert, Klausner, & Szold, 2003) of 11 adolescents, all of whom had previously failed 800 kcal/d diet therapy, the average decrease in BMI was 14.5 kg/m² in 6–36 months ($M = 23$ months) after receiving LAGB. Although all the patients received vitamin and mineral supplementation, 36 percent of the patients still developed anemia, but there were no other complications. In another report (Dolan, Creighton, Hopkins, & Fielding, 2003) of 17 adolescents who were followed 12–46 months (median = 25 months) after LAGB, the average decrease in BMI was 12.0 kg/m² with excess weight loss of 69.3 percent at a two-year follow-up. Complications included band slippage (6%) and leakage of the port (6%). In yet another report (Widhalm, Dietrich, & Prager, 2004), eight adolescents who had failed other therapies (including very low-calorie diet, sibutramine, and orlistat), lost an average of 25 kg at mean follow-up of 10.5 months (range 4–18 months) after undergoing LAGB. In a larger, seven-year retrospective analysis (Angrisani et al., 2005) of 58 adolescents who had undergone LABG after failing ≥ 1 year of medical therapy, BMI decreased by more than 8 kg/m², with more than 40 percent of excess weight loss. The only intraoperative complication was gastric perforation during band positioning (2%). Post-operative complications included band slippage (2%), gastric pouch dilation (3%), and intragastric migration (8%). The band had to be removed because of psychological intolerance in 3 percent, and inadequate weight loss requiring other bariatric surgery occurred in 5 percent.

SUMMARY AND CONCLUSIONS

Intensive therapies that have been used to treat pediatric and adolescent obesity include very low calorie diets, pharmacotherapy, and bariatric surgery. None of these approaches have been reported in sufficient numbers of subjects who have taken part in well-designed experiments with long-term follow-up to demonstrate convincingly their true value for the treatment of pediatric obesity. As the potency of the therapy increases, so do its possible adverse consequences.

Of the aggressive approaches, only bariatric surgery can be said to have even small studies supporting its ability to induce long-lasting (>1 year) effects on body weight in severely obese adolescents. However, bariatric surgery cannot be recommended for any but those at the highest risk for mortality from their obesity. The limited data suggest that pediatric-age patients who undergo RYGB do have large, sustained, weight reductions following the procedure, but they trade the disorders associated with obesity for lifelong medical care for potential nutritional deficiencies. The newer LAGB procedure appears promising in producing gradual but well-sustained weight loss with less risk and much greater reversibility. More clinical trials are necessary before LAGB will replace RYGB as the surgical option of choice in severely obese adolescents who fail all other nonsurgical therapies.

As for medical therapy, the data are also very limited. PSMFs require careful medical supervision and appear to promote only short-term weight loss. Sibutramine and orlistat may be beneficial in the short term, but their long-term impacts on body weight are unclear, and associated side effects may limit their usage. There are insufficient data to support metformin's use in obese children with normoglycemic hyperinsulinism. Octreotide may have some benefits for treating hypothalamic obesity, but larger RCTs are needed to establish its long-term efficacy. Leptin treatment of those rare children who have function-altering mutations of the leptin gene appears justified, but further studies are needed to determine whether leptin therapy is of benefit to nonleptin-deficient children.

Diet, exercise, and behavioral modification remain the foundations to which more intensive treatment may be added. The risks and benefits of intensive weight management therapies should be carefully considered before they are used in pediatric-aged patients. Until further controlled trials become available, aggressive treatments for pediatric obesity should be reserved for only those who have not responded to conventional weight management programs but have significant complications of their obesity. Aggressive approaches should generally be restricted to specialized centers that have experience with those treatments, and should be carried out in the context of a comprehensive weight management program.

REFERENCES

Abu-Abeid, S., Gavert, N., Klausner, J. M., & Szold, A. (2003). Bariatric surgery in adolescence. *Journal of Pediatric Surgery, 38*, 1379–1382.

Andelman, M. B., Jones, C., & Nathan, S. (1967). Treatment of obesity in underprivileged adolescents. Comparison of diethylpropion hydrochloride with placebo in a double-blind study. *Clinical Pediatrics, 6*, 327–330.

Anderson, A. E., Soper, R. T., & Scott, D. H. (1980). Gastric bypass for morbid obesity in children and adolescents. *Journal of Pediatric Surgery, 15*, 876–881.

Angrisani, L., Favretti, F., Furbetta, F., Paganelli, M., Basso, N., Doldi, S. B., et al. (2005). Obese teenagers treated by Lap-Band System: The Italian experience. *Surgery, 138*, 877–881.

Anon. (1979). Liquid Protein Diets. *Center for Disease Control, EPI 78-11-2*.

Anon. (1991). NIH conference: Gastrointestinal surgery for severe obesity. Consensus Development Conference Panel. *Annals of Internal Medicine, 115*, 956–961.

Anon. (1996). Long-term pharmacotherapy in the management of obesity: National Task Force on the Prevention and Treatment of Obesity. *Journal of the American Medical Association, 276*, 1907–1915.

Anon. (1997). Cardiac valvulopathy associated with exposure to fenfluramine or dexfenfluramine: U.S. Department of Health and Human Services interim public health recommendations, November 1997. *Morbity and Mortality Weekly Report, 46*, 1061–1066.

Anon. (2005). Effects of metformin on Energy Intake, Energy Expenditure, and Body Weight in Overweight Children with Insulin Resistance: Accessed November 7, 2005, at http://clinicalstudies.info.nih.gov/detail/A_2000-CH-0134.html.

Apovian, C. M., Baker, C., Ludwig, D. S., Hoppin, A. G., Hsu, G., Lenders, C., et al. (2005). Best practice guidelines in pediatric/adolescent weight loss surgery. *Obesity Research, 13*, 274–282.

Bacon, G. E., & Lowrey, G. H. (1967). A clinical trial of fenfluramine in obese children. *Current Therapeutic Research: Clinical and Experimental, 9*, 626–630.

Barlow, S. E., & Dietz, W. H. (1998). Obesity evaluation and treatment: Expert Committee recommendations. The Maternal and Child Health Bureau, Health Resources and Services Administration and the Department of Health and Human Services. *Pediatrics, 102*, 29.

Berkowitz, R., Fujioke, K., Daniels, S. R., Hoppin, A. G., Owen, S., Perry, A. C., et al. (2006) Effects of sibutramine treatment in obese adolescents: A randomized trial. *Annals of Internal Medicine, 145*, 81–90.

Berkowitz, R. I., Wadden, T. A., Tershakovec, A. M., & Cronquist, J. L. (2003). Behavior therapy and sibutramine for the treatment of adolescent obesity: A randomized controlled trial. *Journal of the American Medical Association, 289*, 1805–1812.

Brolin, R. L., Robertson, L. B., Kenler, H. A., & Cody, R. P. (1994). Weight loss and dietary intake after vertical banded gastroplasty and Roux-en-Y gastric bypass. *Annals of Surgery, 220*, 782–790.

Brown, M. R., Klish, W. J., Hollander, J., Campbell, M. A., & Forbes, G. B. (1983). A high protein, low calorie liquid diet in the treatment of very obese adolescents: Long-term effect on lean body mass. *American Journal of Clinical Nutrition, 38*, 20–31.

Buchwald, H., Avidor, Y., Braunwald, E., Jensen, M. D., Pories, W., Fahrbach, K., et al. (2004). Bariatric surgery: A systematic review and meta-analysis. *Journal of the American Medical Association, 292*, 1724–1737.

Canitano, R. (2005). Clinical experience with Topiramate to counteract neuroleptic induced weight gain in 10 individuals with autistic spectrum disorders. *Brain Development, 27*, 228–232.

Chanoine, J. P., Hampl, S., Jensen, C., Boldrin, M., & Hauptman, J. (2005). Effect of orlistat on weight and body composition in obese adolescents: A randomized controlled trial. *Journal of the American Medical Association, 293*, 2873–2883.

Connolly, H. M., Crary, J. L., McGoon, M. D., Hensrud, D. D., Edwards, B. S., Edwards, W. D., et al. (1997). Valvular heart disease associated with fenfluramine-phentermine. *New England Journal of Medicine, 337*, 581–588.

Cummings, D. E., Weigle, D. S., Frayo, R. S., Breen, P. A., Ma, M. K., Dellinger, E. P., et al. (2002). Plasma ghrelin levels after diet-induced weight loss or gastric bypass surgery. *New England Journal of Medicine, 346*, 1623–1630.

DeFronzo, R. A., & Goodman, A. M. (1995). Efficacy of metformin in patients with non-insulin-dependent diabetes mellitus. The Multicenter Metformin Study Group. *New England Journal of Medicine, 333*, 541–549.

Dolan, K., Creighton, L., Hopkins, G., & Fielding, G. (2003). Laparoscopic gastric banding in morbidly obese adolescents. *Obesity Surgery, 13*, 101–104.

Epstein, L. H., Valoski, A., Wing, R. R., & McCurley, J. (1990). Ten-year follow-up of behavioral, family-based treatment for obese children. *Journal of the American Medical Association, 264*, 2519–2523.

Epstein, L. H., Valoski, A., Wing, R. R., & McCurley, J. (1994). Ten-year outcomes of behavioral family-based treatment for childhood obesity. *Health Psychology, 13*, 373–383.

Farooqi, I. S., Jebb, S. A., Langmack, G., Lawrence, E., Cheetham, C. H., Prentice, A. M., et al. (1999). Effects of recombinant leptin therapy in a child with congenital leptin deficiency. *New England Journal of Medicine, 341*, 879–884.

Farooqi, I. S., Matarese, G., Lord, G. M., Keogh, J. M., Lawrence, E., Agwu, C., et al. (2002). Beneficial effects of leptin on obesity, T cell hyporesponsiveness, and neuroendocrine/metabolic dysfunction of human congenital leptin deficiency. *Journal of Clinical Investigation, 110*, 1093–1103.

Figueroa-Colon, R., Franklin, F. A., Lee, J. Y., von Almen, T. K., & Suskind, R. M. (1996). Feasibility of a clinic-based hypocaloric dietary intervention implemented in a school setting for obese children. *Obesity Research, 4*, 419–429.

Figueroa-Colon, R., von Almen, T. K., Franklin, F. A., Schuftan, C., & Suskind, R. M. (1993). Comparison of two hypocaloric diets in obese children. *American Journal of Diseases of Children, 147*, 160–166.

Fobi, M. A. (1993). Vertical banded gastroplasty vs gastric bypass: 10 years follow-up. *Obesity Surgery, 3*, 161–164.

Fogteloo, A. J., Pijl, H., Frolich, M., McCamish, M., & Meinders, A. E. (2003). Effects of recombinant human leptin treatment as an adjunct of moderate energy restriction on body weight, resting energy expenditure and energy intake in obese humans. *Diabetes Nutrition and Metabolism, 16*, 109–114.

Freemark, M., & Bursey, D. (2001). The effects of metformin on body mass index and glucose tolerance in obese adolescents with fasting hyperinsulinemia and a family history of type 2 diabetes. *Pediatrics, 107*, E55.

Gibson, W. T., Farooqi, I. S., Moreau, M., DePaoli, A. M., Lawrence, E., O'Rahilly, S., et al. (2004). Congenital leptin deficiency due to homozygosity for the Delta133G mutation: report of another case and evaluation of response to four years of leptin therapy. *Journal of Clinical Endocrinology and Metabolism, 89*, 4821–4826.

Godoy-Matos, A., Carraro, L., Vieira, A., Oliveira, J., Guedes, E. P., Mattos, L., et al. (2005). Treatment of obese adolescents with sibutramine: a randomized, double-blind, controlled study. *Journal of Clinical Endocrinology and Metabolism, 90*, 1460–1465.

Golebiowska, M., Chlebna-Sokol, D., Kobierska, I., Konopinska, A., Malek, M., Mastalska, A., et al. (1981). [Clinical evaluation of Teronac (mazindol) in the treatment of obesity in children. Part II. Anorectic properties and side effects (author's transl)]. *Przegl Lek, 38*, 355–358.

Golebiowska, M., Chlebna-Sokol, D., Mastalska, A., & Zwaigzne-Raczynska, J. (1981). [The clinical evaluation of teronac (Mazindol) in the treatment of children with obesity. Part I. Effect of the drug on somatic patterns and exercise capacity (author's transl)]. *Przegl Lek, 38*, 311–314.

Gracious, B. L., Krysiak, T. E., & Youngstrom, E. A. (2002). Amantadine treatment of psychotropic-induced weight gain in children and adolescents: Case series. *Journal of Child and Adolescent Psychopharmacology, 12*, 249–257.

Greenstein, R. J. (1993). Reexploration following vertical banded gastroplasty: Technical observations, and co-morbidity from dentition, smoking and esophageal pathology. *Obesity Surgery, 3*, 265–269.

Greenstein, R. J., & Rabner, J. G. (1995). Is adolescent gastric-restrictive antiobesity surgery warranted? *Obesity Surgery, 5*, 138–144.

Greenway, F. L., De Jonge, L., Blanchard, D., Frisard, M., & Smith, S. R. (2004). Effect of a dietary herbal supplement containing caffeine and ephedra on weight, metabolic rate, and body composition. *Obesity Research, 12*, 1152–1157.

Grugni, G., Guzzaloni, G., Ardizzi, A., Moro, D., & Morabito, F. (1997). Dexfentluramine in the treatment of juvenile obesity. *Minerva Pediatrica, 49*, 109–117.

Hell, E., Miller, K. A., Moorehead, M. K., & Norman, S. (2000). Evaluation of health status and quality of life after bariatric surgery: Comparison of standard Roux-en-Y gastric bypass, vertical banded gastroplasty and laparoscopic adjustable silicone gastric banding. *Obesity Surgery, 10*, 214–219.

Howard, L., Malone, M., Michalek, A., Carter, J., Alger, S., & Van Woert, J. (1995). Gastric bypass and vertical banded gastroplasty- a prospective randomized comparison and 5-year follow-up. *Obesity Surgery, 5*, 55–60.

Hukshorn, C. J., Westerterp-Plantenga, M. S., & Saris, W. H. (2003). Pegylated human recombinant leptin (PEG-OB) causes additional weight loss in severely energy-restricted, overweight men. *American Journal of Clinical Nutrition, 77*, 771–776.

Inge, T. H., Krebs, N. F., Garcia, V. F., Skelton, J. A., Guice, K. S., Strauss, R. S., et al. (2004). Bariatric surgery for severely overweight adolescents: Concerns and recommendations. *Pediatrics, 114*, 217–223.

Inge, T. H., Zeller, M. H., Lawson, M. L., & Daniels, S. R. (2005). A critical appraisal of evidence supporting a bariatric surgical approach to weight management for adolescents. *Journal of Pediatrics, 147*, 10–19.

Inge, T. H., Zeller, M., Garcia, V. F., & Daniels, S. R. (2004). Surgical approach to adolescent obesity. *Adolescent Medicine Clinics, 15*(3), 429–453.

Kay, J. P., Alemzadeh, R., Langley, G., D'Angelo, L., Smith, P., & Holshouser, S. (2001). Beneficial effects of metformin in normoglycemic morbidly obese adolescents. *Metabolism, 50*, 1457–1461.

Komorowski, J. M., Zwaigzne-Raczynska, J., Owczarczyk, I., Golebiowska, M., & Zarzycki, J. (1982). [Effect of mazindol (teronac) on various hormonal indicators in children with simple obesity (author's transl.)]. *Pedicatria Polska, 57*, 241–246.

Kuczmarski, R. J., Ogden, C. L., Grummer-Strawn, L. M., Flegal, K. M., Guo, S. S., Wei, R., et al. (2000). CDC growth charts: United States. *Advance Data from Vital & Health Statistics of the National Center for Health Statistics, 314*, 1–27.

Lawson, M. L., Kirk, S., Mitchell, T., Chen, M. K., Loux, T. J., Daniels, S. R., et al. (2006). One-year outcomes of Roux-en-Y gastric bypass for morbidly obese adolescents: A multicenter study from the Pediatric Bariatric Study Group. *Journal of Pediatric Surgery, 41*, 137–143.

Lee, A., & Morley, J. E. (1998). Metformin decreases food consumption and induces weight loss in subjects with obesity with type II non-insulin-dependent diabetes. *Obesity Research, 6*, 47–53.

Lessig, M. C., Shapira, N. A., & Murphy, T. K. (2001). Topiramate for reversing atypical antipsychotic weight gain. *Journal of the American Academy of Child and Adolescent Psychiatry, 40*, 1364.

Lorber, J. (1966). Obesity in childhood. A controlled trial of anorectic drugs. *Archives of Disease in Childhood, 41*, 309–312.

Lustig, R. H., Hinds, P. S., Ringwald-Smith, K., Christensen, R. K., Kaste, S. C., Schreiber, R. E., et al. (2003). Octreotide therapy of pediatric hypothalamic obesity: A double-blind, placebo-controlled trial. *Journal of Clinical Endocrinology and Metabolism, 88*, 2586–2592.

Lutjens, A., & Smit, J. L. (1977). Effect of biguanide treatment in obese children. *Helvetica Paediatrica Acta, 31*, 473–480.

Malecka-Tendera, E., Koehler, B., Muchacka, M., Wazowski, R., & Trzciakowska, A. (1996). [Efficacy and safety of dexfenfluramine treatment in obese adolescents (author's translation)]. *Pedicatria Polska, 71*, 431–436.

Mathew, G., & Lifshitz, F. (1974). Hyperuricemia in a child: A complication of treatment of obesity. *Pediatrics, 54*, 370–371.

McDuffie, J. R., Calis, K. A., Booth, S. L., Uwaifo, G. I., & Yanovski, J. A. (2002). Effects of orlistat on fat-soluble vitamins in obese adolescents. *Pharmacotherapy, 22*, 814–822.

McDuffie, J. R., Calis, K. A., Uwaifo, G. I., Sebring, N. G., Fallon, E. M., Frazer, T. E., et al. (2004). Efficacy of orlistat as an adjunct to behavioral treatment in overweight African American and Caucasian adolescents with obesity-related co-morbid conditions. *Journal of Pediatric Endocrinology and Metabolism, 17*, 307–319.

McDuffie, J. R., Calis, K. A., Uwaifo, G. I., Sebring, N. G., Fallon, E. M., Hubbard, V. S., et al. (2002). Three-month tolerability of orlistat in adolescents with obesity-related comorbid conditions. *Obesity Research, 10*, 642–650.

Merritt, R. J., Blackburn, G. L., Bistrian, B. R., Palombo, J., & Suskind, R. M. (1981). Consequences of modified fasting in obese pediatric and adolescent patients: Effect of a carbohydrate-free diet on serum proteins. *American Journal of Clinical Nutrition, 34*, 2752–2755.

Michiel, R. R., Sneider, J. S., Dickstein, R. A., Hayman, H., & Eich, R. H. (1978). Sudden death in a patient on a liquid protein diet. *New England Journal of Medicine, 298*, 1005–1007.

Mittendorfer, B., Ostlund, R. E., Jr., Patterson, B. W., & Klein, S. (2001). Orlistat inhibits dietary cholesterol absorption. *Obesity Research, 9*, 599–604.

Molnar, D., Torok, K., Erhardt, E., & Jeges, S. (2000). Safety and efficacy of treatment with an ephedrine/caffeine mixture. The first double-blind placebo-controlled pilot study in adolescents. *International Journal of Obesity and Related Metabolic Disorders, 24*, 1573–1578.

Morrison, J. A., Cottingham, E. M., & Barton, B. A. (2002). Metformin for weight loss in pediatric patients taking psychotropic drugs. *American Journal of Psychiatry, 159*, 655–657.

Norgren, S., Danielsson, P., Jurold, R., Lotborn, M., & Marcus, C. (2003). Orlistat treatment in obese prepubertal children: A pilot study. *Acta Paediatrica, 92*, 666–670.

Ozkan, B., Bereket, A., Turan, S., & Keskin, S. (2004). Addition of orlistat to conventional treatment in adolescents with severe obesity. *European Journal of Pediatrics, 163*, 738–741.

Pavuluri, M. N., Janicak, P. G., & Carbray, J. (2002). Topiramate plus risperidone for controlling weight gain and symptoms in preschool mania. *Journal of Child and Adolescent Psychopharmacology, 12*, 271–273.

Pedrinola, F., Cavaliere, H., Lima, N., & Medeiros-Neto, G. (1994). Is DL-fenfluramine a potentially helpful drug therapy in overweight adolescent subjects? *Obesity Research, 2*, 1–4.

Rand, C. S., & Macgregor, A. M. (1994). Adolescents having obesity surgery: A 6-year follow-up. *Southern Medical Journal, 87*, 1208–1213.

Rauh, J. L., & Lipp, R. (1968). Chlorphentermine as an anorexigenic agent in adolescent obesity. Report of its efficacy in a double-blind study of 30 teenagers. *Clinical Pediatrics, 7*, 138–140.

Rosenbaum, M., Goldsmith, R., Bloomfield, D., Magnano, A., Weimer, L., Heymsfield, S., et al. (2005). Low-dose leptin reverses skeletal muscle, autonomic, and neuroendocrine adaptations to maintenance of reduced weight. *Journal of Clinical Investigation, 115*, 3579–3586.

Samanin, R., & Garattini, S. (1993). Neurochemical mechanism of action of anorectic drugs. *Pharmacology and Toxicology, 73*, 63–68.

Schwartz, T. L., Nihalani, N., Virk, S., Jindal, S., & Chilton, M. (2004). Psychiatric medication-induced obesity: Treatment options. *Obesity Review, 5*, 233–238.

Schwimmer, J. B., Middleton, M. S., Deutsch, R., & Lavine, J. E. (2005). A phase 2 clinical trial of metformin as a treatment for non-diabetic paediatric non-alcoholic steatohepatitis. *Alimentary Pharmacology & Therapeutics, 21*, 871–879.

Soper, R. T., Mason, E. E., Printen, K. J., & Zellweger, H. (1975). Gastric bypass for morbid obesity in children and adolescents. *Journal of Pediatric Surgery, 10*, 51–58.

Sothern, M. S., von Almen, T. K., Schumacher, H. D., Suskind, R. M., & Blecker, U. (1999). A multidisciplinary approach to the treatment of childhood obesity. *Delaware Medical Journal, 71*, 255–261.

Speiser, P. W., Rudolf, M. C., Anhalt, H., Camacho-Hubner, C., Chiarelli, F., Eliakim, A., et al. (2005). Childhood obesity. *Journal of Clinical Endocrinology and Metabolism, 90*, 1871–1887.

Spranger, J. (1965). [Phentermine resinate in obesity. Clinical trial of Mirapront in adipose children (author's translation)]. *Munch Med Wochenschr, 107*, 1833–1834.

Stallings, V. A., Archibald, E. H., Pencharz, P. B., Harrison, J. E., & Bell, L. E. (1988). One-year follow-up of weight, total body potassium, and total body nitrogen in obese adolescents treated with the protein-sparing modified fast. *American Journal of Clinical Nutrition, 48*, 91–94.

Stanford, A., Glascock, J. M., Eid, G. M., Kane, T., Ford, H. R., Ikramuddin, S., et al. (2003). Laparoscopic Roux-en-Y gastric bypass in morbidly obese adolescents. *Journal of Pediatric Surgery, 38*, 430–433.

Stewart, D. A., Bailey, J. D., & Patell, H. (1970). Tenuate dospan as an appetitie suppressant in the treatment of obese children. *Applied Therapeutics, 12*(5), 34–36.

Strauss, R. S., Bradley, L. J., & Brolin, R. E. (2001). Gastric bypass surgery in adolescents with morbid obesity. *Journal of Pediatrics, 138*, 499–504.

Stumvoll, M., Nurjhan, N., Perriello, G., Dailey, G., & Gerich, J. E. (1995). Metabolic effects of metformin in non-insulin-dependent diabetes mellitus. *New England Journal of Medicine, 333*, 550–554.

Sugerman, H. J., Sugerman, E. L., DeMaria, E. J., Kellum, J. M., Kennedy, C., Mowery, Y., et al. (2003) Bariatric sugery for severely obese adolescents. *Journal of Gastrointestinal Surgery, 7*, 102–107.

Suskind, R. M., Sothern, M. S., Farris, R. P., von Almen, T. K., Schumacher, H., Carlisle, L., et al. (1993). Recent advances in the treatment of childhood obesity. *Annals of the New York Academy of Science, 699*, 181–199.

Towbin, A., Inge, T. H., Garcia, V. F., Roehrig, H. R., Clements, R. H., Harmon, C. M., et al. (2004). Beriberi after gastric bypass surgery in adolescence. *Journal of Pediatrics, 145*, 263–267.

Whitlock, E. P., Williams, S. B., Gold, R., Smith, P. R., & Shipman, S. A. (2005). Screening and interventions for childhood overweight: A summary of evidence for the US Preventive Services Task Force. *Pediatrics, 116*, 125–144.

Widhalm, K., Dietrich, S., & Prager, G. (2004). Adjustable gastric banding surgery in morbidly obese adolescents: Experiences with eight patients. *International Journal of Obesity and Related Metabolic Disorders, 28* (Suppl. 3), 42–45.

Yanovski, J. A. (2001). Intensive therapies for pediatric obesity. *Pediatric Clinics of North America, 48*, 1041–1053.

Zelissen, P. M., Stenlof, K., Lean, M. E., Fogteloo, J., Keulen, E. T., Wilding, J., et al. (2005). Effect of three treatment schedules of recombinant methionyl human leptin on body weight in obese adults: A randomized, placebo-controlled trial. *Diabetes Obesity and Metabolic Diseases, 7*, 755–761.

Zhi, J., Melia, A. T., Guerciolini, R., Chung, J., Kinberg, J., Hauptman, J. B., et al. (1994). Retrospective population-based analysis of the dose-response (fecal fat excretion) relationship of orlistat in normal and obese volunteers. *Clinical Pharmacology and Therapeutics, 56*, 82–85.

Zhi, J., Moore, R., & Kanitra, L. (2003). The effect of short-term (21-day) orlistat treatment on the physiologic balance of six selected macrominerals and microminerals in obese adolescents. *Journal of the American College of Nutrition, 22*, pp.357–362.

16

Residential Treatment Programs for Pediatric Obesity

PAUL J. GATELY and CARLTON B. COOKE

Levels of overweight and obesity in children continue to increase despite recognition within the public health agenda, growing levels of media attention, and public debate. Of course the negative physical, psychological, and social consequences of obesity are of major concern to those people involved in tackling this condition. At this time the prevention of obesity is considered the primary objective in efforts to tackle this problem on a national scale (Department of Health, 2004; Institute of Medicine, 2004). However, given the current levels of obesity such a strategy will on average exclude the one in three children that are already overweight to such a degree that their health will be negatively affected. This is a concern given that this group represents a sizable proportion of the population and they are likely to require greater healthcare support in the medium and long term (Haslam, Sattar, & Lean, 2006). Daviglus et al. (2004) concluded that "overweight/ obesity in young adulthood and middle age has long term adverse consequences for health care costs in older age" (p. 2743) with annual health care costs averaging $6,244 for normal weight, $7,653 for overweight, $9,612 for obese and $12,432 for severely obese women. Arterburn, Maciejewski, and Tsevat (2005) have also contributed to this evidence, suggesting healthcare expenditures were 81 percent higher for the morbidly obese than normal weight individuals—equating to more than $11 billion in 2000. Such evidence demonstrates the need for the development and delivery of a range of initiatives to combat this growing epidemic.

PAUL J. GATELY and CARLTON B. COOKE • Leeds Metropolitan University, Leeds, UK.

REVIEW OF GENERAL OBESITY TREATMENT

Despite the clear need for action, reviews of the general treatment of pediatric obesity show that the efficacy of these treatments has been limited (Epstein & Goldfield, 1999; Epstein & Myers, 1998; Jelalian, 1999; Reilly, Wilson, Summerbell, & Wilson, 2002; Summerbell et al., 2003). Studies show some success in some intervention programs, although limitations are evident on closer inspection of the methodologies. Swinburn, Gill, and Kumanyika (2005) question the sole use of the evidence-based medical approach that requires the use of randomized controlled trials within obesity research. Whilst such methodologies may present the most rigorous designs, they have a range of limitations. In addition, few researchers report the specifics of their intervention, limiting the continued evolution of interventions as researchers continue to *reinvent the wheel* (Bewick, Gately, Cooke, Hill, & Walker, 2001; Gutin, Riggs, Ferguson, & Owens, 1999). This is particularly relevant to the use of residential treatment programs, given the significant number of operational processes involved in the delivery of a residential treatment combined with the limited space available within most journal articles—therefore, such information is not made available. One further possible explanation for the poor success of interventions has been the lack of an appropriate and realistic approach. Many researchers have applied the principle of energy balance to develop the fundamental elements of treatment programs. Although such an approach is central to the treatment of this condition, its consideration as a first principle may not fully advance the development of treatment programs. For example, when the determinants of physical activity participation in children are considered, the key determinants are not weight, health, or other such factors—rather, intrinsic motives such as fun, enjoyment, competence and social aspects are regularly highlighted (Dishman, 1994; Fox, 1988; Sallis & Owen, 1997). If we base our interventions simply on what components achieve a negative energy balance, we may continue to develop inappropriate, unrealistic, and unsuccessful treatment programs.

COMPONENTS OF MULTIDISCIPLINARY INTERVENTION PROGRAMS

Diet, physical activity, and behavior modification are components of most interventions typically used to treat obesity in the pediatric population (Barlow & Dietz, 1998; Ebbling, Pawlak, & Ludwig, 2002). In addition to the development of specific treatment components, there is a need to determine the range of treatment options that can be accessed by practitioners and clinicians. Possible interventions for the treatment of pediatric obesity range from general public health information, which is aimed at preventing further development of overweight and obesity, to long-term inpatient (specialist center) treatment programs for long-term morbidly obese children with comorbidities.

RESIDENTIAL TREATMENT PROGRAMS

Barlow and Dietz (1998) suggested that specialist obesity treatment centers may help children who present with complications. They comment that only a few centers are available in the United States, while there are also a limited number of centers globally. The use of more intensive (including residential) approaches is justified given some children have failed in previous attempts to lose weight, their family are unable to provide appropriate support, and/or they have significant levels of obesity or comorbidities. Access to residential treatment programs is limited—the high expense and the lack of centers around the world excludes many children from such facilities. Inspection of the range of treatment options available in such programs demonstrates that they have different objectives, too. Several of the long-term, hospital-based programs attempt to reduce children's body mass to the normal weight range, while summer camp programs or programs of shorter duration attempt to initiate some weight loss, as well as educate participants and their families in behavior modification techniques that can continue in the home environment.

While screening is important on entry to all programs, there are wide variations in the screening practices of intervention programs. The hospital-based programs tend to be much more rigorous in their screening approach. Frelut (2002) briefly reports the screening procedures used by The Theraputic Centre in Margency, France. Admissions require initial screening over the telephone, following self- or physician-led referral. This continues with two half-day sessions over a one-month interval, with a range of medical, psychological, dietetic, and educational assessments being made. In contrast, commercial weight-loss camps in the United States tend to accept children on the basis that they can pay to attend the program. Indeed, a review of the websites of several of the commercial programs did not reveal any exclusion criteria, while most studies reported in the peer-reviewed scientific literature provide some exclusion criteria such as categorization of children as overweight or obese by standard classifications using either national or International Obesity Task Force cut-offs for Body Mass Index (BMI) (Cole, Bellizzi, Flegal, & Dietz, 2000).

The following sections will specifically highlight the range of inpatient treatment program options (residential hospital, research institution environments, and weight-loss camps—commercial or nonprofit) that would be most suitable for morbidly overweight and obese children. According to the criteria used by Reilly et al. (2002), studies of specialist inpatient or residential summer camps are of poor methodological quality. Therefore, a range of studies (with methodological limitations) reported in peer-reviewed journals, obtained from catalogs, databases, and manual searches of reference lists of articles reviewed are used here to discuss the intervention programs that have been undertaken previously.

HOSPITAL-BASED RESIDENTIAL PROGRAMS

A range of researchers and practioners have utilized a variety of inpatient treatment programs (Archibald, Harrison, & Pencharz, 1981; Brown, Klisy, Hollander, Campbell, & Forbes, 1983; Dietz & Schoeller, 1982; Endo et al., 1992; Pena, Bacallao, Barta, Amador, & Johnston, 1989; Stallings, Archibald, & Pencharz, 1988; Wabitsch et al., 1996). The duration of the intervention programs have ranged from 18 days to 12 months. The physical activity components varied considerably in terms of frequency (daily, twice per day, five days per week), time (1–2 hours per day, 20 mins, and five-minutes blocks), and type (aerobic activities, exercise physiotherapy, jogging, muscle training) (Endo et al., 1992), while other recommendations were based on a calorie expenditure. The dietary components also varied considerably and included prescriptions of: high fiber, high-protein/low-calorie liquid diet, protein-sparing modified fast (PSMF), low calorie—or reduction in a specific number of calories—diets. Few of the programs reported the use of behavior modification during treatment.

The outcomes of the treatment programs were impressive, with highly significant weight losses from -8.4 ± 2.4 kg to -15.3 ± 5.3 kg. Of the eight inpatient programs reported, two undertook a follow-up, one reported a maintenance of the reduced percent overweight (% OW) (Stallings et al., 1988), while the other achieved a total reduction of 30.1 kg or a reduction of 61 percent OW (Brown et al., 1983). The variation in methods used and outcomes achieved limits the general applicability of these important intervention programs. It is clear that the interventions highlighted above were not holistic in their nature. The prescription of both the physical activity and the dietary components seem to be simple tools in achieving a negative energy imbalance rather than achieving long-term behavior change. The research questions were also more focused on the assessment of dietary manipulation than the physical activity components. Such an approach, of course, advances the use of this particular strategy, but also demonstrates the infancy of these early inpatient hospital programs.

More recently, hospital inpatient programs have been improved such that greater detail has been provided about these interventions. Important contributions have come from two French groups (Dao, Frelut, Peres, Bourgeois, & Navarro, 2004; Rolland-Cachera et al., 2004) and a group from Belgium (Braet, 2006; Braet, Tanghe, Decaluwé, Moens, & Rosseel, 2004; Braet & Van Winckel, 2000; Deforche, DeBourdeaudhuij, & Bouckaert, 2001; Deforche et al., 2005).

Within the study of Dao et al. (2004), children attended for between six and 12 months, and the program involved progressive submaximal physical activity and a dietary program based on national dietary guidance for this age group. The baseline body mass of the children within this study was high (girls: 100.5 ± 26.3 kg or 38.4 ± 8.0 kg/m^2, boys: 96.5 ± 16.9 kg or 34.5 ± 3.2 kg/m^2) which demonstrates significant obesity in this group. The interventions by Dao et al. also undertook investigations of fat free mass (FFM) changes and fat mass (FM) changes using dual energy x-ray absorptiometry (DXA) as well as changes in aerobic and *anaerobic aptitude.* The anaerobic methods used (hand-grip strength and vertical-jump height) were limited in terms of measuring only one very specific component of anaerobic aptitude, which is not applicable or generalizable to strength in other muscle groups or movements and in terms of dimensions of anaerobic aptitude (i.e., explosive power, anaerobic performance, anaerobic capacity, etc.). In contrast, the DXA and aerobic methodologies (direct measurement of maximal oxygen uptake) are strong, given that the direct measurement of maximal oxygen uptake is a gold standard method, while DXA is also accepted as a valid methodology for the assessment of body composition.

Rolland-Cachera et al. (2004) reported the outcomes of a nine-month inpatient program in which children were exposed to diet and physical activity interventions and psychological support. The children in this study were obese adolescents with a BMI of $36.3\,kg/m^2$ or 4.3 z-scores (2.9 – 5.9). Within this study, participants were randomized to two different dietary groups—a high-protein group in which 19 percent of energy intake was supplied as protein, and a lower-protein group in which approximately 15 percent of energy intake was supplied through protein sources. The physical activity program involved seven hours per week of vigorous sports, seven hours per week of outdoor activities (such as walking or playing), and no opportunity to watch TV within the center. Although the authors report the use of psychological support, they do not state what form it took. Elements of the program, such as no TV and the use of vigorous sports, may not be sustainable for these children in their home environment.

Several additional contributions have been made by researchers from Ghent University. Braet (i.e., Braet, 2006; Braet et al., 2004; Braet & Van-Winkel, 2000) and Deforche (i.e., Deforche et al., 2001, 2005) have both made significant contributions to the evidence base with research carried out at the Zeepreventorium Pediatric Health Center in Belgium. This 10-month inpatient treatment program for obesity—where general education is undertaken at a local school associated with the center—provides some promising evidence associated with residential treatment programs for children. Children were referred by medical doctors following limited outcomes of previous outpatient treatment. The average BMI of children in the Braet et al. study was $32.5\,kg.m^2$, with 31 percent of the children moderately obese (<60%), 28 percent obese (60–80%), and 41 percent were seriously obese (>80% according to the World Health Organization classifications) (WHO, 1998). Children returned home for the weekend twice a month. A multidisciplinary approach using healthy eating, moderate exercise, and cognitive behavioral therapy (CBT) were the components of the program. The dietary program provided energy intakes of 33 percent protein, 53 percent carbohydrates, and 14 percent fat in three meals and two snacks. Children were encouraged to exercise before and after school, with the center offering two hours per day (10 hours per week). In addition, children were encouraged to participate in a range of aerobic activities that were prescribed at an exercise intensity of 20 percent below the each child's maximum heart rate. CBT was provided for 12 weeks. This involved classes on energy balance, lifestyle change, self-regulation skills, monitoring and planning. Parents visited the center every two weeks and were asked to support their children in adopting a new healthy lifestyle at home.

Dao et al. (2004) reported significant reductions in BMI ($34.5 \pm 3.2 \, \text{kg/m}^2$ to $25.5 \pm 2.3 \, \text{kg/m}^2$ for boys and $38.4 \pm 4.1 \, \text{kg/m}^2$ to $28.4 \pm 4.1 \, \text{kg/m}^2$ for girls) as well as significant reductions in FM in the trunk (-63.0 ± 10.1 percent in boys and 51.5 ± 11.4 percent in girls).

Within the study of Rolland-Cachera et al. (2004), significant weight loss was achieved. Children lost $29.3 \pm 9.5 \, \text{kg}$ on average and reduced their BMI by $12.0 \pm 3.7 \, \text{kg/m}^2$. Of interest was the fact that FFM loss represented approximately 40 percent of the reduction in body mass, irrespective of the relatively high protein intake. This demonstrates a significant loss of lean tissue that is of concern, but the authors point out that bio-electrical impedance analysis (BIA) is a problematic methodology and may not accurately reflect the lean tissue loss.

The outcomes of the study by Braet et al. (2004) were that body mass reduced from a pre value of $84.1 \pm 20.0 \, \text{kg}$ to a post value of $63.5 \pm 15.2 \, \text{kg}$ during the 10-month program. Significant improvements in a range of psychological variables were also obtained. Improvements were evident in global self-worth (2.4 ± 0.7 pre to 2.7 ± 0.6 post), athletic competence (2.1 ± 0.5 pre to 2.5 ± 0.6 post) and physical appearance (1.8 ± 0.7 pre to 2.3 ± 0.8 post).

Deforche et al. (2003, 2005) reported the outcomes of a different set of children, within the 2003 study. Body mass was reduced by $23 \, \text{kg}$, while FM was reduced by $17.2 \, \text{kg}$ and FFM was reduced by $5.8 \, \text{kg}$. FFM reduction made up 25 percent of the reduction in body mass. Such a reduction in FFM is acceptable in the context of the overall treatment efficacy, according to Saris (1993). This reduction is 15 percent lower than the data reported by Rolland-Cachera. However, BIA was again used to assess body composition. This method is not accepted as a valid method for the assessment of overweight and obese children and therefore results should be interpreted with caution (Radley, Cooke, et al., 2005).

No follow-up was reported by Dao et al. (2004), but Rolland-Cachera et al. (2004) and the Belgium group both provide follow-up information. Rolland-Cachera et al. reported a significant weight loss followed by a regain such that baseline BMI z-scores went from 4.3 (2.9–5.9) down to 1.7 at the end of treatment and increased to 2.8 (0.8–6.1) two years after treatment. Important analysis of dietary and activity behaviors showed post-intervention energy intake increased and physical activity decreased, demonstrating the challenges of long-term behavior change and some weaknesses in the treatment model. In the Belgium group, follow up data in the Braet et al. (2004) study showed that weight regain did occur but that the mean percent OW value was significantly lower than the baseline value (175.8 $\pm$ 28.0 baseline; 126.8 $\pm$ 17.2 post intervention; and, 144.1 $\pm$ 22.9 14-month follow up). The Deforche et al. (2005) study, using the same program, provided a novel element that was an investigation of the dietary and physical activity behaviors during the follow-up period. All children were interviewed at follow-up about their dietary and physical activity behaviors and, based on this information, children were grouped into four subgroups: healthy eating, healthy physical activity, unhealthy eating, and unhealthy physical activity. The four groups did not differ at baseline, however there were significant differences at follow-up, such that the least healthy group (unhealthy eating and physical activity) had a significantly higher level of percent OW (183 ± 36%) in comparison to the other groups (unhealthy physical activity and healthy eating 150 ± 21%; healthy physical activity and unhealthy eating 156 ± 14%; and the healthy physical activity and healthy eating group 138 ± 16%). The healthiest group had significantly lower levels of percent OW compared to the other groups at follow up.

The most recent study from the Belgium group investigated pretreatment participant characteristics as predictors of success two years following inpatient treatment (Braet, 2006). There are obvious benefits in this approach because it provides useful information to tailor interventions. Braet reported important predictors to be baseline adjusted BMI such that a higher adjusted BMI is associated with a greater weight loss age, such that older children were more successful (total weight loss at two years was 30% for those over 12 years old compared to 23.4% for the younger children). Initial weight loss is important, such that those that lose greater amounts of weight have lower adjusted BMI at two-year follow-up. Braet also highlighted that eating disorder symptoms adversely affect treatment outcomes. However, she suggests further research is required to investigate these complex issues. Information on the cost, as well as more details on such interventions, would be valuable and further process evaluations are necessary as the authors point out. Observations of the intervention components are that the dietary intake of protein seems to be high based on the Institute of Medicine (2005) guidance that protein intake between 10 and 30 percent is an acceptable range for older children. The authors give no reason for this relatively high protein intake. In addition, the physical activity program was based around prescribed aerobic activities, which are associated with the principles of an energy balance model. This approach may not be effective in engaging children in long-term behavioral change. Epstein et al. (1995) demonstrated that reducing sedentary activities was more successful than prescribing exercise classes per se. Given that the activities provided in the residential program are similar to the exercise classes studied by Epstein et al., further consideration of these approaches is warranted. Despite these considerations, this research represents a significant contribution to the literature on efficacious residential/inpatient treatment programs.

In summary, the outcomes of these interventions are similar, they achieve significant weight loss during the intervention period, and weight regain is observed in some children. Like many studies in this field, it is difficult to compare outcomes given a range of differences between interventions, duration, population, outcome measures and their validity—as well as acute and long-term outcomes. Despite this, the evidence demonstrates the interventions used a much more holistic program, incorporating dietary modification, physical activity, and behavior change. Such changes are inline with the reviews by Epstein and Myers (1998) and Summerbell et al. (2003) that a combination of diet, physical activity and behavior change are critical for successful weight loss. Given the limited long-term outcomes, it is necessary to continue these investigations. Weaknesses, such as the physical activity program design, the inpatient nature of the hospital programs, and possible weaknesses in the relevancy to the home environment are important considerations that require further research. Well-designed long-term intervention studies such as the study by Braet (2006), which provides information such as predictors of treatment, is valuable.

RESIDENTIAL SUMMER CAMP PROGRAMS

The other form of specialist treatment program is residential weight-loss summer camp programs (e.g., Barton, Walker, Lambert, Gately, & Hill, 2004; Braet & Van Winckel, 2000; Gately, Cooke, Mackreth, & Carroll, 2000; Gately, Cooke, Knight, & Carroll, 2000; Gately et al., 2005; Holt, Bewick, & Gately, 2005; Nichols, Bigelow, & Canine, 1989; Rohrbacher, 1973; Walker, Gately, Bewick, & Hill, 2003). In addition to the summer camp programs that are documented in the scientific literature, there is a range of commercially run programs that have not been evaluated and will therefore be considered separately. As with the inpatient programs, the duration of interventions varied. The duration of the programs ranged from 10 days (Braet & VanWinkel) to eight weeks (Gately, Cooke, Knight, et al.). The reported components of the physical activity programs included: frequency (consistent given the nature of the camp programs); intensity (ranged from fun-type physical activity to lifestyle activity); time of physical activity (ranged from three to five hours a day); and the types (included lifestyle, sports, aerobic exercise, to skill-based, fun-type physical activity). The dietary components included high protein, low calorie, and low calorie based on estimated basal metabolic rate (BMR). All programs reported some behavior modification in the form of either nutrition education, behavior change, or CBT.

The outcomes of these interventions were equally as impressive as the hospital inpatient programs—they ranged from -13.7 kg (Rohrbacher, 1973), -12.1 kg (Nichols et al. 1989), -4.4 kg/m^2 (Gately, Cooke, Knight, et al., 2000), to -18 percent OW (Braet & VanWinkel, 2000). Some studies did not report a follow-up (Nichols et al., 1989). Where follow-up was available, successful outcomes were reported in all programs (results from baseline): -11.1 kg at six months (Rohrbacher), -2.6 kg/m^2 at one year (Gately, Cooke, Mackreth, et al., 2000), and -15 percent OW at 4.6 years (Braet & VanWinkel).

Gately et al. (2005) recently reported the effects of a six-week nonprofit residential weight-loss camp in the UK. Children were resident in a boarding school environment that provided catering, accommodation, and educational and indoor and outdoor activity facilities. Staff was also housed onsite to ensure full-time care of the children. The program had three components that included physical activity, dietary modification, and lifestyle education using cognitive behavioral techniques. The program's goal was to provide a safe and supportive environment where children could engage in physical activity and lifestyle change during and following the camp. The outcomes of 185 children who attended the weight-loss camp were compared to 94 (38 overweight and 56 normal weight) children who did not attend the summer camp. These data were collated over a four-year period. Children who attended the camp, lost an average of 6 kg, reduced their BMI by 2.4 units, and reduced their BMI SD scores by 0.28. FM decreased significantly (42.7 ± 14.4 kg to 37.1 ± 12.6 kg), while FFM did not change (46.2 ± 10.4 kg to 45.7 ± 10.8 kg). Significant improvements were also recorded in blood pressure (119 ± 8 to 112 ± 9 mmHg systolic and 71 ± 6 to 66 ± 8 mmHg diastolic), aerobic fitness (2.04 ± .52 l/min to 2.28 ± .6 l/min), and self esteem (2.56 ± 0.63 to 2.77 ± 0.58). Multivariate analysis of covariance revealed significant between-group differences across all measures for pre- to post-intervals. During the same period, the comparison groups gained weight, particularly FM.

A positive outcome of the intervention was that 86 percent of the weight loss was due to reductions in FM, which is well above the proportion considered as acceptable during an intervention of this kind (Saris 1993). A subsample of children (n = 28 campers and n = 18 overweight comparison group) were also assessed for intra-abdominal adipose tissue (IAAT) and subcutaneous abdominal adipose tissue (SAAT). Significant between-group by time interactions were evident for both variables. During the intervention, the direction of change within the groups was positive, with improvements in the campers (SAAT decreased by 13%, IAAT decreased by 26%), while an opposite trend in SAAT (↑4%) and no change in IAAT were observed within the comparison group.

A further element of the study was the assessment of sports skills during the six-week camp period (Gately et al., 2005). Data was only collected on the children attending the weight-loss camp, although it demonstrated significant improvements in a range of sports skills, (e.g., badminton serve, basketball shot, soccer dribble, and volleyball volley). Such findings are important given evidence from Walker et al. (2003) within a previous study on the same camp that perceptions of athletic competence and appearance (assessed using Harter's Self Perception Profile for Children; Harter, 1985) significantly improve during the program and that these domains are significant contributors to the improvements in global self-esteem observed at the camp. Although these observations are independent, they have a theoretical basis such that athletic competence is critical to participation in physical activity (Harter, 1978). Therefore, demonstrations of actual and perceived athletic competence contribute to increased global self-worth. Deci and Ryan (1985) have advanced this work, identifying competence as a strong contributor to intrinsic motivation and thus adherence to the associated behavior. Therefore, if programs or interventions are able to promote children's development of intrinsic motivation, they are likely to promote long-term behavior change.

Gately and Cooke (2003) have provided details of their intervention. Figure 16.1 shows the physical activity, dietary, and behavior modification components of their six-week program. It clearly shows that behavior modification is central to the philosophy of the approach as suggested by several reviews (Epstein & Myers, 1998; Summerbell et al., 2003; Barlow & Dietz, 1998). Figure 16.2, also from Gately and Cooke, shows a typical

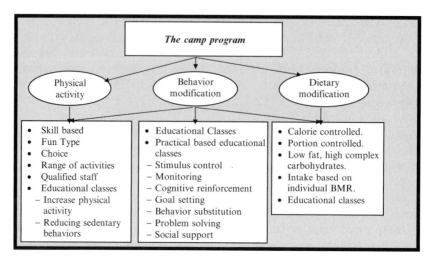

Figure 16.1. Schematic of the Gately et al. (2003) multidisciplinary camp program.

8.00 am	Wake up.
8.30 am	Breakfast.
9.30 am	First period. (Swimming)
10.30 am	Second period (Nutrition)
11.30 am	Third Period (Football)
12.30 p.m.	Lunch
13.30 p.m.	Rest hour
14.15 p.m.	Fourth period (Basketball)
15.30 p.m.	Choice session (Range of activities)
16.15 p.m.	Snack
16.30 p.m.	Choice session (Range of activities)
17.30 p.m.	Dinner
19.00 p.m.	Evening activity (Disco)
21-00 –22.00 p.m.	Bed time.

Figure 16.2. Carnegie International Camp schedule of events (from Gately et al., 2003).

day in the camp program. As well as highlighting the range of activities, it also demonstrates the significant level of control over the participant's behaviors achieved during the camp program. The fact that even sedentary behaviors are programmed into the schedule demonstrates the level of detail and control. This illustrates the potential of residential weight-loss camps as a form of effective treatment. The tight control of the daily schedule is similar to conditions within a laboratory, without the associated feelings of a normal laboratory condition, given that the children see the camp as a holiday-type environment—thus providing both improved internal and ecological validity. We view such control as valuable as we attempt to improve the research quality and evidence base of all our treatment programs.

Finally, the use of rigorous monitoring methodologies within the above studies should be recognized as important in improving the evidence base for understanding the efficacy of these treatment programs. In all the studies by Gately's group, all children were assessed by air displacement plethysmography (i.e., the Bod Pod) (Gately et al., 2005). While Dao et al. (2004) used DXA, which has also been recognized as a valid body composition methodology. Gately et al. (2003) also used MRI—the gold standard methodology for the assessment of SAAT and IAAT. Aerobic fitness was assessed by Gately et al. and Dao et al. using automated indirect calorimetry during a progressive treadmill protocol (also the gold standard methodology for assessment of aerobic fitness). Of course, as effective treatment programs evolve, scientists and health professionals should aspire to use the best research design and assessment methods to achieve greater validity of their findings.

SUMMARY OF RESIDENTIAL TREATMENT PROGRAMS

In summary, the short-term outcomes of these intervention programs are impressive. Despite these positive outcomes, there are a number of limitations of these two forms of specialist centers—they include varied intervention programs, varied methods of assessment (many of which have limited validity), small sample sizes, limited follow-up data, high costs making access prohibitive for many, and participants who tend to be self-selecting and of higher socio-economic status. Finally, a factor that limits their practical reproducibility is the lack of detail provided on the specific nature of the intervention programs when they are reported. Also, given the fact that none of the programs reported here were included in the rigorous review by Reilly et al. (2002) demonstrates a potential for producing biased outcomes.

RESEARCH UNDERTAKEN WITHIN RESIDENTIAL PROGRAMS

A significant benefit of the use of residential programs has been the opportunity to undertaken basic scientific research in a controlled environment. Such research does not address the primary objectives of the intervention or indeed its specific evolution. However, it can make significant contributions to the evidence base in other ways. Examples include research on body composition analysis and appetite, as well as qualitative research associated with behavior change in overweight and obese children.

To assess the efficacy of intervention programs, appropriate and accurate methods are required. However, evidence on the validity of assessment tools for overweight and obese children is limited. Gately et al. (2003), Radley et al. (2003, 2005), and Radley and Carroll (2004) have undertaken several studies on the validity of body composition analysis in overweight and obese children. These studies have compared bio-electrical impedance analysis (BIA), duel energy x-Ray absorptiometry (DXA) and air displacement plethysmography (Bod Pod) against the four-compartment criterion method. These studies showed that the Bod Pod is a valid method for the assessment of body composition for overweight and obese children. The value of obtaining accurate body composition information cannot be understated, given the need to encourage loss of FM and prevent the loss of lean tissue during any weight-loss intervention program. Without such accurate measures, researchers cannot be confident that their intervention is achieving the desired effects.

King, Hester, and Gately (2007) reported the effects of a six-week residential camp program on appetite. The primary outcomes of the paper were that, as expected, body mass and body composition improved during the intervention. In addition, significant increases in hunger and significant decreases in fullness were observed, but these findings require further research given that such feelings would be expected to negatively influence energy intake. An interesting dimension of this study was that morning ratings of hunger were higher at week 6 compared to week 1, and evening meals induced a lower suppression of hunger (see Figure 16.3). Of course, increases in hunger require further investigations (which this group has continued to undertake). However, the study demonstrates that children's subjective appetite sensations are responsive to a medium-term energy imbalance. The fact that children are more hungry at breakfast, and therefore more likely to consume breakfast, may be considered a positive outcome given one of the objectives of the behavior management program on this camp program is the encouragement of children to consume breakfast. Clearly, more research is required on this particular component.

In addition to physiological changes, several researchers have investigated a range of psychological outcomes associated with attendance at a residential summer camp. Barton et al. (2004) investigated cognitive changes given the evidence within both the eating disorder literature and the obesity literature of elevated levels of negative thoughts about

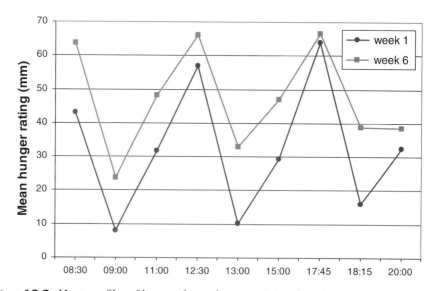

Figure 16.3. Mean profiles of hunger for each time point and week.
Key: 08:30 = Pre-breakfast; 09:00 = Post-breakfast; 12:30 = Pre-lunch; 13:00 = Post-lunch; 17:45 = Pre-dinner; 18:15 = Post-dinner.

shape, weight, food, and eating in comparison to normal weight adults. The study reported that attendance at the camp was associated with change in cognitive content, demonstrated by a reduction in negative—and an increase in positive—thoughts. These changes were also specific to exercise and appearance, with thoughts about exercise becoming less negative and appearance becoming more positive, while thoughts about eating did not change (see Table 16.1). A second finding was that, compared to normal weight children, the obese children who attended the camp had more negative thoughts and dysfunctional beliefs and fewer positive thoughts. At the end of the camp, the number of positive thoughts became normalized, while the dysfunctional beliefs did not change. The authors highlight that the resistance of dysfunctional beliefs to change underscores the level of psychological distress experienced by some adolescents with weight problems. Again, such information is valuable as we continue to develop more effective treatment models.

Holt et al. (2005) reported children's perceptions of attending a residential weight loss camp in the United Kingdom. Through semistructured interviews, children were asked to reflect upon and evaluate their experiences at the camp. The interviews focused on five sections: 1) goals and aspirations; 2) pre-camp concerns; 3) experiences during the first few weeks of camp; 4) experiences during the rest of the camp; and 5) evaluation of strengths and weaknesses of camp. All but one of the children interviewed reported feelings of homesickness during their attendance. A number of management strategies were reported by the children—these included trying to take their mind off the feelings of homesickness and thinking of other things, phoning home, and talking to peers or staff. All children interviewed reported they enjoyed their experience. They reported feelings of peer and staff support, and were pleased with the choice of activities that were provided. This provides an example of an important element of any residential treatment program that is rarely reported by researchers. As part of our treatment programs, we provide staff training

Table 16.1. Mean (SE) number of automatic thoughts about exercise, eating, and appearance at the start and end of camp

	Boys		Girls	
	Start	End	Start	End
Exercise				
Negative	0.55 (0.16)	0.18 (0.14)	0.38 (0.10)	0.03* (0.03)
Positive	0.91 (0.23)	1.91 (0.27)	1.69 (0.19)	2.56*† (0.19)
Eating				
Negative	0.77 (0.21)	0.55 (0.14)	0.69 (0.13)	0.90 (0.13)
Positive	1.05 (0.19)	1.18 (0.22)	1.18 (0.17)	1.46 (0.16)
Appearance				
Negative	2.05 (0.31)	1.18 (0.29)	2.41 (0.20)	1.41* (0.23)
Positive	0.32 (0.19)	1.36 (0.32)	0.33 (0.11)	1.10* (0.22)

* Main effect of time, $p < 0.001$. †Main effects of gender, $p < 0.01$.

on how to effectively deal with homesickness, as well as a number of processes to support staff through the process.

Information Associated with Commercial Residential Weight-Loss Camps

As demonstrated above, the evidence based on residential treatment programs suffers from a number of methodological limitations. This necessitates investigation of other approaches. One such resource for research that is readily available is the commercially run residential programs in the United States. A review of the website that advertises commercial weight-loss camps (www.kidscamps.com) was undertaken to investigate the information they provided about their approach and/or their results. No commercial weight-loss camps identified on this website provided any peer-reviewed evidence to support their approach. It is interesting to note that most of the programs do have an advisory team that includes experts in the fields of medicine, research, nutrition, physical activity, and behavior change. However, with limited peer-reviewed publications, it seems their roles tend to be associated only with program coordination. One camp did provide results of their approach, although there are a range of methodological weaknesses in their study designs, and there are inconsistencies in the results. Such information may be considered more as marketing than evidence of efficacy. It would be more appropriate for such information to fully inform prospective families interested in attending the camp program. Otherwise, they could be misinformed and establish unrealistic expectations. This can be difficult, and requires camp owners to be informed of the appropriate scientific processes, or for people with research skills to be involved. Such a step may be warranted not only to improve practices and program design, but also to appropriately inform potential participants.

Variability in Programs and Procedures

It is clear from the brief descriptions of the interventions above that there is a range of programs involving a variety of practices. Clearly, significant inconsistencies in the physical activity, dietary, and behavior modification elements are apparent across the range of residential treatment programs. It is likely that the multidisciplinary input is varied within interventions, too. Inspection of the methodologies used by researchers demonstrates this, with some interventions more strongly focused on dietary management, while others focused on physical activity or behavior modification. Of course, all researchers use body mass as an outcome variable during the short-term period that the intervention is running. However, for longer-term interventions, or for the collection of follow-up information, other methods are required given the influence of growth. BMI as a measure is not acceptable given that the changes in growth occur not only in stature. Therefore, the common methods used are overweight percentage, standardized BMI, or z-scores. However, given that researchers use a variety of methods, as well as different criteria for the definition of overweight and obesity, it is often difficult to compare the outcomes of interventions.

Informing Practice and Policy

In addition to the development and evolution of treatments per se, the ability to inform practice and policy at micro and macro levels are obvious aspirations that researchers may pursue. Consideration of such issues has been undertaken by Gately and Cooke (2003). Through the use of their residential treatment programs, they have attempted to associate their treatment program with the process of research and the dissemination of the evidence and approach to other parties. Swinburn et al. (2005) have also suggested the use of alternative methods for the development of treatment programs for obesity treatment. Gately and Cooke (2003) suggested a crude model to help the investigation and development of the key ingredients of treatment programs for overweight and obese children, and more importantly their dissemination so that others involved in tackling obesity can engage in their own development, training, and delivery at a local level. The model combines treatment in a residential camp, research, and training/practice. It is currently difficult to implement such a model because the necessary combined expertise for addressing all the issues related to the model exists in only a very few institutions and settings throughout the world. Figure 16.4 shows the elements that are specific to the Carnegie Weight Management Centre (www.carnegieweightmanagement. com) in Leeds, United Kingdom. Other elements can be incorporated into this general model depending upon the specific specialialties of each center. It demonstrates the separate components of treatment within the specialist center, the specific research that is undertaken, and the

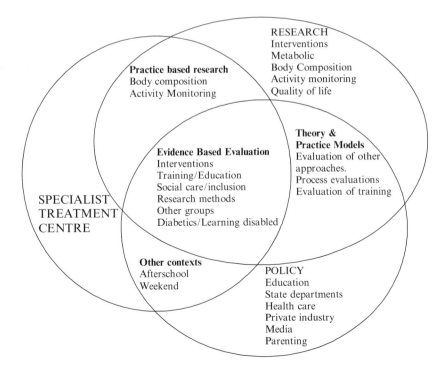

Figure 16.4. Model used by Gately (2003) to develop intervention programs and transfer the key ingredients to other treatment contexts.

dissemination of the information obtained through research and treatment. Not only does each component add independently, but the overlap of each area is important. For example, the overlap between treatment and research elements may answer important questions associated with the validity of monitoring tools within this particular population. The overlap between all three components provides an evidence-based evaluative approach that seeks to triangulate the independent components—overcoming some of the limitations of the evidence-based medical models and evidence-based public health models.

SUMMARY

Inpatient treatment programs and residential summer camp programs have achieved success in terms of short-term outcomes with some reporting success at follow-up. The acceptance of these programs as treatment models is currently restricted by variations in treatment methods, lack of reports on the specifics of the treatment programs, and a range of methodological limitations. Despite this, they may be useful in two very different ways. First, these programs provide an intensive resource for the efficient treatment of the morbidly obese, with associated comorbidities. Second, they provide an environment that can be useful for advancing specific research questions, more appropriate research methodologies, or disseminating models of good practice across a range of groups.

REFERENCES

Archibald, E. H., Harrison, J., & Pencharz, P. (1981). Body composition changes in obese adolescents on a protein sparing modified fast. *Pediatric Research, 15*, 440–445.

Arterburn, D. E., Maciejewski, M. L., & Tsevat, J. (2005). Impact of morbid obesity on medical expenditures in adults. *International Journal of Obesity, 29*, 334–339.

Barlow, S. E., & Dietz, W. H. (1998). Obesity evaluation and treatment: Expert committee recommendations. *Pediatrics, 102*, E29.

Barton, S. B., Walker, L. L. M., Lambert, G., Gately, P. J., & Hill, A. J. (2004). Cognitive change in obese adolescents losing weight. *Obesity Research, 12*, 313–319.

Bewick, B. M., Gately, P. J., Cooke, C. B., Hill, A. J., & Walker, L. (2001). An educational program within a successful residential camp for overweight and obese children. *International Journal of Obesity, 25*, S135.

Braet, C. (2006). Patient characteristics as predictors of weight loss after an obesity treatment for children. *Obesity Research, 14*, 148–155.

Braet, C., Tanghe, A., Decaluwé, V., Moens, E., & Rosseel, Y. (2004). Inpatient treatment for children with obesity: Weight loss, psychological well-being, and eating behavior. *Journal of Pediatric Psychology, 29*, 519 –529.

Braet, C., & VanWinckel, M. (2000). Long-term follow-up of a cognitive behavioral treatment program for obese children. *Behavior Therapy, 31*, 55–74.

Brown, M. R., Klisy, W. J., Hollander, J., Campbell, M. A., & Forbes, G. B. (1983). A high protein, low calorie liquid diet in the treatment of very obese adolescents: Long-term effect on lean body mass. *American Journal of Clinical Nutrition, 38*, 20–31.

Cole, T. J., Bellizzi, M. C., Flegal, K. M., & Dietz, W. H. (2000). Establishing a standard definition for child overweight and obesity worldwide: International survey. *British Medical Journal, 320*, 1240–1242.

Dao, H. H., Frelut, M. L., Peres, G., Bourgeois, P., & Navarro, J. (2004). Effects of a multidisciplinary weight loss intervention on anaerobic and aerobic aptitudes in severely obese adolescents. *International Journal of Obesity, 28*, 870–878.

Daviglus, M. L., Liu, K., Yan, L. L., Pirzada, A., Manheim, L., Manning, W., et al. (2004). Relation of Body Mass Index in young adulthood and middle age to Medicare expenditures in older age. *Journal of the American Medical Association, 292*, 2743–2749.

Deci, E. L., & Ryan, R. M. (1985). The general causality orientations scale: Self-determination in personality. *Journal of Research in Personality, 19*, 109–134.

Deforche, B., DeBourdeaudhuij, I., & Bouckaert, J. (2001). 1.5 year follow-up of obese children after a 10 month residential program. *International Journal of Obesity, 25*, S73.

Deforche, B., DeBourdeaudhuij, I., Tanghe, A., Debode, P., Hills, A. P. & Bouckaert, J. (2005). Role of physical activity and eating behavior in weight control after treatment in severely obese children and adolescents. *Acta Paediatrica, 94*, 464–470.

Department of Health. (2004) *Choosing health: Making healthy choices easier.* Public Health White Paper. London: The Stationery Office.

Dietz, W. H., & Schoeller, D. A. (1982). Optimal dietary therapy for obese adolescents: Comparison of protein plus glucose and protein plus fat. *Journal of Pediatrics, 100*, 638–644.

Dishman, R. K. (1994). *Advances in Exercise Adherence.* Champlain, IL: Human Kinetics.

Ebbling, C. B., Pawlak, D. B., & Ludwig, D. S. (2002). Childhood obesity: Public health crisis, common sense cure. *Lancet, 360*, 473–482.

Endo, H., Takagi, Y., Nozue, T., Kuwahata, K., Uemasu, F., & Kobayashi A. (1992). Beneficial effects of dietary intervention on serum lipid and Apolipoprotein levels in obese children. *American Journal of Diseases of Children, 146*, 303–305.

Epstein, L. H., Valoski, A. M., Vara, L. S., McCurley, J., Wisnioski, L., Kalachian, M. A., Klein, K. R., & Shrager, L. R. (1995). Effects of decreasing sedentary behavior and increasing activity on weight changes in obese children. *Health Psychology, 14*, 1–7.

Epstein, L. H. & Goldfield, G. S. (1999). Physical activity in the treatment of childhood overweight and obesity: Current evidence and research issues. *Medicine Science Sport and Exercise, 31*, S553–S559.

Epstein, L. H., & Myers, M. D. (1998). Treatment of pediatric obesity. *Pediatrics, 101*, 554–571.

Fox, K. (1988). Children's participation motives. *British Journal of Physical Education, 19*, 79–82.

Frelut, M. L. (2002) Interdisciplinary residential management. In W. Burniat, T. Cole, I. Lissau, & E. Poskitt. *Child and Adolescent Obesity: Causes and Consequences, Prevention and Management.* Cambridge: Cambridge University Press.

Gately, P. J., & Cooke, C. B. (2003). The use of a residential summer camp program as an intervention for the treatment of obese and overweight children. A description of the methods used. *Obesity in Practice, 5*, 2–5.

Gately, P. J., Cooke, C. B., Barth, J. H., Bewick, B. M., Radley, D., & Hill, A. J. (2005). Residential weight loss programs can work: A prospective cohort study of acute outcomes for overweight and obese children. *Pediatrics, 116*, 73–77.

Gately, P. J., Cooke, C. B., Knight, C., & Carroll, S. (2000). The acute effects of an 8-week diet, exercise, and educational camp program on obese children. *Pediatric Exercise Science, 12*, 413–423.

Gately, P. J., Cooke, C. B., Mackreth, P., & Carroll, S. (2000). The effects of a children's summer camp program on weight loss, with a 10-month follow up. *International Journal of Obesity, 11*, 1445–1452.

Gately, P. J., Radley, D., Cooke, C. B., Carroll, S., Oldroyd, B., & Truscott, JG. (2003). Comparison of body composition methods in overweight and obese children. *Journal of Applied Physiology, 95*, 2039–2046.

Gutin, B., Riggs, S., Ferguson, M., & Owens S. (1999). Description and process evaluation of a physical training program for obese children. *Research Quarterly, 70*, 65–69.

Harter, S. (1978) Effectance motivation reconsidered: Towards a development model. *Human Development, 21*, 34–48.

Harter, S. (1985). *Manual for the Self-perception Profile for Children.* Denver: University of Denver.

Haslam, D., Sattar, N., & Lean, M. (2006). Obesity – time to wake up. *British Medical Journal, 333*, 640–642.

Holt, N. L., Bewick, B. M., & Gately P. J. (2005). Children's perceptions of attending a residential weight-loss camp in the UK. *Child: Care, Health and Development, 31,* 223–231.

Institute of Medicine of the National Academies. (2004). *Preventing Childhood Obesity: Health in the Balance.* Washington, DC: The National Academies Press.

Institute of Medicine of the National Academies. (2005). *Dietary Reference Intakes. For Energy, Carbohydrate, Fiber, Fat, Fatty Acids, Cholesterol, Protein, and Amino Acids. Food and Nutrition Board.* Washington, DC: The National Academies Press.

Jelalian, E. (1999). Empirically supported treatments in a pediatric psychology: Pediatric obesity. *Journal of Pediatric Psychology, 24,* 223–248.

King, N. A., Hester, J., & Gately, P. J. (2007). Subjective appetite sensations are sensitive to a medium-term activity- and diet-induced energy deficit in obese children. *International Journal of Obesity, 31,* 334–339.

Nichols, J. F., Bigelow, D. M., & Canine, K. M. (1989). Short term weight loss and exercise training effects on glucose-induced thermogenersis in obese adolescent males during hypocaloric feeding. *International Journal of Obesity, 13,* 683–690.

Pena, M., Bacallao, J., Barta, L., Amador, M. & Johnston, F. E. (1989). Fiber and exercise in the treatment of obese adolescents. *Journal of Adolescent Health Care, 10,* 30–34.

Radley, D., Gately, P. J., Cooke, C. B., Carroll, S., Oldroyd, B., & Truscott, J. G. (2003). Estimates of percentage body fat in young adolescents: A comparison of dual-energy X-ray absorptiometry and air displacement plethysmography. *European Journal of Clinical Nutrition, 57,* 1402–1410.

Radley, D., & Carroll, S. (2004). Validity of methods for measurement of body composition in boys. *Obesity Research, 12,* 1034–1035.

Radley, D., Gately, P. J., Cooke, C. B., Carroll, S., Oldroyd, B., & Truscott, J. G. (2005). Percentage fat in overweight and obese children: Comparison of DXA and air displacement plethysmography. *Obesity Research, 13,* 75–85.

Radley, D., Cooke, C. B., Carroll, S., Oldroyd, B., Truscott, J. G., Wright, A., & Gately, P. J. (2005).Validation of fat-free mass estimates using bioelectrical impedance analysis in overweight and obese adolescents. *Obesity Reviews, 6,* 113.

Reilly, J. J., Wilson, M. L., Summerbell, C. D., & Wilson, D. C. (2002). Obesity: Diagnosis, prevention & treatment: Evidence based answers to common questions. *Archives of Disease in Childhood, 86,* 392–395.

Rohrbacher, R. (1973). Influence of a special camp program for obese boys on weight loss, self-concept and body image. *Research Quarterly, 44,* 150–157.

Rolland-Cachera, M. F., Thibault, H., Souberbielle, J. C., Soulie, D., Carbonel, P., Deheeger, M., et al. (2004). Massive obesity in adolescents: Dietary interventions and behaviors associated with weight regain at 2 year follow-up. *International Journal of Obesity, 28,* 514–519.

Sallis, J. F., & Owen, N. (1997). *Physical Activity and Behavioral Medicine.* Los Angeles: Sage.

Saris, W. H. (1993). The role of exercise in the dietary treatment of obesity. *International Journal of Obesity, 1,* S17–21.

Stallings, V. A., Archibald, E. H., & Pencharz, P. B. (1988). Potassium, magnesium and calcium balance in obese adolescents on a protein-sparing modified fast. *American Journal of Clinical Nutrition, 47,* 220–224.

Summerbell, C. D., Ashton, V., Campbell, K. J., Edmunds, L., Kelly, S. & Waters, E. (2003). Interventions for treating obesity in children. *Cochrane Database Systematic Reviews.* CD001872.

Swinburn, B., Gill, T. & Kumanyika, S. (2005). Obesity prevention: A proposed framework for translating evidence into action. *Obesity Reviews, 6,* 23–33.

Wabitsch, M., Braun, U., Heinze, E., Muche, R., Mayer, H., Teller, W., & Fusch, C. (1996). Body composition in 5–18 year-old obese children and adolescents before and after weight reduction as assessed by deuterium dilution and bioelectrical impedance analysis. *American Journal of Clinical Nutrition, 64,* 1–6.

Walker L. M., Gately P. J., Bewick B. M., & Hill A. J. (2003). Children's weight loss camps: Psychological benefit or jeopardy? *International Journal of Obesity, 27,* 748–754.

World Health Organisation. (1998). Obesity: Preventing and managing the global epidemic. *WHO Technical Report Series No 894,.* Geneva.

17

Model Treatment Programs

ANN McGRATH DAVIS and ROCHELLE L. JAMES

Although numerous interventions have been developed to treat child and adolescent obesity, there are relatively few that have strong empirical support in the literature and have the potential for truly affecting patient care on a large-scale basis. This chapter focuses on those model treatment programs that we feel have just such support and potential. School-based programs and inpatient programs—because they are so different from the type of clinic-based programs reviewed below—are not included here. To begin this chapter, components of a model treatment program for pediatric obesity will be discussed. In a review of the literature on multidisciplinary pediatric obesity programs, we identify those components that were noted as key—both those that were included in all programs and those that differentiated between the treatment programs. Next, barriers that are typically faced when implementing treatment programs of this nature are discussed. Finally, we discuss four model treatment programs for child and adolescent obesity that were identified through a literature search and selected for discussion because they encompass the majority of the key components discussed.

Components of a Model Treatment Program

Multidisciplinary. As is the case with many other child and adolescent health problems, child and adolescent obesity is best treated by a multidisciplinary team (Sothern, von Almen, Schumacher, Suskind, & Blecker, 1999). At a minimum, this team should include a nutritionist, exercise physiologist, psychologist, and a physician. The American Academy of Pediatrics Expert Committee recommends that trained nurses, nurse practitioners, nutritionists, physicians, psychologists, and social workers all be part of the multidisciplinary team (Barlow & Dietz, 1998). Each team member has

ANN McGRATH DAVIS • University of Kansas Medical Center, Kansas City, KS 66160.
ROCHELLE L. JAMES University of Kansas, Lawrence, KS 66045.

a unique responsibility that capitalizes upon their expertise. For example, the nutritionist focuses on the dietary aspects of pediatric obesity, concentrating on the *energy in* side of the imbalance that can result in pediatric overweight. Topics they may cover often include reading food labels, increasing fruit and vegetable consumption, snacking, the importance of breakfast, and eating away from home. The exercise physiologist focuses on the *energy out* side of the equation. Exercise can be supervised or simply discussed, and topics may include decreasing sedentary activity, increasing family activity, individual exercise, and group exercise. The psychologist focuses on the behavioral aspects of making these changes—planning with families how to implement these changes in the most successful manner. This includes teaching parents behavioral tools that they can use to help their children be successful, including tracking, goal-setting, proper use of reinforcement, punishment, modeling, and shaping, as well as addressing maintenance issues. The physician focuses on monitoring the general health of the patient, including their BMI, treating any secondary health issues that arise, and referring patients to specialists when necessary.

Individually Tailored. In the literature, there are several factors that have been linked to child and adolescent obesity. However, the factors that cause and maintain obesity in an individual differ from person to person. One area in which this is particularly salient is gender and ethnic differences (Epstein, Myers, Raynor, & Saelens, 1998). For example, Robinson & Killen, (1995) found gender and ethnic differences in adolescents' television viewing, physical activity, and dietary fat intake—factors that are suggested to be related to obesity. Therefore, treatment programs that target child and adolescent obesity should include interventions that are individually tailored to those factors thought to cause and maintain obesity for that particular individual and family (Epstein et al.).

Long-term. There is significant variability in the proposed length of treatment for child and adolescent obesity. The minimal length of treatment seems to be two months (Bacon & Lowrey, 1967; Duffy and Spence, 1993; Gropper & Acosta, 1987) and the maximum is approximately 15 months (Figueroa-Colon, von Almen, Franklin, Schuftan, & Suskind, 1993). Some programs do report that they allow participants to continue to attend intervention throughout their childhood (Sothern et al., 1999), but little research is available on the benefits of this type of long-term treatment. A regression analysis conducted by Goldfield, Raynor, and Epstein (2002) indicates that the number of months of treatment is related to change in percentage of overweight, suggesting that longer treatments have better effects.

Supervised Exercise. Although some child and adolescent obesity interventions are mainly comprised of dietary intervention (Amador, Ramos, Morono, & Hermelo, 1990; Gropper & Acosta, 1987), there is a general consensus in the literature that there should also be a focus on increasing exercise and decreasing sedentary activity. A recent review by Goldfield et al. (2002) addressed this issue, and found that studies that included exercise as part of their intervention were significantly more effective than studies that did not. The authors make the recommendation that future exercise interventions should be modeled after typical child activity patterns (short bouts of strenuous activity), rather than after typical adult physical activity interventions (working out in a gym for 30 minutes or more).

In addition to offering exercise intervention through didactic teaching methods, however, we recommend that exercise facilities be available onsite during child and adolescent obesity interventions, and that all family members in addition to the target child engage in supervised exercise as part of the model treatment intervention. There are very few studies in the literature that include this type of supervised exercise participation as part of their intervention (Eliakim et al., 2002; Sothern, Schumacher, von Almen, Carlisle, & Udall, 2002). However, behavioral principles would indicate that modeling and shaping increased physical activity with the intervention team and entire family would be much more effective than simply telling participants to increase physical activity.

Group and Individual Components. Although it is extremely difficult to find any discussion of this in the literature, pediatric obesity treatment can involve both group and individual components. The majority of intervention programs are primarily focused on group intervention (Brownell, Kelman, & Stunkard, 1983; Golan, Weizman, Apter, & Fainaru, 1998), but several of the model treatment programs described below do contain both a group and an individual component (see Epstein Clinic, Committed to Kids, Healthworks! and Child Health and Sports Center). We hypothesize that including both group and individual components in the same intervention package may be important for several reasons. The group component allows children and families to meet other families like themselves, rely on them for support and advice, and learn from the experiences of others. Other families can also serve as role models and cheerleaders during difficult times, and may help with maintenance after treatment ends, assuming that long-term social relationships are formed.

The individual component allows families to problem-solve individually with members of the treatment team, discussing issues that may pertain solely to their family and not to other families in the intervention group. It also gives families time to discuss private matters with providers, such as personal health issues or mental health issues that may affect treatment. Finally, if families are encountering specific barriers to treatment, these may be helpful to discuss on an individual basis. Providers could potentially also use this time to deliver motivational techniques to families who are having difficulties with motivation, or to otherwise tailor treatment to meet the specific needs of an individual or family. However, as mentioned above, this has yet to be formally investigated in the literature.

Family-Focused. The American Academy of Pediatrics Expert Committee recommends that the whole family, including all caregivers, should be involved in obesity treatment programs for children and adolescents (Barlow & Dietz, 1998). Family-based treatment programs demonstrate considerable success beyond child-only treatments for a number of reasons (Epstein, Valoski, Wing, & McCurley, 1994). For example, if the child must eat differently and do different activities than the rest of the family, the child is likely to feel "deprived, scapegoated, or resentful," and the likelihood that changes will be maintained is diminished (Barlow & Dietz). Family-based treatment programs avoid the view of child as "the patient" by treating the family as a whole (Golan et al., 1998).

In addition, targeting the whole family is especially important in families where both the parent(s) and child(ren) are overweight (Epstein et al., 1994). Parents and primary caregivers have an enduring influence on their young children's dietary and physical activity habits, which may become lifelong (St. Jeor, Perumean-Chaney, Sigman-Grant, Williams, & Foreyt, 2002). Also, dietary habits have been found to cluster within families. For example, children tend to consume a high-saturated fat or a high-cholesterol diet when both of their parents have equally poor diets (Oliveria et al., 1992). Family support for physical activity and parental modeling of physical activity, as well as parents' perceptions of barriers to exercise have been found be key predictors of physical activity levels in school-age children. Thus, families function as central learning environments for children's weight-related behaviors, indicating that targeting the whole family is likely to produce superior, longer-lasting results than simply targeting the child alone (Stucky-Ropp & DiLorenzo, 1993).

When all members of the family are motivated to make changes to the family's eating and exercise habits, the treatment program is more likely to succeed (Goldfield et al., 2002). Conversely, if caregivers, siblings, or other family members do not make changes with the family, they may undermine the effectiveness of the treatment program (Barlow & Dietz, 1998). For example, individuals may keep unhealthy food in the house, reward the child with food, or tease the child about being overweight. These behaviors send opposing messages about the value of healthy habits in weight management. In such situations, the program staff must identify and intervene upon these sources of contradiction. Meetings with the entire family should include education about the causes and maintaining factors of obesity, and discussions of ways to develop environments that promote healthy habits and changes in behavior (Goldfield et al.). Family-based treatment programs should establish realistic and corresponding goals for all family members and promote positive reinforcement (St. Jeor et al., 2002). By involving all family members and other caregivers, the family can institute new healthy dietary and activity behaviors that are consistent with the treatment program's goals for the target child. These changes in the child's environment are necessary for achieving long-term treatment effectiveness (Barlow & Dietz).

The American Academy of Pediatrics Expert Committee recommends that parents receive guidance in parenting skills as part of the treatment to assist them in establishing changes in health behaviors. In addition to general parenting techniques, program staff should stress such practices as praise for positive child behaviors, not rewarding with food, setting times for daily meals and snacks, presenting only healthy choices, removing or reducing unhealthy foods from the home, modeling healthy eating and activity behaviors, and being consistent (Barlow & Dietz, 1998). Israel, Stolmaker, and Andrian (1985) found that teaching parents general child management skills prior to treatment and then continuing to emphasis these skills throughout parent sessions of a weight-reduction program resulted in better maintenance of the child's reduced weight. Parents are the principal agents of change in children's lives (St. Jeor et al., 2002). However, as children become adolescents, parents have less control. Individuals treating adolescents must acknowledge and take into consideration adolescents' increasing independence and control over their own dietary and activity behaviors (Barlow & Dietz, 1998).

Research Component. There are no data available to indicate that child and adolescent obesity programs delivered as part of a program of research are stronger or more efficacious than programs without a research component. However, it is possible that clinics collecting data for publication may be more likely to follow the best measurement techniques and procedures, because they know certain standards must be met for publication. For example, clinics often collect weight on scales that have not been calibrated on a regular basis and only collect single-weight measurements. However, studies published in the literature typically collect weight in triplicate on scales that are regularly calibrated. Above and beyond this hypothesis, however, is the argument that clinics should collect and publish their data simply for the betterment of the field. Because the field of child and adolescent obesity treatment is in its infancy, any contribution to the literature, including process papers or outcome papers, would be welcome additions to the information currently available.

Barriers to Implementing a Model Treatment Program

Efforts to implement treatment programs that incorporate the multiple components discussed above can be met with several obstacles. Many primary care physicians have reported a lack of specialists to whom they can refer overweight children and adolescents for further treatment. This lack of specialists creates a barrier to developing a multidisciplinary team of specialists needed for a model treatment program (Barlow & Dietz, 2002; Jelalian, Boergers, Alday, & Frank, 2003). In addition to specialists, the lack of staff, support services and materials, and exercise facilities can create challenges to implementing a model treatment program (Jelalian et al.; Rhode, Dutton, Kendra, Bodenlos, & Brantley, 2002; Story et al., 2002). Physicians have also reported a lack of time with patients as a constraint to treating child and adolescent obesity (Barlow & Dietz, Jelalian et al.; Rhode et al.; Story et al.). Model treatment programs are intense, as well as long-term, requiring a great deal of time from multiple heathcare providers. The healthcare providers may not be easily compensated for time, given that many insurance companies may not cover obesity treatment as one of their benefits (Schonfeld-Warden & Warden, 1997). Therefore, the lack of insurance reimbursement or other monies to fund obesity treatment can also be a substantial obstacle to launching such treatment programs. Changes need to be made to the policies of insurance companies and managed care organizations to provide incentives for healthcare professionals to treat child and adolescent obesity (Story et al., 2002). In addition, families of children with obesity need to be motivated to participate in obesity treatment programs and adhere to treatment recommendations.

Physicians report a lack of patient and parent motivation as one of the most common barriers to implementing successful treatment programs (Rhode et al.; Story et al.). This lack of motivation by providers and families is an important barrier to overcome when initiating any child and adolescent obesity treatment. However, these factors are even more significant in these intensive treatment programs that require larger commitments of time and effort on the part of both providers and families.

Four Model Treatment Programs

Epstein Clinic (Epstein, Wing, Koeske, & Valoski, 1986). Dr. Leonard H. Epstein is the most well-known pediatric obesity intervention researcher, and his work has resulted in much of the foundation of the child and adolescent obesity treatment literature today. Despite this, it is difficult to find a name or a detailed description of his clinic, the facility, or any discussion of financial solvency issues. However, he has reported his intervention methodology in detail. In general, his treatment targets children 8–12 years of age and includes weekly meetings for 8–12 weeks followed by monthly meetings for another 6–12 months. The nutrition component of these meetings focuses on teaching families the Traffic Light Diet and on reviewing food diaries weekly. The Traffic Light Diet is a very successful dietary intervention developed by Epstein and his team that focuses on categorizing foods as red, yellow, or green, and modifying intake accordingly (Epstein et al., 1986; Valoski & Epstein, 1990). For the behavioral portion of the intervention, behavior modification techniques are taught to parents, although specific techniques vary from study to study. Treatment is individualized in that participants target a 900–1,200 calorie range per day until they are within 10 percent of their goal weight for their height. Families are then taught to increase the calorie intake by 100 calories per day until the child begins to gain weight. Then, participants are asked to remain on the highest calorie intake that did not result in weight gain.

Epstein and his team have manipulated a variety of variables in their treatment studies, resulting in these variables not being a constant part of their clinical treatment. For example, one series of studies examined who should be the target of weight loss—both parent and child, only the child, or use of a nonspecific target (Epstein, Valoski, Wing, & McCurley, 1990; Epstein, Wing, Koeske, Andrasik, & Ossip, 1981; Epstein, Wing, Koeske, & Valoski, 1987). Another series assessed whether diet and lifestyle exercise was more effective than diet alone or a no-treatment control group (Epstein, Wing, Koeske, & Valoski, 1984). Comparing different types of exercise (aerobic, lifestyle, calisthenics) has also been a focus of study (Epstein, Wing, Koeske, & Valoski, 1985). His team has also assessed other situational factors such as how parental weight status affects treatment outcome (Epstein et al., 1986).

Because these and other variables are constantly being manipulated, it is difficult to compare the Epstein Clinic to the other clinics described below. Epstein also uses change in overweight percentage as the primary outcome variable—a measure that is often not reported by others in the literature. However, in one of his review articles (Epstein et al., 1998)

Epstein compares the outcome of a large number of studies (including his own) using body mass index (BMI) and weight in pounds. This review indicates that his interventions typically result in a decreased body weight of approximately five pounds and a decreased BMI of approximately 2.5.

Strengths of the Epstein Clinic include the rigorous methodology, the multidisciplinary nature of the program, and the use of the Traffic Light Diet (an empirically validated treatment). Also, the program lasts from nine months to a year, making it one of the longer clinical intervention programs. The family is always involved in treatment, and sometimes additional family members are even targeted for change, as described above, which increases treatment impact. The program is also individually tailored to each participant, taking into account their degree of weight loss, and determines each child's individual maintenance calorie level needs. The program has an extremely strong research component, which not only serves to improve the clinical intervention they offer to their patients, but also serves to inform the field at large about how to best treat these complicated children and adolescents. Despite the long-term and intensive nature of the program, and the additional research components, it is impressive that the Epstein Clinic typically reports drop-out rates of only 16–20 percent (Epstein et al., 1981).

Despite these many strengths, there is still one potential weakness. The program does not have a supervised exercise component as part of its typical delivery. As described above, telling people how to exercise may be sufficient, but from a behavioral perspective, having family and team members model and directly reinforce exercise participation may be more successful and increase long-term maintenance.

Committed to Kids. (Sothern et al., 1999, 2002). Committed to Kids is an adolescent treatment program for children ages 13–17 years of age. The authors have also reported on a very similar program that targets children 7–17 years of age (Sothern et al., 1999). Their one-year intervention program is very intensive, requiring a two-hour visit per week for the entire year. Team members include medical, psychosocial, nutrition, and exercise personnel. During the two-hour weekly visits, participants are weighed in and engage in the medical portion of their visit for the first 30 minutes. Then, a group session begins where participant accomplishments for that week are reviewed for 15 minutes. For the remaining 75 minutes, the time is shared between nutrition, behavior, and exercise. For example, during the week 3 group session, participants spend 30 minutes engaging in a cooking class on how to make healthy fried chicken, spend the next 20 minutes learning about the behavioral topics of limit-setting and rules for eating, and finally spend the last 40 minutes engaging in aerobic field sports.

There are several strengths to the Committed to Kids program. First, this program is individually tailored to the participant's level of obesity—overweight or mild obesity (85th to 95th BMI percentile and 121–149% IBW), moderate obesity (>95th BMI percentile and 150–200% IBW), and severe obesity (>97th BMI percentile and >200% IBW). Dietary and activity recommendations are made dependant upon the participant's level of obesity, and these recommendations change as the participant's level of obesity changes. Second, participants who complete the one-year intervention are invited to participate in quarterly special events and medical evaluations until their 18th birthday—free of charge. Another strength of Committed to Kids is the involvement of the entire family in the intervention process. Adolescents are encouraged to attend the two-hour sessions with their parents and other relevant family members. Unfortunately, the authors do not present data on how many family members actually attend for each participant. The Committed to Kids program has demonstrated improvements in both self-esteem and self-confidence, and a significant reduction in depression symptoms (Sothern et al., 1999). Finally, BMI changes were achieved in the desired direction and were also maintained over the one-year period, and were fairly large compared to those obtained by other programs (32.3 at baseline to 28.2 at one-year in one study, 33.3 at baseline to 28.3 at one-year in another study) (Sothern et al., 1999, 2002).

As with all clinical intervention programs, Committed to Kids does have some weaknesses. Primarily, only 61 percent of children complete the year-end evaluation, indicating a somewhat significant problem with drop-out. The authors do not present data on the number of sessions attended by these completers, but it was likely a challenge for families to attend such an intensive weekly program for an entire year. This program also does not seem to have a supervised exercise component, and they do not present any data on the fiscal solvency of their program.

HealthWorks! (Hipsky & Kirk, 2002; Kirk et al., 2005). HealthWorks! is a clinic-based behavioral weight management program in Cincinnati, Ohio. Their multidisciplinary team is composed of nutrition, medicine, psychology, nursing, and exercise science experts. They treat children 5–18 years of age with a BMI over the 95th percentile, using both individual and group meetings. A requirement of this program is that at least one adult from the home must attend all meetings with the participant.

The initial meeting is an assessment completed by the physician, psychologist, dietitian, nurse, and exercise physiologist. Following this assessment, children and their families participate in a group meeting with the psychologist that focuses on behavioral aspects of child and adolescent obesity treatment. A treatment plan is then developed by the "care team," which includes all team members and results in family contracts and goal-setting. Once an individualized treatment plan is agreed upon for each participant, a standardized protocol is implemented that includes visits with the dietitian every two weeks for a total of five visits. Participants must also attend weekly exercise groups, where they engage in aerobic activities with other children and trained exercise physiologists. As a final component of this program, parents attend monthly education sessions during the child exercise program that cover a variety of dietary, exercise, and medical topics. After completing their fifth follow-up visit with the dietitian, participants again complete their baseline assessment, and are assessed every six months thereafter. Interestingly, outcome data indicate that it typically takes families just over five months to complete this initial phase of treatment. Data collected on 177 completers of the initial phase indicate that children lose an average of 1.7 in their BMI from baseline (35.6) to post-treatment (33.8), which the authors point out is a statistically significant difference (Kirk et al., 2005).

The main strength of the HealthWorks! program is that it is a clinically based program that is fiscally solvent. Their participants have Medicaid, private insurance, or pay privately, and the clinical revenue generated sustains the clinic without any outside research dollars or grants. Therefore, this is an excellent model for individuals or teams looking to start child and adolescent obesity treatment programs. Other strengths include the multidisciplinary team, the supervised exercise for participants, the individual tailoring of the program to the participant, the inclusion of both group and individual components, and the collection of research data for publication.

HealthWorks! also has several limitations. First, the program seems to be fairly weak on behavioral interventions, covering these topics in only one session prior to the start of the actual intervention. Second, because the program is so individually tailored, it may be difficult for other clinicians around the country to take this program and replicate it based upon what has been published to date. Third, it is unclear why it takes families over five months to move from the initial to the maintenance phases, when the description provided by the team seems to suggest families should move through this phase in about 10 to 12 weeks. Fourth, outcome data indicate that only 45 percent of children and adolescents who begin the program actually complete the initial phase of treatment, resulting in a 55 percent drop out rate. This exceeds the drop-out rate of other programs reviewed here. Finally, the change in BMI—although in the desired direction and comparable to those achieved by the Child Health and Sports Center—is less than some other child and adolescent obesity interventions reviewed here, and seems quite modest for an intensive program of this nature, especially given that it only includes children who complete the program.

Child Health and Sports Center (Eliakim et al., 2002; Nemet et al., 2005). The Child Health and Sports Center is a hospital-based clinic at Tel Aviv University in Israel. This three-month clinic serves children 6–16 years of age. Their intervention is composed of four evening lectures on childhood obesity, general nutrition, a therapeutic nutritional approach for childhood obesity, and exercise, offered over three months for participants and their parents. In addition, participants meet with the team dietitian six times over the three-month period. Who attends these meetings differs by the age of the participant (6–8 yrs–only the parent for first two meetings, child and parents for last four; 9 yrs through adolescence–parents and children invited to all meetings; adolescence–parent and participant to first meeting, parents and adolescent alternate for remaining meetings).

The exercise component of the Child Health and Sports Center is the most intensive part of their program. Participants complete hourly training sessions twice per week over the three-month period at the Child Health and Sports Center gym supervised by individual coaches as well as physicians who were former members of the Israeli national track and field team. Outcome data indicate that children who complete the three-month program lose significantly more weight than controls (who actually gain weight), and that these differences are statistically significant (Eliakim et al., 2002). Mean weight loss is approximately 1 kg (0.7 BMI). Interestingly, the authors have offered an extension of this program out to six months for interested participants, and results indicate that these six-month completers lost significantly more weight than their three-month counterparts (Eliakim et al.). Mean weight loss for the six-month completers was approximately 1.25 kg, compared to 0.58 kg (0.53 BMI vs. 0.95 BMI). A separate one-year outcome study indicates that participants' weight increases from 59.1 kg to 59.7 kg, but that their BMI drops from 27.7 to 26.1 (Nemet et al., 2005).

There are several strengths to the Child Health and Sports Center weight loss program for children. First, the program fits easily into any hospital-based sports facility, with the simple addition of four evening didactic sessions, and the addition of a dietitian who can see the patients for six visits over the three-month period. No data are presented on whether this clinic is financially solvent, but costs are low and mainly include gym membership and the six dietitian visits. Another strength is the willingness of the authors to continue the program for an extended period of time for interested participants. This may help to decrease some of the weight regain that is often seen once intervention ceases. Finally, a definite strength of the program is their low drop-out rates. These range from 13 percent (Eliakim et al., 2002) to 20 percent (Nemet et al., 2005).

Unfortunately, the Child Health and Sports Center did not include any behavioral components or a psychologist—a weakness in terms of being multidisciplinary. Second, their typical program is relatively short in duration (3 months), which may help with decreased drop-out rates, but may also explain their weak findings in terms of weight loss and BMI decrease.

Summary

Model treatment programs for child and adolescent obesity do exist, as evidenced by the four programs described in the this chapter. In fact, it is quite likely that there are several additional programs available that are simply not described in the literature because they are focused on clinical endeavors. However, it is also likely that there are not currently enough programs available to reach all of the children and adolescents who currently need treatment for overweight and obesity. Research suggests that primary care physicians are not well-equipped to handle this demand (Rhode et al., 2002), so additional model treatment programs will need to be developed. Future model treatment programs should ideally include each of the components discussed in this chapter. Some research is also currently emerging on including child-friendly novel approaches as part of weight loss, such as adventure therapy (Jelalian, Mehlenbeck, Loyd-Richardson, Birmaher, & Wing, 2006). If outcomes from these types of programs continue to be promising, future model treatment programs may want to include these additional components in their programs.

We propose several recommendations for clinicians, researchers, and policy-makers in the area of child and adolescent obesity treatment. First, treatment programs should include a multidisciplinary team of providers; interventions individually tailored to children, adolescents, and families; supervised exercise in an onsite exercise facility; and group, as well as individual, components. We recommend that programs are designed to treat participants for at least one year. Perhaps most importantly for children and adolescents with obesity, the whole family needs to be involved in all aspects of treatment, and family-wide health habit changes need to be a target of treatment. We also suggest that parents receive instruction in child behavior management skills to facilitate their children's health habit changes. In addition, programs should actively address potential barriers to treatment success, such as children's and parents' lack of motivation. Second, more formal investigations need to be conducted to determine the ideal length of treatment, as well as when longer treatment should be indicated. Other areas for further research include the additive benefits of including a supervised exercise component and both group and individual treatment components. All child and adolescent obesity treatment programs are encouraged to incorporate data collection into their standard procedures and examine the effectiveness of their programs. Third, insurance companies and managed care organizations policies need to be changed to include the coverage for child and adolescent group treatment for obesity if the general public is to have access to such needed treatment. While there are several model treatment programs that include many of these components, and that show promising empirical support, there are still improvements to be made to these programs, as well as a continuing need to develop more model treatment programs to meet the needs of the growing population of children and adolescent with obesity.

REFERENCES

Amador, M., Ramos, L. T., Morono, M., & Hermelo, M. P. (1990). Growth rate reduction during energy restriction in obese adolescents. *Experimental and Clinical Endocrinology, 96*, 73–82.

Bacon, G. E., & Lowrey, G. H. (1967). A clinical trial of fenfluramine in obese children. *Current Therapeutic Research Clinical Experimental, 9*, 626–630.

Barlow, S. E., & Dietz, W. H. (1998). Obesity evaluation and treatment: Expert committee recommendations. *Pediatrics, 102*, e29.

Brownell, K. D., Kelman, J. H., & Stunkard, A. J. (1983). Treatment of obese children with and without their mothers: Changes in weight and blood pressure. *Pediatrics, 71*, 515–523.

Duffy, G., & Spence, S. H. (1993). The effectiveness of cognitive self-management as an adjunct to a behavioral intervention for childhood obesity: A research note. *Journal of Child Psychology and Psychiatry, 34*, 1043–1050.

Eliakim, A., Kaven, G., Berger, I., Friedland, O., Wolach, B., & Nemet, D. (2002). The effect of a combined intervention on body mass index and fitness in obese children and adolescents - a clinical experience. *European Journal of Pediatrics, 161*, 449–454.

Epstein, L. H., Myers, M. D., Raynor, H. A., & Saelens, B. E. (1998). Treatment of pediatric obesity. *Pediatrics, 101*(Suppl. 3), 554–570.

Epstein, L. H., Valoski, A., Koeske, R., & Wing, R. R. (1986). Family-based behavioral weight control in obese young children. *Journal of the American Dietetic Association, 86*, 481–484.

Epstein, L. H., Valoski, A., Wing, R. R., & McCurley, J. (1990). Ten-year follow-up of behavioral, family-based treatment for obese children. *The Journal of the American Medical Association, 264*, 2519–2523.

Epstein, L. H., Valoski, A., Wing, R. R., & McCurley, J. (1994). Ten-year outcomes of behavioral family-based treatment of childhood obesity. *Health Psychology, 13*, 373–383.

Epstein, L. H., Wing, R. R., Koeske, R., Andrasik, F., & Ossip, D. J. (1981). Child and parent weight loss in family-based behavior modification programs. *Journal Consulting and Clinical Psychology, 49*, 674–685.

Epstein, L. H., Wing, R. R., Koeske, R., & Valoski, A. (1984). Effects of diet plus exercise on weight change in parents and children. *Journal of Consulting and Clinical Psychology, 52*, 429–437.

Epstein, L. H., Wing, R. R., Koeske, R., & Valoski, A. (1985). A comparison of lifestyle exercise, aerobic exercise and calisthenics on weight loss in obese children. *Behavior Therapy, 16*, 345–356.

Epstein, L. H., Wing, R. R., Koeske, R., & Valoski, A. (1986). Effect of parent weight on weight loss in obese children. *Journal of Consulting and Clinical Psychology, 54*, 400–401.

Epstein, L. H., Wing, R. R., Koeske, R., & Valoski, A. (1987). Long-term effects of family-based treatment of childhood obesity. *Journal Consulting and Clinical Psychology, 55*, 91–95.

Figueroa-Colon, R., von Almen, T. K., Franklin, F. A., Schuftan, C., & Suskind, R. M. (1993). Comparison of two hypocaloric diets in obese children. *American Journal of Diseases of Children, 147*, 160–166.

Golan, M., Weizman, A., Apter, A., & Fainaru, M. (1998). Parents as the exclusive agents of change in the treatment of childhood obesity. *American Journal of Clinical Nutrition, 67*, 1130–1135.

Goldfield, G. S., Raynor, H. A., & Epstein, L. H. (2002). Treatment of pediatric obesity. In T. A. Wadden & A. J. Stunkard (Eds.), *Handbook of Obesity Treatment*. New York: Guilford Press.

Gropper, S. S., & Acosta, P. B. (1987). The therapeutic effect of fiber in treating obesity. *Journal of the American College of Nutrition, 6*, 533–535.

Hipsky, J., & Kirk, S. (2002). Health Works! weight management program for children and adolescents. *Journal of the American Dietetic Association, 102*(Suppl. 3), 64–67.

Israel, A. C., Stolmaker, L., & Andrain, C. A. (1985). The effects of training parents in general child management skills on a behavioral weight loss program for children. *Behavior Therapy, 16*, 169–180.

Jelalian, E., Boergers, J., Alday, C. S., & Frank, R. (2003). Survey of physician attitudes and practices related to pediatric obesity. *Clinical Pediatrics, 42*, 235–245.

Jelalian, E., Mehlenbeck, R., Lloyd-Richardson, E. E., Birmaher, V., & Wing, R. R. (2006). 'Adventure therapy' combined with cognitive-behavioral treatment for overweight adolescents. *International Journal of Obesity, 30*, 31–39.

Kirk, S. K., Zeller, M., Claytor, R., Santangelo, M., Khoury, P. R., & Daniels, S. R. (2005). The relationship of health outcomes to improvement in BMI in children and adolescents. *Obesity Research, 13*, 876–882.

Nemet, D., Barkan, S., Epstein, Y., Friedland, O., Kowen, G., & Eliakim, A. (2005). Short- and long-term beneficial effects of a combined dietary-behavioral-physical activity intervention for the treatment of childhood obesity. *Pediatrics, 115*, e443–e449.

Oliveria, S. A., Ellison, R. C., Moore, L. L., Gillman, M. W., Garrahie, E. J., & Singer, M. R. (1992). Parent-child relationships in nutrient intake: The Framingham Children's Study. *The American Journal of Clinical Nutrition, 56*, 593–598.

Rhode, P. C., Dutton, G. R., Kendra, K. E., Bodenlos, J. S., & Brantley, P. J. (2002). *Obesity Management by Primary Care Physicians*. Paper presented at the Association for Advancement of Behavior Therapy, Reno, NV.

Robinson, T. N., & Killen, J. D. (1995). Ethnic and gender differences in the relationships between television viewing and obesity, physical activity, and dietary fat intake. *Journal of Health Education, 26*(Suppl. 2), 91–98.

Schonfeld-Warden, N., & Warden, C. H. (1997). Pediatric obesity: An overview of etiology and treatment. *Pediatric Endocrinology, 44*, 339–361.

Sothern, M. S., Schumacher, H., von Almen, T. K., Carlisle, L. K. & Udall, J. N. (2002). Committed to Kids: An intergrated 4-level approach to weight management in adolescents. *Journal of the American Dietetic Association, 102*, S81–S85.

Sothern, M. S., von Almen, T. K., Schumacher, H. D., Suskind, R. M., & Blecker, U. (1999). A multidisciplinary approach to the treatment of childhood obesity. *Delware Medical Journal, 71*, 255–261.

St. Jeor, S. T., Perumean-Chaney, S., Sigman-Grant, M., Williams, C., & Foreyt, J. (2002). Family-based interventions for the treatment of childhood obesity. *Journal of the American Dietetic Association, 102*, 640–644.

Story, M. T., Neumark-Stzainer, D. R., Sherwood, N. E., Holt, K., Sofka, D., Trowbidge, F. L., et al. (2002). Management of child and adolescent obesity: Attitudes, barriers, skills, and training needs among health care professionals. *Pediatrics, 110*, 210–214.

Stucky-Ropp, R. C., & DiLorenzo, T. (1993). Determinants of exercise in children. *Preventive Medicine, 22*, 880–889.

Valoski, A., & Epstein, L. H. (1990). Nutrient intake of obese children in a family-based behavioral weight control program. *International Journal of Obesity, 15*, 497–498.

18

Cultural Considerations in the Development of Pediatric Weight Management Interventions

DAWN K. WILSON and HEATHER KITZMAN-ULRICH

Over the last 20 years, the prevalence of overweight and obesity have increased dramatically in U.S. adults across racial/ethnic groups, and in both males and females of all age groups (Agudo & Pera, 1999; Center for Disease Control, 1997; Eberhardt et al., 2001; Kuczmarski & Flegal, 2000; Mokad et al., 1999; Ogden et al., 2006). Youth of diverse ethnic backgrounds, in particular, have been negatively impacted by the increasing rate of obesity. For example, national statistics indicate that 31.4 percent of African-American male adolescents, and 42.1 percent of African-American female adolescents are currently overweight (Ogden et al.).

There is a growing interest in the application of ecological models in understanding obesity-related factors and in developing effective interventions. Although a number of different ecological models exist, all share the core belief that behavior is influenced by multiple levels of environmental subsystems (Bronfenbrenner, 1979; Kazak, Rourke, & Crump, 2003; McLeroy, Bibeau, Steckler, & Glanz, 1988; Power, DuPaul, Shapiro, & Kazak, 2003; Sallis, Bauman, & Pratt, 1998). This approach, as outlined by Bronfenbrenner assumes that health and health behaviors are shaped

DAWN K. WILSON and HEATHER KITZMAN-ULRICH • University of South Carolina, Columbia, SC 29208.

This article was support by a grant (R01 HD 045693) funded by the National Institutes of Child Health and Human Development to Dawn K. Wilson, Ph.D.

by environmental subsystems that include the integration of intrapersonal factors (characteristics of the individual), microsystemic factors (families and institutions), mesosystemic factors (interactions between family and institutions), exosystemic factors (communities, policies) and macrosystemic effects (all systems—micro-, meso-, exo-, etc.—related to a culture or subculture). Figure 18.1 presents an ecological model for understanding cultural issues in relation to the prevention and treatment of obesity among minority youth. In this model, concentric circles are used to conceptualize behavioral levels of influence, with the psychobiologic core as the central circle, and distal leverage points as the broadest, outermost circle. Factors such as family and parenting variables are examples of proximal levels of influence. Institutional supports (schools, churches) and policy are distal levels of influence. Specifically, this chapter will provide an integrated review of cultural issues related to obesity prevention and treatment from an ecological perspective. In this chapter, we highlight factors using an ecological approach that are particularly relevant for understanding obesity-related factors (including diet and physical activity) in ethnically diverse pediatric populations. In addition, we provide a summary of the key

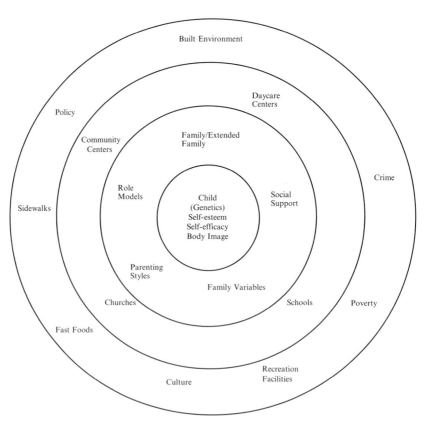

Figure 18.1. Ecological approach to weight management and healthy lifestyles.

obesity prevention and intervention studies that have been implemented for minority children and adolescents, and we propose key priorities for future research.

INDIVIDUAL FACTORS AND OBESITY (INTRAPERSONAL INFLUENCES)

Some important individual factors relating to pediatric weight management include psychosocial variables, such as perceptions of body image, self-efficacy, self-esteem, perceived control, and social norms. A number of investigators have evaluated the relationship between psychosocial factors and diet and physical activity behaviors in minority youth. In a study by Kimm et al. (1997) the relationship between self-esteem and adiposity was evaluated as part of the National Heart, Lung, and Blood Institute (NHLBI) Growth and Health Study of African-American and Caucasian girls. Adiposity was negatively correlated with self-esteem—however, the magnitude of the effect was lower for African-American girls in comparison to Caucasian girls. Another study by Young-Hyman, Schlundt, Herman-Wenderoth, and Bozylinksi (2003) assessed factors related to African-American children's appearance self-esteem and global self-worth. In this study, body mass index (BMI) scores were not significantly related to appearance self-esteem and global self-worth when evaluating the entire sample. Higher BMI scores, however, were related to lower appearance self-esteem in older (8 – 10 years old) children in their study sample. In another study, Motl et al. (2002) examined social cognitive determinants, including intentions, self-efficacy, and perceived behavioral control for physical activity in African-American and Caucasian girls. Self-efficacy was independently related to moderate-to-vigorous activity, and perceived behavioral control was related to vigorous activity in this multiethnic sample of youth.

Several investigators have studied the relationship between body image and ethnicity in adolescents. For example, Perry, Rosenblatt, and Wang (2004) found that African-American girls selected an ideal body size significantly larger than Caucasian adolescents. In a study by Thompson, Corwin, Rogan, and Sargent (1999), African-American adolescents had less body dissatisfaction and weight concerns than Caucasians. In a study by Spruit-Metz, Lindquist, Birch, Fisher, and Goran (2002), parent concerns about their child's weight and pressure for eating were predictive of higher total fat mass after adjusting for socioeconomic status (SES) and energy intake in a multiethnic adolescent population. Additionally, a survey conducted in African-American families found that only 44 percent of caregivers indicated their child's weight was a health risk although approximately 70 percent of the children were classified as overweight or obese (Young-Hyman, Herman, Scott, & Schlundt, 2000). This study also found that adolescent body dissatisfaction and the adolescents' perceptions of family and friends' weight concerns were predictive of adolescents' weight concern regardless of ethnicity. These studies expand on past research by showing that social norms (relating to friends and family members) are predictive of body image satisfaction in multiethnic adolescents.

In summary, previous research has demonstrated that psychosocial factors including body image, self-efficacy, self-esteem, perceived control, and social norms are all important factors in understanding the intrapersonal aspects of minority youth and health behaviors. Future research should integrate these psychosocial theoretical factors into broader ecologically-based studies to test the interactions of individual factors with family- and community-related factors.

FAMILY FACTORS IN OBESITY (MICROSYSTEMIC INFLUENCES)

The immediate family environment also influences adolescents' behavior significantly. According to Baranowski (1997), parents affect their children's health behaviors through a variety of mechanisms such as genetics, direct modeling of behavior, rewarding desirable behaviors while punishing undesirable ones, eliminating or establishing barriers, providing concrete resources to perform certain behaviors, and using authoritative parenting skills to develop children's self-control skills.

Familial relationships are important in the modeling of positive eating behaviors. Through modeling, family members can encourage or discourage certain lifestyle patterns such as overeating (Patterson, Rupp, Sallis, Atkins, & Nader, 1988). Qualitative data supports that adolescents' eating behaviors are influenced by food purchased by the family (Hill, Casswell, Maskill, Jones, & Wyllie, 1998). Although past research supports the "direct modeling hypothesis" (Sallis, Patterson, Buono, & Nader, 1999), more current research underscores the significant role that parental support plays in children's health behaviors (Brustad, 1996; Kohl & Hobbs, 1998; Trost et al. (1997). Parental support has been part of the parental component in many weight-loss interventions targeting youth (Brownell, Kelman, & Stunkard, 1983; Coates, Killen, & Slinkard, 1982; Saelens et al., 2002; Wadden et al., 1990). Increasing parental support may create a more supportive home environment and may increase positive reinforcement and communication between parents and their children.

Several studies have examined the relationship between parental social support, self-efficacy and their child's health behaviors, specifically in minority youth. In a qualitative study, low-income African-American adolescents reported that their parents and grandparents provided positive social support (encouragement) for eating fruits and vegetables, although they did not always provide such foods in the home (Molaison, Connell, Stuff, Yadrick, & Bogle, 2005). Adkins, Sherwood, Story, & Davis (2004) also found that parental social support (tangible) was associated with greater physical activity in African-American girls. Interestingly, parental self-efficacy for supporting daughters to be physically active was also significantly related to higher levels of physical activity in daughters. The relationship between parental social support and health behaviors has been less positive for obese children and adolescents. For example, Zeller & Modi (2006) found that obese multiethnic adolescents reported having higher depressive symptoms and lower perceived general social support (emotional) from family and peers.

Parenting styles among African-American families may also be important in understanding the role of family variables in childhood obesity. Spruijt-Metz et al. (2002) found that African-American mothers' parenting styles consisted of more authoritarian child feeding practices (e.g., rigid and controlling) than Caucasian mothers. However, in one qualitative study by Molaison et al. (2005), low-income African-American adolescents reported that they felt they had input in the decision-making for family purchases of food. In addition, Patrick, Nicklas, Hughes, and Morales (2005) reported that among African-American and Hispanic families, parenting styles that focused on shared decision-making were correlated with healthier eating among young children. In this study, authoritarian parenting practices were negatively correlated with vegetable consumption in these multiethnic youth. In a focus group study by Evans, Wilson, Buck, Torbett, and Williams (2006), African-American adolescents indicated that they wanted their parents to learn new skills for increasing the purchasing of healthy foods, and they wanted to have more input on family food purchases.

Family functioning variables, such as cohesion (i.e., closeness) and connectedness (i.e., nurturance), may also be important in understanding overweight status in adolescents, although few of these studies have included minority youth in their samples. One study assessed cohesion, which is the degree of family closeness or togetherness in a large sample of Caucasian adolescents of varying weight. This study showed a negative association between family cohesion and weight in girls (Mendelson, White, & Schliecker, 1995), indicating that the more closeness there is, the lower the weight of the girls may be. Additionally, in a cross-sectional study of Caucasian girls, lower levels of parental caring and nurturance were found in overweight as compared to normal weight girls (Turner, Rose, & Cooper, 2005). Family connectedness (e.g., nurturance) was also found to be related to adolescent health behaviors (e.g., fruit and vegetable consumption, breakfast eating, physical activity) in a large survey study by Mellin, Neumark-Sztainer, Story, Ireland, & Resnick (2002). In this study, family connectedness was associated with higher rates of eating breakfast, increases in daily fruit and vegetable consumption in girls, and higher levels of physical activity and fruit and vegetable consumption in boys. In addition, in a study involving African-American families, parents' report of family satisfaction was an important mediator for adolescent weight loss (White et al., 2004).

In summary, family variables—including role modeling, parental social support, parental self-efficacy, parenting styles, family cohesion, and connectedness—are important in understanding health behaviors in minority youth. Some evidence seems to suggest that family functioning and parenting styles that are more supportive in nature may be particularly worthy of future investigation. In addition, it may be important for investigators to develop specific intervention components that address parenting issues and barriers for minority families who may have reduced resources for engaging in healthy life style changes.

INTERACTIONS OF FAMILY AND CULTURAL FACTORS (MESOSYSTEMIC INFLUENCES)

Interactions between family and cultural factors are especially important in understanding obesity-related factors in minority youth. An important cultural component to consider in assessing family variables related to weight is the intergenerational aspects of the family. Most family questionnaires measure immediate family domains to assess family functioning variables, although family variables may differ according to ethnicity and may extend into intergenerational or extended family members. For example, Caucasians tend to define family as their immediate or nuclear family. On the other hand, African-Americans tend to define family more broadly to include cousins, godparents, grandparents, aunts, uncles, and close friends (McGoldrick, Giordano, & Pearce, 1996). Intergenerational issues must be adapted to multi-cultural populations to assess the impact of extended family variables on weight-related health outcomes.

Several investigators have examined the relationship between SES and health behavior practices in minorities, and have shown that the relationship of SES to healthy lifestyles may be complex. For example, in a review, Sherwood, Story, and Obarzanek (2004) cited two studies that evaluated dietary intake patterns in African-American and Caucasians adolescents that showed no relationship between parental income (or education) and food consumption. Other investigators have reported, however, that African-Americans living in lower SES environments are less likely to engage in regular physical activity (Wilson, Kirtland, Ainsworth, & Addy, 2004). In a recent study, Gordon-Larsen, Nelson, Page, and Popkin (2006) also reported that lower-SES and high-minority block groups of adolescents had reduced access to facilities, which in turn was associated with decreased physical activity and increased levels of overweight.

Taken together, the studies reviewed above suggest that the interaction of family, environmental factors, and culture are important for enhancing our understanding of factors related to obesity and the prevention and treatment of obesity in minority youth. Future studies are needed to more fully understand the impact of the environment and cultural traditions on the prevalence of obesity in minority youth and their families.

ENVIRONMENTAL FACTORS IN OBESITY (EXOSYSTEMIC INFLUENCES)

There are a variety of environmental factors that may impede weight-control efforts in ethically diverse pediatric populations. For example, community and neighborhood supports for healthy eating and physical activity have been shown to be correlated with BMI (Gordon-Larsen et al., 2006; Johnson, Guthrie, Smiciklas-Wright, & Wang, 1994; Wilson, Ainsworth, & Bowles, 2007). In addition, the home environment may interact with neighborhood and community environments to either hinder or facilitate healthy lifestyle habits related to pediatric weight management.

Some evidence suggests that environmental supports, such as having access to healthy foods, is important for maintaining healthy dietary consumption and that ethnically diverse populations may have increased barriers for consuming such foods. For example, Johnson et al. (1994) reported that living in a rural area and being African-American were significant predictors for higher intake of total fat, saturated fat, cholesterol, and sodium in children. In a focus group study by Molaison et al. (2005), low-income African-American adolescents also reported that grocery stores in their neighborhoods did not supply fresh fruits and vegetables. These adolescents also reported that their home environment was lacking in availability of fresh fruits and vegetables.

Modern technology has also become a barrier in the home environment, which has resulted in increasing rates of sedentary behavior and overeating, and decreasing rates of physical activity. This trend has also been shown to be more prominent in ethnically diverse youth in comparison to Caucasian youth (Brodersen, Steptoe, Williamson, & Wardle, 2005). Previous research has demonstrated that television plays a role in influencing the food choices of American youth. For example, studies that have analyzed the content of advertising targeted at youth have shown that the majority of food advertisements broadcast during prime youth-viewing hours (e.g., Saturday morning and early evenings) are for calorically dense foods with little nutritional value (Byrd-Bredbenner & Grasso, 1999a, 1999b; Kotz & Story, 1999). In one study, Matheson et al. (2004) examined the prevalence of television watching among African-American girls. A total of 40–50 percent of evening meals among African-American girls were consumed while watching television. The investigators reported that a significant proportion of these African American girls consumed food while watching television and the average daily intake of calories consumed increased by 26–35 percent during viewing time.

Several investigators have also examined the relationship between neighborhood safety (e.g., traffic, crime, gangs), access to parks, and physical activity among multiethnic youth (Johns & Ha, 1999; Pate et al., 1997; Romero et al., 2001). In one study (Romero et al.), perceptions of more hazardous traffic and crime, and having a lack of access to parks were significantly associated with lower self-reported physical activity in elementary children. Availability of exercise equipment at home and television watching has also been shown to be significant correlates of physical activity in multiethnic elementary school children (Pate et al.).

In summary, environmental barriers such as limited access to healthy food options, and concerns regarding the safety of neighborhoods for engaging in physical activity, are important factors in understanding health behaviors among minority youth. In addition, the home environment has been shown to have an impact on sedentary behaviors that may increase the risk of obesity in minority youth. Further research is needed at the public policy level to address disparities in these important environmental supports in underserved communities.

INTERVENTION STUDIES IN ETHNICALLY DIVERSE CHILDREN (MACROSYSTEMIC FACTORS)

In this section, we provide an overview of weight gain prevention and weight loss studies in minority youth. Table 18.1 presents a summary of a number of randomized intervention studies and several quasi-experimental studies that have been conducted with minority youth, and highlights the theoretical elements that are relevant to the ecological approach outlined in Figure 18.1. Many of the studies use an approach that includes multiple systems outlined by the ecological model (individual, family, peers, institutions, community) in minority youth and their families.

In general, very little previous research has specifically addressed weight-loss issues in ethnically diverse youth. One study has evaluated the effect of parental participation in overweight female African-American adolescents (Wadden et al., 1990). Thirty-six adolescents received the same 16-week curriculum but were randomized to one of the following parental participation groups: 1) child alone, 2) mother-child together, and 3) mother-child separately. Participants attended one-hour weekly classes and covered material that was adapted from Brownell et al. (1983) that focused on behavioral skills and parental modeling. Mean BMI declined from 35.2 to 33.9 among all three conditions, with no significant differences between treatment conditions. Adolescent weight loss was greater with higher levels of mother attendance.

Another study evaluated a family-based weight-loss intervention delivered through the Internet over six months (White et al., 2004) in 57 adolescent African-American females and their families. Families were randomized to an Internet behavioral group or an education-only comparison condition that received educational information only. The Internet behavioral condition included self-monitoring, goal-setting, problem-solving, behavioral contracting, and relapse prevention. Data at six months demonstrated significantly greater reductions in body fat and weight for the behavioral versus comparison adolescents. Parents' satisfaction with life and family satisfaction were significant mediators of weight loss in adolescents.

A recent study by Resnicow, Taylor, Baskin, and McCarty (2005) was also conducted with African-American girls. Ten churches were randomized to either the high-intensity group or the moderate-intensity group that totaled 147 adolescent girls. The high-intensity group received weekly behavioral sessions that included a behavioral activity, a physical activity, and healthy snacks, a one-day retreat, and messages via telephone or pager based on motivational interviewing. Participants in the moderate-intensity group received six sessions that contained information on barriers and benefits to physical activity, fad diets, and trying new foods. Parents were invited to attend every other group meeting in both group conditions. No significant differences were found between groups, yet participants in the high-intensity group who attended more than 75 percent of sessions had significant reductions in BMI compared to participants who attended less than 75 percent of sessions.

Table 18.1. Weight-loss interventions in minority youth from an ecological approach

Author	Ecological theory construct	Sample	Methods	Primary outcomes	Findings
Beech et al. (2003)	Child/Family	60 African American pre-adolescents	RCT: 1) child-only (12 weekly sessions on physical activity, nutrition, and a take-it home components). 2) parent-only group (12 weekly sessions on physical activity, nutrition, and interactive activities); or 3) self-esteem focused comparison group.	Moderate to vigorous physical activity (MVPA), diet, BMI, waist circumference, body composition	11.7 percent increase in minutes of MVPA, 34.1 percent decrease in servings of sweetened beverages, and 1.5 percent increase in servings of water (combined intervention groups). Parent-only group had trend towards increase in PA and fewer calories from fat.
Engels, Gretebeck, Gretebeck, and Jimenez (2005)	Community (after-school program)/ Family	56 African American preadolescents and 25 parent/guardians	Not RCT: 12-week afterschool program (dance, sport games, fitness activities, nutrition activities, step-counters, and display board within the school.	BMI, body fat, fitness, fruit and vegetable intake	Parents had reductions in BMI, body fat, and improved fitness. Children showed higher intakes of fruits and vegetables.
Fitzgibbon et al. (2005)	Community (Preschool/ Family)	12 preschools (~300 African American preschool children and parents)	RCT: 1) weight control intervention (WCI) 14-week program focused on healthy eating and exercise and parent newsletter or 2) general health intervention (GHI)	BMI, physical activity, food intake	Mean increase in BMI was significantly lower in WCI group vs. GHI at year 1 (0.06 vs 0.59 kg/m^2) and year 2 (0.54 vs. 1.08 kg/m^2).
Frenn et al. (2005)	Community (School)	103 multiethnic sample of adolescents (primarily African American and Hispanic)	Not RCT: 8 sessions of Internet and video-based activities to increase PA and reduce fat intake	MVPA, dietary fat	High attenders (>50 percent) significantly increased MVPA by 22 min. vs. 46min. decrease in control and decreased percent of dietary fat from 30.7 to 29.9.

(continued)

Table 18.1. (continued)

Author	Ecological theory construct	Sample	Methods	Primary outcomes	Findings
Resnicow et al. (2005)	Community (Churches/Family)	147 African American adolescent females in 10 churches	RCT: 1) High Intensity (weekly behavioral sessions, 30 minutes of PA, food prep. retreat) or 2) Moderate Intensity (6 sessions on barriers and benefits of PA). Parents invited to attend every other session.	Adiposity, BMI	No significant differences between groups. High attenders (>75 percent) in High Intensity group had significant reductions in BMI compared to low attenders (<75 percent).
Robinson et al. (2003)	Family/Home	61 African American females (age 8 – 10) and their parents or guardians	RCT: 1) Treatment (dance classes 5 days per week at community centers, 5 in-home lessons on reducing television delivered to participants and a family member, and 5 newsletters mailed to parents/guardians) or 2) control (health education curriculum)	BMI, waist circumference, media use, physical activity	Treatment group reported 23 percent less media use, significant reduction in overall household television viewing compared to controls, and 40 percent decrease in dinners eaten while watching television.
Stolley and Fitzgibbon (1997)	Family	65 African American mother/daughter dyads; preadolescent females	RCT: 1) treatment group (12 culturally tailored sessions on PA and diet) or 2) control. Sessions held at local tutoring center.	Weight, height, percent overweight, diet, parental support and role modeling	Mothers in treatment group had significant positive changes in saturated fat, percent calories from fat, parental support, and role modeling compared to control. Daughters had a significant decrease in percent of calories from fat compared to controls.

Study	Level	Sample	Design/Intervention	Outcomes	Results
Wadden et al. (1990)	Child/Family	36 African American adolescents and parents	RCT: 1) Child Alone, 2) Mother-Child Together, or 3) Mother-Child Separately. Participants attended one-hour weekly classes for 16 weeks.	Weight, BMI	Mean BMI declined from 35.2 – 33.9 (groups combined). No significant differences between groups.
White et al. (2004)	Family	57 adolescent African American females and their families	RCT: 1) Internet behavioral group or 2) control.	BMI, weight, body fat	Adolescents in Internet group lost significantly more fat than those in the control group. For parents, BMI was significantly different between the two groups.
Wilson, Teasley, Friend, Green, and Sica (2002)	Child/Family	53 African American Adolescents and their familes	RCT: 1) behavioral skills plus motivational group or 2) behavioral skills only or 3) General Health Education	Fruit and vegetable intake based on food diaries; min. of moderate-to-vigorous physical activity base on accelerometer estimates	Adolescents in the behavioral skills plus motivation or behavioral skills only showed a significantly greater increase in fruit and vegetable intake as compared to the education only group.
Wilson et al. (2005)	Child/Peers	48 adolescents (83 African American; 83 percent on free or reduced lunch program)	Quasi-experimental design (matched schools): 1) behavioral skills plus motivational group or 2) General Health Education	Moderate-to-vigorous physical activity from accelerometer estimates	Behavioral skills plus motivational intervention resulted in significantly greater physical activity than the general health program.

Note: RCT = Denotes randomized controlled trial

Prevention of weight gain is also an important component for reducing the prevalence of overweight and obesity in minority youth. In a study conducted of primarily African-American and Hispanic children and their parents, 12 preschools were randomly assigned to a weight-control intervention (WCI) or a general health intervention (GHI) (Fitzgibbon et al., 2005). Children in the WCI group participated in a 14-week program focused on healthy eating and exercise. Children in the GHI group participated in a 14-week program focused on general health concepts that did not include information on physical activity and exercise. Parents in both groups received weekly newsletters that included a homework assignment. At one- and two-year follow-ups, the mean increase in BMI was significantly lower in WCI group in comparison to the GHI group. These results indicate that a behavioral school-based program with a correspondent parental component were able to reduce the increase in BMI in minority preschool children.

Beech et al. (2003) evaluated the impact of two ethnically relevant interventions targeting the prevention of weight gain in 60 African-American preadolescents. Participants were randomized to one of three groups: 1) child-only; 2) parent-only; or 3) self-esteem focused comparison. Results showed an 11.7 percent increase in minutes of moderate-to-vigorous physical activity, a 34.1 percent decrease in servings of sweetened beverages, and a 1.5 percent increase in servings of water when combining the two intervention groups. Both intervention groups showed favorable results compared to the comparison group, but the parent-only group demonstrated a trend towards greater improvement in physical activity and fewer calories derived from fat compared to the child-only group. Beech et al. suggest a combined format of both parents and children, allowing for occasional separate sessions, as a promising intervention approach in African-American preadolescents.

Another study examined mother-daughter dyads as part of an obesity prevention program in 65 inner-city, low-income African-American preadolescent girls and their mothers (Stolley & Fitzgibbon, 1997). Mother-daughter dyads were randomized to a treatment or comparison group. The treatment group received a 12-week culturally tailored obesity prevention program—adapted from the Know Your Body Program—targeting healthy eating and physical activity. Parent participation was included to provide support to mothers who have limited access to dietary and physical activity resources. Mothers in the treatment group showed significant decreases in saturated fat and percent calories from fat compared to the no-treatment group. Mothers in the treatment group also showed significant increases in parental support and role modeling for healthy eating compared to the no-treatment group. Daughters showed significant decreases in percent of calories from fat compared to no-intervention. This study demonstrates that culturally tailored obesity prevention in mothers and their preadolescent daughters can have an impact on eating behaviors related to obesity.

Another obesity prevention study targeting African-American girls incorporated dance and reductions in television-viewing in a randomized controlled trial in girls and their parents/guardians (Robinson et al., 2003). Participants were randomized to either a treatment intervention or active control group. The treatment intervention consisted of dance classes, in-home lessons on reducing television delivered to participants and a family member, and five newsletters mailed to parents/guardians. The active control group was a health education program delivered through community health lectures and included mailing newsletters to both participants and their parents/guardians. Both groups incorporated culturally relevant intervention staff. The treatment group reported a significant reduction in overall household television -viewing compared to active controls. Overall, the results indicate the feasibility and acceptance of the dance lessons and reduction in television-viewing as a potential obesity prevention program in African-American girls.

Another study investigated the impact on diet and physical activity of 56 African-American children and 25 parent/guardians after a 12-week afterschool program (Engels et al., 2005). Program components included dance, sport games, fitness activities, nutrition activities, handouts on nutrition and fitness, step counters, and a display board within the school. Participants were asked to log daily fruit and vegetable intake and steps. The program also incorporated a motivational guest appearance from a well-known public figure to the program. Parents had reductions in BMI, body fat, and improved fitness, whereas children showed higher intakes of fruit and vegetables at the end of the program. This study did not incorporate a comparison group, therefore interpretation of these results is limited in demonstrating effectiveness. Further research is needed to replicate these findings in a larger study with a comparison condition.

Frenn et al. (2005) evaluated the effectiveness of a web-based video intervention on increasing physical activity and reducing fat intake in primarily African-American and Hispanic seventh-grade students. The intervention included eight sessions of Internet- and video-based activities. Children who attended at least half of the sessions as part of their science class increased moderate-to-vigorous physical activity by 22 minutes compared with a decrease of 46 minutes for those attending less than half of the sessions. Intervention children who attended at least half of the sessions also decreased dietary fat from 30.7 to 29.9. Much like the above study, this study did not incorporate a comparison group, which limits the conclusions that can be drawn from the study results.

Several studies have specifically evaluated interventions that target dietary intake and physical activity in African-American adolescents, and involve increasing positive family and peer interactions. In one study by Wilson et al. (2002), 53 healthy African-American adolescents and their families were randomized to a 12-week behavioral skills plus motivational intervention, behavioral skills-only, or an education-only group for increasing fruit and vegetable intake and physical activity. Adolescents in the motivational enhancement group also participated in a strategic self-presentation videotape session. Strategic self-presentation involves increasing motivation by creating cognitive dissonance and inducing shifts in self-concept by generating positive coping strategies for engaging friends and family members in making healthy dietary and physical activity changes during a videotaped session. Both intervention groups showed greater increases in fruit and vegetable intake from pre- to post-treatment in comparison to the education-only group. However, correlation analyses revealed that only the behavioral skills plus motivational group showed that self-concept and self-efficacy for behavioral skills were significantly correlated with post-treatment fruit and vegetable intake and change in fruit and vegetable intake.

A quasi-experimental study by Wilson et al. (2005) evaluated the effects of a four-week student-centered intervention to increase physical activity in minority and low-SES adolescents. Twenty-eight students in the intervention school were matched (on race, percentage of free or reduced lunch, gender, and age) with 20 students from another school who served as the comparison group. The intervention emphasized increasing intrinsic motivation and behavioral skills for physical activity. Intervention adolescents took ownership in selecting a variety of physical activities to participate in, and they generated coping strategies for making effective physical activity behavior changes by involving peers and family members in activities. Intervention participants showed greater increases in moderate-to-vigorous physical activity from baseline to week 4 of the intervention than the comparison group. Intervention participants also showed significantly greater increases in physical activity motivation and positive self-concept for physical activity than comparison adolescents.

In summary, the above studies demonstrate that family-based interventions that include parents in the process have been effective in reducing BMI and increasing health behaviors (i.e., nutritious diet and physical activity) to prevent obesity in minority youth. Factors that have been studied to date include participation of parents—either directly, or indirectly through mailings. In addition, studies that increase adolescent self-concept and intrinsic motivation for health behaviors are promising. As Figure 18.1 denotes, interventions for pediatric weight management issues in ethnically diverse youth will need to consider all levels of the ecological approach if long-term lifestyle change is the goal.

FUTURE DIRECTIONS

Many of the skills needed to prevent weight gain or promote weight loss in ethnically diverse children can be difficult for families, and even more difficult for those struggling with family problems. It is probably easier for some families to provide positive support or develop skills through interventions than others. It would be valuable to assess family risk and protective factors for ethnically diverse youth who achieve better outcomes in weight-loss programs (Kazak, 2002). For example, if adolescent weight loss increased with the mother's attendance in the intervention, then the mother's attendance could signify protective factors, including support for the adolescent's weight-loss efforts or learning appropriate modeling behaviors. Also, measures of parenting styles and family functioning may also be important predictors of weight loss. These studies outlined in this chapter point to the importance of parental and family support as factors that increase healthy behaviors in overweight adolescents. In general, future research should focus on understanding how ecological factors may interact with family-related factors (e.g., child perceptions, peer groups, institutions, environment, and culture) to prevent obesity and promote healthy life style in ethnically diverse youth.

REFERENCES

Adkins, S., Sherwood, N., Story, M., & Davis, M. (2004). Physical activity among African-American girls: The role of parents and the home environment. *Obesity Research, 12*(Suppl.), 38–45.

Agudo, A., & Pera, G. (1999). Vegetable and fruit consumption associated with anthropometric, dietary and lifestyle factors in Spain. *Public Health Nutrition, 2,* 263–271.

Baranowski, T. (1997). Families and health actions. In D. Gochman (Ed.), *Handbook of Health Behavior Research: Personal and Social Determinants* (pp. 179–206). New York: Plenum Press.

Beech, B., Klesges, R., Kumanyika, S., Murray, D., Klesges, L., McClanahan, B., et al. (2003). Child- and parent- targeted interventions: The Memphis GEMS pilot study. *Ethnicity & Disease, 13*(Suppl. 1), 40–53.

Brodersen, N., Steptoe, A., Williamson, S., & Wardle, J. (2005). Sociodemographic, developmental, environmental, and psychological correlates of physical activity and sedentary behavior at age 11 to 12. *Annals of Behavioral Medicine, 29,* 2–11.

Bronfenbrenner, U. (1979). *The Ecology of Human Development.* Cambridge, MA: Harvard University Press.

Brownell, K. D., Kelman, J. H., & Stunkard, A. J. (1983). Treatment of obese children with and without their mothers: Changes in weight and blood pressure. *Pediatrics, 71,* 515–523.

Brustad, R. (1996). Attraction to physical activity in urban school children: Parental socialization and gender influences. *Research Quarterly for Exercise and Sport, 67,* 316–323.

Byrd-Bredbenner, C., & Grasso, D. (1999a). A comparative analysis of television food advertisements and current dietary recommendations. *American Journal of Health Studies, 15,* 169–180.

Byrd-Bredbenner, C., & Grasso, D. (1999b). Prime-time health: An analysis of health content in television commercials broadcast during programs viewed heavily by children. *International Journal of Health Education, 2,* 159–169.

Center for Disease Control. (1997, March 7). Update: Prevalence of overweight among children, adolescents, and adults–United States 1988–1994. *Morbidity and Mortality Weekly Report, 46,* 199–202.

Coates, T. J., Killen, J. D., & Slinkard, L. A. (1982). Parent participation in a treatment program for overweight adolescents. *International Journal of Eating Disorders, 1,* 37 – 48.

Eberhardt, M. S., Ingram, D. D., Makuc, D. M., Pamuk, E. R., Freid, V. M., Harper, S. B., et al. (2001). *Urban and Rural Health Chartbook.* (NCHS Publication No. 76-641496). Hyattsville, MD: National Center for Health Statistics.

Engels, H., Gretebeck, R., Gretebeck, K., & Jimenez, L. (2005). Promoting healthful diets and exercise: Efficacy of a 12-week after-school program in urban African Americans. *Journal of the American Dietetic Association, 105,* 455–459.

Evans, A. E., Wilson, D. K., Buck, J., Torbett, H., & Williams, J. (2006). A qualitative analysis of barriers and motivators for healthy eating among underserved adolescents. *Journal of Family and Community Health, 29,* 17–27.

Fitzgibbon, M., Stolley, M., Schiffer, L., Van Horn, L., Kaufer-Christoffel, K., & Dyer, A. (2005). Two-year follow-up results for Hip-Hop to Health Jr.: A randomized controlled trial for overweight prevention in preschool minority children. *Journal of Pediatrics, 146,* 618–625.

Frenn, M., Malin, S., Brown, R., Greer, Y., Fox, J., Greer, J., et al. (2005). Changing the tide: An internet/video exercise and low-fat diet intervention with middle-school students. *Applied Nursing Research, 18,* 13–21.

Gordon-Larsen, P., Nelson, M. C., Page, P., & Popkin, B. M. (2006). Inequality in the built environment underlies key health disparities in physical activity and obesity. *Pediatrics, 117,* 417–424.

Hill, L., Casswell, S., Maskill, C., Jones, S., & Wyllie, A. (1998). Fruit and vegetables as adolescent food choices in New Zealand. *Health Promotion International, 13,* 55–65.

Johns, D. P., & Ha, A. S. (1999). Home and recess physical activity of Hong Kong children. *Research Quarterly for Exercise and Sport, 70,* 319–323.

Johnson, R. K., Guthrie, H., Smiciklas-Wright, H., & Wang, M. Q. (1994). Characterizing nutrient intakes of children by sociodemographic factors. *Public Health Reports, 109,* 414–420.

Kazak, A. E. (2002). Challenges in family health intervention research. *Families, Systems, & Health, 20,* 51–59.

Kazak, A. E., Rourke, M. T., & Crump, T. A. (2003). Families and other systems in pediatric psychology. In M. C. Roberts (Ed.), *Handbook of Pediatric Psychology* (3rd ed.). New York: Guilford Press, pp. 150–175.

Kimm, S., Barton, B., Berhane, K., Ross, J., Payne, G., & Schreiber, G. (1997). Self-esteem and adiposity in black and white girls: The NHLBI growth and health study. *Annals of Epidemiology, 7,* 550–560.

Kohl, H., & Hobbs, K. (1998). Development of physical activity behaviors among children and adolescents. *Pediatrics, 101,* 549–554.

Kotz, H., & Story, M. (1999). Food advertisements during children's Saturday morning television programming: Are they consistent with dietary recommendations? *Journal of the American Dietetic Association, 94,* 1296–1300.

Kuczmarski, R. L., & Flegal, K. M. (2000). Criteria for definition of overweight in transition: Background and recommendations for the United States. *American Journal of Clinical Nutrition, 72,* 1074–1081.

Matheson, D., Wang, Y., Klesges, L., Beech, B., Kraemer, H., & Robinson, T. (2004). African-American girls' dietary intake while watching television. *Obesity Research, 12*(Suppl.), 32–37.

McGoldrick, M., Giordano, J., & Pearce, J. K. (Eds.). (1996). *Ethnicity and Family Therapy, (2nd ed.).* New York: Guilford Press.

McLeroy, K. R., Bibeau, D., Steckler, A., & Glanz, K. (1988). An ecological perspective on health promotion programs. *Health Education Quarterly, 15,* 351–377.

Mellin, A. E., Neumark-Sztainer, D., Story, M., Ireland, M., & Resnick, M. D. (2002). Unhealthy behaviors and psychosocial difficulties among overweight adolescents: The potential impact of familial factors. *Journal of Adolescent Health, 31,* 145–153.

Mendelson, B. K., White, D. R., Schliecker, E. (1995). Adolescents' weight, sex, and family functioning. *International Journal of Eating Disorders, 17,* 73–79.

Mokad, A. H., Serdula, M. K., Dietz, W. H., Bowman, B. A., Marks, J. S., & Koplan, J. P. (1999). The spread of obesity epidemic in the United States, 1991–1998. *Journal of the American Medical Association, 282,* 1519–1522.

Molaison, E., Connell, C., Stuff, J., Yadrick, K., & Bogle, M. (2005). Influences on fruit and vegetable consumption by low-income black American adolescents. *Journal of Nutrition Education and Behavior, 37,* 246–251.

Motl, R., Dishman, R., Saunders, R., Dowda, M., Felton, G., Ward, D., & Pate, R. (2002). Examining social-cognitive determinants of intention and physical activity among black and white adolescent girls using structural equation modeling. *Health Psychology, 21,* 459–467.

Ogden C. L., Carroll M. D., Curtin L. R., McDowell, M. A., Tabak, C. J., & Flegal, K. M. (2006). Prevalence of overweight and obesity in the United States, 1999–2004. *Journal of American Medical Association, 295,* 1549–1555.

Pate, R. R., Trost, S. G., Felton, G., Ward, D., Dowda, M., & Saunders, R. (1997). Correlates of physical activity behavior in rural youth. *Research Quarterly for Exercise and Sport, 68,* 241–248.

Patrick, H., Nicklas, T. A., Hughes, S. O., & Morales, M. (2005). The benefits of authoritative feeding style: Caregiver feeding styles and children's food consumption patterns. *Appetite, 44,* 243–249.

Patterson, T., Rupp, J., Sallis, J. F., Atkins, C., & Nader, P. (1988). Aggregation of dietary calories, fats, and sodium in Mexican American and Anglo families. *American Journal of Preventive Medicine, 4,* 75–82.

Perry, A., Rosenblatt, E., & Wang, X. (2004). Physical, behavioral, and body image characteristics in a tri-racial group of adolescent girls. *Obesity Research, 12,* 1670–1679.

Power, T., DuPaul, G., Shapiro E., & Kazak, A. (2003). *Promoting Children's Health: Integrating School, Family, and Community.* New York: Guilford Press.

Resnicow, K., Taylor, R., Baskin, M., & McCarty, F. (2005). Results of Go Girls: A weight control program for overweight African-American adolescent females. *Obesity Research, 13,* 1739–1748.

Robinson, T., Killen, J., Kraemer, H., Wilson, D., Matheson, D., Haskell, W. L., et al. (2003). Dance and reducing television viewing to prevent weight gain in African-American girls: The Stanford GEMS pilot study. *Ethnicity & Disease, 13*(Suppl. 1), 65–77.

Romero, A. J., Robinson, T. N., Kraemer, H. C., Erickson, S. J., Haydel, K. F., Mendoza, F., et al. (2001). Are perceived neighborhood hazards a barrier to physical activity in children? *Archives of Pediatric Adolescent Medicine, 155,* 1143–1148.

Saelens, B., Sallis, J. F., Wilfley, D. E., Patrick, K., Cella, J. A., & Buchta, R. (2002). Behavioral weight control for overweight adolescents initiated in primary care. *Obesity Research, 10,* 22–32.

Sallis, J. F., Bauman, A., & Pratt, M. (1998). Environmental and policy interventions to promote physical activity. *American Journal of Preventive Medicine, 15,* 379–397.

Sallis, J., Patterson, T., Buono, M., & Nader, P. (1999). Relation of cardiovascular fitness and physical activity to cardiovascular disease risk factors in children and adults. *American Journal of Epidemiology, 127,* 933–941.

Sherwood, N., Story, M., & Obarzanek, E. (2004). Correlates of obesity in African-American girls: An overview. *Obesity Research, 12*(Suppl.), 3–5.

Spruit-Metz, D., Lindquist, C., Birch, L., Fisher, J., & Goran, M. (2002). Relation between mothers' child-feeding practices and children's adiposity. *American Journal of Clinical Nutrition, 75,* 581–586.

Stolley, M., & Fitzgibbon, M. (1997). Effects of an obesity prevention program on the eating behavior of African American mothers and daughters. *Health Education & Behavior, 24,* 152–164.

Thompson, S., Corwin, S., Rogan, T., & Sargent, R. (1999). Body size beliefs and weight concerns among mothers and their adolescent children. *Journal of Child and Family Studies, 8,* 91–108.

Trost, S., Pate, R., Saunders, R., Ward, D., Dowda, M., & Felton, G. (1997). A prospective study of the determinants of physical activity in rural fifth grade children. *Preventive Medicine, 26,* 257–263.

Turner, H. M., Rose, K. S., & Cooper, M. J. (2005). Schema and parental bonding in overweight and non-overweight female adolescents. *International Journal of Obesity and Related Metabolic Disorders, 29,* 381–7.

Wadden, T. A., Stunkard, A. J., Rich, L., Rubin, C. J., Sweidel, G., & McKinney, S. (1990). Obesity in black adolescent girls: A controlled clinical trial of treatment by diet, behavior modification, and parental support. *Pediatrics, 85,* 345–352.

White, M. A., Martin, P. D., Newton, R. L., Walden, H. M., York-Crowe, E. E., Gordon, S. T., et al. (2004). Mediators of weight loss in a family-based intervention presented over the Internet. *Obesity Research, 12,* 1050–1059.

Wilson, D. K., Ainsworth, B. E., & Bowles, H. (2007). Body mass index and environmental supports for physical activity in active and inactive residents of a U.S. Southeastern County. *Health Psychology, 26,* 710–717.

Wilson, D. K., Evans, A. E., Williams, J., Mixon, G., Minette, C., Sirad, J., et al. (2005). A preliminary test of a student-centered intervention on increasing physical activity in underserved adolescents. *Annals of Behavioral Medicine, 30,* 119–124.

Wilson, D. K., Friend, R., Teasley, N., Green, S., & Sica, D. A. (2002). Motivational versus social cognitive interventions for promoting and physical activity habits in African-American adolescents. *Annals of Behavioral Medicine, 24,* 310–319.

Wilson, D. K., Kirtland, K., Ainsworth, B., & Addy, C. L. (2004). Socioeconomic status and perceptions of access and safety for physical activity. *Annals of Behavioral Medicine, 28,* 20–28.

Young-Hyman, D., Herman, L., Scott, D., & Schlundt, D. (2000). Caregiver perceptions of children's obesity-related health risk: A study of African American families. *Obesity Research, 8,* 241–248.

Young-Hyman, D., Schlundt, D., Herman-Wenderoth, L., & Bozylinksi, K. (2003). Obesity, appearance, and psychological adaptation in young African-American children. *Journal of Pediatric Psychology, 28,* 463–472.

Zeller, M., & Modi, A. (2006). Predictors of health-related quality of life in obese youth. *Obesity, 14,* 122–130.

Section V

Prevention of Pediatric Obesity

19

Prevention of Childhood Obesity in Childcare Settings

BARBARA A. DENNISON and MYLES S. FAITH

This chapter addresses the topic of childhood obesity prevention in child-care (i.e., preschool and daycare) settings. Despite the increasing interest and attention to childhood obesity prevention, interventions in child-care settings are few. None-the-less, these settings offer great potential because they can reach children at young ages and may influence the development of dietary habits, physical activity, and television (TV) viewing patterns.

The chapter begins by providing the rationale for targeting preschool-age children and childcare settings. Next, viable behavioral targets and programs in daycare or preschool settings are reviewed. Finally, challenges to modifying childcare settings and potential opportunities and/or gaps requiring further research are discussed.

RATIONALE FOR TARGETING PRESCHOOL AGE CHILDREN

Childhood obesity is a national and worldwide public health problem. In the United States in 2003–2004, 26.2 percent of children aged two through five years, and 37.2 percent of children aged six through 11 years were either overweight or obese (i.e., had a body mass index [BMI] at or above the sex-specific 85th BMI-for-age percentile) (Ogden et al., 2006).

BARBARA A. DENNISON • University of Albany – SUNY, Rensselaer, NY 12144; New York State Department of Health Albany, NY 12204. **MYLES S. FAITH** • University of Pennsylvania, Philadelphia, PA 19104.

The rates of obesity in the United States have nearly tripled over the past 35 years. While most studies find that the prevalence of obesity (BMI > 95th reference percentile) is higher among Hispanics than non-Hispanic blacks or non-Hispanic whites, a recent study among low-income preschoolers found that between 1989 and 2003, the rates of increase were parallel for the three groups (Edmunds et al., 2006).

Childhood obesity is not just a cosmetic problem. The adverse consequences associated with obesity are significant—both in dollars and impaired health. These include, but are not limited to, hyperlipidemia and cardiovascular disease, insulin resistance, glucose intolerance and diabetes mellitus, cholelithiasis, hypertension and stroke, sleep apnea, and numerous orthopedic complications (Pi-Sunyer, 1993). Furthermore, obese individuals have higher mortality rates (National Institutes of Health, 1998). In children and adolescents, the adverse psychological consequences and lower self-esteem associated with obesity have long been recognized (French, Story, & Perry, 1995; Strauss, 2000). Increasingly, medical complications, including hypertriglyceridemia and low HDL-cholesterol levels, hypertension, sleep apnea, glucose intolerance, and type II diabetes mellitus are being reported at younger and younger ages (Dietz, 1998; Gidding et al., 1996; Must et al., 1999). In addition, childhood obesity tends to track over time into adulthood (Guo, Wu, Chumlea, & Roche, 2002; Magarey, Daniels, Boulton, & Cockington, 2003; Whitaker, Wright, Pepe, Seidel, & Dietz, 1997). Among children aged three through five years, having a BMI above the 85th percentile conferred an odds ratio of 4.1 for adult overweight, while having a BMI above the 95th percentile conferred an odds ratio of 7.9 (Whitaker et al.,). Mounting evidence suggests that dietary, physical activity, and TV- viewing behaviors have their origins in childhood, track over time, and influence subsequent adiposity (Dennison, Straus, Mellits, & Charney, 1988; Klesges, Klesges, Eck, & Shelton, 1995; Moore, Nguyen, Rothman, Cupples, & Ellison, 1995; Stein, Shea, Basch, Contento, & Zybert, 1991). A review study by Serdula et al. (1993) concludes that the obese child is at significant risk for becoming the obese adult.

The preschool child is an ideal target for prevention strategies for developmental reasons. Biologically, the period prior to the adiposity rebound appears to be a critical period in the development of obesity (Bouchard, 1996; Whitaker, Pepe, Wright, Seidel, & Dietz, 1998). Parents and caretakers are truly gatekeepers for young children, controlling not only the foods offered to the child, but also the environmental context in which food is offered and consumed. These adult role models may also provide opportunities for active play and movement. Psychologically, preschool-age children are very imitative, copying the dietary behaviors, food preferences, and eating patterns—in addition to exercise or TV-viewing habits (Birch, 1980; Dennison, Jenkins, & Chen, 1996). Young children's food preferences are quite malleable because they are influenced by the social-affective context in which foods are offered (Birch, Zimmerman, & Hind, 1980). Thus, interventions might be more successful if implemented at the time when food preferences and lifestyle behaviors are developing, rather than after they are already established.

RATIONALE FOR TARGETING CHILDCARE SETTINGS

Childcare centers provide unique opportunities to reach young children. Sixty-five percent of mothers with children under six years are in the labor force (Bachu & O'Connell, 2000). In 1999, only 23 percent of all families with children under six years had one parent who stayed home (U.S. Census Bureau, 2007). In 2002, two-thirds of U.S. preschool children participated in an average of 32 hours/week in regular childcare programs (Overturf & Johnson, 2005).

Head Start, a federally-funded, comprehensive, early childhood development program, was developed to foster school readiness by providing educational, health, nutritional, social, and other services to enrolled children and their families. It serves more than 900,000 low-income preschool children and their families each year (Head Start Bureau, 2007). Because of the Head Start program, low-income and minority children are more likely to attend childcare. They are also more likely to be overweight. Thus, childcare settings (including Head Start programs) offer great potential for obesity prevention initiatives.

BEHAVIORAL TARGETS FOR OVERWEIGHT PREVENTION INITIATIVES

Research suggests several potential policy, environmental, and behavior-change initiatives for childcare settings. These include: a) changes in the availability, variety, and portion sizes of foods and beverages; b) increased opportunities, time, and vigor of physical activity; c) reduced sedentary activities (including TV and other recreational media); d) enhanced social cues to foster healthier eating and more physical activity; e) satiety training with children; and f) parent skills training. These are reviewed below.

Changing the Availability, Variety, and Portion Sizes of Foods and Beverages

Increased vegetable intakes are associated with lower obesity rates. Among adults, McCrory et al. (1999) found that consuming a greater variety of vegetables was associated with decreased energy intake per kilogram of body weight ($r=-0.28$, $p<0.05$), and with decreased percentages of body fat ($r=-0.31$, $p=0.008$). A study among preschoolers found lower obesity rates with increased frequency of consuming carrots (odds Ratio = 0.85, $p<0.005$; Dennison, Jenkins, Erb, Rockwell, & Gregg, 2000). Among Native Canadian Cree students, youth who were obese consumed significantly fewer fruits and vegetables than nonobese children (Bernard, Lavallee, Gray-Donald, & Delisle, 1995).

Fruit juice variety and availability has increased dramatically over the past 20–30 years, resulting in increased fruit juice consumption. The highest juice intakes are seen among preschoolers, especially low-income children participating in public health nutrition programs that provide or subsidize with fruit juice. A number of studies have found that excess fruit juice intake may contribute to obesity (Dennison, Rockwell, & Baker, 1997; Skinner, Carruth, Moran, Houck, & Coletta, 1999; Smith & Lifshitz, 1994), or to further excess weight gain among children who are already overweight (Faith, Dennison, Edmunds, & Stratton, 2006; Welsh et al., 2005). These concerns contributed to the recommendations of the American Academy of Pediatrics (2001b) Committee on Nutrition that fruit juice intake be limited to no more than 4–6 oz/day for children one to six years of age.

The increase in sugar-sweetened soft drink consumption in the United States is even more striking than the increases in fruit juice, with intakes more than doubling between 1977–78 and 1994–96 (Tippets & Cleveland, 1999). In a recent study of preadolescents, both baseline consumption of sugar-sweetened drinks and the change in intakes over two years were associated prospectively with obesity risk (Ludwig, Peterson, & Gortmaker, 2001).

The sizes of ready-to-eat prepackaged foods and beverages have increased dramatically, as have the quantities of food served in restaurants (French, Story, & Jeffery, 2001). In an effort to sell customers "value meals," fast food restaurants are increasingly offering ever-larger "super-sized" meals. The size of candy bars—and even the size of standard dinner and salad plates used in restaurants—have increased dramatically since the 1950s. Rolls and colleagues (2000) found that while younger children (aged 3.0 through 4.3 years) consumed similar amounts of macaroni and cheese when served three different-sized portions, older preschoolers (aged 4.3 through 6.1 years) consumed proportionately larger amounts of food as the serving size increased (Rolls, Engell, & Birch, 2000).

Studies show that caloric intake from a given food group is increased when a greater variety of foods from that group are available (McCrory et al., 1999; Rolls et al., 1981). Children typically eat more vegetable servings per day when vegetables are served more frequently (i.e., at more meals/snacks during the day) (Dennison, Rockwell, & Baker, 1998). Children consume more fruit and vegetable servings for lunch when schools offer a greater variety of fruits and vegetables (Hearn et al., 1998).

Taken together, these studies suggest a series of possible intervention targets for childcare settings in terms of dietary factors. These include increasing fruit and vegetable intake, reducing sweet beverage intake, and reducing total caloric intake by manipulating the size of portions served and the variety of foods offered.

Increasing Opportunities, Time for Physical Activity

Physical activity levels tend to track over time (Dennison et al., 1988; Pate, Baranowski, Dowda, & Trost, 1996), and reduced physical activity is associated prospectively with greater weight status (Klesges et al., 1995; Moore et al., 1995; Takahashi et al., 1999). The guide *Active Start: A Statement of Physical Activity Guidelines for Children, Birth to Age Five Years* (2002) recommends that "preschoolers accumulate at least 60 minutes daily of structured physical activity" and that they "engage in at least 60 minutes and up to several hours of daily of unstructured physical activity and should not be sedentary for more than 60 minutes at a time except when sleeping." Brown et al. (2006) observed and coded children's activity at three preschools. They were sedentary more than 80 percent of the time, and engaged in moderate to vigorous physical activity less than 5 percent of the time.

Reducing Sedentary Behavior

TV viewing (hours/day) has been associated cross-sectionally and prospectively with the prevalence of childhood obesity (Andersen, Crespo, Bartlett, Cheskin, & Pratt, 1998; Dietz, Jr. & Gortmaker, 1985; Gortmaker, Dietz, Jr., & Cheung, 1990). In elementary school-based studies, reductions in TV viewing by girls (Gortmaker et al., 1999) and reductions in TV viewing by both boys and girls (Robinson, 1999) were associated with decreases in obesity measures. Among preschool children, Dennison, Erb, & Jenkins (2002) noted that the prevalence of obesity was related to the number of hours the children viewed TV. Each one hr/week increase in TV viewing was associated with a 6 percent increase in the prevalence of obesity (p<0.004). In addition, children with a TV in their bedroom watched more hours/week of TV (17.3 vs. 12.8 hours/week, p<0.0001) and were more likely to be overweight than children without a TV in their bedroom.

Children who watch more TV, and those with a TV in their bedroom, also snack more frequently (Dennison, Erb, Gregg, & Jenkins, 2001), as do adults (Maras, 1997). Snacking during TV viewing tends to involve higher-fat items, while children who routinely eat while viewing TV consume fewer fruits and vegetables, less milk—and more pizza, snack foods, and soda—which is consistent with the foods advertised on TV (Coon, Goldberg, Rogers, & Tucker, 2001; Fitzpatrick, Edmunds, & Dennison, 2007; Jeffery & French, 1998). The amount of time a child watched TV was correlated with the child's dietary total fat intake and saturated fat intake, after adjustment for parental educational attainment (Dennison et al., 1996).

Epidemiological studies have established that TV viewing as a risk factor for obesity in preschool children (Jago, Baranowski, Baranowski, Thompson, & Greaves, 2005). Cross-sectional studies find a positive association between hours spent viewing TV and obesity risk (Dennison et al., 2002), particularly among children viewing more than two hours/day (Lumeng, Rahnama, Appugliese, Kaciroti, & Bradley, 2006).

There are two primary mechanisms by which TV viewing is hypothesized to influence weight status. First, TV viewing is a sedentary activity, which displaces more vigorous physical activities that expend greater amounts of energy. The evidence supporting this relationship, however, is mixed with weak associations (DuRant, Baranowski, Johnson, & Thompson, 1994; Gortmaker et al., 1999; Robinson, 1999). TV viewing also influences weight status through increased caloric intake (Blass et al., 2006; Francis, Lee, & Birch, 2003; Snoek, van Janssens, & Engels, 2006; Stroebele & de Castro, 2004). TV advertisements appear to influence increased consumption of snack foods and sweets—i.e., low nutrient, high-energy foods. More than half of all commercials aired during children's TV programming are for food-related items, and the vast majority of these are promoting foods high in sugar, fat, or salt, and low in nutritional value (Kotz & Story, 1994; Story & Faulkner, 1990).

Experimental studies with children have demonstrated the direct effects of exposure to advertising for high-energy foods on actual snack-food choices and consumption (Borzekowski & Robinson, 2001; Galst, 1980; Goldberg, Gorn, & Gibson, 1978). A prospective, observational study demonstrated that for each hour increase in TV viewing, children consumed an additional 167 kcal/d from increased consumption of foods commonly advertised on TV (Wiecha et al., 2006).

The American Academy of Pediatrics (2001a) issued recommendations that parents not permit children under two years of age to watch any TV or videos, and that children over two years of age should be limited to no more than one to two hours per day of total media time, and that this should be limited to quality, educational, nonviolent programming. Child-care settings could support these goals by limiting access to TV or other media, and by teaching parents about alternative activities to TV viewing at home.

Enhancing Social Cues that Foster Healthier Eating and More Physical Activity

The imitative nature of young children can be used to advantage to encourage children to try novel foods through social learning (Birch, 1980; Harper & Sanders, 1975; Hertzler, 1983), especially with repeated exposures (Birch, 1979).

Satiety Training

Greater attention may be given to help children recognize internal feelings of hunger and fullness, which can lead to better energy intake regulation (Johnson, 2000), as opposed to external cues to eat. This can be achieved in part through a variety of training and educational materials (Birch & Fisher, 1998; Dietz, Stern, & American Academy of Pediatrics, 1999; Faith, Kermanshah, & Kissileff, 2002; Keller et al., 2006; Satter, 1987, 1991).

If children do not want to eat a food, they should not be bribed or rewarded, as studies show that rewarding the consumption of a food (a contingency) devalues the food and decreases the liking for that food (Birch, Birch, Marlin, & Kramer, 1982). Nor should children be praised for eating all of a food or cleaning their plate (Klesges et al., 1983). Parental encouragements to eat were associated with an increased likelihood that the child would eat and prompts to eat were associated with children's weight status (Klesges, Mallot, Boschee, & Weber, 1986).

Parent and Caregiver Skills Training

Most parents of overweight children fail to recognize that their child is overweight (Baughcum, Chamberlin, Deeks, Powers, & Whitaker, 2000; Dennison, Jenkins, Erb, & Rockwell, 2000a, 2000b). Dietz (1983) found that parents of overweight children tended to have difficulty setting limits with respect to food and other areas. In a cross-sectional study, Johnson and Birch (1994) noted that mothers of overweight preschool children tended to be more controlling of their children's food intake—specifically limiting how much food their child ate. However, Davison and Birch (2000) reported that overweight girls whose fathers were more restrictive (i.e., more frequently limited the amount of food) tended to gain less weight over time. In sum, parents who are overly controlling may contribute to obesity, while imposition of some limits (in response to parental perception that the child is overweight) may help slow continued weight gain.

Approximately two-thirds of parents reported using food as a reward and withholding food, usually dessert, as a punishment (Dennison et al., 2000a; Eppright et al., 1972). When young children were allowed to choose freely from a selection of foods, they selected many non-nutritious foods. When children were told that their mother was going to review the foods selected, they chose fewer non-nutritious foods. When mothers modified their children's choices, they focused on reducing foods lowest in nutritional value rather than increasing foods highest in nutritional value (Klesges, Stein, Eck, Isbell, & Klesges, 1991).

Little research has investigated the role of childcare providers. Yet, the majority of young children spend time in out-of-home childcare before beginning elementary school. The attitudes and behaviors of these caregivers also play an important, but often overlooked, role in children's development of eating habit and food preferences.

FINDINGS FROM EXISTING CHILDCARE INTERVENTION STUDIES

Only a limited number of behaviorally-based chronic disease prevention interventions have been conducted in the childcare setting. We review these below.

Healthy Start

Healthy Start was a nonrandomized, controlled, multicomponent intervention conducted in nine Head Start centers in upstate New York (Williams, Strobino, Bollella, & Brotanek, 2004; Williams et al., 2002). It was designed to promote heart-healthy behaviors and decrease cardiovascular disease risk factors among preschoolers from low-income families. Healthy Start had three groups of centers—a control group, a group where the school food was modified, and a third group where the school food was modified plus the children and parents received a nutrition education curriculum. The goals of the project were to modify the children's dietary intakes—primarily, decrease the saturated fat content, and secondarily, reduce dietary cholesterol and total fat content—to decrease their serum cholesterol levels. The food service staff at Head Start Centers were provided with in-service training sessions in purchasing and preparing heart-healthy meals and snacks. In each of the two years of the study, the

Healthy Start program was successful in reducing the total fat and saturated fat content of school snacks and meals. In the first year, there were
reductions of 3.4 percent and 2.2 percent in the percentages of calories from
total fat and saturated fat, respectively, and in the second year, additional
reductions of 2.6 percent and 2.3 percent in the percentages of calories
from total fat and saturated fat, respectively, were seen in school meals
and snacks (Williams et al., 2004). There were no changes, however, in the
children's diets consumed at home, which represented about two-thirds
of their daily intakes, and no changes or differences in the children's daily
dietary intakes. The addition of the Healthy Start skills-based, develop-
mentally-appropriate nutrition curriculum, which included take-home
materials and parent meetings, had no additional effect on the children's
diets or their serum cholesterol levels. Children attending the centers
where the school meals and snacks were modified, however, did experience a reduction—relative to children attending the control centers—in
their serum cholesterol levels (−6.0 vs. −0.4 mg/dL, or a difference of −5.6
[95 percent CI −9.9, −1.3]) (Williams et al.).

Hip Hop to Health, Jr.

Hip-Hop to Health Jr. was a randomized, controlled dietary and physical
activity intervention evaluated in 24 Head Start programs in Chicago, Illinois
(Fitzgibbon, Stolley, Dyer, VanHorn, & KauferChristoffel, 2002). The 14-
week curriculum was administered three times a week by early childhood
educators. Each session included a 20-minute interactive session targeting
healthy eating or reduced TV viewing, as well as 20 minutes of moderate-
to-vigorous aerobic physical activities. The intervention has been evaluated in Head Start sites serving predominantly minority children—either
predominantly black children or predominantly Latino children. At 12
Head Start Centers with predominantly black children (81 percent black
at the six control sites and 99 percent black at the six intervention sites),
the children in the intervention group—at one-year and two-years post-
intervention—had significantly smaller increases in BMI, adjusted for age
and sex, than did the control group; difference = −.53 kg/m^2 (95 percent
CI [−0.91, −0.14]) at one year and difference = −.54 kg/m^2 (95 percent CI
[−0.98, −0.10]) at two years (Fitzgibbon et al., 2005). While dietary saturated fat intake was lower among children in the intervention group vs.
the control group at one year post-intervention, these changes were not
sustained. All other dietary measures, as well as exercise frequency and
intensity and hours of TV viewed per day were similar among children in
the intervention and control groups at both the one-year and two-year
follow-up time points (Fitzgibbon et al.).

The Hip-Hop to Health Jr. Curriculum was culturally adapted for use
with Latino children by adding cultural-specific messages and translating
materials into Spanish (Fitzgibbon et al., 2002). The adapted intervention was taught in both English and in Spanish by two early childhood teachers to classes of predominantly Hispanic children (73 percent Hispanic at
six control centers and 89 percent Hispanic at six intervention centers).
At one and two years post-intervention, there were no significant differences

in children's dietary intakes, physical activity, or obesity measures. Unlike the trial among predominantly black children, the culturally-adapted Hip-Hop to Health Jr. program was not effective in preventing excessive weight gain among Latino preschool-age children (Fitzgibbon et al., 2006). The reasons for these differences are not known, but warrant further exploration.

Brocodile the Crocodile

Brocodile the Crocodile was a 39-week health promotion curriculum evaluated in 16 childcare (preschool and daycare) centers in upstate New York (Dennison, Russo, Burdick, & Jenkins, 2004). It was integrated into the standard preschool curriculum and taught by a two-person team (an early childhood educator and a music teacher) who visited each childcare center once a week. Each session included 30 minutes of musical movement activities, using the KinderMusic program (MusicBox), a 10-minute healthy snack session, and 20 minutes of interactive educational lessons about healthy eating (32 weeks) or reduced TV viewing (7 weeks). The curriculum was influenced by Bandura's social learning theory, which emphasizes constructs of modeling, retention, and reinforcement (Bandura, 1976). For example, the classroom curriculum was designed to allow the children to observe and model targeted behaviors, such as turning off the TV, selecting, and participating in an alternative activity. Take-home components included a weekly newsletter with suggested activities for the child to directly engage the parent. Families were encouraged to eat dinner as a family with the TV turned off, to read regularly to the children, and to provide alternatives—from a suggested list generated by the children—to watching TV, including physical activity options.

Children in the intervention group compared to the control group had a significant reduction in TV/video viewing of 4.7 hours per week over the course of the study. Children in the intervention group had small, but insignificant reductions in BMI of $-0.36\,\text{kg/m}^2$ (95 percent CI [-1.22, 0.5]) and in triceps skinfold thickness of $-0.41\,\text{mm}$ (95 percent CI [-3.5, 2.7]) compared to the control group (Dennison et al., 2004).

Spark-E

The *Sports, Play, and Active Recreation for Kids* (SPARK) program was developed for use by classroom teachers in elementary schools. It has been associated with increased levels of physical activity during physical education classes, and with improved cardiovascular endurance among girls (Sallis et al., 1997). These same researchers developed and field-tested a comprehensive physical activity program for younger children in the preschool setting. The curriculum promotes the development of basic movement and manipulative skills, engages physical activity and movement through games, and promotes positive social and personal skills.

Regular childcare staff, after participating in two training sessions led by SPARK staff, implemented the SPARK-EC curriculum following detailed lesson plans using music CDs, manipulatives, and resource materials. Although the impact of the SPARK-EC curriculum on children's physical activity levels and/or obesity levels has not been fully evaluated, preliminary findings are promising. The program has been well-received and there has been fairly widespread dissemination of the curriculum in many childcare centers, including Head Start programs.

OTHER STRATEGIES TO AFFECT CHILDCARE ENVIRONMENTS

Nutrition and Physical Activity Self-Assessment in Childcare.

The *Nutrition and Physical Activity Self-Assessment for Childcare* (NAP SACC, 2007) is an environment and policy intervention that employs health educators to assist childcare center staff in implementing policy, practice, and environmental changes to improve the childcare nutrition and physical activity environments. Implementation of the program requires that health educators participate in a half-day training session led by NAP SACC staff. This intervention is based on the social cognitive theory. It includes a self-assessment instrument, which is completed by center directors with assistance from trained health educators (Ward, Saunders, & Pate, 2007). The self-assessment was developed based on national recommendations, research data, and/or expert opinion. It consists of nine nutrition and six physical activity areas that have been found to be associated with childhood obesity (Ammerman et al., 2007). Following the self-assessment, the health educator helps center staff identify specific areas for improvement and develop an action plan. Ongoing technical assistance is provided for approximately six months to help the center staff meet their targeted goals. In addition to the self-assessment, the NAP SACC program provides a consultation guide for the health educator, materials for five workshops (conducted by the health educator), and handouts for the center staff and parents. These workshops include: 1) Childhood Overweight; 2) Nutrition for Young Children; 3) Physical Activity for Young Children; 4) Personal Health and Wellness for Staff; and 5) Working with Families to Increase Healthy Weight Behaviors. Results from a pilot study of the NAP SACC are promising (Benjamin, Ammerman, Sommers, Dodds, & Ward, in press) and a larger evaluation in 96 childcare centers in North Carolina has been recently completed. These results demonstrate improvements to childcare center nutrition environments following the six-month intervention period (Ward, personal communication). Additional evaluation is underway to assess changes in knowledge and behaviors of childcare staff, and to assess changes in children's behaviors and/or weight status.

Local or City Policy or Regulatory Change

In 2006, the New York City Department of Health and Mental Hygiene amended Article 47 of the New York City Public Health Code affecting group daycare centers in New York, NY (New York City Board of Health, 2006). This amendment requires that children participate in at least 60 minutes per day of physical activity (which is prorated for children attending less than full-day programs). It states that during inclement weather, active play should be encouraged and supported in safe indoor play areas. TV, video, and other visual recordings are not to be used with children under two years of age. For children over two years of age, viewing of TV, video, and other visual recordings is to be limited to no more than 60 minutes of educational programming. Juice shall be limited to no more than 6 fl oz per day. In addition, the regulation specifies that juice shall not be given to children under eight months of age, juice shall not be provided in a bottle, and that only 100 percent fruit and/or vegetable juice is permitted. The implementation, compliance, and impact of this regulation on children's nutritional intakes, physical activity levels, and risk of developing obesity have yet to be determined.

Public Health Nutrition Programs

In the United States, children up to five years of age, who are at nutritional risk and residing in low-income families (i.e., household income < 185 percent poverty levels), may receive supplemental food and beverages, nutrition education, and referral to medical care through the Special Supplemental Nutrition Program for Women, Infants, and Children (WIC). The WIC program is federally-funded, administered by states, and heavily regulated by the U.S. Department of Agriculture. The foods and beverages provided to families and children are based on nutritional needs determined in the 1960s–1970s that have since changed. Overnutrition leading to obesity is the major nutritional challenge facing today's children, rather than micronutritional deficiencies and failure to thrive from inadequate calories. In response to growing calls for reforms, the Institute of Medicine (IOM) recently provided recommendations to the U.S. Department of Agriculture to improve the food packages offered (Institute of Medicine, Food and Nutrition Board, and Committee to Review the WIC Food Packages, 2005). Specific changes include reducing the amount of juice provided and adding fruits and vegetables to the package. Some states make limited amounts of fruits and vegetables available to participants through farmers market programs during the summer months, or provide vouchers—on a limited basis, specifically for the purchase of fruits and vegetables. In general, these programs are well-received and utilized by participants.

Another large federally-funded program—The Child and Adult Care Food Program (CACFP)—reimburses participating childcare providers for meals served to eligible children (i.e., household income < 185 percent federal poverty level) (U.S. Department of Agriculture, Food and Nutrition Service, 2006). Nationally, 2.9 million children are served daily through CACFP. In New York State, which has the third largest CACFP program in the country, more than 95 percent of providers serve infants and children. This funding provides reimbursement to Head Start programs and other childcare centers serving very low-income populations in all states.

The U.S. Department of Agriculture sets nutritional standards for reimbursable foods and beverages served at each meal or snack. Standards are guided by concerns of undernutrition and nutrient deficiencies, not obesity. Because standards are set for each meal, rather than daily offerings, centers can be reimbursed for serving fruit juice multiple times during the day. Because fruit juice is cheaper and easier to purchase, prepare, and serve than fruit, it is not surprising that children in many centers reimbursed by CACFP receive two or more servings of fruit juice per day. Nationally, nearly half of CACFP centers offer breakfast, lunch, and one snack while 25 percent offer breakfast, lunch, and two snacks—providing more than 60 percent of the RDA for calories for a preschool child. Thus, many children attending childcare centers receive the majority of their daily dietary intake while at daycare, placing daycare staff as the primary role models for healthful eating behaviors.

CHALLENGES TO INTERVENTION IN CHILDCARE SETTINGS

The determinants of obesity are multifactorial and the current obesity epidemic is largely driven by societal changes and market forces. The increased availability of highly processed, high-fat, high-sugar, high-calorie foods at lower relative costs, combined with decreased opportunities for physical activity and an increased variety of sedentary activities—such as TV viewing and video games—has shifted the energy balance sheet. The net result for a growing number of American children is excessive weight gain relative to linear growth, resulting in increased rates of obesity.

As the enrollment of young children in childcare programs has expanded, so has their potential role in contributing to, or preventing, the development of obesity-promoting dietary and lifestyle behaviors. The majority of childcare programs, however, are subject to economic pressures that limit staffing, programming, and menu planning. Program staff often report it is the cost of purchasing, storing, and preparing fruits and vegetables that is the limiting factor, not a lack of knowledge about their health benefits. Similarly, providing moderate-to-vigorous physical activity programs rather than offering TV or video viewing has the associated costs of staff training and implementation in addition to the costs of providing facility space (i.e., gymnasium space). A limitation of childcare-specific interventions (or school-based interventions) is that they primarily impact the childcare (or school) environment, and—to a lesser degree (if parents are reached through the intervention)—the home environment. This may partly explain the modest effects that interventions to address childhood obesity in childcare settings have had. Community-based interventions that target multiple sectors, including the childcare centers, the home, and other community partners and organizations may be more successful in changing behaviors and social norms, as well as being more sustainable (Baker et al., 2007).

CONCLUSIONS

Young children rely on parents and caregivers to create their food and activity environments. Parents and caregivers influence the availability and accessibility of foods, the structure of meals, meal socialization patterns, and the modeling of eating and dietary behaviors. These early years are a critical time for establishing lifetime healthy eating habits. Many children attending childcare centers consume a significant portion of their daily dietary intake while at childcare, placing childcare staff in the role of modeling healthful behaviors, in addition to providing opportunities for children to be physically active.

Childcare settings offer potential opportunities to help foster the development of healthy eating patterns and active lifestyles. At present, however, their potential is largely untapped and not fully evaluated. As the childhood obesity epidemic continues to expand—affecting even younger children—it is imperative that obesity prevention efforts begin before birth (by promoting optimal maternal weight gain during pregnancy), during infancy (by supporting breast feeding during the first year of life), and through the preschool years (by ensuring health-promoting, obesity-preventing home, childcare, and community environments). Additional and longer, controlled intervention studies for obesity prevention delivered in childcare settings are needed—they would fill a major void in the existing literature.

REFERENCES

American Academy of Pediatrics. (2001a). Children, adolescents, and television. *Pediatrics, 107*, 423–426.

American Academy of Pediatrics. (2001b). The use and misuse of fruit juice in pediatrics (RE0047). *Pediatrics, 107*, 1210–1213.

American Alliance for Health, Physical Education, Recreation & Dan (AAHPERD), Active start: A statement of physical activity guidelines for children, birth to age five years (2002). [On-line]. Retrieved from: http://www.aahperd.org/NASPE/ns_active.html

Ammerman, A., Ward, D., Benjamin, S., Ball, S., Sommers, J., Molloy, M. et al. (2007). An intervention to promote healthy weight: Nutrition and Physical activity Self-Assessment for Child Care (NAPSACC). *Preventing Chronic Disease: Public Health Research, Practice, and Policy.*

Andersen, R. E., Crespo, C. J., Bartlett, S. J., Cheskin, L. J., & Pratt, M. (1998). Relationship of physical activity and television watching with body weight and level of fatness among children: Results from the Third National Health and Nutrition Examination Survey. *The Journal of the American Medical Association, 279*, 938–942.

Bachu, A. & O'Connell, M. (2000). Fertility of American women: June 1998. *Rep. No. Current Population Report P20-526.* Washington, DC: U.S. Census Bureau.

Baker, I. R., Dennison, B. A., Boyer, P. S., Sellers, K. F., Russo, T. J., & Sherwood, N. A. (2007). An asset-based community initiative to reduce television viewing in New York state. *Preventive Medicine.*

Bandura, A. (1976). *Social Learning Theory, (1st ed.).* Englewood Cliffs, NJ: Prentice-Hall.

Baughcum, A. E., Chamberlin, L. A., Deeks, C. M., Powers, S. W., & Whitaker, R. C. (2000). Maternal perceptions of overweight preschool children. *Pediatrics, 106*, 1380–1386.

Benjamin, S., Ammerman, A., Sommers, J., Dodds, J., & Ward, D. (in press). Improving nutrition and physical activity environments in child care: Results from the NAP SACC pilot project. *Journal of Nutrition Education and Behavior.*

Bernard, L., Lavallee, C., Gray-Donald, K., & Delisle, H. (1995). Overweight in Cree schoolchildren and adolescents associated with diet, low physical activity, and high television viewing. *Journal of the American Dietetic Association, 95*, 800–802.

Birch, L. L. (1979). Dimensions of preschool children's food preferences. *Journal of Nutrition Education, 11*, 77–80.

Birch, L. L. (1980). Effects of peer model's food choices and eating behaviors on preschoolers food preferences. *Child Development, 51,* 489–496.

Birch, L. L., Birch, D., Marlin, D. W., & Kramer, L. (1982). Effects of instrumental consumption on children's food preference. *Appetite, 3,* 125–134.

Birch, L. L. & Fisher, J. O. (1998). Development of eating behaviors among children and adolescents. *Pediatrics, 101,* 539–549.

Birch, L. L., Zimmerman, S. I., & Hind, H. (1980). The influence of social-affective context on the formation of children's food preferences. *Child Development, 51,* 856–861.

Blass, E. M., Anderson, D. R., Kirkorian, H. L., Pempek, T. A., Price, I., & Koleini, M. F. (2006). On the road to obesity: Television viewing increases intake of high-density foods. *Physiology and Behavior, 88,* 597–604.

Borzekowski, D. L. & Robinson, T. N. (2001). The 30-second effect: An experiment revealing the impact of television commercials on food preferences of preschoolers. *Journal of the American Dietetic Association, 101,* 42–46.

Bouchard, C. (1996). Can obesity be prevented? *Nutrition Reviews, 54,* S125–S130.

Brown, W. H., Pfeiffer, K. A., McIver, K. L., Dowda, M., Almeida, M. J., & Pate, R. R. (2006). Assessing preschool children's physical activity: The Observational System for Recording Physical Activity in children-preschool version. *Research Quarterly for Exercise and Sport, 77,* 167–176.

Coon, K. A., Goldberg, J., Rogers, B. L., & Tucker, K. L. (2001). Relationships between use of television during meals and children's food consumption patterns. *Pediatrics, 107,* E7.

Davison, K. K. & Birch, L. L. (2000). Predictors of change in girls' Body Mass Index between ages 5 to 7 years. *Obesity Research, 8*(Suppl 1), 18S.

Dennison, B. A., Erb, T. A., Gregg, D. J., & Jenkins, P. L. (2001). Child obesity related to TV viewing, TV in bedroom, and snacking while watching TV. *Pediatric Research, 49,* 160A.

Dennison, B. A., Erb, T. A., & Jenkins, P. L. (2002). Television viewing and television in bedroom associated with overweight risk among low-income preschool children. *Pediatrics, 109,* 1028–1035.

Dennison, B. A., Jenkins, P. L., & Chen, T. (1996). Excess TV viewing by preschoolers is associated with high fat and SFA diets. *Circulation, 94,* I–578.

Dennison, B. A., Jenkins, P. L., Erb, T. A., & Rockwell, H. (2000a). Early childhood obesity not recognized by most parents. *Pediatric Research, 47,* 25A.

Dennison, B. A., Jenkins, P. L., Erb, T. A., & Rockwell, H. (2000b). Moms who breast-feed report healthier child feeding practices: A possible link to lower obesity rates. *Pediatric Research, 47,* 146A.

Dennison, B. A., Jenkins, P. L., Erb, T. A., Rockwell, H. L., & Gregg, D. J. (2000). Increased frequency of eating carrots is significantly associated with reduced prevalence of child obesity in a low-income population. *Obesity Research, 8,* 40S.

Dennison, B. A., Rockwell, H. L., & Baker, S. L. (1997). Excess fruit juice consumption by preschool-aged children is associated with short stature and obesity. *Pediatrics, 99,* 15–22.

Dennison, B. A., Rockwell, H. L., & Baker, S. L. (1998). Fruit and vegetable intake in young children. *Journal of the American College of Nutrition, 17,* 371–378.

Dennison, B. A., Russo, T. J., Burdick, P. A., & Jenkins, P. L. (2004). An intervention to reduce television viewing by preschool children. *Archives of Pediatric and Adolescent Medicine, 158,* 170–176.

Dennison, B. A., Straus, J. H., Mellits, E. D., & Charney, E. (1988). Childhood physical fitness tests: Predictor of adult physical activity levels? *Pediatrics, 82,* 324–330.

Dietz, W. H., Jr. (1983). Childhood obesity: Susceptibility, cause, and management. *Journal of Pediatrics, 103,* 676–686.

Dietz, W. H. (1998). Health consequences of obesity in youth: Childhood predictors of adult disease. *Pediatrics, 101,* 518–525.

Dietz, W. H., Jr. & Gortmaker, S. L. (1985). Do we fatten our children at the television set? Obesity and television viewing in children and adolescents. *Pediatrics, 75,* 807–812.

Dietz, W. H., Stern, L., & American Academy of Pediatrics (1999). *American Academy of Pediatrics guide to your child's nutrition.* NewYork: Villard Books.

DuRant, R. H., Baranowski, T., Johnson, M., & Thompson, W. O. (1994). The relationship among television watching, physical activity, and body composition of young children. *Pediatrics, 94,* 449–455.

Edmunds, L. S., Woelfel, M. L., Dennison, B. A., Stratton, H., Pruzek, R. M., & Abusabha, R. (2006). Overweight Trends among Children Enrolled in the New York State Special Supplemental Nutrition Program for Women, Infants, and Children. *Journal of the American Dietetic Association, 106,* 113–117.

Eppright, E. S., Fox, H. M., Fryer, B. A., Lamkin, G. H., Vivian, V. M., & Fuller, E. S. (1972). Nutrition of infants and preschool children in the North Central Region of the United States of America. *World Review of Nutrition and Dietetics, 14,* 269–332.

Faith, M. S., Dennison, B. A., Edmunds, L. S., & Stratton, H. H. (2006). Fruit juice intake predicts increased adiposity gain in children from low-income families: Weight status-by-environment interaction. *Pediatrics, 118,* 2066–2075.

Faith, M. S., Kermanshah, M., & Kissileff, H. R. (2002). Development and preliminary validation of a silhouette satiety scale for children. *Physiology and Behavior, 76,* 173–178.

Fitzgibbon, M. L., Stolley, M. R., Dyer, A. R., VanHorn, L., & KauferChristoffel, K. (2002). A community-based obesity prevention program for minority children: Rationale and study design for Hip-Hop to Health Jr. *Preventive Medicine, 34,* 289–297.

Fitzgibbon, M. L., Stolley, M. R., Schiffer, L., Van, H. L., KauferChristoffel, K., & Dyer, A. (2005). Two-year follow-up results for Hip-Hop to Health Jr.: A randomized controlled trial for overweight prevention in preschool minority children. *Journal of Pediatrics, 146,* 618–625.

Fitzgibbon, M. L., Stolley, M. R., Schiffer, L., Van, H. L., KauferChristoffel, K., & Dyer, A. (2006). Hip-Hop to Health Jr. for Latino preschool children. *Obesity (Silver.Spring), 14,* 1616–1625.

Fitzpatrick, E., Edmunds, L. S., & Dennison, B. A. (2007). Positive effects of family dinner are undone by television viewing. *Journal of the American Dietetic Association, 107,* 666–671.

Francis, L. A., Lee, Y., & Birch, L. L. (2003). Parental weight status and girls' television viewing, snacking, and body mass indexes. *Obesity Research, 11,* 143–151.

French, S. A., Story, M., & Jeffery, R. W. (2001). Environmental influences on eating and physical activity. *Annual Review of Public Health, 22,* 309–335.

French, S. A., Story, M., & Perry, C. L. (1995). Self-esteem and obesity in children and adolescents: A literature review. *Obesity Research, 3,* 479–490.

Galst, J. P. (1980). Television food commercials and pro-nutritional public service announcements as determinants of young children's snack choices. *Child Development, 51,* 935–938.

Gidding, S. S., Leibel, R. L., Daniels, S., Rosenbaum, M., Van, H. L., & Marx, G. R. (1996). Understanding obesity in youth. A statement for healthcare professionals from the Committee on Atherosclerosis and Hypertension in the Young of the Council on Cardiovascular Disease in the Young and the Nutrition Committee, American Heart Association. Writing Group. *Circulation, 94,* 3383–3387.

Goldberg, M. E., Gorn, G. J., & Gibson, W. (1978). TV messages for snack and breakfast foods: Do they influence children's preference? *Journal of Consumer Research, 5,* 81.

Gortmaker, S. L., Dietz, W. H., Jr., & Cheung, L. W. (1990). Inactivity, diet, and the fattening of America. *Journal of the American Dietetic Association, 90,* 1247–52, 1255.

Gortmaker, S. L., Peterson, K., Wiecha, J., Sobol, A. M., Dixit, S., Fox, M. K. et al. (1999). Reducing obesity via a school-based interdisciplinary intervention among youth: Planet Health. *Archives of Pediatric and Adolescent Medicine, 153,* 409–418.

Guo, S. S., Wu, W., Chumlea, W. C., & Roche, A. F. (2002). Predicting overweight and obesity in adulthood from body mass index values in childhood and adolescence. *American Journal of Clinical Nutrition, 76,* 653–658.

Harper, L. V., & Sanders, K. M. (1975). The effect of adults' eating on young children's acceptance of unfamiliar foods. *Journal of Experimental Child Psychology, 20,* 206–214.

Head Start Bureau (2007). *Head Start Program Fact Sheet Fiscal Year 2006* Washington, DC: U.S. Department of Health and Human Services.

Hearn, M. D., Baranowski, T., Baranowski, J. C., Doyle, C., Smith, M., Lin, L. S. et al. (1998). Environmental influences on dietary behavior among children: Availability and accessibility of fruits and vegetables enable consumption. *Journal of Health Education, 29*, 26–32.

Hertzler, A. A. (1983). Children's food patterns–a review: II. Family and group behavior. *Journal of the American Dietetic Association, 83*, 555–560.

Institute of Medicine (U.S.), Food and Nutrition Board, & Committee to Review the WIC Food Packages (2005). *WIC Food Packages: Time for a Change.* Washington, DC: The National Academies Press.

Jago, R., Baranowski, T., Baranowski, J. C., Thompson, D., & Greaves, K. A. (2005). BMI from 3–6y of age is predicted by TV viewing and physical activity, not diet. *International Journal of Obesity (Lond), 29*, 557–564.

Jeffery, R. W., & French, S. A. (1998). Epidemic obesity in the United States: Are fast foods and television viewing contributing? *American Journal of Public Health, 88*, 277–280.

Johnson, S. L. (2000). Improving Preschoolers' self-regulation of energy intake. *Pediatrics, 106*, 1429–1435.

Johnson, S. L., & Birch, L. L. (1994). Parents' and children's adiposity and eating style. *Pediatrics, 94*, 653–661.

Keller, K. L., Assur, S. A., Torres, M., Lofink, H. E., Thornton, J. C., Faith, M. S. et al. (2006). Potential of an analog scaling device for measuring fullness in children: Development and preliminary testing. *Appetite, 47*, 233–243.

Klesges, R. C., Coates, T. J., Brown, G., Sturgeon-Tillisch, J., Moldenhauer-Klesges, L. M., Holzer, B. et al. (1983). Parental influences on children's eating behavior and relative weight. *Journal of Applied Behavior Analysis, 16*, 371–378.

Klesges, R. C., Klesges, L. M., Eck, L. H., & Shelton, M. L. (1995). A longitudinal analysis of accelerated weight gain in preschool children. *Pediatrics, 95*, 126–130.

Klesges, R. C., Mallot, J. M., Boschee, P. F., & Weber, J. M. (1986). The effects of parental influences on children's food intake, physical activity, and relative weight. *International Journal of Eating Disorders, 5*, 335–346.

Klesges, R. C., Stein, R. J., Eck, L. H., Isbell, T. R., & Klesges, L. M. (1991). Parental influence on food selection in young children and its relationships to childhood obesity. *American Journal of Clinical Nutrition, 53*, 859–864.

Kotz, K., & Story, M. (1994). Food advertisements during children's Saturday morning television programming: Are they consistent with dietary recommendations? *Journal of the American Dietetic Association, 94*, 1296–1300.

Ludwig, D. S., Peterson, K. E., & Gortmaker, S. L. (2001). Relation between consumption of sugar-sweetened drinks and childhood obesity: A prospective, observational analysis. *Lancet, 357*, 505–508.

Lumeng, J. C., Rahnama, S., Appugliese, D., Kaciroti, N., & Bradley, R. H. (2006). Television exposure and overweight risk in preschoolers. *Archives of Pediatric and Adolescent Medicine, 160*, 417–422.

Magarey, A. M., Daniels, L. A., Boulton, T. J., & Cockington, R. A. (2003). Predicting obesity in early adulthood from childhood and parental obesity. *International Journal of Obesity Related Metabolic Disorders, 27*, 505–513.

Maras, E. (1997, October). Consumers note what is important in buying snacks. *Automatic Merchandiser,* 64–68.

McCrory, M. A., Fuss, P. J., McCallum, J. E., Yao, M., Vinken, A. G., Hays, N. P. et al. (1999). Dietary variety within food groups: Association with energy intake and body fatness in men and women. *American Journal of Clinical Nutrition, 69*, 440–447.

Moore, L. L., Nguyen, U. S., Rothman, K. J., Cupples, L. A., & Ellison, R. C. (1995). Preschool physical activity level and change in body fatness in young children. The Framingham Children's Study. *American Journal of Epidemiology, 142*, 982–988.

Must, A., Spadano, J., Coakley, E. H., Field, A. E., Colditz, G., & Dietz, W. H. (1999). The disease burden associated with overweight and obesity. *The Journal of the American Medical Association, 282*, 1523–1529.

National Institutes of Health (1998). Clinical guidelines on the identification, evaluation, and treatment of overweight and obesity in adults: The evidence report. *Rep. No. NIH publication no. 98-4083.* Washington, D.C.: National Heart, Lung, and Blood

Institute (in cooperation with the National Institute of Diabetes and Digestive and Kidney Diseases).

New York City Board of Health. (2006). Notice of adoption of amendments to Article 47 of the New York City Health Code. *Article 47, 47.35–47.37. Day Care Services.* Ref Type: Statute

Nutrition and Physical Activity Self Assessment for Child Care (2007). NAPSACC [On-line]. Retrieved from: www.napsacc.org

Ogden, C. L., Carroll, M. D., Curtin, L. R., McDowell, M. A., Tabak, C. J., & Flegal, K. M. (2006). Prevalence of overweight and obesity in the United States, 1999–2004. *The Journal of the American Medical Association, 295,* 1549–1555.

Overturf, Johnson, J. (2005). Who's minding the kids? Child care arrangements: Winter 2002. *Rep. No. Current Population Report P70-101.* Washington, DC: U.S. Census Bureau.

Pate, R. R., Baranowski, T., Dowda, M., & Trost, S. G. (1996). Tracking of physical activity in young children. *Medicine and Science in Sports and Exercise, 28,* 92–96.

Pi-Sunyer, F. X. (1993). Medical hazards of obesity. *Annals of Internal Medicine, 119,* 655–660.

Robinson, T. N. (1999). Reducing children's television viewing to prevent obesity: A randomized controlled trial. *The Journal of the American Medical Association, 282,* 1561–1567.

Rolls, B. J., Engell, D., & Birch, L. L. (2000). Serving portion size influences 5-year-old but not 3-year-old children's food intakes. *Journal of the American Dietetic Association, 100,* 232–234.

Rolls, B. J., Rowe, E. A., Rolls, E. T., Kingston, B., Megson, A., & Gunary, R. (1981). Variety in a meal enhances food intake in man. *Physiology and Behavior, 26,* 215–221.

Sallis, J. F., McKenzie, T. L., Alcaraz, J. E., Kolody, B., Faucette, N., & Hovell, M. F. (1997). The effects of a 2-year physical education program (SPARK) on physical activity and fitness in elementary school students. Sports, Play and Active Recreation for Kids. *American Journal of Public Health, 87,* 1328–1334.

Satter, E. (1987). *How to Get Your Kid to Eeat – But Not too Much.* Palo Alto, CA: Bull Publishing Co.

Satter, E. (1991). *Child of Mine: Feeding with Love and Good Sense.* Palo Alto, CA: Bull Publishing Co.

Serdula, M. K., Ivery, D., Coates, R. J., Freedman, D. S., Williamson, D. F., & Byers, T. (1993). Do obese children become obese adults? A review of the literature. *Preventive Medicine, 22,* 167–177.

Skinner, J. D., Carruth, B. R., Moran, J., Houck, K., & Coletta, F. (1999). Fruit juice intake is not related to children's growth. *Pediatrics, 103,* 58–64.

Smith, M. M. & Lifshitz, F. (1994). Excess fruit juice consumption as a contributing factor in nonorganic failure to thrive. *Pediatrics, 93,* 438–443.

Snoek, H. M., van, S. T., Janssens, J. M., & Engels, R. C. (2006). The effect of television viewing on adolescents' snacking: Individual differences explained by external, restrained and emotional eating. *Journal of Adolescent Health, 39,* 448–451.

Stein, A. D., Shea, S., Basch, C. E., Contento, I. R., & Zybert, P. (1991). Variability and tracking of nutrient intakes of preschool children based on multiple administrations of the 24-hour dietary recall. *American Journal of Epidemiology, 134,* 1427–1437.

Story, M. & Faulkner, P. (1990). The prime time diet: A content analysis of eating behavior and food messages in television program content and commercials. *American Journal of Public Health, 80,* 738–740.

Strauss, R. S. (2000). Childhood obesity and self-esteem. *Pediatrics, 105,* e15.

Stroebele, N. & de Castro, J. M. (2004). Television viewing is associated with an increase in meal frequency in humans. *Appetite, 42,* 111–113.

Takahashi, E., Yoshida, K., Sugimori, H., Miyakawa, M., Izuno, T., Yamagami, T. et al. (1999). Influence factors on the development of obesity in 3-year-old children based on the Toyama study. *Preventive Medicine, 28,* 293–296.

Tippets, K. S. & Cleveland, L. E. (1999). How current diets stack up: comparison with dietary guidelines. In E. Frazao (Ed.), *America's Eating Habits: Changes and Consequences* (pp. 51–70). U.S. Department of Agriculture, Economic Research Service, Food and Rural Economics Division. Agriculture Information Bulletin No. 750.

U.S. Census Bureau (2007). Money income in the United States: 1999. *Rep. No. Current Population Report P60-209.* Washington, DC: U.S. Government Printing Office.

U.S. Department of Agriculture, Food and Nutrition Service (2006). Child & Adult Care Food Program. U.S. Department of Agriculture [online]. Retreived from: http://www.fns.usda.gov/cnd/care/CACFP/aboutcacfp.htm

Ward, D. S., Saunders, R. P., & Pate, R. R. (2007). *Physical Activity Interventions in Children and Adolescents.* Champaign, IL: Human Kinetics.

Welsh, J. A., Cogswell, M. E., Rogers, S., Rockett, H., Mei, Z., & Grummer-Strawn, L. M. (2005). Overweight among low-income preschool children associated with the consumption of sweet drinks: Missouri, 1999–2002. *Pediatrics, 115,* e223–e229.

Whitaker, R. C., Pepe, M. S., Wright, J. A., Seidel, K. D., & Dietz, W. H. (1998). Early adiposity rebound and the risk of adult obesity. *Pediatrics, 101,* E5.

Whitaker, R. C., Wright, J. A., Pepe, M. S., Seidel, K. D., & Dietz, W. H. (1997). Predicting obesity in young adulthood from childhood and parental obesity. *The New England Journal of Medicine, 337,* 869–873.

Wiecha, J. L., Peterson, K. E., Ludwig, D. S., Kim, J., Sobol, A., & Gortmaker, S. L. (2006). When children eat what they watch: Impact of television viewing on dietary intake in youth. *Archives of Pediatric and Adolescent Medicine, 160,* 436–442.

Williams, C. L., Bollella, M. C., Strobino, B. A., Spark, A., Nicklas, T. A., Tolosi, L. B. et al. (2002). "Healthy-start": Outcome of an intervention to promote a heart healthy diet in preschool children. *Journal of the American College of Nutrition, 21,* 62–71.

Williams, C. L., Strobino, B. A., Bollella, M., & Brotanek, J. (2004). Cardiovascular risk reduction in preschool children: The "Healthy Start" project. *Journal of the American College of Nutrition, 23,* 117–123.

20

Obesity Prevention Programs for School-aged Children and Adolescents

DAVID M. JANICKE, BETHANY J. SALLINEN,
and JESSICA C. WHITE PLUME

Obesity is a critical public health epidemic (U.S. Department of Health and Human Services, 2000). The most recent data from the National Health and Nutrition Examination Survey shows that over 33 percent of children between the ages of two and 19 years are either at-risk for overweight status (between the 85th and 95th percentile for body mass index [BMI] based on age and gender) or overweight (above the 95th percentile for BMI based on age and gender) (Ogden et al., 2006). Childhood obesity is linked to a variety of negative health and mental health consequences for children and adolescents (Freedman, Dietz, Srinivasan, & Berenson, 1999; Zametkin, Zoon, Klein, & Munson, 2004). Moreover, childhood and adolescent obesity are significant predictors of overweight status in adulthood and further health complications as an adult (Field, Cook, & Gillman, 2005; Freedman et al., 2005). Obesity-associated annual hospital costs specific to children ages six to 17 have increased threefold over the last 20 years (Wang & Dietz, 2002). Not surprisingly, reducing the proportion of the U.S. population that is overweight or obese is a primary goal of Healthy People 2010 (U.S. Department of Health and Human Services).

With the increasing recognition of the obesity epidemic, its tremendous health consequences for individuals, and the cost associated with treatment, funding organizations and researchers have begun to devote significant resources to reducing obesity. While a number of factors related to the

---

DAVID M. JANICKE, BETHANY J. SALLINEN, and JESSICA C. WHITE PLUME • University of Florida, Gainesville, FL 32610.

obesogenic environment impact obesity, most experts agree that the fundamental proximal issue is an imbalance in the energy equation in which caloric intake exceeds calorie expenditure (Schmitz & Jeffery, 2002). However, the fact that obesity is overtly or inadvertently supported across social, cultural, institutional, and physical environments makes effectively changing obesity trends a significant challenge. While the treatment of children and adolescents who are obese is a critical step to improving the health of children across the world, reducing and maintaining weight loss is difficult. Ultimately, stemming the tide of this epidemic may rest in prevention strategies that decrease the development of obesity in children and adolescents (Gill, 1997).

Primary, Secondary, and Tertiary Prevention

The NIH Obesity Research Task Force has described three levels of obesity prevention (U.S. Department of Health and Human Services, 2004). Primary prevention involves preventive efforts and interventions for all children in a given population, regardless of weight or risk status. Secondary prevention involves interventions for children who are not currently overweight, but have a known risk factor for the development of obesity (e.g., an obese parent, a parent with type II diabetes). Secondary prevention programs are not delivered to all children in a given population, but rather only those with selected risk factors. Tertiary, or *targeted* prevention involves prevention of weight gain, weight loss, or the management of comorbid health issues (i.e., hyperlipidemia, hypertension, or type II diabetes) in children who are already overweight or obese. All levels of intervention are critical to improving the quality of life of children, and the successful management of this epidemic. However, there is a growing sentiment that—due to limited healthcare resources, the cost of treatment programs, and the less than ideal long-term maintenance of weight loss for people of all ages—prevention-focused programs (primary and secondary prevention) ultimately offer the best chance of stemming the tide of the epidemic.

Settings for Preventive Interventions

Efforts to address the obesity epidemic occur at many levels. Public health approaches attempt to intervene at the population level. These include, but are not limited to, advocacy and media campaigns to influence healthy dietary habits and physical activity, taxation of various food products, efforts to reduce portion sizes and increase healthy menu options on restaurants, healthy changes in the built environment, prohibiting fast food and soft drink sales in schools, and funding for school lunch and physical education programs (Frank, Andresen, & Schmid, 2004; Horgen & Brownell, 2002; Wadden, Brownell, & Foster, 2002). These approaches are addressed in greater breadth and depth in other sections of this handbook.

Obesity prevention may also take a more educational and behavioral change approach that includes direct contact and training with children rather than strictly modifications to supportive environments or community-wide education. While individuals are targeted, such preventive programs may include components of environmental change in systems serving the targeted population that support individual behavior change indirectly through modifying the availability of healthy lifestyle opportunities. In school-based intervention programs, this may involve working with targeted schools to modify the foods served in the cafeteria, or the physical education curriculum. For example, the Child and Adolescent Trial for Cardiovascular Health program (CATCH) (Leupker et al., 1996) worked with schools to decrease the percent of energy from fat in foods served in school lunches, and the amount of moderate-to-vigorous activity built into the physical education curriculum.

The most common venue—and indeed where one finds the greatest volume of published data on obesity prevention programs—is the school environment (Gortmaker et al., 1999; Sahota et al., 2001). Children consume approximately one third of their daily calories at school and schools provide significant time and opportunities for energy expenditure. Moreover, school programs allow for the use of existing organization, communication, and social structures (Schmitz & Jeffery, 2002). However, prevention programs are not, and should not be, limited to the school environment (Center for Disease Control and Prevention, 1997). Targeting children and adolescents through community organizations or settings (Baranowski et al., 2002, 2003), as well as addressing the important influence of the family unit and parent-child interactions are also critical venues and domains for obesity prevention.

Targeted Outcomes for Prevention Programs

Three categories of outcome measures have been generally reported in the literature on preventive intervention programs. Weight status outcomes such as body mass index (BMI), waist circumference, and body composition variables (e.g., skinfold thickness, percentage body fat) provide the most direct measure of weight status change. Other biological markers (i.e., blood pressure, cholesterol) provide adjunctive information, but important measures of health status change have also been included in some trials.

As preventive intervention programs attempt to impact weight and health status outcomes, a second category of outcome variables focuses on the behavioral factors that theoretically are most directly linked to weight status. Three areas of focus are often the primary behavior targets of preventive interventions and include reductions in energy intake, increases in physical activity, and reductions in sedentary activity. Reductions in energy intake have been addressed through a variety of strategies by targeting increases in fruit and vegetable intake, decreases in high-fat and high-sugar foods, and decreases in high-sugar beverages. Increases in physical activity have been addressed by targeting increases in competitive or organized sports, organized school and social activities, general play activities, and increased activity in everyday activities of life. Finally, as children are spending more and more time each day in sedentary activities (e.g., watching television, playing video games, and surfing the

Internet), more interventions are targeting reductions in media use as ways to increase time available for physical activity, and reduce exposure to stimuli associated with increased food consumption.

A third category of outcome variables includes knowledge, attitudes, and psychosocial functioning variables. Theoretically, each of these factors is more distally related to weight and health status change through their impact on individual dietary intake and physical activity patterns. Knowledge variables often focus on guidelines for healthy eating habits and physical activity, nutrition content of foods, and strategies for managing dietary intake. Attitude variables may include self-efficacy for making healthy lifestyle changes, health behavior preferences and intentions, perceived support for lifestyle behaviors, and motivation for change.

The remainder of this chapter reviews the state of the literature and provides examples of preventive intervention programs for school-aged children and adolescents. This review and discussion is limited to primary or secondary obesity prevention programs that involve some form of direct contact with children and adolescents, and identify weight status and behavior change variables as primary outcome measures. Different aspects of preventive programs in schools and communities are discussed by first examining comprehensive programs intended to prevent obesity via a variety of simultaneously operating health behavior channels. Then, we review programs that have targeted intervention resources via a single risk factor identified as potentially salient for obesity prevention.

Prevention Programs Targeting Multiple Risk Factors

To effectively facilitate children and families overcoming the many obstacles to maintaining healthy weight, researchers have created programs that target the basic obesity mechanisms such as caloric intake, dietary quality, and physical activity, via interventions that acknowledge and incorporate the multiple influences on children's health behaviors. A number of groundbreaking intervention trials were conducted in the 1980s and 1990s that targeted the critical mechanisms of obesity (Killen et al., 1989; Leupker et al., 1996) in the context of identified health targets such as cardiovascular disease. While these were not obesity prevention programs per se, they were clearly instrumental in the evolution of obesity prevention programs, and are therefore noted here.

A cardiovascular risk reduction trial that resulted in positive changes in weight status was the Stanford Heart Health program (Killen et al., 1989). Approximately 1,500 tenth grade students from four high schools participated in this randomized control, multicomponent program to reduce risk factors associated with cardiovascular disease. Physical activity and nutrition were addressed in the seven-week program, along with other risk factors including cigarette smoking, managing stress, and problem-solving. At post-treatment, adolescents in the intervention group showed significant improvements in BMI, as well as triceps skinfold and subscapular skinfold thickness (Killen et al.).

Another excellent example of an early, large-scale, school-based program is CATCH (Leupker et al., 1996). CATCH was initially a comprehensive, three-year, randomized controlled intervention trial implemented with 3rd - 5th graders in 96 public schools across California, Louisiana, Minnesota, and Texas. Environmental change objectives addressed the nutritional quality of food service offerings by working closely with food service staff, and similarly increasing the amount of moderate-to-vigorous physical activity in physical education (PE) programs by working closely with PE staff. Classroom education modules that included activities to promote healthy eating and physical activity were delivered across 3rd, 4th, and 5th grades. Teachers attended training annually and received monetary incentives for developing innovative ideas to promote the CATCH goals. At post-intervention, there were no differences between intervention and control schools in weight status outcomes. However, intervention schools were successful in decreasing the percent of calories from fat and saturated fat served to and consumed by children, and in increasing time dedicated to vigorous activity in PE classes. Furthermore, these changes persisted at the three-year follow-up (Nader et al., 1999). While this program failed to lead to significant changes in weight status, CATCH served as a model for future programs by demonstrating how a large-scale, multicomponent intervention program can successfully change school environments, and highlighted the importance of contributions by school personnel in building school-based programs. With evaluation-based revisions, CATCH was well-received by communities and continues to be implemented in schools across Texas (Coordinated Approach to Child Health, 2006).

School-Based Obesity Prevention Programs. A number of recent school-based intervention programs targeted multiple risk factors and identified obesity-related outcomes as primary endpoints (Caballero et al., 2003; Donnelly et al., 1996; Gortmaker et al., 1999; Neumark-Sztainer, Story, Hannan, Stat, & Rex, 2003; Sahota et al., 2001; Stolley & Fitzgibbon, 1997; Warren, Henry, Lightowler, & Perwaiz, 2003). Two programs serve as excellent examples and are emphasized to illustrate how multiple complex health goals are operationalized in comprehensive programs. One of the only programs in this category to demonstrate positive changes in weight status is Planet Health—a two-year, school-based intervention designed to reduce obesity in middle school youth (Gortmaker et al.). Ten middle schools in Massachusetts were randomized to the Planet Health Program or a control condition. Intervention targets included an increase in moderate-to-vigorous physical activity, reductions in TV time, increases in consumption of fruits and vegetables, and a decrease in consumption of high-fat foods. Sixteen 45-minute classroom modules addressing the goals of the program were delivered by classroom teachers across math, language arts, science, and social studies classes in both year 1 and year 2. Physical activity education was delivered in PE classes and organized into 30 five-minute units per year.

Results demonstrated the prevalence of obesity (composite measures of BMI and triceps skinfolds ≥ 85th percentile based on gender and age) for females in intervention schools dropped from 23.6 percent to 20.3 percent over the two-year intervention, while in the control schools the prevalence increased from 21.5 percent to 23.7 percent (odds ratio [OR], 0.47; 95% CI, 0.24–0.93; p = .03). There were no significant differences for males across school groups. Thirty percent of participants were African-American adolescents, and the largest intervention effects were seen among girls in this group (OR 0.14; 95% CI, 0.04–0.48; p< .01). Female participants in the interventions schools also reported a greater increase in fruit and vegetable consumption and lower total energy intake than females in control schools. A unique aspect of this intervention was the fact that it included reduced TV time as a specific target behavior. Both male and female participants in the intervention schools reported greater reductions in the number of TV hours per day, with reductions in TV time mediating the change in weight status for females. The Planet Health program was also one of the first to report on the incidence of restrictive dietary behaviors for children in the program. Child participants in the Planet Health intervention schools were half as likely to endorse the use of restrictive dietary behaviors at post-treatment relative to those in control schools at post-treatment (Gortmaker et al., 1999). This was primarily due to a fewer *new onset* cases of restrictive dieting in the intervention versus control schools.

Because the risk for obesity and associated adverse health outcomes is higher in some underserved and ethnic minority groups (Freedman et al., 2005; Hannon, Rao, & Arslanian, 2005; Hedley et al., 2004), addressing obesity prevention in diverse populations is critical. Pathways (Caballero et al., 2003) was the first large-scale multicomponent school-based intervention designed to prevent obesity in Native American children. The three-year intervention program, developed in collaboration with participating tribal communities, was delivered in 41 schools in seven Native American communities. Classroom curricula were delivered via two 45-minute lessons per week for 12 weeks during 3rd and 4th grade, and eight weeks during 5th grade. Food service was improved to comply with U.S. Department of Agriculture (USDA) School Lunch and Breakfast Program requirements. Physical education programming included a minimum of three 30-minute sessions per week of moderate-to-vigorous physical activity. Short exercise breaks were also designed to promote physical activity in the classroom. Families were included via family action packs that included information on Pathways activities and tips for preparing healthy snacks at home.

Process evaluation showed that participation and implementation quality was high for schools and moderate for parents. Unfortunately, there were no statistically significant changes in measures of obesity and body composition. School lunch observations did show reduced fat intake and 24-hour recall showed significantly lower total daily energy intake (1892 vs. 2157 kcal/d) and percentage of energy from total fat (31.1 percent vs. 33.6 percent) for children in the intervention relative to control schools. Statistically significant increases in self-reported physical activity were present in the intervention group, but changes in physical activity as measured by accelerometer were not present.

Overall, many multitargeted school-based programs have reported significant changes in self-reported dietary intake and physical activity, as well as improved attitudes and knowledge regarding health domains related to obesity. However, most have not led to significant changes in weight status outcomes. The lack of success in this area—despite significant support from schools and communities and improved behavioral intentions of participants in many studies—is troubling and emphasizes the magnitude of the challenges and barriers experienced by researchers, community stakeholders, and families who wish to effect positive change in this area.

Community-based Programs. While schools offer an excellent venue to address obesity prevention, the challenges identified in many school trials— as well as the multiple environmental factors contributing to the obesity epidemic—suggest that preventive programs in alternative settings are also warranted. The Girls' Health Enrichment Multisite Studies (GEMS) is a current and sophisticated example of these. In an innovative research format, investigative teams from four centers (Baylor College of Medicine, University of Memphis, University of Minnesota, and Stanford University School of Medicine) collaborated to share common measurement protocols and timelines in identifying effective obesity prevention strategies for African-American girls (Rochon et al., 2003). Each research team independently conducted formative research that informed the development of four unique pilot programs to meet the needs and challenges of their respective communities. The results of these 12-week pilot programs concluded Phase 1 of GEMS and are reviewed here. Phase 2 is ongoing and will evaluate the outcomes of a two-year full-scale trial of the four programs. For all GEMS centers, participants were 8- to 10-year old African-American females. Participants were above the 25th (Memphis and Minnesota) or the 50th (Stanford and Baylor) percentiles for age- and sex-specific BMI (Rochon et al.). The Baylor GEMS included a four-week, summer day-camp program for participants, plus an eight-week Internet-based follow-up program focusing on specific dietary and physical activity goals (Baranowski et al., 2003). The intervention camp incorporated a variety of interactive multimedia activities, such as a mystery-solving game in which children used senses of touch, taste, and smell to discover fruits and vegetables—or an activity in which girls created cheers that served as mnemonics for decision-making, problem-solving, and asking behaviors. Each day included several opportunities for physical activity and ended with behavioral goal-setting.

Participants in the Memphis GEMS (Beech et al., 2003) were randomized into one of three group interventions: a) a girls-only intervention (n = 21); b) a parents- or guardians-only intervention (n = 21); or c) a girls-only control group that focused only on self-esteem improvement (n = 18). The GEMS child-targeted intervention sessions included one hour devoted to active participation in physical activities and food activities, such as taste-testing, food art, food preparation, and basic label reading. Physical activity time focused primarily on hip-hop aerobics. For the parent-targeted group, each session was divided into three segments of 25 minutes each for physical activity, didactic nutrition education, and interactive nutrition activity.

The Minnesota GEMS approach consisted of one-hour afterschool "club meetings" for girls twice per week for 12 weeks (Story et al., 2003). The sessions were led by trained African-American GEMS staff and were aimed to be fun and interactive. For example, to learn to drink more water than soda, girls were provided chilled bottled water at each meeting, measured the amount of sugar in different size containers of soda, created a rap about drinking water, and set personal water-drinking goals. Each meeting included fun physical activities, as well as incentives for attendance, reaching short-term goals, and completing activities. Minnesota GEMS included a family component that reinforced meeting activities. This included family packets, family-night events, phone calls to follow up on family activity and nutrition goals, and organized neighborhood walks.

The Stanford GEMS (Robinson et al., 2003) intervention aimed to increase physical activity through dance classes and reduce sedentary activity through a television-viewing reduction program. Both components have been successfully utilized in previous interventions (Flores, 1995; Robinson, 1999). Each participant received five in-home sessions of a television intervention that included TV-time reduction strategies (e.g. "budgeting"). Sessions were delivered by female African-American women who served as role-models and discussed the impact of TV within cultural and social contexts as well as in consideration of holistic health. In addition, dance sessions were provided five days per week to encourage social and cultural efficacy while also replacing sedentary behavior with moderate-to-vigorous physical activity. Sessions were available at three community centers, and daily participation in the program was encouraged rather than required.

Overall, none of the GEMS site programs reported significant changes in anthropometric measures, which was expected given the brief 12-week intervention period. However, differences often emerged in expected directions and significant changes in potential mediating factors were evident. When programs set specific behavioral goals and provided incentives contingent on effort and goal achievement, changes in health behaviors were often observed (e.g., TV time, physical activity). Moreover, the Stanford GEMS program (Robinson et al., 2003) highlights the importance of structuring and introducing intervention components in a manner that is acceptable and attractive to adolescents. Stanford GEMS results suggest that emphasis on personally important concepts such as cultural reasons to dance and avoid television, as opposed to motivation for weight reduction per se, may lead to greater participation and investment by adolescents. As pilot programs, these interventions and assessments aimed to guide the feasibility of larger-scale evaluations. The ongoing GEMS Phase 2 is guided by the pilot results and should provide rich data regarding obesity prevention in high-risk children.

As research progresses with GEMS and other multicomponent programs, the assessment of feasibility, cost-effectiveness, and the ability to generalize results in future evaluations will be crucial. For example, some GEMS interventions utilized existing infrastructure such as school space and busses for afterschool meetings. Similarly, programs with open revolving participation led by college students may be more cost-effective than programs with a fixed number of sessions available only to the initially participating cohort. While the focus on individual goal-setting is a critical element of the program, it is also time-intensive and may limit the volume of participants that can be impacted at one time. Cost-effectiveness and feasibility are potentially key points of comparison between the multitargeted interventions just described, and the programs reviewed below.

Single-component Prevention Programs

The obesity prevention programs reviewed above feature multiple program components (e.g., classroom education, PE classes, and school lunch modification) and multiple behavioral targets. In contrast, the selected single component obesity prevention programs reviewed in this section each target a specific risk factor, such as reducing media use (Robinson, 1999), increasing physical activity (Flores, 1995; Yin et al., 2005), or improving dietary intake (Epstein et al., 2001; James, Thomas, Cavan, & Kerr, 2004). While not as comprehensive, these programs have the advantage of providing greater depth of coverage and thus a more focused intervention that may lead to greater impact on targeted outcomes.

Programs Addressing Television Use. Robinson (1999) targeted reducing television, videotape, and video game use in 3rd and 4th graders enrolled in two public elementary schools in San Jose, California. Classroom teachers incorporated 18 30- to 50-minute lessons into their curriculum during the first several months of the school year. Children were taught to self-monitor media use and budget media time during the six-month program. Electronic television time managers were distributed to all homes to assist families with budgeting media use. All children participated in a television turnoff for 10 days, and thereafter were encouraged to limit media use to seven hours per week. Newsletters were sent home to parents with suggestions for limiting media use for the entire family. Post-intervention results indicated that children in the intervention group had significant decreases in BMI, triceps skinfold thickness, waist circumference, and waist-to-hip ratio in comparison to children in the control group. Both parents and children in the intervention group reported significantly decreased television viewing, with children also reporting a significant decrease in the use of video games. Children in the intervention condition also decreased the frequency of eating meals while watching television.

It is noteworthy that targeting a reduction in media use only—without substituting physical activity—resulted in a significant relative decrease in measures of adiposity. Multiple studies have included reduction in television time as one component of multiple component programs that suggest promising impacts on adiposity. As noted previously, Planet Health (Gortmaker et al., 1999) found that significant reductions in TV time mediated change in weight status for females, but not for males. The Stanford GEMS program targeted reduction in TV time with the results suggesting a trend toward significant changes in adiposity. While it is impressive that targeting reduction in media use results in significant positive impacts on measures of adiposity, it is important to better understand the specific mechanisms that lead to this change (Robinson, 1999). Clearly, nutrition and physical activity are important variables, and their relationship to reductions in media use should be explored. Given these promising results, targeting reduction in media use may be a cost-effective and feasible option for school districts to consider, because it can more easily be incorporated into existing curriculum, does not overburden teachers, and does not require hiring multiple highly trained staff members to deliver the program.

Programs Addressing Physical Activity. There are a number of multiple component programs that target physical activity in combination with additional variables of interest (e.g., Caballero et al., 2003; Gortmaker et al., 1999; Leupker et al., 1996). Other prevention programs focus on physical activity exclusively (Flores, 1995; Pangrazi, Beighle, Vehige, & Vack, 2003; Yin et al., 2005). For a comprehensive review of school-based physical activity programs, please see Kahn et al. (2002). In general, while many prevention programs are successful with increasing levels of physical activity during the program, change in weight status is seldom reported. Innovative single-component programs that report important gains in fitness or adiposity markers will be detailed below.

Yin and colleagues (Yin et al., 2005) reported on the Georgia FitKid Project—an eight-month afterschool obesity prevention program for third-grade students. Program sessions were two hours in length and consisted of a 40-minute academic enrichment period (i.e., students received homework assistance and engaged in academic enrichment activities), a healthy snack, and an 80-minute physical activity period. FitKid instructors were teachers and staff from the intervention schools. Average attendance for students was approximately 3.5 days per week. Unfortunately, no significant differences were reported in BMI, waist circumference, blood pressure, or cholesterol from pre- to post-treatment. However, follow-up analysis of students in the intervention group with at least 40 percent attendance showed a significant decrease in percent body fat (26.5% to 25.8%), and greater gains in bone mineral density ($0.86 g/cm^2$ to $0.89 g/cm^2$) and cardiovascular fitness (159.1 bpm to 154.5 bpm). The Georgia FitKid Project represents a novel afterschool program that incorporates both academic enrichment activities and physical activity. Given the positive gains in important health-related and fitness variables, this program appears promising, and highlights the importance of considering other fitness-related variables in addition to BMI and waist circumference.

In an innovative fitness program that served as a precursor to the Stanford GEMS project, Flores (1995) reported on Dance for Health—a 12-week school-based aerobic exercise program for African-American and Hispanic 7th graders. Students in the Dance for Health program participated in the dance-oriented physical activity curriculum instead of the control group's regular physical education program. All students met three times per week for 50 minutes. Students in the Dance for Health program also participated in a health education program twice per week for 30 minutes. At the end of the 12-week program, girls in Dance for Health significantly decreased their BMI (intervention: 22.9 to 22.1; control: 22.2 to 22.5; $p < .05$) and heart rate (intervention: 83.7 to 72.7; control: 79.0 to 78.9; $p < .01$) relative to the control group. There were no significant reductions for males in the program. The development of a culturally sensitive approach to increasing physical activity in minority girls emphasizes the value of tailoring interventions that are culturally relevant to the targeted population.

Programs Addressing Dietary Intake. Many multiple component programs have included dietary intervention as one aspect of prevention programs (e.g., Caballero et al., 2003; Gortmaker et al., 1999; Leupker et al., 1996). Other programs have focused solely on making positive dietary changes (e.g., Baranowski et al., 2002; Epstein et al., 2001; James et al., 2004; Stolley & Fitzgibbon, 1997). Although both types single- and multiple-component programs make positive changes in children's dietary habits, the impact of these programs on adiposity is negligible. Selected single-component programs targeting changes in dietary intake are described below.

James and colleagues (James et al., 2004) reported on a 12-month, school-based education program designed to reduce the consumption of carbonated beverages and weight status in children 7 to 11 years old in England. In this randomized controlled trial, the intervention consisted of four, one-hour class lessons across the year, including promotion of drinking water, tasting fruit to learn about the sweetness of natural products, a music competition to produce a song with a healthy message, an art presentation, and a classroom quiz. After one-year, there was no significant change in BMI or BMI-z scores. However, the mean percentage of overweight and obese children in the control condition increased by 7.5 percent compared with a decrease in the intervention group of 0.2 percent. Moreover, after one year, children in the intervention group showed a significantly greater decrease in self-reported consumption of carbonated beverages over three days relative to children in the control group (a reduction of 0.6 glasses per day [250 milliliters] versus an increase of 0.2 glasses per day).

Epstein and colleagues (Epstein et al., 2001) reported on a parent-focused behavioral weight-control program that targeted either increasing fruit and vegetable (IFV) intake or decreasing high-fat/high-sugar (DFS) food intake. Participants were obese parents with a non-obese child between the ages of six and 11 years. The six-month treatment consisted of eight weekly sessions, four biweekly sessions, and two monthly sessions. Child-oriented workbook materials were sent home with parents at each session. Parent and child workbooks included the following components: introduction to weight-control and prevention, developing a healthy eating and activity environment for children, behavior change techniques, and maintenance of behavior change. After one year, consumption of high-fat/high-sugar foods significantly decreased for children across both conditions, while only children of parents in the IFV group showed a trend toward a greater consumption of fruits and vegetables in comparison to children of parents in the DFS group. While at the one-year follow-up parents in the IFV group showed greater decreases in percentage overweight than parents in the DFS group, children's overweight percentage was stable for both groups. While there was no impact of child weight status at post-treatment, targeting parents only may be a cost-effective option for prevention programs, because one parent can influence change in multiple family members.

Of the single-component programs reviewed above, the programs focusing on media use reduction appear to have the most impact on weight status in comparison to programs targeting dietary intake or physical fitness. Although single-component programs are not as comprehensive as multiple-component programs, these results suggest that targeting a specific risk factor, such as media use, can lead to positive changes in measures of adiposity. There are potential advantages associated with single-component programs—such as increased cost-effectiveness, and greater sustainability and generalizabilty—although these factors have not been examined closely in the literature to date. Although greater topic depth can be achieved in single-component programs, multiple-component programs provide greater breadth and acknowledge multiple influences on the development and maintenance of obesity in children. Obviously, effective prevention efforts will require making changes in multiple domains, such as dietary intake, physical activity, and sedentary behavior. Ultimately, isolating components in single-component programs may allow for greater examination of the specific mechanisms that are responsible for producing change, and inform the development of even more effective multiple-component programs.

Conclusions

Overall, data regarding the prevention of pediatric obesity is scarce relative to the prominence of obesity in the causes of morbidity and mortality facing populations in industrialized countries (Summerbell et al., 2005). While advances in public health research have led to the recognition that an ecological approach to obesity prevention is the most fitting, programs directly intervening with children continue to be a prevention domain with significant potential (Eriksen, 2005; Mercer et al., 2003). Despite limited research in this area, a variety of excellent programs targeting nutrition and physical activity in children and adolescents have led to positive changes in obesity related knowledge, attitudes, and behavioral outcomes. Unfortunately, these positive outcomes have not often translated into significant improvements in weight status.

A number of factors likely contribute to the rarity of significant changes in weight status. Most notably, limitations inherent to current school settings may contribute to the lack of significant improvement in weight status in this environment. Despite efforts to include fun, moderate-to-vigorous physical activity for all children in school-based programs, the total amount of time spent in physical activity within the school day is limited by the time allocated to PE classes and the number of PE classes per week. The best school-based programs thus far may successfully increase children's activity level to 30 minutes, three times per week—an amount that should have numerous health benefits, but may not be enough to reduce BMI. Similarly, time allowed in classrooms for additional health-related curriculum is limited. Adding health behavior curriculum may be a burden or even time-prohibitive for teachers. To an extent, limitations such as these are a natural consequence of the school setting. However, structural changes to the larger school systems to expand the potential impact of obesity prevention (e.g., extended PE requirements, editing existing academic curricula and materials to include behavioral health education, and altering vending and food service policies) are possible, but dependent on social, political, and financial support.

Given the opportunity for a public health approach to prevention via school systems, it would be premature to conclude that school-based programs are ineffective in preventing obesity. Rather, there are likely key implementation and program factors that are yet to be maximized. For example, after several years of evolving, some school-based tobacco use prevention programs were successful in achieving smoking reductions that were maintained in controlled, long-term follow-up evaluations. One of the most successful of these programs—Life Skills Training—teaches children a combination of social resistance skills and general life skills, with the inclusion of active role-playing during lessons (Botvin, Baker, Dusenbury, Botvin, & Diaz, 1995). The educational program rests on children learning to critique and resist the social influences (such as advertising and peer pressure) contributing to unhealthy choices. Perhaps school-based obesity prevention programs could similarly benefit from an increased emphasis on the process of making healthy lifestyle choices and the behavioral practice of concrete skills (e.g., declining unhealthy food portions offered by family or restaurants; requesting alternative healthy food options; structuring their environment to promote healthy choices; setting specific, gradual goals for behavior change; rewarding goal achievement).

Behavioral psychology indicates that children's behavioral patterns are most likely to change when the consequences of these behaviors are consistent across settings and individuals to which they are exposed. Therefore, the collaboration and coordination of staff approaches and environments within schools—a challenge certainly—may be crucial. Similarly, individual behaviors are most likely to change when target behaviors are clear, specific, and immediately and appropriately reinforced. While school-based programs have been relatively comprehensive in including health targets, additional layers (e.g., media, teacher and staff health promotion) and the depth of *school culture* change may be achievable. When health messages and reinforcements infuse all aspects of the school, including staff experiences and modeling, schools may be a more powerful contributor to obesity prevention efforts.

The duration and intensity of preventive programs may also impact long-term results. While self-reported changes in physical activity and dietary intake have been reported in numerous studies, it may ultimately take programs of longer duration and intensity to establish changes in healthy lifestyle behaviors that are maintained throughout childhood and adolescence. Consistent, long-term changes in these lifestyle behaviors may be necessary to produce changes in weight status that are detectable in larger samples, with children of varying weight status. For example, it might be beneficial for nutrition education to be a formal component of school curriculum beginning in kindergarten and extending into the adolescent years. More research examining the feasibility, effectiveness, and long-term maintenance of programs of greater duration is needed. From 2000 to 2004, only three published studies described prevention programs of at least 12 months duration (Summerbell et al., 2005). There are multiple projects of longer duration currently underway, such as GEMS Phase II and the Trial of Activity for Adolescent Girls (TAAG)—a trend that will need to continue in the future.

Lack of significant changes in weight status variables may also be influenced by the moderating effect of anthropometric and demographic variables. For example, Gortmaker et al. (1999) reported that females, but not males, demonstrated changes in weight status in the Planet Health intervention. In addition to gender, another variable that may impact treatment outcome is baseline weight status. Relative to nonoverweight children, those who are overweight may exhibit fewer positive lifestyle habits, hold different attitudes about their body and motivation to change (Pesa, Syre, & Jones, 2000), and experience different barriers to healthier dietary habits (Zabinski, Saelens, Stein, Hayden-Wade, & Wilfley, 2003). As a result, they may respond differently to prevention programs in comparison to children who are not already obese. Consideration of baseline weight status, gender, or other variables as potential moderators of physiological and behavioral outcomes may elucidate positive effects on subgroups of children, as well as inform future preventive interventions.

Future Directions

Although preventive programs to date have demonstrated limited success in changing the overall weight status of child and adolescent participants, they should ultimately inform the development of new, more effective preventive programs. One area for improvement in preventive programs involves greater family involvement. A number of programs have included components for impacting parent involvement and the family environment. However, in most cases either the proposed intensity of the family intervention, or the actual follow-through by parents, has been limited (Baranowski et al., 2002; Caballero et al., 2003; Leupker et al., 1996). More recently, some of the GEMS pilot programs (Beech et al., 2003; Story et al., 2003) incorporated greater parent and family involvement, but the short-term, pilot nature of the programs limited potential effects on child outcomes. Greater family and parent involvement can affect change through parental purchasing and preparation of food, modeling of healthy lifestyle behaviors, and helping to create a positive and supportive environment to motivate children to adopt healthy lifestyle behaviors. Intervention research focusing on weight status change in overweight children has demonstrated that parent involvement is critical to weight status change in children (Epstein, Valoski, Wing, & McCurley, 1994; Golan & Crow, 2004). Along with educational components addressing nutrition and physical activity, these interventions include strong behavioral training in which group leaders work directly with parents to help create strategies to motivate and support their children. However, for the most part, prevention programs have not duplicated the intensity of parent involvement found in these programs. Clearly, one limitation is that such intensive parental involvement is time and labor intensive for both program leaders and parents. Incorporation of such a module in an all-inclusive setting may not be practical. One possibility is to focus more intensive family-based interventions on children at greater risk for obesity, such as those who have a parent who is obese or has type II diabetes. These family programs or modules could be particularly fruitful by positively impacting the health of the entire family.

There continues to be a need for greater focus on the development of community-based programs, with greater access to collaboration with community partners. More partners and community involvement may result in greater ideas, more comprehensive, multilevel intervention components, and greater access to community resources. Expanding community-based programs will also provide more opportunities for family involvement. For example, community and schools can work together to open facilities with healthful activities for children and families. An example is the Stanford GEMS project with community centers open for dancing five days per week. Opening more venues can be a wonderful adjunct to prevention programs—providing fun and safe opportunities to children when other options are limited. As researchers work with communities in developing programs, publication of structured formative research efforts would also be extremely useful.

The adaptation of successful programs for diverse populations also is critical. In a recent review of obesity prevention programs, Schmitz and Jeffery (2002) noted that prevention programs conducted in less diverse settings (predominately working with children from the same ethnic background) were more likely to show significant obesity-related treatment effects, although whether or not this is due to greater acceptability, addressing differential environment barriers, or other factors, is uncertain. Certainly, the continued development of culturally sensitive programs—possibly in conjunction with targeting children at greater risk (i.e., secondary prevention)—is warranted. GEMS and Pathways are examples of two such programs. However, given the reality of our multicultural society, we also need programs that can effect positive change in settings with children from multiple, diverse backgrounds (Schmitz & Jeffery).

There are a number of other recommendations that may benefit future research in this area. Given that many children in these programs are not overweight, as well as the limited reliability and validity of self-report measures of dietary intake and physical activity, reliably detecting changes in weight status and other primary outcomes is difficult. Thus, it would be beneficial for researchers to incorporate additional, more objective, measures of secondary health outcomes. These may include assessment of cardiovascular fitness or bone mineral density—such as in Georgia Fitkids (Yin et al., 2005)—muscle mass, or muscle strength. In addition, because prevention programs emphasize the adoption of healthier eating habits, there is potential for participants to adopt overly restrictive dietary behaviors or excessive exercise programs. Conversely, curricula in preventive programs may help limit the use of these more extreme weight control behaviors. This remains an empirical question. As such, it is increasingly important that future prevention and weight-loss programs build curriculum to address these issues, as well as incorporate appropriate assessment protocols to monitor these behavioral outcomes (Irving & Neumark-Sztainer, 2002).

Another critical question that researchers and program developers must consider is whether programs are sustainable by school or community groups. If the preventive program does not ultimately address the most relevant concerns of the participants and community (Summerbell et al., 2005), if the level of training for those to implement that protocol is too great, or the costs to fund and maintain the program are too high, the program will not succeed over the long-term. Although the specific issues and considerations effecting sustainability are unique to each setting and often evolve throughout the course of a study, they ultimately must be addressed by program developers and researchers.

Given the budget limitations of school districts, granting agencies, and the limitations placed on preventive health care programs by managed care, it is surprising that more researchers have not considered cost-effectiveness in their analyses. Future efforts in this area—especially focusing on long-term cost-effectiveness—will be critical to providing the data to influence potential partners, stakeholders, and policy-makers of the financial feasibility and impact of these programs. Correspondingly, expanded involvement of relevant stakeholders (families, schools, and community organizations) in the design, implementation, assessment, and modification of obesity prevention programs is recommended (Summerbell et al., 2005). Involvement of community stakeholders is instrumental for the continued improvement, long-term success and sustainability of these programs (Srinivasan & Collman, 2005).

There are a number of innovative prevention programs in school and community settings. It will be important to continue to fully evaluate these interventions, as well as the program components, to determine the critical elements impacting outcomes (Koplan, Liverman, & Kraak, 2005). Similarly, assessment of treatment integrity is also critical, because even the best-designed programs are likely to have limited effect if not implemented as planned. The greatest successes in public health history have blossomed with public support movements (e.g., motor vehicle safety, safer workplaces). Because the public is affected by the information environment, it behooves researchers to disseminate their results to other in forms that will allow maximal support of solutions to the obesity epidemic (Eriksen, 2005). For example, regular correspondence with appropriate media outlets should elicit increased public support for prevention programming. To aid this effort, results disseminated to the public and decision makers will need to be clear and meaningful for all consumers (e.g., number of children that will not develop diabetes or die prematurely as a result of the program).

Closing

Overall, the limited success of preventive programs to demonstrate positive impacts on child and adolescent weight status speaks to the multiple environmental determinants of obesity. Efforts to address environmental, organizational, and system changes throughout schools and communities are needed in conjunction with efforts to address individual and family behavior changes, if we expect to see long-term changes in child and adolescent health behaviors and weight status (Summerbell et al., 2005). Beyond individual and community targeted efforts, population-based ecological approaches, such as changes to the built environment (Frank et al., 2004), shifts in popular mass media (Huhman et al., 2005), regulations on advertising and food labeling (Wadden et al., 2002), and limitations on fast food and soft drink sales in schools (Wadden et al., 2002)—just to name a few—will also be necessary to significantly slow the upward curve of obesity prevalence. While the increase in rates of obesity has been dramatic, it has occurred over a number of years. Reversing this trend will therefore take time, patience, and collaborative efforts across multiple levels of society.

REFERENCES

Baranowski, T., Baranowski, J., Cullen, K., deMoor, C., Rittenberry, L., Hebert, D., et al. (2002). 5 a day achievement badge for African American boy scouts. *Preventive Medicine, 34*, 353–363.

Baranowski, T., Baranowski, J., Cullen, K., Thompson, D., Nicklas, T., Zakeri, I., et al. (2003). The Fun, Food, & Fitness Project: The Baylor GEMS pilot study. *Ethnicity and Diseases, 13*, S30–39.

Beech, B., Klesges, R., Kumanyika, S., Murray, D., Klesges, L., McClanahan, B., et al. (2003). Child & parent-targeted interventions: The Memphis GEMS study. *Ethnicity and Disease, 13*, S40–S53.

Botvin, G. J., Baker, E., Dusenbury, L., Botvin, E. M. & Diaz, T. (1995). Long-term follow-up results of a randomized drug abuse prevention trial in a White middle-class population. *Journal of the American Medical Association, 273*, 1106–1112.

Caballero, C., Clay, T., Davis, S., Ethelbah, B., Rock, B., Lohman, T., et al. (2003). Pathways: A school-based, randomized controlled trial for the prevention of obesity in American Indian schoolchildren. *American Journal of Clinical Nutrition, 78*, 1030–1038.

Center for Disease Control and Prevention. (1997). Guidelines for school and community programs to promote lifelong activity among young people. *Morbidity & Mortality Weekly Report, 46*, 1–36.

Coordinated Approach To Child Health: The Catch Mission. (n.d.) Retrieved February, 2006 from: http://www.sph.uth.tmc.edu/catch/about.htm

Donnelly, J., Jacobsen, D., Whatley, J., Hill, J., Swift, L., Cherrington, A., et al. (1996). Nutritional and physical activity program to attenuate obesity and promote physical and metabolic fitness in elementary school children. *Obesity Research, 4*, 229–243.

Epstein, L., Gordy, C., Raynor, H., Beddome, M., Kilanowski, C., & Paluch, R. (2001). Increasing fruit and vegetable intake and decreasing fat and sugar intake in families at risk for childhood obesity. *Obesity Research, 9*, 171–178.

Epstein, L., Valoski, A., Wing, R., & McCurley, J. (1994). Ten-year outcomes of behavioral family-based treatment for childhood obesity. *Health Psychology, 13*, 373–383.

Eriksen, M. P. (2005). Lessons learned from public health efforts and their relevance to preventing childhood obesity. In J. Koplan, C. Liverman, & V. Kraak (Eds). *Preventing Childhood Obesity: Health in the Balance.* Institute of Medicine, The National Academies of Sciences Press, Washington, D.C.

Field, A., Cook, N., & Gillman, M. (2005). Weight status in childhood as a predictor of becoming overweight or hypertensive in early adulthood. *Obesity Research, 13*, 163–169.

Flores, R. (1995). Dance for Health: Improving fitness in African American and Hispanic adolescents. *Public Health Reports, 110*, 189–193.

Frank, L. D., Andresen, M.A., & Schmid, T. L. (2004). Obesity relationships with community design, physical activity, and time spent in cars. *American Journal of Preventive Medicine, 27*, 87–96.

Freedman, D., Dietz, W., Srinivasan, S., & Berenson, G. (1999). The relation of over-weight to cardiovascular risk factors among children and adolescents: The Bogalusa heart study. *Pediatrics, 103,* 1175–1182.

Freedman, D., Khan, L., Serdula, M., Dietz, W., Srinivasan, S. & Berenson, G. (2005). Racial differences in the tracking of childhood BMI to adulthood. *Obesity Research, 13,* 928–935.

Gill, T. (1997). Key issues in the prevention of obesity. *British Medical Bulletin, 53,* 359–388.

Golan, M., & Crow, S. (2004). Targeting parents exclusively in the treatment of child-hood obesity: Long-term results. *Obesity Research, 12,* 357–361.

Gortmaker, S., Peterson, K. Wiecha. J. Sobol, A., Dixit, S., Fox, M., et al. (1999). Reduc-ing obesity via a school-based interdisciplinary intervention among youth: Planet Health. *Archives of Pediatric and Adolescent Medicine, 153,* 409–418.

Hannon, T., Rao, G., & Arslanian, S. (2005). Childhood obesity and type 2 diabetes mel-litus. *Pediatrics, 116,* 473–480.

Hedley, A. A., Ogden, C. L., Johnson, C. L., Carroll, M. D., Curtin, L. R., & Flegal, K. M. (2004). Prevalence of overweight and obesity among U.S. children, adolescents, and adults, 1999–2002. *Journal of the American Medical Association, 291,* 2847–2850.

Horgen, K., & Brownell, K. (2002). Confronting the toxic environment: Environment and public health actions in a world crisis. In T.A. Wadden & A.J. Stunkard (Eds.), *Handbook of Obesity Treatment.* New York, NY: Guilford Press.

Huhman, M., Potter, L., Wong, F., Banspach, S., Duce, J., & Heitzler, C. (2005). Effects of a mass media campaign to increase physical activity among children: 1-year results of the VERB campaign. *Pediatrics, 116,* e277–e284.

Irving, L., & Neumark-Sztainer, D. (2002). Integrating the prevention of eating disorders and obesity: Feasible or futile? *Preventive Medicine, 34,* 299–309.

James, J., Thomas, P., Cavan, D., & Keer, D. (2004). Preventing childhood obesity by reduc-ing consumption of carbonated drinks. *British Medical Journal, 328,* 1236–1241.

Kahn, E. B., Ramsey, L. T., Brownson, R. C., Heath, G. W., Howze, E. H., Powell, K. E., et al. (2002). The effectiveness of interventions to increase physical activity: A sys-tematic review. *American Journal of Preventive Medicine, 22*(suppl. 4), 73–107.

Killen, J., Robinson, T., Telch, M., Saylor, K., Maron, D., Rich, T., et al. (1989). The Stan-ford Adolescent Heart Health Program. *Health Education Quarterly, 16,* 263–283.

Koplan, J., Liverman, C., & Kraak, V. (Eds.). (2005). *Preventing Childhood Obesity: Health in the Balance.* Institute of Medicine: The National Academies of Sciences Press, Washington, D.C.

Leupker R., Perry, C., McKinley, S. Nader P., Parcel, G., Stone, E., et al. (1996). Out-comes of a field trial to improve children's dietary patterns and physical activity: The child and adolescent trail for cardiovascular health (CATCH). *Journal of the American Medical Association, 275,* 768–776.

Mercer, S., Green, L., Rosenthal, A., Husten, C., Khan, L., & Dietz, W. (2003). Possible lessons from the tobacco experience for obesity control. *American Journal of Clinical Nutrition, 77,* 1073S–1082S.

Nader, P., Stone, E., Lytle, L., Perry, C., Osganian, S., Kelder, S., et al. (1999). Three-year maintenance of improved diet and physical activity: The CATCH cohort. *Archives of Pediatric and Adolescent Medicine, 153,* 695–704.

Neumark-Sztainer, D., Story, M., Hannan, P. J., Stat, M., & Rex, J. (2003). New Moves: A school based obesity prevention program for adolescent girls. *Preventive Medicine, 37,* 41–51.

Ogden, C. L., Carroll, M. D., Curtin, L. R., McDowell, M. A., Tabac, C. J., & Flegal, K. M. (2006). Prevalence of overweight and obesity in the United States, 1999 – 2004. *Journal of the American Medical Association, 295(13),* 1549–1555.

Pangrazi, R., Beighle, A., Vehige, T., & Vack, C. (2003). Impact of Promoting Lifestyle Activity for Youth (PLAY) on children's physical activity. *Journal of School Health, 73,* 317–321.

Pesa, J., Syre, T., & Jones, E. (2000). Psychosocial differences associated with body weight among female adolescents: The importance of body image. *Journal of Ado-lescent Health, 26,* 330–337.

Robinson, T. (1999). Reducing children's television viewing to prevent obesity: A randomized controlled trial. *Journal of the American Medical Association, 282*, 1561–1567.

Robinson, T., Killen, J., Kraemer, H., Wilson, D., Matheson, D., Haskell, W., et al. (2003). Dance and reducing television viewing to prevent weight gain in African-American girls: The Stanford GEMS pilot study. *Ethnicity and Disease, 13*, S65–S77.

Rochon, J., Klesges, R., Story, M., Robinson, T., Baranowski, T., Obarzanel, E., et al. (2003). Common design elements of the Girls health Enrichment Multi-site Studies (GEMS). *Ethnicity and Disease, 13*, S6–S14.

Sahota, P., Rudolf, M., Dixey, R., Hill, A., Barth, J., & Cade, J. (2001). Randomized controlled trial of primary school based intervention to reduce risk factors for obesity. *British Medical Journal, 323*, 1029–1032.

Schmitz, K., & Jeffery, R. (2002). Prevention of obesity. In T. A. Wadden & A. J. Stunkard (Eds.), *Handbook of Obesity Treatment*. New York, NY: Guilford Press.

Srinivasan, S., & Collman, C. (2005). Evolving partnerships in community. *Environmental Health Perspectives, 113*, 1814–1816.

Stolley, M., & Fitzgibbon, M. (1997). Effects of an obesity prevention program on the eating behavior of African American mothers and daughters. *Health Education and Behavior, 24*, 152–164.

Story, M., Sherwood, N., Himes, J., Davis, M., Jacobs, D. Jr., Cartwright, Y., et al. (2003). An after-school obesity prevention program for African-American girls: The Minnesota GEMS pilot study. *Ethnicity and Disease, 13*, S54–S64.

Summerbell, C. D., Waters, E., Edmunds, L. D., Kelly, S., Brown, T., & Campbell, K. J. (2005). Interventions for preventing obesity in children. Cochrane Database of Systematic Reviews, *3*, Article CD001871.

U.S. Department of Health & Human Services (2004). *Strategic Plan for NIH Obesity Research*. Washington, D.C.: National Institutes of Health.

U.S. Department of Health & Human Services (2000). *Healthy People 2010: National Health Promotion and Disease Prevention Objectives*. Atlanta, GA: Centers for Disease Control and Prevention.

Wadden, T., Brownell, K., & Foster, G. (2002). Obesity: Responding to the global epidemic. *Journal of Consulting and Clinical Psychology, 70*, 510–525.

Wang, G., & Dietz, W. (2002). Economic burden of obesity in youths aged 6 to 17 years: 1979–1999. *Pediatrics, 109*, E81.

Warren, J., Henry, C., Lightowler, H., & Perwaiz, S. (2003). Evaluation of a pilot school program aimed at the prevention of obesity in children. *Health Promotion International, 18*, 287–296.

Yin, Z., Gutin, B., Johnson, M., Hanesm J. Jr., Moore, J., Cavnar, M., et al. (2005). An environmental approach to obesity prevention in children: Medical College of Georgia FitKid Project year 1 results. *Obesity Research, 13*, 2153–2161.

Zabinski, M., Saelens, B., Stein, R., Hayden-Wade, H., & Wilfley, D. (2003). Overweight children's barriers to and support for physical activity. *Obesity Research, 11*, 238–246.

Zametkin, A., Zoon, C., Klein, H., & Munson, S. (2004). Psychiatric aspects of child and adolescent obesity. *Journal of American Academy of Child & Adolescent Psychiatry, 43*, 134–150.

21

Preventing Childhood Obesity through Collaborative Public Health Action in Communities

VICKI L. COLLIE-AKERS
and STEPHEN B. FAWCETT

Obesity, including among children, is a global public health problem that has grown dramatically over the last several decades (Wang & Lobstein, 2006). The rising prevalence of overweight and obesity in the population, and its dramatic implications for health care costs, requires collaborative public health action (Institute of Medicine, 2003). Obesity is caused by an imbalance of energy intake—too many calories consumed in food and drink in relation to energy used or calories burned in daily activity (Goran, Reynolds, & Lindquist, 1999). It is "a multi-factoral condition with wide-ranging causes, including genetic, social, cultural, and behavioral factors" (Parsons, Power, Logan, & Summerbell, 1999).

Obesity prevention efforts focus on the personal and environmental factors that affect the key behaviors of physical activity and healthy nutrition (Dietz & Gortmaker, 2001). Personal factors include: a) *knowledge and skill*, such as knowledge of healthy food choices and skills in physical activity; b) *experience and history*, such as a history of positive consequences of engaging in physical activity; and c) *biology/genetics*,

VICKI L. COLLIE-AKERS and STEPHEN B. FAWCETT • University of Kansas, Lawrence, KS 66045.

including a family history or predisposition to obesity. The "prominent predictor" of obesity among children is overweight in early childhood (Salbe, Weyer, Lindsay, Ravussin, & Tataranni, 2002).

Environmental factors related to the behaviors of healthy nutrition and physical activity include: a) *access, barriers, and opportunities*, such as the availability of healthy snacks in preschools; b) *support and services*, including nutrition counseling and public recreational services; c) *consequences of actions*—for example, social consequences from peers of food choices or engaging in sports activities; and d) *policies and living conditions*, such as school policies regarding soft drinks in vending machines. For instance, French, Story, and Jeffery (2001) reported dramatic trends in the availability of healthy and less-healthy food choices. They noted the increased availability of soft drinks, such as those in vending machines, has led to a decrease in milk consumption—a healthier food choice. Similarly, the availability of fast food restaurants that promote eating away from home has increased dramatically since the 1970s, with resulting increases in portion size and fat content of meals (French et al.). Exposure to television advertising has been linked to consumption of higher-fat foods (Jeffery & French, 1998); and, conversely, community-wide media campaigns to promote fruit and vegetable intake may be a protective factor. Similarly, widespread availability of television and computers, for instance, make sedentary activity more likely (French et al.), as does the automobile transport of children instead of walking. Conversely, better-designed public spaces, such as safe and accessible parks and walkways, might increase the likelihood of physical activity among children and adolescents (Goran et al., 1999).

To address these multiple and interrelated factors affecting physical activity and healthy eating for all children requires collaborative public health action in communities. Community health interventions are marked by the involvement of multiple sectors—such as schools and youth organizations—in creating environments that promote healthy behaviors (Fawcett et al., 2000; Institute of Medicine, 2003). In its knowledge synthesis related to preventing childhood obesity, the Institute of Medicine (2005) noted that evidence of community interventions is derived less from interventions that specifically target obesity than from earlier population-level efforts to reduce risk for cardiovascular diseases—for instance, the Stanford Three Community Study, the Stanford Five-City Project, Minnesota Heart Health Program, the Pawtucket Heart Health Program, and the North Karelia project. These population health efforts "demonstrated the feasibility of community-based approaches to promoting physical activity and changes in dietary intake" (Institute of Medicine).

This chapter provides a brief review of evidence suggesting the potential for community health interventions to prevent childhood obesity. We outline a framework for collaborative public health action to prevent childhood obesity and its implications for community health interventions and related research. Finally, we conclude with a discussion of challenges and opportunities for such approaches, and make recommendations for research and practice on community efforts for preventing obesity among children and adolescents.

A BRIEF REVIEW OF COMMUNITY INTERVENTIONS
TO PREVENT CHILD AND ADOLESCENT OBESITY

A number of community interventions have attempted to reduce risk for obesity and chronic diseases for which obesity is a risk factor, by promoting healthy nutrition and physical activity. Consistent with an analysis of personal and environmental factors, these interventions used single forms or combinations of five behavior-change strategies. First, some interventions involved *providing information and enhancing skills*, for instance, using public service announcements to promote fruit and vegetable intake (Beech et al., 2003). Other efforts implemented a specific curriculum in school settings designed to provide information about physical activity (Paine-Andrews et al., 1997). Second, interventions *enhanced services and support*, for instance, by offering afterschool clubs to promote healthy eating (Story et al., 2003), or by engaging volunteers from different organizations across the community to build on the services that were generally offered in high school physical education classes—such as training in water aerobics, yoga, and kickboxing.

Third, some interventions involved *modifying access, barriers, and opportunities*, for example, by installing physical fitness stations in each classroom (Harris et al., 1997) or by providing prompts for children to walk up stairs in shopping centers rather than riding escalators (Task Force on Community Preventive Services, 2001). In one study, Cullen, Bartholomew, and Parcel (1997) used a randomized-control group design to examine whether fruit and vegetable consumption could be increased among Junior Girl Scouts through a multicomponent intervention that included having the girls sample different fruits and vegetables for taste. Fourth, some community interventions *changed the consequences* of key behaviors, for example, promoting the use of budgets for television-watching time to reduce the time spent in sedentary activities (Robinson et al., 2003). Other community interventions used price reduction in super markets to promote the purchase of lower-fat foods (Paine-Andrews, Francisco, Fawcett, Johnston, & Coen, 1996) or incentives to maintain key behaviors of healthy eating (Luepker et al., 1994). Fifth, the strategy of *modifying policies and broader systems* has been used, for example, to change school policies to lower fat content in school lunch menus (Harris et al.).

Many of these community interventions used a combination of strategies. For instance, the Minnesota Heart Health Program was a 10-year community trial project that occurred in three communities. The study used two comparison communities for each of the three communities that received the intervention. Intervention components included mass media communications (e.g., about the health benefits of healthier diets), incentives for behavior change at the individual level, and services including screenings to reduce risk for cardiovascular diseases (Luepker et al., 1994). Researchers reported "modest and time-limited improvements in exposure to coronary heart disease risk-reducing messages and activities and in coronary heart disease risk factors" (Luepker et al., p. 1391) for the experimental communities. Similarly, the Kansas LEAN project—a statewide coalition to promote healthy eating that included the state health department and other organizations—implemented media campaigns (providing information and enhancing support), modification of school menus (modifying access, barriers, and opportunities), and provision of instore coupons for healthier foods (changing consequences) (Harris et al., 1997; Johnston, Marmet, Coen, Fawcett, & Harris, 1996; Paine-Andrews et al., 1996).

Reviews of published interventions suggest varying degrees of success. The Cochrane Collaboration (www.cochrane.org) conducted a systematic review of evidence-based interventions to address childhood obesity that used randomized control trials (Summerbell et al., 2005). Although many interventions focused on schools as the setting, a few effective interventions were at the community level. For instance, the Girls' Health Enrichment Multisite Study (GEMS) used different community intervention among African-American girls across four sites (Rochon et al., 2003). One of the sites recruited African-American girls from a low-income neighborhood to participate in a dance class held at a local community centers and an at-home health education program that emphasized a reduction in television watching. The researchers reported a significant reduction in television-watching as a result of the intervention (Robinson et al., 2003). Another GEMS site used afterschool clubs and parent take-home packets to emphasize physical activity and nutrition (Story et al., 2003). Results reported from the four sites indicated changes in several key behaviors (e.g., reduced consumption of sweetened drinks, reduced television watching, increased healthy eating). In another community intervention study, researchers examined the effects of implementation of the Know Your Body program—designed to promote physical activity and healthy nutrition among low-income African-Americans (Stolley & Fitzgibbon, 1997). Key variables were determined to be increased access to healthy food choices, including healthy food items that could be obtained in nearby businesses, and safe walking areas in local neighborhoods. Results indicated that there was a significant difference between the body mass index (BMI) of those that received the intervention and those that did not.

A third study identified by the Cochrane Collaboration specifically targeted childhood obesity among Native Americans. This community intervention involved the use of peer educators to deliver a parenting program in the homes of families with children (Harvey-Berino & Rourke, 2003). Participants were separated into two groups—those that received a general parenting skills curriculum and those that received a parenting skills curriculum that included lessons focused on "how parenting skills could facilitate the development of appropriate eating and exercise behaviors" (Harvey-Berino & Rourke, p. 607). Researchers noted a corresponding change in energy intake—a decrease among participants in the parenting program and an increase among control participants. These three community interventions did not specifically target individual participants who were already obese, but rather used universal approaches to reduce the risk of obesity among all children in the community. Findings of the Cochrane Collaboration suggest that many controlled studies focused on the school sector—settings that provided easier and more intensive access to children. Although research is limited, there is some evidence that multisector initiatives in communities can contribute to preventing childhood obesity (Institute of Medicine, 2005).

The U.S. Centers for Disease Control and Prevention's Guide to Community Preventive Services (www.thecommunityguide.org) also provide systematic reviews of interventions to reduce risk for chronic diseases and to promote the key behaviors of physical activity and healthy nutrition. Although the reviews for obesity and nutrition are not yet available, reviews for interventions to promote physical activity have been completed. Criteria for inclusion in the CDC Community Guide included studies that showed effects when comparing groups of people exposed to the intervention with groups of people not exposed (either concurrently or before and after comparison) (Task Force on Community Preventive Services, 2001). Of the six intervention approaches rated as *recommended*—meaning that robust evidence was available for the efficacy of the intervention—four were interventions that took place in community settings (Task Force for Community Preventive Services).

First, the CDC Community Guide recommended the use of community-wide campaigns for promoting physical activity. These multicomponent campaigns included broad media campaigns and other components such as "self-help groups; risk factor screening, counseling, and education about physical activity in worksites, schools, and other settings; and environmental or policy changes such as the creation of walking trails" (Kahn et al., 2002). A second recommended strategy was implementation of point-of-decision prompts. This involved placing signs in locations such as staircases and elevators to prompt people to take the route that maximized the energy used through physical activity. Interventions used posters with differing messages, including signs that emphasized heart health and others that emphasized weight control (Andersen, Franckowiak, Snyder, Bartlett, & Fontaine, 1998; Kerr, Yore, Ham, & Dietz, 2004). For instance, Andersen et al. compared the effects of two different types of signage in a Baltimore shopping mall—one to use the stairs to promote heart health, and the other to enhance weight control. Researchers determined that both signs created a statistically significant increase in physical activity.

A third recommended intervention was social support in community settings. Intervention activities included establishing walking clubs and setting up buddy systems to promote physical activity. Some of the reviewed studies involved providing support in group settings, such as developing working groups to engage in physical activity and discussing the participants' efforts (Gill, Veigl, Shuster, & Notelvitz, 1984). Other effective approaches provided support individually, such as a study in which research staff provided 10-minute telephone contacts with participants to increase maintenance of physical activity programs (King, Taylor, Haskell, & Debusk, 1988). The final community intervention that was *recommended* in the CDC Community Guide was "to create or provide access to places and facilities where people can be physically active" (Kahn et al., 2002). Access may be through worksites, schools, and other settings; including the design of publicly available walking paths or designing the built environment to assure opportunities for physical activity.

A FRAMEWORK FOR COLLABORATIVE PUBLIC HEALTH ACTION TO PREVENT CHILDHOOD OBESITY

Collaborative partnerships—alliances among individuals and organizations in common purpose—can leverage resources and mobilize communities to address childhood obesity (Institute of Medicine, 2005). A framework

to guide such efforts can help target activities to personal and environmental factors related to the goals of the initiative. Based on the work of
Fawcett and colleagues (2000), and the U.S. Centers for Disease Control
and Prevention (2002), the Institute of Medicine (2003) developed a framework to guide collaborative public health action in communities. Adapted
for childhood obesity prevention, Figure 21.1 displays the five phases in
the framework: 1) assessing, prioritizing, and planning; 2) implementing
targeted action and preventive interventions; 3) community and system
change; 4) achieving widespread change in behavior and risk factors (e.g.,
physical activity, healthy nutrition); and 5) improving population-level
outcomes in childhood obesity.

Assessment, Prioritizing, and Planning

This phase involves several activities that provide the foundation
for subsequent phases. A community health initiative would begin with an
assessment of the prevalence of childhood obesity and related behavioral
risk factors, and a prioritizing of potential target groups (e.g., groups
of children from populations with disparities in health outcomes). For
instance, school records might be reviewed to assess the prevalence of
overweight children. Similarly, behavioral surveys could be conducted with
school children to determine how many consume five or more servings
of fruits or vegetables, or how many spend more than two hours a day
in sedentary activities (e.g., watching television). Based on the assessment, the community health initiative can prioritize the issues (e.g., too
little physical activity) and target groups (e.g., children in schools with
higher BMI). An analysis of the problem can help to identify the personal
and environmental factors to be addressed (e.g., modifying access and
opportunities for physical activity; changing policies for school lunches),
among whom, and through what channels of influence (e.g., schools;
media; business). For instance, the assessment might suggest that children
between the ages of 8 and 10 in a particular community are experiencing
a higher prevalence of obesity among children and should receive more
intensive efforts through elementary schools, youth organizations, and

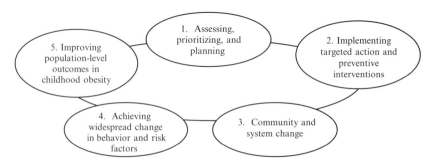

Figure 21.1. Framework for collaborative public health action to prevent childhood obesity
(Adapted from Institute of Medicine, 2003; Center for Disease Control and Prevention, 2002;
Fawcett et al., 2000).

faith communities. The GEMS study, focusing on African-American girls, illustrated the use of assessments to determine the population to be targeted (Robinson et al., 2003). Strategic planning consists of developing a vision, mission, objectives, strategies (e.g., using the five behavior-change strategies), and related action steps. As with the Kansas LEAN effort, for instance, the action plan should culminate in a targeting of community and system changes (i.e., new or modified program, policies, or practices) to be sought in each sector (e.g., schools, government, business), and decisions about who will do what by when to bring about targeted changes in the environment (Paine-Andrews et al., 1997).

Implementing Targeted Action and Preventive Interventions

The second phase of the framework involves initial implementation of the strategic and action plan developed during Phase One. Targeted activities and evidence-based preventive interventions are intended to create an environment that makes healthy behaviors—such as physical activity and healthy eating—easier and more likely. This may include coalition building or arranging partnerships to facilitate a new afterschool recreational program, advocating for a change in school policy to increase vending machine choices for healthy foods, or the implementation of a practice change in faith communities to promote physical activity as part of religious services. The resulting comprehensive community intervention, with multiple components influencing multiple sectors of a community, would likely include selected evidence-based programs and policies, such as those identified in the Cochrane Collaboration and CDC Community Guide, and other promising approaches for which there is yet to be a sufficient evidence base for a strong recommendation.

Community and System Change

This phase consists of the implementation of new or modified programs (e.g., a youth program that promotes physical activity, a *walking school bus* in particular neighborhoods), policies (e.g., policies among Girl and Boy Scout leaders about providing fresh fruits as snacks at scouting functions, school policies banning soft drinks in school buildings), or practices (e.g., daycare provider's practice of walking to field trips instead of driving). Because there is limited evidence that any single intervention will effect population-health improvement in diverse contexts, effective community interventions will likely consist of hundreds of changes in programs, policies, and practices (community and system changes) distributed in the multiple settings that can influence child behavior (Fawcett, Carson, Lloyd, Collie-Akers, & Schultz, 2005; Fawcett et al., 2000; Paine-Andrews et al., 1997).

Achieving Widespread Change in Behavior and Risk Factors

The fourth phase involves continual monitoring and promotion of behaviors, and attention to risk/protective factors to assure that the initiative is being successful. An initiative may use archival records, direct observation, or self-reporting in school surveys to monitor behaviors; including consumption of fruits and vegetables, time spent being sedentary or watching television, engagement in physical activity, or (more specifically) use of stairs as opposed to elevators or escalators. The aim of this phase is to assure widespread change in the behaviors of key actors—in this context, children, parents, and community decision-makers.

Improving Population-level Outcomes in Childhood Obesity

The final phase requires monitoring of the population-level outcomes of interest, such as the prevalence of overweight or obesity among children. This might be accomplished by working with pediatricians or school nurses to assure measurement of the height and weight of the children they serve, or conducting a survey among parents about whether they have been informed by a healthcare provider that their child is overweight or obese.

This framework for collaborative public health action is intended to be both *interactive* and *iterative* (repeating) (Fawcett et al., 2000; Fawcett, Francisco, Schultz, 2004). As an interactive model, if a community partnership sets a priority on increasing fruit and vegetable intake among preschool-aged children in Phase One, the targeted action and community changes implemented in Phases Two and Three might create opportunities for preschool-aged children to consume fruits and vegetables or decrease opportunities to consume other less nutritious foods. In an iterative approach, if assessment of the prevalence of obesity and physical activity among children (assessed in Phases Four and Five) yielded unsatisfactory results, members of the initiative should return to previous phases (Phases One and Two) to plan, take action, and implement different interventions (Phase Three) to change the community and system to maximize the potential for success in effecting behavior change (Phase Four) and improvement in population-level outcomes (Phase Five).

This Framework for Collaborative Public Health Action provides an orienting guide for community members and practitioners to use in local efforts to prevent childhood obesity. Key community processes or mechanisms, such as assessment and action planning, may be critical to creating community and system changes sufficient enough to effect widespread behavior change and improvement in population-level outcomes (e.g., Roussos & Fawcett, 2000). Using available evidence from empirical research, mul-tiple case studies, and review papers, 12 *best processes* have been identified as important in effecting change and improvement in healthy communities' efforts (Community Tool Box, http://ctb.ku.edu). Roussos & Fawcett (2000) outlined seven of these factors or evidence-based processes including: a) developing a clear vision and mission, b) engaging in action planning, c) building leadership, d) provision of documentation and feedback, e) provision of technical assistance, f) arranging for community mobilizers, and e) making outcomes matter (e.g., provision of bonus grants for improved outcomes). Further research suggests that additional commmunity processes may be important including: a) analyzing information about the problem or goal (Goodman, Steckler, Hoover, & Schwartz, 1993; Shortell et al., 2002); b) defining an organizational structure and operational mechanism

(Israel, Schultz, Parker, & Becker, 1998; Ploeg et al., 1996); c) developing a model of change (Merzel & D'Afflitti, 2003; Ploeg et al.); d) implementing effective interventions (Kreuter, Lezin, & Young, 2000; Sorensen, Emmons, Hunt, & Johnston, 1998); and e) planning for sustainability (Merzel & D'Afflitti; Sorensen et al.).

Implications for Comprehensive Community Interventions to Prevent Childhood Obesity

The guidance provided by the Framework for Collaborative Public Health Action has practical implications for those designing community interventions to prevent child and adolescent obesity. Engaging individuals and organizations from multiple sectors, the action plan developed during Phase One serves as a map of the components and elements of an emerging comprehensive community intervention. Such interventions should use multiple behavior-change strategies (e.g., modifying access and opportunities; changing policies) to address targeted behaviors (e.g., physical activity, healthy nutrition) in multiple contexts (e.g., schools, youth organizations, businesses, etc.).

Table 21.1. Illustrative components and elements (by sector) of a comprehensive community intervention to prevent child and adolescent obesity

Intervention component	Illustrative intervention elements by sector
Providing Information and Enhancing Skills	• Provide local faith organizations with a list of physically-active games to play during youth activities. (Faith Communities)
Enhancing Services and Support	• Link school nurses with registered dieticians to whom parents may be referred. (Schools and Health Organizations) • Expand existing youth programs to include components on physical activity and nutrition. (Youth Organizations)
Modifying Access, Barriers, and Opportunities	• Engage grocery stores in developing displays at children's height that offer a selection of fruits and vegetables. (Business) • Offer discounted rates at the YWCA and YMCA for children who use the facilities. (Community Organizations)
Changing the Consequences	• Recognize restaurants that make healthy options easily identifiable in the local newspapers. (Business and Media) • Provide coupons on fruits and vegetables to families who use city recreational facilities. (Business and Government)
Modifying Policies and Broader Conditions	• Implement a policy of serving only healthy food items at functions of churches and synagogues. (Faith Communities) • Implement city policy requiring publicly-funded youth programming to use 15 percent of program time participating in physical activity. (Youth Organizations and Government)

Table 21.1 displays illustrative components and elements (by sector) that may define an emerging community intervention to prevent childhood obesity (Fawcett et al., 2005).

A Prospective Research Program for Studying Community-Level Prevention of Childhood Obesity

While providing direction for the activities of a community initiative, the Framework for Collaborative Public Health Action also suggests several key research questions for examining the effects of comprehensive community initiatives to prevent child and adolescent obesity. Such questions, and related research methods, can guide community-based participatory research (CBPR) to understand and improve such efforts (Fawcett, Schultz, Carson, Renault, & Francisco, 2003; Minkler & Wallerstein, 2003).

Research Question #1: Is the initiative serving as a catalyst for community/system change related to childhood obesity? This question can be addressed by examining evidence of community and system change (i.e., discrete instances of new or modified programs, policies, or practices) facilitated by the effort and related to the mission of preventing childhood obesity (Fawcett et al., 2000). (See Table 21.1 for nine illustrative instances of community/system change.) Documenting the number and type of community/system changes helps to examine the unfolding of the independent variable (the comprehensive intervention) over time. Community change can be viewed as a product of particular behaviors of group members; including planning, advocacy, organizing, and mobilizing community members to take action. A cumulative graph displaying the distribution of community/ system changes over time is particularly helpful in examining the question of whether an initiative is serving as a catalyst for change—that is, whether it is transforming the environment with intervention elements such as noted in Table 21.1. Based on earlier research with partnerships for healthy nutrition (e.g., Harris et al., 1997; Paine-Andrews et al., 1997), a hypothetical example of such a graph can be viewed in Figure 21.2.

The graph displays the cumulative total of changes in the environment facilitated by a hypothetical community initiative to prevent childhood obesity. When graphed as a cumulative record, each new change in the environment is added to all the prior ones to make salient the discontinuities in the rate of change. In a cumulative record, a marked increase in slope during a certain period of time reflects a higher rate of change; and a flatter line indicates a lower rate. Consistent with a CBPR process, researchers and community members should be regularly engaged in assessing whether the initiative is facilitating change in the environment consistent with the mission.

Research Question #2: What factors or processes are associated with the rate of community/ system change? The discontinuities (marked increases or decreases) identified in Question #1 present an opportunity to identify candidate factors that may have an impact on the rate of change. Candidate processes and factors associated with these discontinuities, such as hiring a community mobilizer, can be identified from reviews of

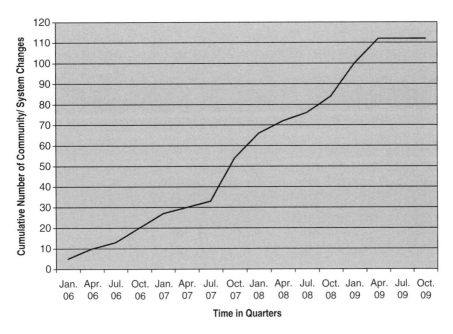

Figure 21.2. Hypothetical community partnership to prevent childhood obesity.

records or qualitative interviews with key informants who are part of the community health effort. Figure 21.2 displays data from a hypothetical community partnership to prevent childhood obesity. Several points of discontinuity and candidate factors (e.g., marked increases following action planning; marked decreases after loss of leadership) can be seen from these example data. As knowledge of best processes emerges, community efforts can use these mechanisms to enhance the rate of change—for instance, by renewing the action plan annually or by assuring the presence of community mobilizers to stimulate change efforts.

Research Question #3: How do the community/ system changes contribute to changes in population-level outcomes related to childhood obesity? Documentation of community and system changes should include a secondary analysis of characteristics that help to understand and enhance the type and potential penetration of the environmental changes. A secondary analysis might include coding of each community/ system change by: a) goal (i.e., physical activity, healthy nutrition), b) intensity of behavior change strategy (i.e., providing information, modifying access), c) duration (i.e., one-time event, more than once, and ongoing), d) sector (e.g., schools, business), e) prioritized population (e.g., preschool children, parents), and f) place of the event (i.e., neighborhood or school). Reflection on the distribution of community/system change can help initiative members to recognize how their activities may be contributing to improvement in population-level outcomes. For example, if members of a childhood obesity

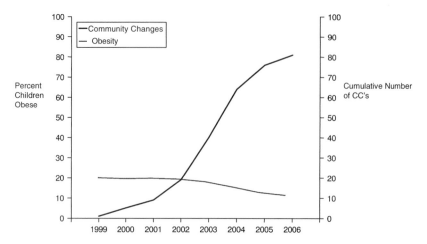

Figure 21.3. Hypothetical Association of community/System Changes with population-health Improvement.

initiative prioritize objectives related to both nutrition and physical activity, the distribution of the initiative's community changes should reflect this prioritization. If 85 percent of the changes are related to nutrition, the group can anticipate that indicators of population-level outcomes related to physical activity may not experience the same improvement as nutrition. Such systematic analysis of the contribution of community changes can be used by an initiative to see how to adjust the comprehensive intervention efforts to maximize improvement in population-level outcomes.

Research Question #4: Are the community/ system changes associated with improvements in population-level outcomes? Ongoing assessment of population-level outcomes (e.g., prevalence of overweight or obesity among children and adolescents) is critical to answering this question. Members of the initiative should consider whether the population-level indicators have changed since the onset of the community intervention. A method for examining whether the efforts of an initiative are associated with improvement in population-level outcomes is to overlay a graph displaying indicators of population-level outcomes with the unfolding of community changes over time. Although stronger experimental designs—such as RCTs or interrupted time series designs—are required to attribute cause and effect, examining possible associations of environmental change and improvement in population-level outcome can be instructive. If the display does not suggest an association, the initiative may consider how adjusting their efforts could increase the likelihood of population-level impact.

CONCLUSION AND DISCUSSION

The Framework for Collaborative Public Health Action suggests some opportunities to understand and improve community efforts to prevent childhood obesity. Despite the promise of comprehensive community approaches, there are many challenges to research and practice. First, study design choices are limited when the unit of analysis is the whole community (e.g., all children in a zip code). Although the widely-accepted standard of good design and randomized control trials (RCT) is beneficial in ruling out threats to internal validity, it may be less feasible and appropriate for evaluation of comprehensive community interventions. Some researchers (e.g., Victora, Habicht, & Bryce, 2004) argue that RCTs may have limited external validity because they may not capture the unique features of community interventions, including their multiple components and the complexity and variation of interventions in context. Additionally, Thompson, Coronado, Snipes, and Puschel (2003) make the case that RCTs are less effective in involving community members—a factor in assuring sustainability of the intervention. Alternative designs, such as an interrupted time series design with multiple communities, can be effective in determining the efficacy of community interventions (Biglan, Ary, & Wagenaar, 2000). Less expensive and more appropriate to the varied research questions guiding community interventions, interrupted time-series experiments involve two or more communities, the collection of common measures repeatedly over time, and the staggered implementation of the intervention in one community at a time.

A second research challenge is measuring the dose of an intervention received by members of the community being targeted, and determining which aspects of the intervention may have contributed to observed changes. Because community interventions are often *multi-faceted*, it is likely that not all of the facets of an intervention are received by all people in the community (Thompson et al., 2003). For instance, a particular group of children may be more (or less) likely to experience aspects of the community intervention—such as access to healthier foods or opportunities for physical activity—if these elements are more (or less) prominent in the particular schools, youth organizations, and neighborhoods they frequent. Obtaining estimates of the *dose* of the intervention—what intervention components and elements are actually experienced—is an important and difficult consideration in examining the impact of the community intervention for different groups.

Several advantages can be noted for using the collaborative framework related research questions. First, the focus of the model is on the intermediate outcome of community/system change (i.e., new or modified programs, policies, or practices), or how the environment is changing related to risk for childhood obesity. Improvements in population-level outcomes—such as reduced prevalence of obesity among children—may take several years or more to achieve. Focus on an intermediate outcome that documents (monthly) changes in the environment related to the reduced risk for childhood obesity may lead to more sustained efforts. Second, the iterative framework prompts users to consider whether outcomes (both intermediate and longer-term) are being met, and whether adjustments in the unfolding intervention are indicated. The iterative nature attempts to assure that targeted actions and interventions are grounded in an appropriate assessment and analysis of the problem. Third, the first few phases—from assessment to targeted action to environmental change— enable community members to build a foundation for their efforts. Often, the group may have a proposed solution, such as a training program for children in healthy food choices, but later has knowledge about the scope of the problem, for whom this is a particular problem, or the root causes of the problem (e.g., beyond information, to more influential environmental factors related to access, consequences, and policies). For population-level improvement, a single-intervention approach, such as a healthy food curriculum in one school, is less likely to be effective than a comprehensive intervention grounded in an assessment of the problem and the conditions that affect the problem.

Several recommendations for research emerge from these considerations about challenges in community efforts to prevent childhood obesity. First, the research question should guide the choice of research designs. For example, simple time-series designs involving empirical case studies—such as illustrated by Figures. 21.2 and 21.3—may be appropriate for pilot interventions in whole communities. However, if researchers are testing the efficacy of an established community intervention, a randomized control trial or a multiple time-series design across communities may be used to demonstrate a more convincing relationship between the comprehensive intervention and the population-level outcomes of interest.

Second, consistent with recommendations from the Institute of Medicine's report of progress on reducing childhood obesity (2007), research on comprehensive community interventions should collect multiple measures to monitor the effects of community interventions and develop evidence of their effectiveness. Documentation of community/system changes (i.e., the unfolding of program, policies, and practices) can help discern what elements of the intervention were actually implemented. Similarly, an analysis of contribution (i.e., amount of community changes by goal, behavior change strategy, etc.) can help estimate the anticipated dose of the intervention received by the priority population. Measurement of different population-level outcomes (e.g., prevalence of overweight and obesity, prevalence of related co-morbidities) may show the varied ways the intervention had an impact.

A third recommendation is to structure investigations to assure a long-enough period of intervention to effect longer-term outcomes. Outcomes related to obesity or chronic diseases often have a lengthy period over which they develop. Thus, multiyear studies will be required to capture changes in environments, widespread behaviors changes, and desired improvements in population-level outcomes. Finally, it is critical to engage those experiencing the problem—including children and adults—and those contributing to the problem (e.g., businesses, schools) in planning for how to solve the problem. This can be done by using a process of community-based participatory research (CBPR) framework (Fawcett, Boothroyd, et al., 2003).

With a CBPR framework, members of research institutions, community organizations, and those experiencing the problem can be equal partners in: a) developing the research questions, b) identifying the strategies used to address the problem, c) deciding what design and methods to use, and d) analyzing the results of community efforts. CBPR methods have the advantage of increased vested interest from community members in the effort, thereby increasing the likelihood of sustained, longer-term efforts to bring about key changes in communities and systems. They permit the coupling of specialized knowledge of outside experts—such as that regarding evidence-based interventions—with the experiential knowledge that community members bring. CBPR methods can also increase the validity of chosen intervention strategies and methods, such as when children and parents help to adapt community interventions to fit the local culture and context.

Several recommendations for practice can enhance community efforts to prevent childhood obesity. First, thorough assessments and analyses of the problem can help guide local efforts. For instance, an analysis of natural contingencies that maintain the behaviors of eating high-calorie or high-fat foods can provide a strong foundation for interventions that attempt to improve population-level outcomes. Should an analysis of the problem indicate that young children typically obtain unhealthy foods outside of the home, interventions to address parents' skills in selecting and preparing foods in the home may be less responsive to the situation. By contrast, the community intervention may focus on reducing access to unhealthy snacks and sampling of healthier food choices in daycare and other settings frequented by children. Further, an analysis of the problem can reveal promising channels of influence—for instance, to reach young children the key channels of influence may include daycare centers and preschools and parents' worksites. Among children ages 11–13, however, the key channels of influence may be peers, schools, and businesses such as convenience stores adjacent to schools.

Second, although many of the interventions reviewed attempted to reach everyone in the community (a universal approach), comprehensive community initiatives may consider using both universal and targeted approaches. Primary prevention of childhood obesity should be focused on the population in general, because all children are at risk. However, some more intensive efforts could profitably target those at particular risk for obesity (e.g., children with parents who are obese). Using both approaches may be beneficial since this may help assure the appropriate intensity needed for the population at large, and for those experiencing specific risk factors.

Third, community interventions should address the behavior of both proximate targets—those experiencing the problem (e.g., children who are overweight or obese), and thoses whose behavior may contribute to the problem (e.g., parents, youth organization leaders). Although many research studies focus only on school settings, an ecological approach would seek change in all of the contexts and environments in which children come in contact (Parcel, Green, & Bettes, 1988). Public health approaches are multisectoral; they engage members of all relevant sectors in developing and implementing elements of the intervention. It is important to identify key sectors and appropriate representatives from those sectors; including those interested in the issue and those able to leverage resources.

Childhood obesity is a significant public health problem, both globally and locally. The potentially damaging impact of childhood obesity on the lifelong health of millions of children and adults demands effective community interventions. Collaborative public health action would focus on creating environments that promote healthy behaviors—such as physical activity and healthy eating—that prevent the onset of overweight among children. To insure health-promoting environments, it will require hundreds of changes in the variety of settings in which children live, learn, and play—in their homes, schools, youth organizations, faith organizations, and neighborhoods. Using a framework for collaborative public health action can optimize the environments for obesity prevention among children and adolescents. Such systematic community-level efforts recognize our responsibility to the next generation—assuring the health and well-being of *all* our children.

ACKNOWLEDGEMENTS

We appreciate the consultation and feedback on this chapter from our colleagues, Valorie Carson and Terri Mathews, as well as the support of other KU Work Group colleagues in the development of this chapter.

REFERENCES

Andersen, R. E., Franckowiak, S. C., Snyder, J., Bartlett, S. J., & Fontaine, K. R. (1998). Can inexpensive signs encourage the use of stairs? Results from a community intervention. *Annals of Internal Medicine, 129*, 363–369.

Beech, B. M., Klesges, R. C., Kumanyika, S. K., Murray, D. M., Klesges, L., McClanahan, B., et al. (2003). Child- and parent-targeted interventions: The Memphis gems pilot study. *Ethnicity and Disease, 13*, S40–S53.

Biglan, A., Ary, D., & Wagenaar, A. C. (2000). The value of interrupted time-series experiments for community intervention research. *Prevention Science, 1*, 31–49.

Center for Disease Control and Prevention. (2002). Syndemics overview: What procedures are available for planning and evaluating initiatives to prevent syndemics? Retrieved February 24, 2004 from http://www.cdc.gov/syndemics

Cullen, K., Bartholomew, L., & Parcel, G. (1997). Girl scouting: An effective channel for nutrition education. *Journal of Nutrition Education, 92*, 86–91.

Dietz, W. H., & Gortmaker, S. L. (2001). Preventing obesity in children and adolescents. *Annual Review of Public Health, 22*, 337–353.

Fawcett, S. B., Boothroyd, R., Schultz, J. A., Francisco, V. T., Carson, V., & Bremby, R. (2003). Building capacity for participatory evaluation within community initiatives. *Journal of Prevention and Intervention in the Community, 26*, 21–36.

Fawcett, S. B., Carson, V. L., Lloyd, J., Collie-Akers, V. L., & Schultz, J. A. (2005). *Promoting healthy living and preventing chronic disease: An action planning guide for communities.* Lawrence, KS: University of Kansas.

Fawcett, S. B., Francisco, V. T., Hyra, D., Paine-Andrews, A., Schultz, J. A., Russos, S., et al. (2000). Building healthy communities. In A. Tarlov & R. S. Peters (Eds.), *Society and population health: A state perspective.* New York, NY: New Press.

Fawcett, S. B., Francisco, V. T., & Schultz, J. A. (2004). Understanding and improving the work of community health and development. In J. R. Burgos (Ed.), *Theory, basic and applied research, and technological applications in behavior science* (pp. 209–242). Guadalajara, Mexico: Universidad de Guadalajara.

Fawcett, S. B., Schultz, J. A., Carson, V., Renault, V., & Francisco, V. T. (2003). Using internet based tools to build capacity for community-based participatory research and other efforts to promote community health and development. In M. Minkler &

N. Wallerstein (Eds.), *Community-based participatory research for health* (pp. 155–178). San Francisco: Jossey-Bass.

French, S. A., Story, M., & Jeffery, R. W. (2001). Environmental influences on eating and physical activity. *Annual Review of Public Health, 22,* 309–335.

Gill, A. A., Veigl, V. L., Shuster, J. J., & Notelovitz, M. (1984). A well woman's health maintenance study comparing physical fitness and group support programs. *Occupational Therapy Journal of Research, 4,* 286–308.

Goodman, R. M., Steckler, A., Hoover, S., & Schwartz, R. (1993). A critique of contemporary community health promotion approaches: Based on a qualitative review of six programs in Maine. *American Journal of Health Promotion, 7,* 208–220.

Goran, M. I., Reynolds, K. D., & Lindquist, C. H. (1999). Role of physical activity in the prevention of obesity in children. *International Journal of Obesity and Related Metabolic Disorders, 23,* S18–S33.

Harris, K., Paine-Andrews, A., Richter, K., Lewis, R., Johnston, J., James, V., et al. (1997). Reducing elementary school children's risks for chronic diseases through school lunch modifications, nutrition education, and physical activity interventions. *Journal of Nutrition Education, 29,* 196–202.

Harvey-Berino, J., & Rourke, J. (2003). Obesity prevention in preschool native-american children: A pilot study using home visiting. *Obesity Research, 11,* 606–611.

Institute of Medicine. (2003). *The future of the public's health in the 21st century.* Washington, DC: The National Academies Press.

Institute of Medicine. (2005). *Preventing childhood obesity: Health in the balance.* Washington, DC: The National Academies Press.

Institute of Medicine. (2007). *Progress in preventing childhood obesity: How do we measure up?* Washington, DC: The National Academies Press.

Israel, B., Schultz, A., Parker, E., & Becker, A. (1998). Review of community-based research: Assessing partnership approaches to improve health. *Annual Review of Public Health, 19,* 173–202.

Jeffery, R. W., & French, S. A. (1998). Epidemic obesity in the United States: Are fast foods and television viewing contributing? *American Journal of Public Health, 88,* 277–280.

Johnston, J., Marmet, P. F., Coen, S., Fawcett, S. B., & Harris, K. J. (1996). Kansas lean: An effective coalition for nutrition education and dietary change. *Journal of Nutrition Education, 28,* 115–118.

Kahn, E. B., Ramsey, L. T., Brownson, R. C., Heath, G. W., Howze, E. H., Powell, K. E., et al. (2002). The effectiveness of interventions to increase physical activity. A systematic review. *American Journal of Preventive Medicine, 22,* 73–107.

Kerr, N. A., Yore, M. M., Ham, S. A., & Dietz, W. H. (2004). Increasing stair use in a worksite through environmental changes. *American Journal of Health Promotion, 18,* 312–315.

King, A. C., Taylor, C. B., Haskell, W. L., & Debusk, R. F. (1988). Strategies for increasing early adherence to and long-term maintenance of home-based exercise training in healthy middle-aged men and women. *American Journal of Cardiology, 61,* 628–632.

Kreuter, M. W., Lezin, N. A., & Young, L. A. (2000). Evaluating community-based collaborative mechanisms: Implications for practitioners. *Health Promotion Practice, 1,* 49–63.

Luepker, R. V., Murray, D. M., Jacobs, D. R., Jr., Mittelmark, M. B., Bracht, N., Carlaw, R., et al. (1994). Community education for cardiovascular disease prevention: Risk factor changes in the Minnesota heart health program. *American Journal of Public Health, 84,* 1383–1393.

Merzel, C., & D'Afflitti, J. (2003). Reconsidering community-based health promotion: Promise, performance, and potential. *American Journal of Public Health, 93,* 557–574.

Minkler, M., & Wallerstein, N. (2003). *Community-based participatory research for health.* San Francisco: Jossey-Bass.

Paine-Andrews, A., Francisco, V. T., Fawcett, S. B., Johnston, J., & Coen, S. (1996). Health marketing in the supermarket: Using prompting, product sampling, and price reduction to increase customer purchases of lower-fat items. *Health Marketing Quarterly, 14,* 85–99.

Paine-Andrews, A., Harris, K. J., Fawcett, S. B., Richter, K. P., Lewis, R. K., Francisco, V. T., et al. (1997). Evaluating a statewide partnership for reducing risks for chronic diseases. *Journal of Community Health, 22,* 343.

Parcel, G. S., Green, L. W., & Bettes, B. A. (1988). School-based programs to prevent or reduce obesity. In N. A. Krasnegor, G. D. Grave & N. Kretchmer (Eds.), *Childhood obesity: A biobehavioral perspective* (pp. 143–157). Caldwell, NJ: Telford Press.

Parsons, T. J., Power, C., Logan, S., & Summerbell, C. D. (1999). Childhood predictors of adult obesity: A systematic review. *International Journal of Obesity and Related Metabolic Disorders, 23,* S1–S107.

Ploeg, J., Dobbins, M., Hayward, S., Ciliska, D., Thomas, H., & Underwood, J. (1996). Effectiveness of community development projects. Retrieved May 16, 2002 from http://web.cche.net/ohcen/groups/hthu/95-5abs.htm

Robinson, T. N., Killen, J. D., Kraemer, H. C., Wilson, D. M., Matheson, D. M., Haskell, W. L., et al. (2003). Dance and reducing television viewing to prevent weight gain in African-American girls: The Stanford gems pilot study. *Ethnicity and Disease, 13,* S65–S77.

Rochon, J., Klesges, R. C., Story, M., Robinson, T. N., Baranowski, T., Obarzanek, E., et al. (2003). Common design elements of the girls health enrichment multi-site studies (gems). *Ethnicity and Disease, 13,* S6–S14.

Roussos, S. T., & Fawcett, S. B. (2000). A review of collaborative partnerships as a strategy for improving community health. *Annual Review of Public Health, 21,* 369–402.

Salbe, A. D., Weyer, C., Lindsay, R. S., Ravussin, E., & Tataranni, P. A. (2002). Assessing risk factors for obesity between childhood and adolescence: I. Birth weight, childhood adiposity, parental obesity, insulin, and leptin. *Pediatrics, 110,* 299–306.

Shortell, S. M., Zukoski, A. P., Alexander, J. A., Bazzoli, G. J., Conrad, D. A., Hasnain-Wynia, R., et al. (2002). Evaluating partnerships for community health improvement: Tracking the footprints. *Journal of Health Politics, Policy, and Law, 27,* 49–91.

Sorensen, G., Emmons, K., Hunt, M. K., & Johnston, D. (1998). Implications of the results of community intervention trials. *Annual Review of Public Health, 19,* 379–416.

Stolley, M. R., & Fitzgibbon, M. L. (1997). Effects of an obesity prevention program on the eating behavior of African American mothers and daughters. *Health Education and Behavior, 24,* 152–164.

Story, M., Sherwood, N. E., Himes, J. H., Davis, M., Jacobs, D. R., Jr., Cartwright, Y., et al. (2003). An after-school obesity prevention program for African-American girls: The Minnesota gems pilot study. *Ethnicity and Disease, 13,* S54–S64.

Summerbell, C. D., Waters, E., Edmunds, L. D., Kelly, S., Brown, T., & Campbell, K. J. (2005). Interventions for preventing obesity in children. *Cochrane Database Systematic Review, (3),* CD001871.

Task Force on Community Preventive Services. (2001). Increasing physical activity. A report on recommendations of the task force on community preventive services. *Morbidity and Mortality Weekly Reports Recommendations Report, 50,* 1–14.

Thompson, B., Coronado, G., Snipes, S. A., & Puschel, K. (2003). Methodologic advances and ongoing challenges in designing community-based health promotion programs. *Annual Review of Public Health, 24,* 315–340.

Victora, C. G., Habicht, J. P., & Bryce, J. (2004). Evidence-based public health: Moving beyond randomized trials. *American Journal of Public Health, 94*(3), 400–405.

Wang, Y., & Lobstein, T. (2006). Worldwide trends in childhood overweight and obesity. *International Journal of Pediatric Obesity, 1,* 11–25.

Section VI

Future Directions

22

The Role of Public Policy in Addressing the Pediatric Obesity Epidemic

PATRICIA B. CRAWFORD,
GAIL WOODWARD-LOPEZ, SUZANNE RAUZON,
LORRENE RITCHIE, and MAY C. WANG

It is widely believed that broad societal changes and major shifts in worldwide nutrition and physical activity are driving the current epidemic of obesity (World Health Organization, 2003). Prevention strategies based solely on individual and family responsibility for change will not be maximally effective and must be supported by broader-based environmental programs that provide a counterbalance to the societal trends that are contributing to escalating obesity rates. Environmental policy has a proven track record in public health amelioration efforts. The reduction in U.S. smoking rates is partially attributed to excise taxes and regulation, auto fatalities were reduced by seat belt laws and mandated airbags, and local restrictions on selling handguns have reduced gun-related violence and fatalities.

This chapter will discuss environmental forces contributing to the problem, and how a community-based policy approach plays a necessary role in the prevention of childhood overweight in the United States. A specific focus on environmental change within school systems will be examined through a case study of a school nutrition policy change at the state and local levels. Such a community-based approach can make use of public policy to address structural disparities and inequities in the distribution of open space, enhance opportunities for physical activity, and increase accessibility to a variety of high quality, nutritious foods that promote health.

PATRICIA B. CRAWFORD, GAIL WOODWARD-LOPEZ, SUZANNE RAUZON, LORRENE RITCHIE, and MAY C. WANG • University of California, Berkeley, CA 94720.

IS INDIVIDUAL CHANGE POSSIBLE IN AN UNSUPPORTIVE ENVIRONMENT?

The prevailing ideology in the United States is one of individualism. Our political and social systems are based upon a belief in the efficacy and importance of individual choice, individual freedom to act, and individual responsibility for one's choices and actions. And, to a great extent, our approaches to healthcare—including the treatment of obesity —have accepted this paradigm of individual responsibility, focusing on dieting advice, fitness coaching, and nutrition education messages that hold parents and children solely responsible for behavior change after the overweight problem has developed.

Social and economic forces, shaped by collective individual desires for safety, prosperity, and pleasure, have contributed to the unhealthy environment we live in today. However, if major causes of the acknowledged obesity epidemic have been environmental in nature, then it follows that a focus on broad-based environmental rather than individualistic responses is needed to effectively halt the epidemic. It is not productive, and may be counterproductive, to expect an individual child or family to change its behaviors within the context of a community milieu that is inhospitable to the healthier lifestyle required to achieve and maintain a normal weight.

Changes to the overall environment send powerful messages and create social conditions that can initiate readiness for individual change. External controls in the home, office, or school environment can reduce exposure to cues that encourage overeating and underactivity, and improve access to health-supporting foods and activities. For example, in the United States we spend 13 percent of our annual budgets on food—the third largest financial outlay behind housing and transportation (United States Department of Labor & Bureau of Labor Statistics 2003). Our desire for convenience and affordability, coupled with aggressive marketing and access to large *value* portion sizes where we live, work, and play results in the combination of motivation, opportunity, and encouragement to engage in behaviors counter to healthy weight maintenance. In the future, preferences are more likely to shift if calorie-dense, low-nutrient foods are less readily available or affordable, and fresh produce, whole grain products, low-fat protein sources, and other low-calorie, nutrient-rich foods are more easily accessible.

ENVIRONMENTAL CHANGE THROUGH PUBLIC POLICY

Developing an environmental approach to the prevention of obesity involves persuading policy makers to take steps to influence the environment or behavioral context in ways that are conducive to, and supportive of, individual change. There are many opportunities and examples of environmental policy change that can contribute to reducing the occurrence of childhood overweight. Influencing the direction of public spending on transportation, parks, or safety, for example, can impact the opportunities for movement, activity, and play among children. Farm subsidies can affect access to fresh foods and the integration of more variety into eating patterns. Zoning and planning policy can affect the number and location of fast food restaurants and can encourage spatial configurations conducive to walking. Legislation can be passed requiring fast food and chain restaurants to post point-of-purchase nutrition information such as caloric, fat, and sugar content on menus. Laws that limit food marketing and advertising of low-nutrient/high-calorie items aimed at children can be enacted. These and other initiatives are being debated in various jurisdictions throughout the country.

Public Policy Affecting the Food and Activity Environment

Public policy can be formulated at many levels—international, national, state, or local (in community settings, neighborhoods, or school districts). There are many examples of efforts under way at all of these levels to shape environments that increase both access to a variety of nutritious foods reasonable in portion size and caloric content, and opportunities for physical activity.

Internationally, the World Health Organization (WHO) has recognized the influence of world-wide changes in diet and physical activity; it has adopted wide-ranging recommendations for the prevention of noncommunicable diseases, such as chronic conditions that may result from a lifetime of overweight. The WHO Global Strategy on Diet, Physical Activity and Health contains several objectives to increase awareness of the effects of diet and exercise, support the development of multilevel policies in many sectors of society, and establish monitoring and evaluation efforts in this area (WHO, 2003).

The lives of individuals, including their weight, are impacted by a multitude of national and state-level policy decisions regarding funding in areas, for example, of transportation, parks, public safety, school lunch programs, and farm subsidies (Dorfman, Wilbur, Lingas, Woodruff, & Wallack, 2005). One of the earliest U.S. national initiatives to prevent obesity, emanating from the 1969 White House Conference on Food, Nutrition and Health, recommended the promotion of physical activity, expansion of school physical education programs, development of community recreation facilities, and implementation of a mass media activity campaign. Since then, the Public Health Service has initiated a system of issuing 10-year health goals for the nation entitled "Healthy People Goals." While these goals emphasize regular exercise, good nutrition, and the need to reduce the prevalence of obesity, they provide little in the way of specific programmatic steps or funding to operationalize the goals.

In 2004, President George W. Bush signed the Child Nutrition and Women, Infant, and Children (WIC) Reauthorization Act into law, with the goal of creating an appropriate balance between encouraging healthy environments to address the childhood obesity epidemic while preserving local control for states, communities, and schools (Committee on Education and Workforce, 2004). The Act requires that local wellness policies be developed in school districts participating in the National School Lunch Program, affecting the majority of public schools in the country. This broad-reaching law will result in schools across the country setting goals for nutrition education and physical activity, establishing nutrition guidelines for foods served on campus, monitoring their wellness activities, and involving the community in policy development. This poses an opportunity for health professionals to become involved in local efforts to participate in environmental prevention efforts to reduce childhood overweight.

Schools: An Ideal Focus for Environmental Change

On the local level, schools are prime areas for local policy impacting the development of childhood overweight. Schools are generally responsive to the communities they serve and are a primary source of modeling and care for children outside the home. Increasing and improving physical education, and improving the nutritional content of foods served on campus have been the main goals of local policy initiatives to date.

During the last several years, the strongest antiobesity environmental focus has been to change individual behavior through modifying institutional practices within the schools. The concentrated effort on school policy change developed, in part, because children spend many hours in school each weekday, in a standardized environment that encompasses all children (overweight, normal weight, and underweight alike). Relatively easy access to such a controlled environment, to which children are exposed regularly, provides an excellent opportunity to influence behaviors that play a role in energy imbalance and contribute to increased rates of overweight among children.

School Nutrition and Related Policies. More than half of U.S. youth eat one of their three major daily meals in school, and more than 10 percent eat two of their three main meals there (Dwyer, 1995). Schools further influence students' eating patterns by what is or is not taught in the classroom, and by what is or is not sold and promoted on campus. With their mandate to educate and care for children during an extended part of each weekday, schools are well-suited to take steps to improve the healthfulness of the foods served on campus. First, foods that foster poor nutritional health can be removed. Second, nutritious and appetizing foods can become more widely available for consumption.

Schools can influence students' eating patterns by setting criteria, including nutritional guidelines, for what can be sold and promoted on campus (Centers for Disease Control and Prevention, 1996). Health advocates have targeted items sold in vending machines, snack bars and carts because most of these foods and beverages are not subject to USDA regulation and tend to consist primarily of sweetened beverages and high-fat and/or sugar snack foods (U.S. Department of Agriculture, 2002). According to the United States General Accounting Office (2003), 43 percent of elementary schools, 74 percent of middle schools, and 98 percent of high schools have vending machines, school snack bars, and/or other food services outside of the school lunch and breakfast programs. The National Dairy Council (2004) found that 71 percent of schools surveyed allow students to use vending machines or to purchase minimal nutritional value foods via snack bars and other a la carte sales during the lunch period. A study of 251 schools in 24 states found that

75 percent of beverages and 85 percent of food options in school vending machines were of poor nutritional quality (Center for Science in the Public Interest, 2004).

School food service departments in the United States are caught between the competing responsibilities of serving children nutritious foods and running a fiscally solvent food service business. School food services are typically required to be self-supporting—they do not usually receive subsidies from the school general fund. They do receive a federal reimbursement through the USDA School Lunch and Breakfast programs, but this is usually insufficient to cover the actual costs of feeding children. The rates of reimbursement may be adjusted each year, and vary in some states, but generally are 22–30 cents for a full-price lunch, 1.92–2.09 dollars for a reduced price meal, and 2.32–2.49 dollars for a free meal provided to children based on income eligibility (USDA, 2005). Consequently, many school food service departments in the United States rely heavily on sales of unregulated foods—foods sold a la carte to generate the additional income needed to offset the inadequate federal and state reimbursement received (Fox, Crepinsek, Conner, & Battaglia, 2001; Vargas, Woodward-Lopez, Kim, & Crawford, 2005; Woodward-Lopez, Vargas, et al., 2005). A study of 16 middle and high schools in California found that a la carte sales accounted for an average of 31 percent of food service department revenues (range of 3.5 to 66%) (Woodward-Lopez, Vargas, et al.). Twelve other school districts reported that a la carte sales accounted for 25 to 80 percent of their food service department's operating budget (Vargas et al.; Woodward-Lopez, Kim, et al., 2005).

Additional school-based groups, such as special training programs, athletic departments, and associated student bodies, have come to depend upon the sales of unregulated foods and beverages to support their programs (Vargas et al., 2005; Woodward-Lopez, 2004; Woodward-Lopez, Kim, et al., 2005; Woodward-Lopez, Vargas et al., 2005). These so-called *competitive* foods typically compete with the meal service, further reducing school revenues from meal reimbursement (Vargas et al.; Woodward-Lopez, Kim, et al.; Woodward-Lopez, Vargas, et al.). These foods are also commonly high in fat, sugar, sodium, and calories, and low in nutritional value (California Center for Public Health Advocacy, 2002). Schools across the nation have come to rely heavily on the sale of sweetened beverages and foods such as pizza, cookies, candy, chips, and french fries (CCPHA; California State Legislature, 2003). However, a USDA analysis of dietary intake data for children who ate meals provided by the National School Lunch Program (NSLP) demonstrated that they had higher intakes of vegetables, milk and other dairy products, protein-rich foods and many nutrients, and lower intakes of added sugars than children who did not eat the NSLP meals (Gleason & Suitor, 2001).

Several programs demonstrate promising nutrition policy changes that do not negatively impact school food service revenues. Studies have shown that when snack foods and highly sweetened beverages have been limited on school campuses, students choose healthier options if they are available. In San Diego, California (2001), the Vista Unified School District installed 17 vending machines selling healthy food and beverage choices, including granola bars, juice, and milk, as part of a pilot program to improve student health. Despite the fact that soda was still sold on campus, the new vending machines were profitable and provided an additional $15,000 in commissions for the school district—a 67 percent increase over *soda only* sales (LaFee, 2003). At the Folsom Cordova Unified School District in Sacramento County, California, high school lunch sales skyrocketed when the district food service director substituted low-fat salads, teriyaki chicken, sushi rolls, and sandwiches for burgers, pizzas, and soda. Sales at two high schools actually increased from 85 and 125 school lunches sold to 700 and 800, respectively (LaFee). Also in California, the 16 middle and high schools that participated in the pilot testing of nutrition standards for competitive foods as specified in SB 19 found that students began eating more meals and fewer competitive foods, to the financial benefit of school food service departments (Woodward-Lopez, Vargas, et al., 2005). Similar trends were reported or observed in other studies (McCarthy, 2006; Vargas et al., 2005; Woodward-Lopez, Kim, et al., 2005).

Internationally, efforts are also taking place to make environmental policy changes at the school level. A report of a study in Great Britain indicated that schools that removed soda machines were extremely effective in reducing obesity among school children (Press conference, Associated Press, 2004). Many communities in Canada have taken action that resulted in the removal of high-caloric carbonated drinks in elementary and middle schools (Reuters, 2004). In France, the Parliament voted to ban all vending machines that sell candy and soft drinks in schools (de Pommereau, 2004).

School Physical Education and Related Policies. Supporters of change in school physical education (PE) feel that the moderate amount of activity needed for health benefits could easily be accommodated in school physical education classes (Cline, Spradlin, & Plucker, 2005). Schools today provide one of the few supervised locations where children can be physically active. Research has demonstrated that daily physical education at school can significantly reduce overweight and improve cardiovascular fitness (U.S. Department of Health and Human Services, 1996). One recent report concluded that adding one hour per week of physical education time for first-graders could significantly reduce body mass index (BMI) for overweight and at-risk-for-overweight girls (National Institute Health Care Management Foundation, 2004). The Centers for Disease Control and Prevention also states that physical activity does not need to be strenuous to be beneficial. Even brisk walking is a recommended mode of increasing physical activity. The impact of having schools promote physical activity would be substantial, because most children between the ages of six and sixteen attend school and would thus benefit from such a policy (DHHS).

Reduced opportunities for physical activity outside of school make restoration of daily physical activities in school a high priority. Some states require daily PE in elementary schools, but requirements in virtually all states decline at the high school level. Until recently, students in most states had to take a year or two of PE in high school to graduate.

However, Minnesota does not mandate any number of credits to graduate, and a new Florida law allows high school students to graduate in three years by skipping PE and some electives (National Association for Sport and Physical Education and American Heart Association, 2006). Roughly one-third of all high schools give students another out—if they participate in band, cheerleading, school sports teams, or similar activities, they are exempt from physical education.

Illinois is currently the only state to mandate daily PE from kindergarten through 12th grade. However, physical education classes are not a certainty, even in Illinois. A recent survey estimated that fewer than 10 percent of the state's elementary schools comply with the law. Even California's relatively tough requirements—whereby elementary schools must offer an average of 20 minutes of PE per day, middle and high schools must offer an average of 40 minutes per day, and high school students must take PE for two years to graduate—have produced disappointing results. Only 27 percent of the state's fifth-, seventh- and ninth-graders met minimal physical fitness standards in the 2004/05 school year, and it is widely acknowledged that few elementary schools comply with the state's minimum requirements due to competing priorities and lack of qualified staff (Vargas et al., 2005; Woodward-Lopez, 2004; Woodward-Lopez, Kim, et al., 2005). Clearly, more efforts are needed.

Mandated student-teacher ratios for PE classes can minimize the number of students standing on the sidelines for extended periods waiting their turn, resulting in an increase in student participation in activities. The optimal staffing level is reported to be lower than 25 to 1 (DiMassa, 2003). However, currently, in California, the average student-teacher ratio is 43 to 1. In Los Angeles, classes average 55 to 65 students per class, with some gym classes exceeding 70 students per teacher.

Suggested policy changes to improve school physical education opportunities for students include:

- Enact and enforce policies requiring physical education for all students (grades K–12).
- Provide monitoring, incentives, and support for compliance with existing requirements, especially at the elementary level.
- Increase active participation by all students in physical education classes.
- Establish joint-use agreements to increase access to community-based spaces for physical activity during the school day and access to school facilities after school hours.
- Increase funding for school physical education programs to decrease physical education class size; improve curricula, facilities and equipment; and provide teacher training and support.

Examples of State and Local School Policy Initiatives

Physical Education. Some state governments have implemented innovative new school policies. With the goal of promoting students' physical well-being, Massachusetts now requires PE at all grade levels (Byrne, 2003).

Other states, such as Georgia, have created committees to study physical education within their schools (Carl Vinson Institute of Government, 2005). Forty-eight states continue to require physical education in schools, but the scope of the requirement varies. In 2005, 35 states considered legislation related to physical activity or physical education in schools, and at least eight of those states enacted legislation, including Arizona, Colorado, Kansas, Kentucky, Louisiana, Montana, South Carolina, and Texas.

Some states have focused on refining or increasing physical education requirements or encouraging positive physical activity programs for students during and after the school day. Both the cost of physical education programs and an emphasis on academics are perceived barriers to increasing physical education in schools. Connecticut enacted legislation in 2005 to require a daily recess period to encourage physical activity by school children without incurring additional costs for physical education programs. Recognition is growing that physical activity during the school day is feasible and may even contribute to an increase in student achievement.

Nutrition. There are encouraging signs that significant changes are being attempted to modify the school food environment. The last five years have seen dramatic increases in school nutrition legislation. In 2001 and 2002, three states passed legislation related to nutrition education, school nutrition policy, and the school food environment. Ten states passed similar legislation in 2003, twelve in 2004, and twenty-six in 2005. During this five-year period, a total of 31 states passed one or more pieces of legislation related to school food. Twenty-four of the states passed legislation mandating or regulating school food standards or policies. Seventeen of the states passed legislation on nutrition education. Twelve states passed legislation to prohibit or limit unhealthy foods. Fewer states passed legislation to promote healthy foods or to restrict vending contracts.

Kentucky enacted the most expansive piece of school nutrition and physical education legislation to date in 2005. In addition to strict food and beverage standards, it calls for penalties to be assessed if any school violates the standards, in the following manner:

- For the first violation, a fine of no less than one week's revenue from the sale of competitive food.
- For subsequent violations, a fine of at least one month's revenue from the sale of competitive food.
- For "habitual violations," defined as more than five violations within a six-month period, a six-month ban on competitive food sales.
- Money collected from these fines will be transferred to the local school district's food service fund.

The Education Department of West Virginia, a state with an especially high rate of obesity, implemented statewide nutrition standards prohibiting the sale in schools of foods that are more than 40 percent sugar by weight, and all fruit juice drinks that contain less than 20 percent real fruit juice. In addition, all other foods available on West Virginia campuses must contain fewer than eight grams of fat per one-ounce serving (West Virginia Department of Education, 2004).

Many local school districts are also taking the initiative to establish nutrition policies. In 2002, the Los Angeles Unified School District took the lead by voting to ban all soft drinks from all schools in the district—schools may only provide water, milk, beverages that contain at least 50 percent juice and no added sweeteners, and sports drinks with less than 42 grams of added sweetener per 20 ounces (Samuels, Craypo, Boyle, Stone-Francisco, & Schwarte, 2006). Also in 2002, the Oakland Unified School District voted to ban all soft drinks and other highly sweetened beverages, as well as candy, from their campuses. Many other school districts across California have developed and implemented similar nutrition policies (Woodward-Lopez, 2004; Vargas et al., 2005; Woodward-Lopez, Kim, et al., 2005; Woodward-Lopez et al., 2006).

The Impact of School Environmental Change: A Case Study Evaluating California School Legislation

Background. The state of California led the nation in initiating legislative changes in the school environment. Table 22.1 outlines the numerous bills concerning school nutrition that have been introduced or passed in California since 2001. Initially, the California legislature passed (but did not fund) Senate Bills 19 and 56, establishing nutrition standards for *competitive* foods and beverages (categorized as *snacks*) sold at public schools outside

Table 22.1. California legislation addressing school a la carte foods and beverages

Year	Title	Description	Status
2001	SB 19 and SB 56: The Pupil Nutrition, Health, and Achievement Act of 2001	Set minimum nutrition standards for a la carte foods and beverages sold in elementary and middle schools. State to give each school 10 cents reimbursement per meal served.	Passed and signed into law by the Governor but never implemented as funding resources not available.
2003	SB 677	Set nutrition standards for beverages sold in elementary and middle schools, essentially eliminated soda sales.	Passed and went into effect in July 2004.
2004	SB 1566	Set nutrition standards (same as SB 19) for a la carte foods sold in elementary and middle schools.	Defeated.
2005	SB 12	Set nutrition standards (same as SB 19) for a la carte foods sold in schools K–12. No funding requirements included.	Passed and signed into law by the Governor.
2005	SB 965	Extended the ban on the sale of soda and other sweetened beverages to include high schools.	Passed and signed into law by the Governor.
2005	SB 281	Provided a framework to implement the $18.2 million in the Governor's budget to include more fresh fruits and vegetables in school meal programs.	Passed and signed into law by the Governor.

of the federally reimbursed school meal program. Subsequently, several bills were passed that built upon and strengthened this early legislation, resulting in some of the most comprehensive and stringent legislation of this type in the country.

In the same year that SB 19 and SB 56 were passed, a program called Linking Education, Activity, and Food (LEAF) was created, and $4 million in funding was provided to support a 21-month pilot project to test the feasibility of SB 19 and SB 56 in 16 middle and high schools located in nine demographically varied California school districts. Six reports detailing the findings are available in full at www.cnr.berkeley.edu/cwh/activities/LEAF.shtml#eval. The LEAF program evaluation results demonstrate how an environmental approach can have a positive effect on the nutritional habits of children, while balancing established school interests and shaping change through institutionally acceptable methods. The following is a summary of findings from the LEAF program evaluation.

Nutrient Standard, Advisory Council and Nutrition/Physical Activity Policy Implementation. Of the 16 schools involved in the LEAF pilot study, 15 achieved complete or near-complete campus-wide compliance with the new 2001 nutrition standards for competitive foods and beverages. School meal services were improved by increased variety and appeal of healthy options, as well as by modifications in the cafeteria environment. The number of points of service was increased, reducing students' wait time for meals. This is particularly important because meal service time has been reduced over the years in favor of increasing classroom time. The majority of districts assembled diverse and well-represented Child Nutrition and Physical Activity Advisory Councils. All nine participating districts successfully adopted nutrition policies and all but one adopted physical activity policies. Most of the LEAF schools created additional nutrition education classes or enhanced existing ones. In addition, many LEAF schools built or renovated campus fitness centers, weight rooms, or similar facilities and equipment. New activities were added to some of the PE classes.

Impact on attitudes and behaviors. The primary behavioral change was increased student participation in the meal program, as measured by school meal participation rates maintained by food service personnel. The purchase of competitive foods and beverages decreased due to reduced access. Students' understanding of the importance of physical activity increased, although their activity levels did not appear to change. Conversely, students' nutrition behavior did improve, even though their level of knowledge did not increase. Most teachers, parents, and students agreed on the need for fresh foods, increased variety, and sufficient quantity to satisfy student demand. However, many parents and students remained dissatisfied with menu offerings, cafeteria ambience, and the brevity of meal periods. Teachers were more likely than parents to support nutrition restrictions on competitive foods, and to recognize the school's role in supporting healthy eating.

Impact on Food and Beverage Sales. The most significant initial barrier to policy implementation was the perception that there would be a loss of revenue from food and beverage sales. However, even though schools' food services saw a decrease in student purchase of foods and beverages sold a la carte, there was a concomitant increase in school meal purchases. These reported gains appeared to result from three factors: 1) improved variety and appeal of meals, 2) improved attractiveness and efficiency of dining areas, and 3) reduced appeal of and access to competitive foods and beverages. Some higher meal service costs were reported and were associated primarily with menu changes, such as increased fresh produce, rather than with SB 19 compliance, per se. Although, in most cases, the sales gain experienced by food services from meals was at the expense of the other venues (such as vending machines and student stores), at two schools these other venues *also* experienced increases in sales. In both these schools, the other venues made changes similar to those in food services, demonstrating that nutrient guidelines such as those in SB 19 can result in an increased revenue flow for both meal services and other venues when there is a concerted effort to provide and promote high quality items that appeal to students.

Lessons Learned in California: Key Steps to Change in the Nutrition Environment in Schools

The evaluation of the LEAF program, which piloted early legislation to change the school environment in California, reveals the potential for this approach and provides insight into the important steps that health professionals, policy advocates, and community groups can take. LEAF findings were substantiated by other findings from studies conducted in California over a similar time period (Crawford, 2006; McCarthy, 2006; Samuels et al., 2006; Vargas et al., 2005; Woodward-Lopez, 2004; Woodward-Lopez, Kim, et al., 2005). These findings point to the following seven steps as important ingredients in a successful environmental change:

Step 1: Find a champion. A single individual or champion of the policy was instrumental in convincing key district leaders to support the new policy. This person was either a school board member, a food service director, a parent, or a district level administrator whose desire to pass the new policy stemmed from a strong personal interest in the health of the district's children.

Step 2: Build a strong base of school district (internal) support; form a Child Nutrition and Physical Activity Advisory Council. Child Nutrition and Physical Activity Advisory Councils (CNPAACs) were the most common means by which key stakeholders were brought into the process. The CNPAAC also serves as a vehicle for ensuring the issues stay on the front burner.

Support from key internal (school-based) stakeholder groups—such as school administrators, school food service personnel, and program advisors—involved in the sale of foods and beverages is essential. Parents and community groups can be especially important when internal stakeholders are not readily on board. Once school administration and school food service personnel are on board, resistance from other stakeholders is usually easily addressed. Educational efforts for the wider community, parents, and students help garner support for the policy and ensure its successful passage and implementation.

Step 3: Gather data, conduct a pilot, and devise a local policy. Presenting data and convincing research to the school board and other stakeholders was essential to passing a school district nutrition policy. Compelling data on the health consequences of dietary practices and physical activity levels, the weight and fitness status of a district's students, and information on rates of childhood obesity, diabetes, and other associated health problems were instrumental in gaining support for a district nutrition policy. Data specific to a district's student population, such as BMI, fitness test results, or dietary intake studies was especially compelling to school opinion leaders. Many school districts found that the process of conducting an assessment of their schools' nutrition and physical activity environment was very useful because it helped get everyone on the same page and provided an objective basis for establishing policy priorities. Several school districts first piloted the nutrient standards at one or two schools in the district. The data from these pilots, especially the data on school food sales, was used to convince school board members of the feasibility of implementing a district-wide nutrition policy. Evidence of the success of the pilot program was instrumental in the school board's decision to pass the policy.

Step 4: Address the budgetary concerns of students, parents, and administrators. School districts are concerned about changes that may be costly to the school district. Many student- and parent-run school groups rely on sales of calorie-dense, low-nutrient foods to support student activities and sports teams. School food services worry that changing foods and beverages will negatively impact their sales—a worry based on the fear that students will not buy the healthier foods and beverages. Some schools have addressed these concerns by conducting small, short-term changes and evaluating the impacts on sales and other operating costs. Almost all stakeholders felt it was important to make changes slowly, in a stepwise fashion, to allow time for adjustment to shifts in revenues and expenditures as well as adjustments in student preferences. Throughout the process, it is important to monitor sales and operating costs using standardized accounting practices so that decisions are based on accurate data. Alternative, nonfood fundraisers should be considered to meet the financial needs of school-based programs. Student involvement in the selection and promotion of healthy options is critical for ensuring adequate sales.

Step 5: Identify and address students' concerns; involve them in the change process. According to stakeholders, student resistance to changes in nutrition and physical activity policies varied greatly, ranging from no resistance at all to highly vocal concern, and even temporary boycotts. The majority of stakeholders felt that student resistance was temporary, and could be overcome by keeping them informed and involved. Some students were concerned about loss of their favorite foods or beverages and others were primarily concerned about loss of funding for their favorite programs and clubs. It is vital to conduct interviews or sessions with students to learn what their perceptions are and address their concerns and interests before a change takes place. Involving students or student leadership groups in the change is also important.

Step 6: Enlist support from key individuals throughout the school community. School districts have found that winning support from students, parents, teachers, and board members helped to pass a policy and get it implemented smoothly. Without the support of influential individuals, strong opposition to policies can arise from well-meaning parents and students voicing concerns about *freedom of choice* rights, or expressing the belief that it is the role of the home and not the school to address health behaviors. They may also spread the perception that new policies will negatively impact school clubs, teams, and food services operations. Engaging key supporters throughout the school community early in the process of change can prevent policies from being undermined.

Step 7: Use media coverage, legislative efforts, and advocacy efforts to raise awareness and influence support. National media coverage of the childhood obesity epidemic, including stories of the school's role in feeding children and providing nutrition education, pressured school decision-makers to take action, particularly in the Hemet, Oakland, Los Angeles, and San Francisco unified school districts. An analysis of the media coverage surrounding the passage of the policies in Los Angeles and Oakland (Lingas & Dorfman, 2005) found that important strategies for advocates included focusing on a few key points related to the policy, understanding the opposition to the policy, and creating—as well as responding to—news. Likewise, the passage of state legislation (e.g., SB 19 and SB 677 in California) motivated school districts to pass and implement or even enact their own local food and beverage policies that were broader than the bills themselves, before these new laws went into effect. In Los Angeles, San Francisco, and Oakland, strong grassroots community organizing, complemented by the policy expertise of statewide advocacy groups, helped garner local support for district policies. A number of community members, including parents, played essential roles in the passage and implementation of the district policies.

Factors That Sustain School Environmental Change Policies

The success of a health policy that makes changes to our environment relies to a great extent on continued monitoring and enforcement. Clear public support for a policy and sufficient resource appropriation are crucial for sustained, successful policy implementation. In the San Francisco Unified School District, for example, parents were deeply involved in committees that were instrumental in developing the district nutrient standards. Even after the standards were developed, the committees continued to meet, addressed barriers, and monitored compliance. In the Los Angeles Unified School District, following a clear mandate from the school board, administrators in the district oversaw the implementation and continued adherence to the policy. The policy was monitored and reported on annually. In the Hemet Unified School District, resources were allocated by the beverage vending company to help the district transition the beverages sold on school campuses.

In contrast, some schools or districts that did not have plans to sustain the changes felt it was not feasible to continue changes without additional external funding. Other districts discovered that the school community stakeholders had not been engaged in policy development, passage, and implementation, and felt that without this engagement it would not be possible to sustain the changes. Stakeholders from many districts felt that long-term sustainability was dependent upon local monitoring and enforcement, complemented by monitoring and enforcement at the state level. Administrators, in particular, felt that those issues for which they are accountable to the state tend to become top priorities (Woodward-Lopez et al., 2006). State-level involvement also serves to *level the playing field* so that no one district, school, or department within a school feels it is experiencing an undue burden. State-level accountability also helps ensure sustainability by reducing the dependency of policy adherence on a few charismatic individuals who championed the policy.

SUMMARY

Addressing the problem of childhood overweight through changes in the environment can be effective, as evidenced by successes of school districts that have implemented environmental policy changes. This approach can be an important component to establishing healthful changes in social norms. Future steps to link health education in schools with environmental school policy changes will likely increase the effectiveness of these efforts.

Policy changes in the areas of nutrition and physical activity to prevent overweight are increasingly occurring in the school setting. Passage of the National Child Nutrition and WIC Reauthorization Act of 2004 has ensured continued effort and new opportunities for health professionals to become involved in this area. Through this bill, Congress established a *requirement* that any school district receiving federal funding for school meals must develop and implement a *wellness policy* addressing nutrition and physical activity by autumn of 2006. This regulation ensures that *all* schools establish nutrition guidelines for *all* foods served on school campuses.

An understanding of the impact of environmental policy is urgently needed to provide policy-makers with information on successful strategies that improve feasibility, acceptability, and effectiveness of short-term goals, and enhance the sustainability of these efforts. The contributions of long-term policy changes to reducing the child obesity epidemic will take years to materialize. In the meantime, provision of healthful environments optimal for support and learning is a worthy goal. No one can argue that children should go to school with an environment that is antagonistic to making healthy choices. If we know what a healthful food and activity environment is for children, it is indefensible not to provide it in our societal institutions for them. Children must not be held solely responsible for making food and activity choices that will have detrimental effects on their future health.

REFERENCES

Associated Press. (2004, April 23). Schools that can soda cut obesity. *CBSNEWS.com.* Retrieved September 21, 2006 from www.cbsnews.com/stories/2004/04/23/health/main613336.shtml

Byrne, D. (2003). *Physical education. 2003 Health Policy Tracking Service, National Conference of State Legislatures,* 1–22. Falls Church, VA: Netscan.

California Center for Public Health Advocacy (CCPHA). (2002). National Consensus Panel on School Nutrition: Recommendations for competitive food standards in California schools. Davis, CA. Retrieved September 21, 2006 from http://www.publichealthadvocacy.org/PDFs/school_food_stan_pdfs/standards.pdf

California State Legislature. (2003, February). Senate Bill No. 677: Introduced February 21, 2003. Retrieved September 21, 2006 from http://info.sen.ca.gov/pub/03-04/bill/sen/sb_0651-0700/sb_677_bill_20030917_chaptered.html

Carl Vinson Institute of Government. (2005). Peach State Poll – October 21, 2005: Public opinions on obesity and possible policy options to address childhood obesity. Retrieved September 21, 2006 from www.cviog.uga.edu/peachpoll/2005-10-21.pdf

Center for Science in the Public Interest (CSPI). (2004). *Dispensing junk: How school vending undermines efforts to feed children well.* Washington, DC: CSPI.

Centers for Disease Control and Prevention (CDC). (1996). Guidelines for school health programs to promote lifelong healthy eating. *Morbidity and Mortality Weekly Report, 45*(RR-9). Retrieved September 21, 2006 from http://www.cdc.gov/mmwr/preview/mmwrhtml/00042446.htm

Cline, K. P., Spradlin, T. E., & Plucker, J. A. (2005). Child obesity in Indiana: A growing public policy concern. *Center for Evaluation & Education Policy: Education Policy Brief, 3(1).*

Committee on Education and Workforce. (2004). Child nutrition and WIC Reauthorization Act. Retrieved September 21, 2006 from http://edworkforce.house.gov/issues/108th/education/childnutrition/billsummaryfinal.htm

Crawford, P. B. (2006). *Soda out of schools study (SOS).* Center for Weight and Health, University of California, Berkeley, and Samuels and Associates (preliminary findings).

de Pommereau, I. (2004). French schools' new bête noire: Vending machines. *The Christian Science Monitor.* Retrieved September 21, 2006 from www.csmonitor.com/2004/1008/p01s02-woeu.html

DiMassa, C. M. (2003, November 19). Campus crowding can make P.E. a challenge, *L. A. Times,* B.2.

Dorfman, L., Wilbur, P., Lingas, E., Woodruff, K., Wallack, L. (2005). Accelerating policy on nutrition: Extracting lessons from tobacco alcohol, firearms, and traffic safety. *Berkeley Media Studies Group,* March 2005. Retrieved September 21, 2006 from www.bmsg.org/pdfs/BMSG_AccelerationReport.pdf

Dwyer, J. (1995). The school nutrition dietary assessment study. *American Journal of Clinical Nutrition,* 61(Suppl 1), 173S–177S.

Fox, M. K., Crepinsek, M. K., Conner, P., & Battaglia, M. (2001). *School nutrition dietary assessment study II: Final report.* Alexandria, VA: U.S. Department of Agriculture, Food and Nutrition Service, Special Nutrition Programs Report No. CN-01-SNDAI-IFR. Retrieved September 21, 2006 from http://www.fns.usda.gov/oane/MENU/Published/CNP/FILES/SNDAIIfindsum.htm

Gleason, P., & Suitor, C. (2001, March). *Food for thought: Children's diets in the 1990s.* Princeton, NJ: Mathematica Policy Research. Document No. PR01-12. Retrieved September 21, 2006 from http://www.mathematica-mpr.com/publications/PDFs/childdiet.pdf

LaFee, S. (2003). Healthy choices, healthy budgets: California schools find ways to bolster the lunch line bottom line. *California Schools,* 61(4), 16–20, 42, 48.

Lingas, E. O., & Dorfman, L. (2005). Obesity crisis or soda scapegoat? The debate over selling soda in schools. *Berkeley Media Studies Group,* Issue 15. Retrieved September 21, 2006 from www.bmsg.org/pdfs/Issue15.pdf

McCarthy, W. (2006). *Evaluation of SB 19 Pupil Nutrition Act (SB, 19).* WestEd, University of California, Los Angeles, Center for Weight and Health, University of California, Berkeley, and Samuels and Associates (preliminary findings).

National Association for Sport and Physical Education (NASPE) and American Heart Association (May, 2006). *Shape of the nation.* Retrieved September 21, 2006 from www.aahperd.org/naspe/shape of the nation.

National Dairy Council. (2004). *Creating a healthy school environment for children.* Retrieved September 21, 2006 from http://www.nationaldairycouncil.org/ NationalDairyCouncil/Health/Digest/dcd73-6Page1.htm

National Institute for Health Care Management (NIHCM) Foundation. (2004). Obesity in young children: Impact and intervention. *Research brief.* Washington, DC: NHIHCM.

Reuters. (2004, January 7). Soda gets the axe in Canada school crackdown. *CNN.com.* Retrieved September 21, 2006 from www.cnn.com/2004/EDUCATION/01/07/ canada.sodas.reut

Samuels, S., Craypo, L., Boyle, M., Stone-Francisco, S., & Schwarte, L. (2006). Improving school food environments through district level policies: Findings from Six California Case Studies. Samuels and Associates, Oakland, CA. Prepared for California Endowment and Robert Wood Johnson Foundation. Retrieved February 8, 2008 from www.calendow.org/collection_publications.aspx?coll_id=16&ItemID=304.

U.S. Department of Agriculture (USDA). (2002). State competitive foods policies. *National school lunch program.* Retrieved September 21, 2006 from http://www.fns.usda. gov/cnd/Lunch/CompetitiveFoods/state_policies_2002.htm

U.S. Department of Agriculture (USDA). (2005). National school lunch, special milk, and school breakfast programs; National average payments/maximum reimbursement rates, *Federal Register*, 70, 136.

U.S. Department of Health and Human Services (DHHS). (1996). *Physical activity and health: A report of the surgeon general.* Atlanta, GA: U.S. Department of Health and Human Services, Centers for Disease Control and Prevention, National Center for Chronic Disease Prevention and Health Promotion. Retrieved September 21, 2006 from http://www.cdc.gov/nccdphp/sgr/pdf/sgrfull.pdf

U.S. Department of Labor, Bureau of Labor Statistics. (2003). *Consumer Expenditure Survey 2003.* Retrieved September 21, 2006 from http://www.bls.gov/cex/csxann03.pdf

U.S. General Accounting Office (GAO). (2003). School lunch program: Efforts needed to improve nutrition and healthy eating. *GAO report number 03-506.* Washington, DC: General Accounting Office. Retrieved September 21, 2006 from http://www.gao. gov/new.items/d03506.pdf

U.S. Surgeon General David Satcher, U.S. Department of Health and Human Services. (2001). *The surgeon general's call to action to prevent and decrease overweight and obesity.* Available from: US GPO, Washington. Retrieved September 21, 2006 from http://www.surgeongeneral.gov/topics/obesity/calltoaction/toc.htm

Vargas, A., Woodward-Lopez, G., Kim, S., & Crawford, P. B. (2005). *In-depth interviews with SHAPE California schooldistricts.* Prepared for Nutrition Services Division, California Department of Education by the Center for Weight and Health, University of California, Berkeley.

West Virginia Department of Education. (2004). *Executive summary—standards for school nutrition policy.* Retrieved September 21, 2006 from http://wvde.state. wv.us/policies/p4321.1.html

Woodward-Lopez, G. (2004). *Model school nutrition/physical activity policy grants: Cross-site evaluation report.* Prepared for Nutrition Services Division, California Department of Education by the Center for Weight and Health, University of California, Berkeley.

Woodward-Lopez, G., Kim, S., & Crawford, P. B. (2005). *Survey of SHAPE California school districts.* Prepared for Nutrition Services Division, California Department of Education by the Center for Weight and Health, University of California, Berkeley.

Woodward-Lopez, G., Vargas, A., Kim, S., Proctor, C., Hiort-Lorenzen, C., Diemoz, L., & Crawford, P. B. (2005). *LEAF cross-site evaluation: Fiscal impact report.* Center for Weight and Health, University of California, Berkeley. Retrieved September 21, 2006 from http://www.cnr.berkeley.edu/cwh/PDFs/LEAF_Fiscal_Report.pdf

Woodward-Lopez, G., Vargas, A., Kim, S., Proctor, C., Hiort-Lorenzen, C., Diemoz, L., & Crawford, P.B. (2006). LEAF cross-site evaluation: Report on participant assessment of the adequacy of SB 19. Center for Weight and Health, University of California, Berkeley. Retrieved September 21, 2006 from http://www.cnr.berkeley. edu/cwh/PDFs/LEAF_Adequacy_Report.pdf

World Health Organization (WHO). (2003). *Obesity and overweight information sheet.* Retrieved September 21, 2006 from http://www.who.int/dietphysicalactivity/ publications/facts/obesity/en/.

23

Application of Innovative Technologies in the Prevention and Treatment of Overweight in Children and Adolescents

DEBORAH F. TATE

Internet and other technology-based interventions have increasingly been developed and evaluated for behavior change. Recently, two review papers have been published evaluating Web- or computer-based interventions for chronic disease compared with non-Web-based or no-treatment controls (Wantland, Portillo, Holzemer, Slaughter, & McGhee, 2004; Murray, Burns, See, Lai, & Nazareth, 2005). One review of 24 randomized controlled trials (RCTs) pooled across 3,000 child and adult participants, found that interactive health communication applications (e.g., computer or Internet-based packages that combine health information with social, decision, or behavior change support) had significantly positive effects on changing patient knowledge, perceived social support, and key behavioral and clinical outcomes when compared with non-Web-based control programs (Murray et al.). Effect sizes in the meta-analytic review ranged from -.01 to .75, but results were more favorable for patients assigned to the Web-based interventions compared with control groups. The reviews included several interventions developed for pediatric chronic illnesses, such as asthma self-management and type-I diabetes. Because these

DEBORAH F. TATE • University of North Carolina, Chapel Hill, NC 27599.

reviews compared Web-based programs to non-Web-based interventions or controls, they do not enable much delineation of the components of such programs that lead to greater efficacy. In fact, few hypotheses about the way in which these technologies are best developed or applied have been explicitly tested, but to date, most of the research on using technology for child or adolescent overweight suggests initial feasibility with some limited outcome evaluations.

Children and adolescents are increasingly exposed to a wide variety of technologies at younger ages than in prior decades. Technologies that are commonly used by this age group include computers, mobile phones, portable music players, video and portable electronic games, TV, and others. This chapter will review and discuss promising directions for using technology with children and adolescents with a particular focus on application of prevention or treatment of overweight.

Availability of Technology to Children and Adolescents

The changing landscape of modern society over the past 20 years has made the use of technology a part of daily life—even for young children. From the early 1980s to 2003, the percent of American households with at least one computer rose from only 8 percent to 62 percent (U.S. Census; Computer and Internet Use 2003). The prevalence of home computers is the greatest in households with a school-age child—76 percent of households with a child age 6–17 have one or more computers compared with 57 percent of those without children living in the household (U.S. Census; Computer and Internet Use 2003). The pattern is similar for Internet access. Sixty-seven percent of homes with a school-age child had Internet access in 2003 compared with 50 percent of homes without children. Children also have access to computers and the Internet at school. When both home and school access is considered, only 7 percent of children enrolled in grades K-12 did not use a computer in any location in 2003. Compared to adults, computer use was greater among children, as compared to adults (U.S. Census, 2003).

Teens are also avid users of a variety of media including computers and Internet, cell phones, personal digital assistants, and new emerging devices. About 87 percent of teens aged 12–17 report using the Internet, and half of those are daily users (Lenhart, Madden, & Hitlin, 2005). Among home Internet users, one of every two report that they have a broadband connection. Teens enjoy a wide variety of online activities, but the most frequently cited activities are sending/reading email, visiting websites for entertainment or sports, playing games, getting news, and sending/receiving instant messages. Although teens still report using e-mail, they prefer communicating with friends and even parents via instant messaging (Lenhart et al.). It has been estimated that almost half (43 percent) of teens in 2005 owned a cellular or mobile phone, and more than a third of teens report having used their phone to send text messages (Lenhart et al.).

In sum, youth have unprecedented access and familiarity with varied technologies ranging from computers and the Internet to video games and cell phones. Access extends to both school and home, making the use of technology in interventions with this age group, if not yet unquestionable, at least worthy of strong consideration and future development.

Conceptual Frameworks for Technological Interventions

Developers and researchers interested in using technology to reach children and adolescents hypothesize that not only are these technologies part of life for youth around the world, but such systems have particular appeal because they can make delivery of educational content and behavioral skills training more interactive and engaging. The Elaboration Likelihood Model (ELM, Petty & Cacioppo, 1986) suggests that if technology affords greater interactivity and tailoring of content, then kids will pay more attention to key messages, result in greater central-route cognitive processing, and lead to more lasting attitudinal change. CD-Rom, computer-based, and Internet interventions have most commonly relied on theoretical frameworks involving ELM, and social cognitive theory (SCT) constructs (Baranowski et al., 2003; Patrick et al., 2001), such that the game or program includes opportunities for developing behavioral capability and enhancing self-efficacy through skills training and mastery experiences—modeling, goal setting, reinforcement, and feedback. The transtheoretical model (Prochaska, Diclemente, & Norcross, 1992) has also been applied to technology-based systems with tailored information and program recommendations matched to the child's stage of readiness in specific behavioral domains (Patrick et al.). Winett, Tate, Anderson, Wojcik, and Winett (2005) and Hurling, Fairley, and Dias (2006) provide detailed descriptions and examples of how specific SCT, ELM, and the principles of computer-human interaction are used to design specific components of Internet programs.

As noted above, theoretical constructs are used in the design of technology-based interventions, but technology may also be used to strengthen the application of behavioral principles underlying standard interventions. For example, pediatric weight control historically has relied heavily on behavioral theory and behavior modification techniques (Epstein, Roemmich, & Raynor, 2001), and emerging technologies may allow us to apply behavioral techniques with greater ease and fidelity. Several studies have used technology in supporting behavioral economics paradigms such that access to highly desired video games or television is made contingent on completing physical activity or other weight regulation behaviors (Faith et al., 2001; Goldfield et al., 2006; Saelens & Epstein, 1998). Other technologies could support maintaining or changing energy balance by making the recording of behaviors easier (e.g., PDA or cell-phone recording), and perhaps someday, eliminating the need to physically enter monitoring information because the device is sophisticated enough to collect and transmit the data without involving the child. It is easy to imagine this with physical activity using accelerometers to collect and wirelessly transmit frequent reports of physical activity monitoring data so that reinforcement can be provided more proximally to the behavior. Feedback could be preprogrammed for immediate delivery based on achieving certain activity levels, and provided throughout the week rather than when the treatment provider can review activity diaries at a weekly session. Similarly, detection of noncompliance with behavioral goals or targets could trigger problem-solving via an automated feature, a phone call, or an e-mail exchange during the week or after a few missed exercise opportunities rather than at the next treatment encounter. Many such uses of technologies to enhance standard treatment are emerging.

Using Technology in Prevention and Treatment of Overweight

Using technology for self-management of many chronic illnesses raises fewer concerns than using technology in the fight against childhood overweight. The argument is often presented that modern societal trends involving technology are responsible for significant daily energy savings, and that using technology or developing technology-based interventions will increase time spent in sedentary behaviors, further exacerbating the problem rather than contributing to the solution. Recent studies in this area demonstrate that the relationship between technology use and energy balance is not straightforward. A cross-sectional study of Finnish adolescents age 14–18 found that the relationship between screen time and BMI depends on the type of screen time, and was inconsistent for boys and girls (Kautiainen, Koivuslita, Lintonen, Virtanen, & Rimplea, 2005). Television viewing and computer use was associated with overweight in girls but not in boys, and no relationship was found between video-game playing and overweight among boys or girls (Kautiainen et al.). A large meta-analysis found that the relationship between TV viewing and body fatness, although statistically significant, was a small effect and of questionable clinical significance (Marshall, Biddle, Gorely, Cameron, & Murdey, 2004).

The association between screen time and sedentary behavior could be caused by reductions in energy expenditure as screen time use increases. However, studies also suggest a role for increasing caloric intake and snacking while viewing TV (Utter, Scragg, & Schaaf, 2006; Wiecha et al., 2006). Other studies find a mixed relationship between TV viewing and energy intake. In a laboratory examination of preschool children's caloric intake while watching TV, Francis and Birch (2006) showed that when lunch and snack were provided in the laboratory with or without a TV, children consumed significantly less in the TV condition. There were no effects of sex or weight status, however the effects were moderated when home TV viewing and eating practices were considered. Children who viewed more daily hours of TV at home, and who had a higher frequency of eating meals while viewing TV, ate significantly more in the TV condition.

Experimental studies do not find a universal relationship across types of screen time, suggesting that some media may be more *active* than others. Studies of video-game playing in boys aged 7–10 years (Wang & Perry, 2006), and in 16–25 year olds (Segal & Dietz, 1991), have shown that physiologic responses and metabolic equivalents during traditional video-game playing are greater than sedentary behavior and television viewing. In Wang and Perry's study, they estimate the average caloric expenditure to be about one calorie per minute of video game playing for an average nine-year old boy. However, they state that such games, while contributing to overall expenditure, were not at an intensity level sufficient to promote cardiovascular conditioning. Other video games directly produce physical activity during game play. These are referred to as activity-based video games (e.g., dance, tennis, boxing, etc.) and typically result in substantially more caloric expenditure. In a controlled study, a dance-based video game produced energy expenditure levels of 91 kcal/hr above resting energy expenditure, and was roughly equivalent to watching television while walking on a treadmill at 1.5 miles/hr (Lanningham-Foster et al., 2006). Evidence from a recent intervention trial also points to the potential weight gain prevention effects of a comprehensive computer game that was not an activity-based game. A well-designed theory-based multimedia computer game used in a comprehensive school-based intervention slightly increased overall activity and reduced BMI among girls (Goran & Reynolds, 2005).

The sum of this evidence suggests that computers and other screen time may not universally promote inactivity, and that the thoughtful use of these technologies can be part of our toolbox of intervention strategies. It is also important to note that participants are fairly sedentary when they interact with most of our commonly used psycho-educational intervention modalities (e.g., reading print materials, sitting in treatment group meetings, driving to and from treatment clinics, or sitting in school classrooms). Thus, harnessing the power of these technologies to extend the reach of clinical care to actively engage youth in physical activity, or to create engaging behavior change programs, may be an important direction for reaching this target age group.

Technology Programs targeting Nutrition and/or Activity in Schools

Early attempts to use technology as standalone programs with children used multi-media based programs. Originally, these interventions were delivered via CD-Rom on a local computer, but because broadband Internet access has increased their application, Web-based intervention is also now feasible and being investigated. Most of these interventions have been conducted by incorporating the technology as part of a school-based intervention, and have been supplemented with in-class activities led by the classroom teacher. Table 23.1 provides an overview of school-based nutrition interventions using technology for dietary behavior change or physical activity promotion, and separates those with additional classroom components from standalone interventions.

One of the most comprehensive, multi-level interventions (Goran & Reynolds, 2005) was the Interactive Multimedia for Promoting Physical Activity program (IMPACT) on a CD-Rom. The IMPACT study evaluated fourth-grade students at four elementary schools in which students played an interactive social cognitive theory-based game for 45 minutes once per week for eight weeks. The game was supplemented by four classroom lectures and four homework assignments designed to link the school intervention to home with family education and involvement. Overall, the intervention showed more positive outcomes for girls than boys. After eight weeks, girls increased time spent in light physical activities by an

Table 23.1. Summary of school-based CD-Rom or Internet nutrition interventions

Authors	Technology used	Study design	Sample size and age	Theoretical components	Intervention duration and contact time	Outcomes
Intervention Plus a Classroom and or Family Component						
Goran and Reynolds (2005)	Multimedia CD-Rom	? Randomized or Quasi-experimental	4 Schools n =202 4th Graders age 9.5 ±.4yrs	SCT: Self-monitoring Goal Setting Targeted SE and OE	1. 8 multi-media sessions 43(45min each)	Differential efficacy for boys and girls.
		1. IMPACT multimedia cd-rom (2 schools)		Classroom activities also SCT reinforcing concepts introduced in CD-rom Targeted Self-efficacy embedding opportunities for mastery, modeling, repetition, and feedback.	4 Classroom lessons (45min each) 4 Family homework assignments (45min each) 12 hours total contact time	Increase in light PA in girls (~20min/d)
						Slight decrease in moderate PA for both girls and boys.
		2. Control (2 Schools)			2. No contact 1. 3 WWW modules (5 hours) plus 10 hours of NCI and ACS classroom curriculum over 1 month 15 hours total contact time	CD-rom game resulted in 0.2kg lower post intervention body weight vs. control girls.
Long and Stevens (2004)	Internet	Quasi-experimental Assigned to 1) Intervention (4 classrooms) or 2) Control	Two schools N =121 age 12–16		2. Standard course of study in health, science, home economics classes with nutrition content estimated at ≤3 hours	Intervention students had greater self-efficacy for healthy eating and dietary knowledge at post test compared to controls.
						No differences in self-reported intake via FFQ.

Standalone interventions without supplemental classroom component

	Technology	Design	Sample	Theory/Content	Intervention	Results
Baronowski et al. (2003)	Multimedia CD-Rom	Randomized 2 group 1. Squire's Quest PEMT (14 schools) 2. Control (14 Schools)	26 Schools n =1,578 4th Graders	SCT: Goal setting Skills training (virtual kitchen, problem solving, decision making)	1: 10 Multimedia Sessions (25min each) delivered over 5 weeks ■ 4.2 hours of total contact time 2: No contact	Game Resulted in 1 greater serving of Fruits, Juice or Vegetables compared with Controls
Frenn et al. (2005)	Internet/video	Quasi-experimental in 1 middle school assigned to 1) science class control (3 classrooms) or 2) intervention (3 classrooms)	1 school N = 178 age 12–14 years	Trans-theoretical Model Reinforcement	1. 8 session blackboard platform incorporating 2–3 minute videos delivered over 1 month 2. regular science class meetings	Students in the intervention who completed more than 50 percent of the sessions had a greater decrease in percent dietary fat compared with controls.
Turnin et al. (2001)	Multimedia CD-Rom	Randomized 2 group post-test only	16 Schools N =1,876 age 7–12	None explicitly stated. Knowledge building exercises.	1. 10 sessions (60min each) delivered over 5 weeks	Self-reported nutrition knowledge significantly greater in game group compared with control at post.

(continued)

Table 23.1. (continued)

Authors	Technology used	Study Design	Sample size and age	Theoretical components	Intervention duration and Contact Time	Outcomes
		1. Nutrition Ed Game (8 schools) 2. Standard Teacher Led Nutrition Education (8 schools)			10 hours of total contact time 2. same schedule?	No differences in self-reported child diet intake via 3 day recall.
Winett et al. (1999)	Internet	Quasi-experimental 1) Internet Intervention (2 classes) 2) Controls- Standard Nutrition curriculum (2 classes)	1 school n =180 girls 4 classes 9th -10th grade 14–16	SCT modeling, behavioral prescriptions, individualized mastery steps with personalized goal setting, and feedback	1. 5 modules delivered over 5 weeks (20 minutes per module) <2 hours of contact time 2. standard class curriculum	Girls in Internet intervention showed greater self-reported behavior changes in increasing regular meals, fruits and vegetables, and fiber and decreasing the consumption of regular sodas. No consistent evidence that the program was effective decreasing r consumption of high-fat snacks or high-fat dairy.

average of 20 minutes per day. Importantly, the intervention produced slight decreases in body weight (age-adjusted BMI z-scores), corresponding to about −0.2 kgs.

It is difficult to evaluate the specific efficacy of the computer game component in the Goran and Reynolds (2005) study, but a few studies have evaluated a standalone multimedia intervention in schools without changing or adding any classroom components. In one of the largest RCTs to date, Baranowski and colleagues (2003) developed and evaluated an SCT-based multimedia game called "Squire's Quest" designed to increase the fruit and vegetable consumption of 4th graders. The intervention was an RCT with 26 schools involving over 1,500 children. Students in schools assigned to receive the game played 10 sessions for 25 minutes each over five weeks. There were no additional classroom or family components. Students randomized to receive the intervention increased their fruit, juice, or vegetable servings by one serving per/day in comparison to students in control schools after the five week intervention. Similarly, Winett and colleagues (Russ et al., 1998; Winett et al., 1999) developed and evaluated (in a quasi-experimental study) an interactive Internet intervention designed as a teen magazine delivered in five modules during a health education class. Compared with standard nutrition education, girls receiving the Web-based nutrition and physical activity program had more self-reported regular meal consumption, increased fruit and vegetable servings, decreased regular soda consumption, and increases in aerobic activity.

Overall, these early school-based interventions have demonstrated initial feasibility of these approaches, although they have generally been short in duration—ranging from five to eight weeks on average—and have used self-reported diet changes (Goran as the exception) as the primary outcomes.

Standalone Internet-based Behavioral Interventions for Obesity

Several randomized trials for obesity in adults have evaluated specific components of Internet programs that lead to greater efficacy of Internet programs (Tate, Wing, & Winett, 2001; Tate, Jackvony, & Wing, 2003, 2006). Internet behavioral weight loss interventions that include professional support during the behavior change process improve the efficacy of the Internet approach compared with self-directed Internet programs that include *all* other behavioral elements. Recently, this work was extended to evaluate another way of providing behavior change support via a computer-tailored automated counseling system in adults (Tate et al., 2006). In this study, adults were randomized to receive a self-directed website, or a behavioral Web-based program, that included computerized weekly feedback or the same Web program with human counselor weekly feedback via e-mail. At three months, participants receiving computer-automated counseling support had lost significantly more weight as compared with those using an Internet program with no ongoing behavior change support, and the weight losses were equivalent in magnitude to participants receiving e-mail counseling from a trained weight-loss professional. At six months, participants followed by human e-mail counselors continued to lose additional weight and had better overall outcomes, but the weight losses achieved in the group given the computer expert systems support were approximately 5 percent of initial body weight, suggesting a promising direction to explore in the development of less costly behavior change support mechanisms.

In one of the longest Internet interventions for adolescents, Williamson and colleagues (2005) recruited overweight adolescent African-American girls aged 11–15 to evaluate the effects of providing an Internet behavioral weight-loss program with ongoing e-mail support compared with an Internet health education program and were followed over two years. Girls were enrolled with an overweight or obese parent and given access to an interactive behavior change website. At six months, the Internet behavioral program, with ongoing support from a treatment professional via e-mail, produced more favorable reductions in body fat and dietary fat intake among girls, and also produced reductions in body weight among parents, compared to the health education program (Williamson et al.). However, these effects were not maintained at the two-year follow-up—in part due to reduced utilization of the Internet program (Williamson et al., 2006). Our ability to understand the level of engagement needed, and the amount of new content and value added feedback required, to engage users of Internet or other technology-based programs over long periods of time is one of our great challenges.

Technology Programs as Adjunct to Clinical Care

There are many ways in which technology can be used to augment standard face-to-face treatment programs for child or adolescent overweight. Extending treatment contact has been shown to improve adult weight management outcomes (Perri, Nezu, Patti, & McCann, 1989). Electronic communication via e-mail, text messaging, or chat groups may be used to communicate between sessions, and the Web, cell phones, or personal digital assistants (PDAs) can be used to collect self-monitoring data. Adjunctive computer-based approaches can also be used to deliver part of the treatment, thereby decreasing the total number of therapist or medical office visit contact hours needed.

In pediatric medicine, technology-based interventions delivered via CD-Rom or the Internet have demonstrated great potential for extending care and reducing costs. For example, two studies involving a total of over 330 patients with pediatric asthma have shown that providing additional self-management intervention via multimedia or game-based programs—as compared with standard patient education—results in significant self-reported improvements and more objective indicators, such as reduced steroid use, reduced medical visits, and fewer missed days of school (Krishna et al., 2003; McPherson, Glazebrook, Forster, James, & Smyth, 2006). Another strategy, particularly useful for younger children, is to deliver interventions directed at the parent using the Internet or other technology. As an adjunct to standard care for pediatric encopresis (Ritterband et al., 2003), parents were given access to a parent-focused interactive multi-media Internet intervention with structured behavioral treatment delivered with no other human contact. Compared with standard care, children whose parents were randomized to the adjunctive Internet intervention showed greater symptom improvement. Research also suggests that most parents will follow through when provided with a *prescription* from their physician to visit a specific behavioral-oriented website to help inform their child's treatment. In a busy pediatric medical specialty clinic, researchers investigated whether parents would follow through on a *prescription* to visit a website with specific treatment information given by the attending physician (Ritterband et al., 2005). A written prescription to visit a study-specific website was provided to parents with a unique login identifier for the website. Half of the families were randomized to receive a reminder to visit the website sent two days after the clinic visit. In the email reminder group, 77 percent of families visited the website within one week of the original clinic visit. Taken together, these studies suggest that in areas of pediatric medicine, where behavioral interventions have been shown to be effective, extending brief clinic encounters with fully automated Internet or multimedia interventions is feasible, acceptable to families, and can significantly improve medical outcomes with great potential to scale with little incremental cost.

Multimedia computer programs have also been used as adjuncts to physician counseling for activity and nutrition in adolescents. Patient-Centered Assessment and Counseling for Exercise plus Nutrition (PACE+) consisted of a multimedia-based adjunct to a physician counseling intervention to promote dietary changes and physical activity for adolescents ages 11– 18 (Patrick et al., 2001). The interactive computer program was designed to assess the adolescent's current physical activity and nutrition behaviors, compare them with recommended levels, and create tailored action plans using the transtheoretical model. Each adolescent received feedback on their behavior compared to the recommended guidelines, and was encouraged to choose one activity and one nutrition behavior that were below recommended levels to consider changing. Adolescents selected a target behavior, created an action plan, printed out their plan, and had a discussion with their care provider. The study compared the use of the office-based computer program alone, compared with using the program coupled with follow-up phone calls (frequent vs. infrequent) and found that at four months, all groups increased physical activity with no between-group differences. Because no group received standard care, the effects of the computer program could not be determined, but contrary to their hypothesis, follow-up phone calls did not increase efficacy.

To explore the potential for an adjunctive Internet intervention to improve over and above an abbreviated clinic-based adolescent obesity intervention, our research team recently investigated the use of an adjunctive Internet intervention for overweight adolescent girls (ages 14–17) coupled with an abbreviated form of standard behavioral weight-control treatment. The abbreviated treatment was delivered in nine face-to-face group sessions over six months rather than a more typical 16–24 session program. The combined Internet plus nine face-to-face sessions program was compared with the nine face-to-face sessions alone

(Tate, Jelalian, Ferguson, & Wing, 2005). The content of the face-to-face sessions was identical between the groups, adapted for adolescents from Epstein et al. (2001), and delivered weekly for the first month (four sessions) and then one session per month for months 2–6. Parents were included in a separate parent group session in months 1, 4, and 9, and were encouraged to support their teen's behavior changes. Both treatment groups received an identical reinforcement program for weight-loss behaviors. Points were given for attending face-to-face group sessions, submitting a diary, any weekly weight loss, and meeting the standard physical activity goal, with a bonus point for achieving a higher physical activity goal. Points were redeemable at any time during the study for gift certificates to local merchants of interest to teens. The Internet intervention (received by only one group) was designed to provide on-going contact in between the monthly sessions. The Internet intervention was comprised of a colorful, attractive interactive website that included new weekly content; a links library to age-appropriate material related to eating, activity, and body image, etc.; a place for messages and communication with peers; a monitoring diary; and an interactive virtual map that tracked the physical activity of the girls in that group and showed progress through virtual cities in the United States based on their logged miles. The Internet intervention also included a weekly chat group meeting led by a trained weight management professional and an email follow-up about the self-monitoring diary during the weeks in between monthly visits. After six months, both the face-to-face only, and the face-to-face plus Internet groups had significant reductions in BMI compared to baseline, with no differences between the treatment groups (Tate et al. 2005). These results suggest that in the short term, adding an additional Internet component to a robust face-to-face intervention did not produce any additional benefit.

Methods for Self-Monitoring

Other promising directions for integrating or using technology with children or adolescents include making monitoring of diet or activity less obtrusive and onerous, perhaps more fun, and ultimately more accurate. In adults, handheld devices—typically PDAs—have been used for self-monitoring a variety of behaviors. A review reporting on randomized trials comparing paper and portable electronic diaries in adults showed that portable electronic diaries were preferred by patients and resulted in the collection of more timely data (Lane, Heddle, Arnold, & Walker, 2006). Similar findings were observed in children ages 8–16 years, when paper diaries for chronic pain self-monitoring were compared with electronic dairies (Palermo, Valenzuela, & Stork, 2004). Children rated electronic diaries as easy to use and showed significantly greater compliance and accuracy in recording with the e-diaries in comparison with paper. Interestingly, there was a gender effect—boys were more compliant with electronic format compared with paper diaries.

PDAs have also been used to collect frequent reports of physical activity in youth (Dunton, Whalen, Jamner, Henker, & Floro, 2005). High-school students were alerted via the alarm function on the PDA every 30 minutes during waking hours on four consecutive days, and were asked to report the primary activity they were doing at that time. Adolescents generally complied with the rigorous protocol with 73 percent of students responding to the prompt within three minutes on 75 percent of the occasions. Self-reported intensities of activities were also distinguishable with heart rate monitoring data also collected during the same interval. Despite a willingness to use handheld devices, and the potential benefits of more discrete recording, estimating dietary intake is still problematic. Yon, Johnson, Harvey-Berino, and Gold (2006) found that adults enrolled in a weight management intervention were no more accurate in using their PDA-monitoring methods than when using traditional paper diaries. Accepting that dietary monitoring data is fraught with inaccuracies, one benefit of such technologies is that the electronic information can be transferred via upload to a treatment provider without having to retype the information or wait for it to be received via postal mail—thus reducing patient burden and enabling a quicker response from the provider.

Given the increasing prevalence of cell or mobile phone technology in both adults and children (Lenhart et al., 2005), the portability of the devices, and the ever increasing functionality of small screens, many of the monitoring, messaging, and behavior change applications originally designed for the computer and the Internet can be integrated with or perhaps delivered exclusively with mobile devices in the future. Studies suggest that adolescents are receptive to follow-up care using cell phone text messaging. In the study "R U OK 2 TXT 4 RESEARCH," 91 percent of 16–24 year old Australian general practice patients had mobile phones and were receptive to receiving follow-up questions after an office visit via text messages (Haller, Sanci, Sawye, Coffey, & Patton, 2006)—suggesting widespread adoption of mobile phones among this age group, and willingness to have contact with health providers via this mechanism.

There is also potential to impact parent-child coregulation of health behaviors with such technologies. For example, a pilot study with 9- to 15-year olds with type-I diabetes and their parents showed that regular transference of child glucose monitor readings to the parent's cell phone was well-received by both parents and children, and reduced parental intrusions among well-controlled children (Gammon et al., 2005). However, among children who were not well-controlled or who were not monitoring on schedule, it increased parental reminders or *nagging*.

In sum, there is great potential to easily send data to care professionals or parents with emerging technologies. However, these findings highlight the potential for the function to either promote compliance or increase conflict, and underscore the need for such surveillance and communication systems to be part of a comprehensive intervention that addresses these issues.

Challenges and Considerations for the Future

Despite the promise that technology offers for extending clinical care and for developing standalone interventions with greater reach, several challenges deserve consideration as we build on the early studies reviewed here and design for the future.

Engagement and adherence to technology-based interventions over time is a problem; but one that may be attributable, at least in part, to the ways in which we have used technology thus far. In early studies, systems were designed with the expectation that people will use these systems the way they use traditional face-to-face psychotherapy or class sessions in school settings (e.g., once per week interactions). It is likely that as individuals change their behavior, they experience periods when they need more frequent support and feedback, and other times when they can go for several weeks with minimal help. Thus far, Internet- and other technology-based interventions have followed traditional weekly contact schedules likely derived from traditional psychotherapy, medical, and school models. It is not clear what schedule of intervention is optimal in this new treatment format and whether the optimal interaction frequency differs by individual factors such as motivation level, behavioral capability, ease of skill acquisition, or phase of behavioral adoption (e.g., early adoption, maintenance, etc.).

We know that static Web pages with little variation in form or content and collection of monitoring data are not engaging enough to promote long-term use in youth, or even among adult populations. Youth are particularly savvy users of media and, in some of the early studies of technology-based interventions, less-than-optimal computer interfaces (including platforms like Blackboard) have been reported (Frenn et al., 2005). While familiar to academic researchers, inexpensive, and easy to develop, these systems are very limited in form and function, academic in nature, and may not be engaging enough to promote use of them when they are outside of a controlled school environment. Adolescent girls who were interviewed following a semi-automated text-messaging intervention for bulimia (Robinson et al., 2006) had high expectations, requesting a high degree of personal relevance from automated messages, prompt responses to text entries, and a range of preferences for actual human input.

Future research is needed to explore design elements that promote ongoing engagement. In an innovative three-group pilot study, Hurling and colleagues (2006) found that a more interactive Internet physical activity promotion website was more engaging and utilized over time than a control website with the same look, feel, content, and basic functionality but with less-interactive behavior change tools (see Figure 23.1). It should be noted that the control site was not at all static. Importantly, the interactive components were carefully selected and designed based on behavior change theory and human-computer interaction principles, and differences in interactivity were somewhat subtle but theoretically important distinctions. In their discussion, the authors state a point worth repeating: "An engaging system with ineffective behaviour change tools is as useless as a nonengaging system with effective behaviour change tools." (Hurling et al., p. 12). More studies with additive designs are needed to begin to explore these issues.

It is equally important to consider the impact that the intervention setting might have on adherence and attention. There are different levels of forced attention that are inherent in the setting chosen for intervention that might contribute to utilization. When a child or teen is brought by

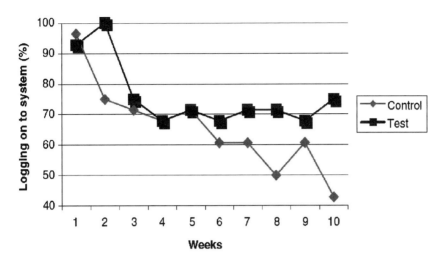

Figure 23.1. Percent of participants logging in to various Internet physical activity promotion websites by week (from Hurling, Fairley, & Dias (2006).

the parent to a treatment setting—even if they are not interested in paying attention to the discussion—the demand characteristics of sitting with a treatment provider or other group members will force a certain level of attention. Similarly, a Web-based or CD-Rom intervention delivered in the classroom may be considered a diversion from regular school activities and may capture attention in that setting. However, if the same intervention is delivered in the home, competing demands from other more valued activities, such as television, instant messaging with friends, or playing favorite video games with no underlying health agenda, may lead to less utilization of the health intervention when delivered in this setting.

Finally, emerging research indicates that adolescents may not process Web-based information in the same way that they process print or other modalities. Despite a stated preference for digital media, a recent study of adolescent girls randomized to receive either an interactive website or a content and format-matched interactive print booklet promoting physical activity, found that at two weeks, girls had greater behavioral intention and self-reported physical activity after interacting with the interactive print booklet than after using the website (Marks et al., 2006)—due in part to greater cognitive processing and utilization of the print-based materials. This underscores the need to optimize intervention designs to include technologies chosen for a specific purpose and with regard to user preference. Future interventions may include multiple technologies or communications channels, and give users a choice about how they wish to have follow-up—for example, SMS text messaging to the phone or e-mail (i.e., Hurling et al., 2006) or submitting self-monitoring information via a Web diary or an automated touch-tone phone system (i.e., Wing, Tate, Gorin, Raynor, & Fava, 2006).

SUMMARY

Although the data on using technology in the prevention and treatment of overweight in children and adolescents is in its infancy, early indicators from technology-based interventions with adults, other areas of pediatric behavioral medicine, and in nutrition and physical activity promotion, show that the feasibility and initial efficacy has been demonstrated. Because youth are one of the fastest growing users of a wide variety of technologies, continued research on how to best utilize technology in obesity prevention and treatment for youth is needed. Many challenges exist for next generation programs to be engaging, yet with careful application of behavioral theory, where use of technology is well-matched to functional goals (e.g., monitoring devices are portable, information provision is easy to read), and where user preferences and use patterns are considered.

REFERENCES

Bandura, A. (1986). *Social foundations of thought and action.* Englewood Cliffs, NJ: Prentice-Hall.

Baranowski, T., Baranowski, J., Cullen, K. W., Marsh, T., Islam, N., Zakeri, I., et al. (2003). Squire's quest! Dietary outcome evaluation of a multimedia game. *American Journal of Preventative Medicine, 24,* 52–61.

Dunton, G. F., Whalen, C. K., Jamner, L. D., Henker, B., & Floro, J. N. (2005). Using ecologic momentary assessment to measure physical activity during adolescence. *American Journal of Preventative Medicine, 29,* 281–287.

Epstein, L. H., Roemmich, J. N., & Raynor, H. A. (2001). Behavioral therapy in the treatment of pediatric obesity. *Pediatric Clinics of North America, 48,* 981–993.

Faith, M. S., Berman, N., Heo, M., Pietrobelli, A., Gallagher, D., Epstein, L. H., et al. (2001). Effects of Contingent-TV on physical activity and TV-Viewing in obese. Children. *Pediatrics, 107,* 1043–1048.

Francis, L. A., & Birch, L. L. (2006). Does eating during television viewing affect preschool children's intake? *Journal of the American Dietetic Association, 106,* 598–600.

Frenn, M., Malin, S., Brown, R. L., Greer, Y., Fox, J., Greer, J., et al. (2005). Changing the tide: An internet/video exercise and low-fat diet intervention with middle-school students. *Applied Nursing Research, 18,* 13–21.

Gammon, D., Årsand, E., Walseth, O. A., Andersson, N., Jenssen, M., & Taylor, T. (2005). Parent-child interaction using a mobile and wireless system for blood glucose monitoring. *Journal of Medical Internet Research, 7,* e57.

Goran, M. I., & Reynolds, K. (2005). Interactive multimedia for promoting physical activity (IMPACT) in children. *Obesity Research, 13,* 762–771.

Haller, D., Sanci, L., Sawyer, S., Coffey, C., & Patton, G. (2006). R u ok 2 txt 4 research? Feasibility of text message communication in primary care research. *Australian Family Physician, 35,* 175–176.

Hurling, R., Fairley, B. W., & Dias, M. B. (2006). Internet-based exercise interventions: Are more interactive designs better? *Psychology & Health, 21,* 757–772.

Kautiainen, S., Koivusilta, L., Lintonen, T., Virtanen, S. M., & Rimpela, A. (2005). Use of information and communication technology and prevalence of overweight and obesity among adolescents. *International Journal of Obesity (London), 29,* 925–933.

Krishna, S., Francisco, B. D., Balas, E. A., König, P., Graff, G. R., & Madsen, R. W. (2003). Internet-enabled interactive multimedia asthma education program: A randomized trial. *Pediatrics, 111,* 503–510.

Lane, S. J., Heddle, N. M., Arnold, E., & Walker, I. (2006). A review of randomized controlled trials comparing the effectiveness of hand held computers with paper methods for data collection. *BMC Medical Informatics and Decision Making, 31,* 23.

Lanningham-Foster, L., Jensen, T. B., Foster, R. C., Redmond, A. B., Walker, B. A., Heinz, D., et al. (2006). Energy expenditure of sedentary screen time compared with active screen time for children. *Pediatrics, 118*, e1831–e1835

Lenhart, A., Madden, M., & Hitlin, P. (2005). *Teens and technology: Youth are leading the transition to a fully wired and mobile nation.* Pew Internet and American Life Project. Retrieved from http://www.pewinternet.org/pdfs/PIP_Teens_Tech_July2005web.pdf

Long, J. D., & Stevens, K. R. (2004). Using technology to promote self-efficacy for healthy eating in adolescents. *Journal of Nursing Scholarship, 36*, 134–139.

Marks, J. T., Campbell, M. K., Ward, D. S., Ribisl, K. M., Wildemuth, B. M., & Symons, M. J. (2006). A comparison of web and print media for physical activity promotion among adolescent girls. *Journal of Adolescent Health, 39*, 96–104.

Marshall, S. J., Biddle, S. J., Gorely, T., Cameron, N., & Murdey, I. (2004). Relationships between media use, body fatness and physical activity in children and youth: A meta-analysis. *International Journal of Obesity and Related Metabolic Disorders, 28*, 1238–1246.

McPherson, A. C., Glazebrook, C., Forster, D., James, C., & Smyth, A. (2006). A randomized, controlled trial of an interactive educational computer package for children with asthma. *Pediatrics, 117*, 1046–1054.

Murray, E., Burns, J., See, T. S., Lai, R., & Nazareth, I. (2005). Interactive health communication applications for people with chronic disease. Cochrane Database of Systematic Reviews, 19, CD004274.

Palermo, T. M., Valenzuela, D., & Stork, P. P. (2004). A randomized trial of electronic versus paper pain diaries in children: Impact on compliance, accuracy, and acceptability. Pain, 107, 213–219.

Patrick, K., Sallis, J. F., Prochaska, J. J., Lydston, D. D., Calfas, K. J., Zabinski, M. F., et al. (2001). A multicomponent program for nutrition and physical activity change in primary care: PACE+ for adolescents. *Archives of Pediatric and Adolescent Medicine, 155*, 940–946.

Perri, M. G., Nezu, A. M., Patti, E. T., & McCann, K. L. (1989). Effect of length of treatment on weight loss. *Journal of Consulting and Clinical Psychology, 57*, 450–452.

Petty, R. E., & Cacioppo, J. T. (1986). The elaboration likelihood model of persuasion. *Advances in Experimental Social Psychology, 19*, 123–205.

Prochaska, J. O., DiClemente, C. C., & Norcross, J. C. (1992). In search of how people change: Applications to additive behaviors. *American Psychologist, 47*, 1102–1114.

Ritterband, L. M., Borowitz, S., Cox, D. J., Kovatchev, B., Walker, L. S., Lucas, V., et al. (2005). Using the internet to provide information prescriptions. *Pediatrics, 116*, e643–e647.

Ritterband, L. M., Cox, D. J., Walker, L. S., Kovatchev, B., McKnight, L., Patel, K., et al. (2003). An internet intervention as adjunctive therapy for pediatric encopresis. *Journal of Consulting and Clinical Psychology, 71*, 910–917.

Robinson, S., Perkins, S., Bauer, S., Hammond, N., Treasure, J., & Schmidt, U. (2006). Aftercare intervention through text messaging in the treatment of bulimia nervosa-Feasibility pilot. *International Journal of Eating Disorders, 39*, 633–638.

Russ, C. R., Tate, D. F., Whitely, J. A., Winett, R. A., Winett, S. G., & Pfleger, J. (1998). The effects of an innovative www-based health behavior program on the nutritional practices of tenth grade girls: Preliminary report on the eat$_4$ life program. *Journal of Gender, Culture, & Health, 3*, 121–128.

Saelens, B. E., & Epstein, L. H. (1998). Behavioural engineering of activity choice in obese children. *International Journal of Obesity, 22*, 275–277.

Segal, K. R., & Dietz, W. H. (1991). Physiologic responses to playing a video game. *American Journal of Diseases of Children, 145*, 1034–1036.

Stone, A. A., & Shiffman, S. (2002). Capturing momentary, self-report data: A proposal for reporting guidelines. *Annals of Behavioral Medicine*, 24, 236–243.

Tate, D. F., Jackvony, E. H., & Wing, R. R. (2003). Effects of internet behavioral counseling on weight loss in adults at risk for Type 2 diabetes: A randomized trial. *Journal of the American Medical Association, 289*, 1833–1836.

Tate, D. F., Jackvony, E. H., & Wing, R. R. (2006). A Randomized trial comparing human e-mail counseling, computer automated tailored counseling, and no counseling in an internet weight loss program. *Archives of Internal Medicine, 166*, 1620–1625.

Tate, D. F., Jelalian, E., Ferguson, E., & Wing, R. R. (2005). Combining face-to-face and internet channels in the treatment of overweight adolescent girls. *Obesity, 13,* A3.

Tate, D. F., Wing, R. R., & Winett, R. A. (2001). Using internet technology to deliver a behavioral weight loss program. *Journal of the American Medical Association, 285,* 1172–1177.

Turnin, M. C., Tauber, M. T., Couvaras, O., Jouret, B., Bolzonella, C., Bourgeois, O., et al. (2001). Evaluation of microcomputer nutritional teaching games in 1,876 children at school. Diabetes and Metabolism, 27, 459-464.

U.S. Census Bureau. (2005). Computer and internet use in the United States: 2003, current population reports. October 2005.

Utter, J., Scragg, R., & Schaaf, D. (2006). Associations between television viewing and consumption of commonly advertised foods among New Zealand children and young adolescents. *Public Health Nutrition, 9,* 606–612.

Wang, X., & Perry, A. C. (2006). Metabolic and physiologic responses to video game play in 7- to 10-year-old boys. *Archives of Pediatric and Adolescent Medicine, 160,* 411–415.

Wantland, D. J., Portillo, C. J., Holzemer, W. L., Slaughter, R., & McGhee, E. M. (2004). The effectiveness of web-based vs. non-web-based interventions: A meta-analysis of behavioral change outcomes. *Journal of Medical Internet Research, 6,* e40.

Wiecha, J. L., Peterson, K. E., Ludwig, D. S., Kim, J., Sobol, A., & Gortmaker, S. L. (2006). When children eat what they watch: Impact of television viewing on dietary intake in youth. *Archives of Pediatric & Adolescent Medicine, 160,* 436–442.

Williamson, D. A., Martin, P. D., White, M. A., Newton, R., Walden, H., York-Crowe, E., et al. (2005). Efficacy of an internet-based behavioral weight loss program for overweight adolescent African-American girls. *Eating & Weight Disorders, 10,* 193–203.

Williamson, D. A., Walden, H. M., White, M. A., York-Crowe, E., Newton, R. L., Jr, Alfonso, A., et al. (2006). Two-year internet-based randomized controlled trial for weight loss in African-American girls. *Obesity (Silver Spring), 14,* 1231–1243.

Winett, R. A., Roodman, A. A., Winett, S. G., Bajzek, W., Roviniak, L. S., & Whiteley, J. A. (1999). The effects of the *Eat4Life* internet-based health behavior program on the nutrition and activity practices of high school girls. *Journal of Gender, Culture & Health, 4,* 239–254.

Winett, R. A., Tate, D. F., Anderson, E. S., Wojcik, J. R., & Winett, S. G. (2005). Long-term weight gain prevention: A theoretically based internet approach. *Preventive Medicine, 41,* 629–641.

Yon, B. A., Johnson, R. K., Harvey-Berino, J., & Gold, B. C. (2006). The use of a personal digital assistant for dietary self-monitoring does not improve the validity of self-reports of energy intake. *Journal of the American Dietetic Association,* 106(8), 1256–1259.

24

Motivational Interviewing and Pediatric Obesity

ROBYN S. MEHLENBECK
and YANA MARKOV WEMBER

The prevalence of pediatric overweight continues to increase, with the most recent estimates indicating that approximately 19 percent of children and 17 percent of adolescents in the United States are overweight, as defined by a BMI greater than or equal to the 95th percentile for age and gender (Ogden et al. 2006). Other studies have indicated that 37 percent of children and 34 percent of adolescents are either at risk for, or are, overweight (BMI >=85th percent) (Ogden et al.). Childhood obesity is associated with a significant number of short- and long-term health consequences, psychosocial risks, and an increased risk for obesity in adulthood (Freedman, Dietz, Srinivasan, & Berenson, 1999; Ludwig & Ebbeling, 2001; Whitaker, Wright, Pepe, Seidel, & Dietz, 1997). Given these long-standing implications and risks, Healthy People 2010 lists the reduction in prevalence of overweight among children as a key indicator of national health (U.S. Department of Health and Human Services, 2000).

Interventions to treat overweight children and adolescents are varied in their results. Most group-based interventions for children include a parent component, dietary restrictions (e.g., traffic light diet, reduced calorie diet), and a physical activity prescription (e.g., increase physical activity, decrease sedentary activity), as well as behavioral components targeting implementation of recommendations. With school-age children, family-based cognitive-behavioral group intervention is effective for weight loss (Epstein, Valoski, Wing, & McCurley, 1994), and has demonstrated long-term efficacy. There

ROBYN S. MEHLENBECK and YANA MARKOV WEMBER • The Warren Alpert Medical School of Brown University and Rhode Island Hospital/Bradley Hasbro Children's Research Center, Providence, RI 02903.

is less empirical evidence demonstrating efficacy of psychosocial weight-management interventions in adolescents (Jelalian & Saelens, 1999), and it remains unclear as to whether parents should participate in a group treatment program, and within what format. Even when a group format is available, it is not clear that group treatment is an effective intervention, particularly for adolescents. In addition, few people have access to group treatment for pediatric weight loss. Therefore, to reach more people and to continue to find effective treatments, consideration of treatment options for pediatric overweight is a priority (Dietz, 2006; Kirk, Scott, & Daniels, 2005).

Despite success with specific interventions, it is clear that many professionals remain frustrated regarding the treatment of pediatric overweight. One aspect of this may be the motivation (or lack thereof) of the child, adolescent, and/or their parents. Motivational interviewing (MI) has become an increasingly popular intervention to help people make changes in their lives by enhancing motivation. While developed and traditionally applied to problem drinking behaviors, forms of MI have been adapted for use in a variety of settings and for many health behaviors—including adolescent substance use, smoking, diet/exercise behaviors, and treatment adherence. Given its efficacy in other health- related areas, MI could not only enhance existing pediatric weight-loss interventions, but could be applied in a variety of settings (Resnicow, Davis, & Rollnick, 2006). The advantages of MI intervention approaches may include enhanced motivation for both children and their parents, increased adherence to recommendations, potential for administration by a wide variety of professionals, brevity and cost-effectiveness, and applicability in primary care settings. The goals of this chapter are to describe MI, review research that supports its use as an intervention, and offer practical recommendations for application to pediatric weight loss.

Motivation for change is considered to be a key factor in the success of interventions geared toward changing any health behavior. MI is a viable technique for enhancing motivation for behavior change and is defined as "a client-centered, directive method for enhancing intrinsic motivation to change by exploring and resolving ambivalence" (Miller & Rollnick, 2002, p 25). MI techniques incorporate four basic principles: a) expressing empathy, b) developing discrepancy, c) rolling with resistance and d) supporting self-efficacy (Miller & Rollnick). It is important to note that in many extant studies and commentaries on the use of MI techniques, it is clear that *pure* MI is not always used. Rather, protocols refer to adaptations of MI (AMI) that preserve the basic tenets of MI but differ from MI in the number of sessions conducted, actual techniques employed, and target audience. Much of the literature uses MI and AMI interchangeably. For the purpose of this chapter, and given the range of interventions that apply MI principles, it is assumed that all interventions reviewed are AMIs unless it is clearly indicated that the study involved a pure MI intervention (Miller & Rollnick). All of the AMIs reviewed did incorporate the four basic principles of MI that are presented in further detail below.

Although it is a basic component of MI, the first principle (i.e., expression of empathy) is not always utilized by clinicians. This principle suggests that the provider should actively listen and seek to understand the patient's point of view without judging, criticizing, blaming, or approving of behavior. Ambivalence is seen as normal, and reluctance to change is expected. The expression of empathy can be a powerful first step in working with families who have struggled with longstanding weight issues and have felt criticism from both family members and professional providers. Even a simple, sincere acknowledgement of the potential frustration and difficulty of making long-term changes in diet and exercise can help the family feel more understood and less defensive.

In developing discrepancy, the pros and cons of both current behaviors and new (i.e., healthier) behaviors are explored from the patient's perspective. In doing so, providers are able to highlight discrepancies between current behaviors and future goals. Behavior is unlikely to change if a person does not feel that such a change is more important and beneficial than maintaining their current behavior patterns. Rather than directing a person to change their behavior, this allows patients and families to increase consideration of—and motivation for—change. The following hypothetical example illustrates this principle. A parent is frustrated that her daughter will not stop eating junk food at home, yet continues to have this food available for consumption. One intervention technique is to ask the mother to stop buying junk food. However, using the MI principle of creating discrepancy may be more effective. For example, the provider could assist the mother in identifying ways in which the purchase of unhealthy food may help or hurt the daughter's weight-loss efforts. Additionally, the provider could assist the mother in exploring the effects of her actions within the broader family context.

Utilizing the third principle (rolling with resistance), providers maintain respect for their patients, reframe resistance and ambivalence as *normal*, and collaboratively problem-solve around barriers to change. When following this principle, the idea of *noncompliance* is eliminated. By understanding and normalizing resistance, this technique can help decrease frustration in both providers and patients and actually help increase motivation to change. For example, a child might state that he wants to lose weight, but refuses to forgo high-calorie desserts. The child would likely expect the provider to tell him he has to give up dessert to lose weight. The child may also expect the provider to express disappointment in the child if he refuses, stating that if he really wanted to lose weight, he would stop eating sweets. Following the *roll with resistance* principle of MI, the provider would normalize the child's resistance to change and highlight the child's wish to lose weight. The provider might also enlist the child in helping identify what he does want to do to lose weight and how the adults around him may help or hinder these efforts. Rather than starting an argument, the provider has opened up an aura of acceptance that can lead to problem-solving and increased self-efficacy for making changes for the client. Ultimately, the child might suggest on his own that he needs help cutting out dessert, or that he could choose healthier options (e.g., fruit) for dessert.

Finally, it is critical to support the patient's self-efficacy by enhancing a patient's personal responsibility and ability to carry out behavior change. Reflecting relevant positive attributes is also important to boost the patient's self-confidence in achieving the goals he/she has set. Social cognitive theory (Bandura, 1977) posits that perceived self-efficacy—or the confidence to change behavior—is a major determinant of whether behavior is initiated, the amount of effort expended, and how long a person will persist in the face of adverse circumstances. If a patient lacks confidence in his/her ability to change, success is unlikely. For children trying to lose weight, it is important to consider both the child's own self-efficacy and the family's belief that the child can be successful. Interventions should be designed to increase efficacy in both areas.

HOW THE TRANSTHEORETICAL MODEL OF CHANGE FITS WITH MI

MI interventions are often linked to the transtheoretical model of change (TTM)—a model developed by Prochaska and DiClemente (1982) to describe the process of behavior change. According to this model, there are five stages of change through which a person progresses during behavior change. These include: 1) precontemplation, or not even thinking about changing the behavior within the next six months; 2) contemplation, or thinking about changing the behavior in the next six months; 3) preparation, or planning to change in the next month; 4) action, or currently making health-relevant changes in the behavior; and 5) maintenance, or maintaining the behavior change for at least six months (Prochaska & DiClemente, 1982). A key assumption of this model is that effective interventions need to be matched to the individual's specific stage of change. Thus, it would make sense that when utilizing an adaptation of a motivational intervention, it would be more effective when an identified stage of change is utilized as a baseline. However, it is important to note that there is no consistent empirical support tying the transthoretical model of change and MI together (Wilson & Schlam, 2004). Despite this lack of empirical evidence, most studies continue to link these two concepts. Many studies suggest that *readiness to change* does not occur progressively through predefined and linear stages (as suggested in TTM), but is better defined as a state that fluctuates (Britt, Hudson, & Blampied, 2004).

What is consistent in both the TTM model and MI interventions is the concept of meeting the patient and/or family where they are. This clearly applies to pediatric weight loss, in that *readiness to change* will dictate what a child and/or family is ready to do. Any clinician who has tried to encourage a child to exercise when that child has no interest in weight loss will verify that this intervention will not work. A parent who is ready to alter the entire family's meal plan is likely to have more success with her/his child's weight loss. Clearly, further studies are needed to assess the effects of matching AMIs to the identified stage of change. Additionally, research that addresses the stages of change across interventions would be valuable.

WHAT DOES A TYPICAL INTERVENTION BASED ON PRINCIPLES OF MI LOOK LIKE?

As indicated by the studies below, there is wide variety in the application of MI principles to treatment protocols. Some studies presented stand alone AMI treatments, while others used AMI as a prelude or adjunct to other clinical interventions. Actual minutes of AMI employed in the reviewed interventions ranged from 15 to 240 minutes, depending on the study (Burke, Arkowitz, & Menchola, 2003). The settings included general medical practices, outpatient clinics, specialty clinics (e.g., substance abuse clinic), hospitals, and study laboratories (more traditional research settings). There have been many iterations of the MI model, making it difficult to identify a *typical* MI intervention.

Another issue regarding the delivery of MI is the training of the interventionists. Proponents of MI argue that adequate training provided by experts is critical in delivering an appropriate intervention. For example, Resnicow et al. (2006) highlights that in one intervention all interventionists went through a two day training prior to implementing the intervention, and participated in ongoing supervision. This training piece also contributes to whether an intervention is considered a MI or AMI. The reader is referred to the website: *www.motivationalinterview.org* for a list of expert trainers and where training is provided.

WHAT DO WE KNOW ABOUT MI AND AMIs FOR ADULTS?

Since its inception, MI or AMIs have been used for a variety of clinical problems, and the empirical research with adults has blossomed. As mentioned previously, MI was initially developed for substance abuse interventions. Three landmark studies have demonstrated the efficacy of MI in this context (Miller, Benefield, & Tonigan, 1993; Project MATCH, 1997; Stephens, Roffman, & Curtin, 2000).

Several meta-analyses have been conducted to examine the efficacy of AMI interventions on various health behaviors involving alcohol, drugs, smoking, asthma, diabetes, HIV-risk behaviors, eating disorders, and diet and exercise (Dunn, Deroo, & Rivara, 2001; Burke et al., 2003; Burke, Dunn, Atkins, & Phelps, 2004; Rubak, Sandbaek, Laurizen, & Christensen, 2005). Within these areas, several treatment outcomes have been used to measure the effectiveness of AMI interventions. These outcomes include objective medical findings (e.g., blood pressure, weight loss, Hemoglobin A1C), adherence to treatment (attendance), and behavioral factors (e.g., cigarettes/day, drinks/day). Burke et al.'s (2003) findings suggest that, when compared to a no-treatment or placebo control group, AMIs are efficacious for substance use and changes to diet and exercise, but not for smoking cessation and HIV-risk behaviors. In comparison to other active treatments, AMIs were comparable in efficacy but were considerably briefer—likely making AMIs more cost-effective. Rubak et al. reported similar findings, with significant effects found for MI for body mass index (BMI), total blood cholesterol, systolic blood pressure, blood alcohol concentration, and standard ethanol content, while combined effect estimates for cigarettes per day and for Hemoglobin A1C (HbA1C) were not significant. The reader is referred to these two meta-analyses for additional details on specific studies.

WHAT DO WE KNOW ABOUT USE OF MI AND AMIs FOR OVERWEIGHT ADULTS?

In the two aforementioned meta-analyses of AMI interventions, the outcomes being targeted by the intervention were not always clear. Burke's meta-analysis included five studies targeting diet (Woollard et al., 1995; Mhurchu, Margetts, & Speller, 1998; Smith, Heckemeyer, Dratt, & Kehryl, 1997), exercise (Harland et al., 1999), and/or eating disorders (Treasure et al., 1999). While there were significant effects for some outcomes, including blood pressure and increased physical activity, no significant effect was found for BMI (Burke et al., 2003). However, only one of the five studies reported BMI outcomes—likely limiting the ability to generalize of this finding.

Rubak et al. (2005) identified 10 studies measuring weight loss and/or changes in physical activity. They found that 80 percent of the studies demonstrated a significant effect utilizing AMIs. Although results suggested a statistical and clinical decrease in BMI among studies measuring this variable, it was unclear how many of the studies targeted weight loss or BMI as an outcome. For example, one study utilized AMI for patients with hypertension (Woollard et al., 1995), and found significant decreases in both weight and blood pressure over 18 weeks.

Only one study to date has utilized AMI to specifically target weight management in adults (Smith et al., 1997). Adult women with non-insulin dependent diabetes (NIDDM) who received a three-session AMI intervention attended more weight management group meetings, completed more food diaries, and recorded blood glucose significantly more often than women who had not received this intervention. Adding MI to the weight-control program did not result in significantly greater weight loss. However, these findings suggest that MI can increase adherence to a weight management program. Description of the AMI (with sample dialogue) can be found in DiLillo, Siegfried, and West (2003). Two other randomized studies have indicated that adding an MI component can both increase fruit and vegetable consumption (Resnicow, Jackson, & Wang, 2001) and lower fat intake (Bowen, Ehret, & Pedersen, 2002)—supporting the use of AMIs in attempts to modify diet among adults (VanWormer & Boucher, 2004).

While there are few studies attempting to intervene directly on motivation, several studies have attempted to evaluate what motivational factors are related to weight loss in adult samples. One study examined the role of autonomous motivation as a predictor of weight loss (Williams, Grow, Freedman, Ryan, & Deci, 1996). Results suggest that adults' autonomous motivation to participate in a weight-loss program is positively related to their staying in the program, losing weight in the program, and maintaining weight loss one year after completion of the program. Goldberg and Kiernan (2005) utilized AMI techniques prior to randomization in a behavioral weight loss trial to increase retention. While it was not possible to isolate the effects of the AMI intervention because other retention strategies were employed simultaneously, the group reported a 94 percent retention rate at an 18-month follow-up, which is considerably higher than that reported by many other weight-loss studies. Another study reported increased adherence to a treatment designed to increase physical exercise for adults who received some motivational intervention (Harland et al., 1999). To date, only one published randomized study utilizing motivational interventions found no differences in diet and/or exercise for the AMI group in comparison to the standard intervention (Mhurchu et al., 1998).

Interestingly, MI or AMI have rarely been utilized to enhance the efficacy of adult weight management interventions in empirical studies, despite the strong suggestion that motivational techniques can help increase exercise (Biddle & Fox, 1998), promote changes to diet (Resnicow et al., 2001), and affect other medical factors related to overweight (Rubak et al., 1995; Woollard et al., 2005).

WHAT DO WE KNOW ABOUT MI AND AMIs FOR ADOLESCENTS?

The developmental characteristics of adolescence may make MI interventions particularly appropriate when seeking to promote health behavior change within this population. For adolescents, ambivalence regarding behavior change is developmentally typical. One benefit of MI is that ambivalence is normalized and adolescents are assisted in moving through the ambivalence in a nonconfrontational manner. MI seems particularly suited for adolescents because it is brief, accepting, empathic, and collaborative when developing options for change. It also addresses ambivalence about change. Furthermore, because adolescents are less likely to self-refer to treatment than adults, demonstrate lower motivation to change health behaviors than adults (Melnick, Deleon, Hawke, Jainchill, & Kressel, 1997), and may engage in health behaviors with significant physical and mental health risks, strategies to enhance motivation are critical.

To date, most randomized MI and AMI interventions conducted with adolescents, both in medical and community settings, have targeted substance use behaviors such as drinking and smoking. For example, in a study of adolescent smokers recruited in a hospital clinic setting, 22 percent of those receiving a 30-minute MI intervention had quit smoking at follow-up in comparison to 10 percent of those in an *advice-only* control group (Colby et al., 1998). Another study demonstrated that older adolescents who received a motivational enhancement intervention in the emergency department after an alcohol-related event had significantly lower incidence of drinking and driving, traffic violations, alcohol-related injuries, and alcohol-related problems when compared to adolescents who received a standard care intervention (Monti et al., 1999). Spirito et al., (2004) replicated these findings with adolescents as young as 13.

Adolescent MI interventions have also been successful in enhancing diabetes control, increasing treatment adherence, and decreasing health risk behaviors. For example, three pilot studies that targeted adolescents with type I diabetes reported promising results, suggesting that AMIs can be beneficial in improving glycemic control and diabetes perception (Channon, Smith, & Gregory, 2003; Knight et al., 2003; Viner, Christie, Taylor, & Hey, 2003). Channon and colleagues assigned 22 adolescents who were identified as being in the contemplation stage of change to the motivation intervention condition. These adolescents received an average of 4.7 individual sessions over a six-month period. MI techniques focused on dietary adherence, alternatives, problem-solving, making choices, goal-setting, and the avoidance of confrontation. Results indicated that the participants had a 1.1 percent greater decrease in serum HbA1C during the intervention in comparison to a matched control sample.

Similarly, participation in a pilot group-based intervention incorporating elements of MI and solution-focused therapy was associated with improved glycemic control in 21 diabetic adolescents, ages 11–17 (Viner et al., 2003). Adolescents who were identified as either in the contemplation or action stage of change attended six weekly sessions in a small group divided by age. Results indicated a 1.5 percent decrease in HbA1C compared to no change in matched controls. Finally, Knight and colleagues (2003) enrolled six adolescents with diabetes, ages 13–16, in a six-week, group-based MI intervention to address metabolic control. When compared to a matched *usual care* control group, the adolescents who had received the intervention reported more positive shifts in their attitudes toward their diabetes—particularly increased views of control and acceptance. This study did not report on any physiological outcomes. While these preliminary results are promising, these early studies lack sufficient scientific rigor to support more generalized conclusions.

WHAT DO WE KNOW ABOUT MI AND AMIs FOR PEDIATRIC WEIGHT LOSS?

The extant research has shown that AMI interventions can help adolescents initiate treatment or change health behaviors, suggesting that this technique may be a useful adjunct to enhance pediatric weight-control programs. An excellent review by Resnicow et al. (2006) highlights not only the current evidence for AMIs in pediatric weight management, but conceptual issues to be taken into consideration in designing randomized controlled trials. Consistent with the adult literature, few studies have been conducted using MI or AMIs to target pediatric weight loss. The Go Girls study (Resnicow, Taylor, & Baskin, 2005) is the only randomized controlled trial utilizing MI as part of the active intervention targeting weight loss in adolescents. The Go Girls study was a church-based nutrition and physical activity intervention for overweight African-American females, comparing interventions of moderate and high intensity. The moderate intensity intervention included six sessions of culturally-sensitive behavioral group intervention. Each session included a behavioral activity, physical activity, and preparation and tasting of healthy foods. The high-intensity program involved 20–26 group sessions, plus four to six motivational interviewing telephone calls designed to enhance each participant's plans and progress regarding topics discussed in group sessions. Results indicated no significant differences for change in BMI between groups or any significant association between number of MI calls and change in BMI (Resnicow et al.).

Resnicow also reports on a pilot study in progress utilizing MI delivered by pediatricians and registered dieticians to prevent overweight in children ages three to seven (Schwarz, unpublished data 2006). Children who were either between the 85th and 95th BMI percentile—or between the 50th and 85th BMI percentile and had an obese parent—were randomized to either a control condition, a minimal intervention (one pediatrician-led MI session), or an intensive intervention (two pediatrician- and two registered dietician-led MI sessions). Preliminary results indicate high parent satisfaction with the counseling. However, outcome results for BMI and weight-related behaviors are not yet available.

Finally, while not directly targeting weight, one study has examined the effectiveness of a brief, individually-focused AMI intervention in promoting dietary adherence among adolescents with high cholesterol levels (Berg-Smith et al., 1999). The purpose of the intervention was to target barriers to dietary adherence in preadolescent children. Both children and their parents participated in the intervention. At a three-month follow-up, consumption of calories from fat as well as cholesterol intake had decreased. This study demonstrated that participants' readiness to change increased over the course of the intervention. Although these results are promising, the study lacked a control group, limiting conclusions regarding efficacy and the ability to generalize results. Clearly, additional research is needed to identify ways in which AMI could enhance pediatric weight-management interventions. Furthermore, AMI may be a beneficial adjunct in family-based interventions for overweight children—targeting both unhealthy eating and physical activity patterns.

CONSIDERATIONS IN USING MI IN PEDIATRIC POPULATIONS

The previous studies have highlighted many issues to consider when applying MI to a pediatric population, particularly for pediatric weight loss. The first involves questions regarding the target of the intervention. In all the adolescent studies reported, the adolescent was clearly the target of the motivation intervention. However, in one reviewed prevention study, the parent was the target of the intervention. In examining what is known about successful pediatric weight management, the target of the intervention is not always clear (child, parent, or both). Thus, future studies will need to take this into consideration when developing motivational interventions.

Second, even if the child or adolescent is the target of the intervention, children live within a family whose influence must be considered when attempting to help the child change health behaviors. Motivation across family members is rarely uniform, even if all members have a common goal of helping a child lose weight. The actions of a parent or sibling may affect the home environment. Thus, when applying MI interventions for pediatric weight loss, the role of other family members will need to be accounted for. The idea of applying MI techniques to the family is not unique. For example, Dishion and Kavanaugh (2003) developed a brief, three-session motivational intervention called the Family Check-Up (FCU) for parents of at-risk youth. Preliminary studies found that families participating in the FCU reported significantly fewer behavioral problems in their adolescents in comparison to a wait-list control group, as well as improved family perceptions of management of behavior issues at home (Dishion, Nelson, & Kavanaugh, 2003). A model similar to the FCU may be very useful for pediatric weight loss.

Finally, one advantage of MI is that a variety of professionals can be trained to administer the intervention, rather than relying solely on psychologists, pediatricians, or dieticians. Given the paucity of research applying MI to pediatric weight loss, it remains unclear whether the most efficacious intervention is to add MI to existing behavioral group-based interventions or if the pediatrician's office is the most efficacious context. Once the target of the intervention is decided upon, other treatment settings could also be considered. For example, MI interventions targeting adolescents could be administered in the school setting or other places that adolescents gather naturally.

In summary, while more empirical research is clearly needed, MI techniques may be an important addition to pediatric weight-management interventions. Sindelar, Abrantes, Hart, Lewandes, and Spirito (2004) provided an excellent overview of applying the principles of MI to pediatric practice in general. A brief, motivational intervention can support a child and his/her family by increasing their current level of motivation, enhancing the match between a parent's and child's interest in losing weight, and helping each family member identify individual steps to achieve pediatric weight management. AMIs can be delivered within multiple settings, including primary care, and help promote an alliance between providers and clients. AMIs may be more cost-effective than longer-term interventions because they can be delivered by many different service providers at various levels and are much briefer interactions. Finally, receiving appropriate, formal training in motivational interviewing may be viewed as an excellent time investment given the broad application of MI interventions within the healthcare setting.

CASE APPLICATIONS

The following section presents two cases illustrating the application of MI in pediatric weight management. Several techniques are employed, but both cases keep the guiding principles in mind. Some of these techniques include using open-ended questions, reflective listening, affirmations, highlighting self-motivational statements, addressing concerns, exploring ambivalence, and summarizing (see Table 24.1 for examples of each). In putting these principles and techniques into practice, the reader is also referred to Rollnick, Mason, and Butler (1999) as well as the motivational interviewing website: *www.motivationalinterview.org.*

Table 24.1. Examples of techniques used in MI

Technique	Description	Example statement
Open-Ended Questions	Questions that cannot be answered with 'yes' or 'no' can help develop rapport and gain a clearer understanding of your client's perspective	"Tell me what you have been up to since our last meeting?" "What have you tried in the last month?"
Reflective Listening	A brief restatement of what your client has said to show that you are closely listening to their perspective and to give your client the chance to hear out loud what he/she said	"You are frustrated that no one understands how hard it is for you to lose weight" "You want your mother to take walks with you, but not to "nag" about your weight"
Affirmations	Positive statements regarding your client's strengths in a sincere, genuine manner can help with rapport, self-efficacy and motivation	"Clearly you have put a lot of thought into this and even tried a few things on your own" "You have shown that you can go without potato chips for a week – that takes a lot of willpower when they are sitting in the cabinet at home!"
Highlighting Self-Motivational Statements	Reinforcing what the client states about his/her own motivation including recognizing a problem, concerns, intention to change and optimism for change	"Although your mother is more worried about your weight, you would like to be able to run faster when you play basketball" "It is impressive that you have decided you want to do something about your weight and are asking fwwor some help with that!"
Addressing Concerns	A chance to identify ongoing concerns and problem solve barriers to change in a nonconfrontational manner, but still giving appropriate feedback	"You are worried it will be too hard to lose weight. I wonder what step might feel doable that would affect your weight?" "Your father likes to eat junk food at home. I wonder if we could come up with any ideas to help you with this issue?"
Exploring Ambivalence	Giving the client permission to be ambivalent can be a powerful intervention alone, as well as taking the opportunity to explore the pros/cons of making the behavior change without judgment	"We know that there are good and not so good things about trying to lose weight – let's talk about both the good things and the not so good things." "It makes sense that your child does not always worry about their weight."
Summarizing	A longer version of reflective listening, where the provider is able to restate back to the client what the discussion has been about, with emphasis on the self-motivational and self-efficacious statements made by the client	"So, in meeting today, we have discussed your concerns about your child's weight, his/her concerns and how much conflict there is in the family around this issue. Both of you would love to fight less. Both of you would like to feel better about yourselves in different ways. Since you both agree on the importance of feeling better and making home a happier place, I wonder if we can agree on one goal to work on – some options might include taking more walks together or mom buying healthier foods for everyone."

Case 1

John (age 16) presents to a weight-loss treatment program accompanied by his mother. While John has agreed to participate in this teen weight-management program to "get his mother off his back," he does mention that he is interested in getting in better shape for football. However, despite being moderately overweight, he is not too concerned about his weight. His mother, who is also moderately overweight, is anxious for John to lose weight. She is worried about John's health because he has a family history of diabetes, hypertension, and high cholesterol. John's mother has been trying to get John to lose weight for the last couple of years.

In meeting with John alone to discuss his interest in the program, it becomes clear that John came with his mother to appease her and to help her "worry less." If John attempts to lose weight for his mother, he is less likely to succeed. Rather, the leader empathizes with John concerning the difficulty of parents worrying about their teens. She then comments on how much John must care about his mother to be willing to consider trying to lose weight to help decrease her worry. While John shrugs this off, the leader asks him if he has any worries about his weight. John acknowledges that he would like to lose a few pounds to be able to run faster and improve his football performance. The leader then reinforces that, for most people, being overweight can hinder sport performance and that he is already "ahead of the game" in recognizing that losing some weight is likely to improve his performance. Additionally, John mentions that he feels that losing some weight would make it easier to get a date. The leader highlights that John has clearly thought about some benefits of losing weight on his own. The leader then prompts John about the disadvantages (i.e., "cons") of trying to lose weight. John replies that there are no disadvantages, but notes that weight loss is difficult. The leader agrees with John that losing weight is a very difficult thing to do, and asks if he has tried in the past to lose weight. John acknowledges that he tried to cut back on junk food for a week and because he does love to play football, he often exercises outside of practice during football season. He also acknowledges that he usually loses some weight during football season, but then gains more over the rest of the year. The leader praises John's efforts and comments on how he is already aware of the things that are successful for him—notably, increasing his exercise activity. He also knows that while it is difficult for him to cut back on the junk food for the long term, he is very successful at this in the short term. He is then encouraged to think about what he likes about football and the extra activity he does during football season. John's mood brightens as he discusses the teamwork and the game, highlighting that when he does go for jogs, he is often thinking of football plays. The leader then states that she is impressed by how much he has already accomplished and recognized about himself. She also comments on how what he has said suggests that he would like to take control of his weight to improve his football. Additionally, the leader emphasizes that John has already identified weight control strategies that have been successful for him—all without his mother's input. John appears a little surprised and begins to ask more questions about the weight management program.

In this case example, John's mother was the primary instigator to seek weight-loss treatment. John initially appeared reluctant to consider changing his health behaviors, attending the interview simply to appease his mother. The leader used several motivational techniques to help John consider that the weight-management treatment might be a good thing from his own perspective (not his mother's). These techniques included expressing empathy, listening reflectively, emphasizing the client's perspective (notice that there were no comments about his health, as this is rarely motivating to a teenager), and increasing confidence by highlighting past success. Any signs of resistance were met with an empathetic comment rather than a contradiction or challenge. Had John been clearly uninterested, a motivational intervention might have focused on supporting John in telling his mother that he currently had no desire to participate in weight-loss treatment while emphasizing John's knowledge of what might work in future weight loss attempts. The leader might then suggest a follow-up appointment to "check in" and promote additional opportunity for motivational intervention.

Case 2

Cindy (age 10) presents to her pediatrician's office. The pediatrician is concerned because her weight has been steadily increasing over the past several years and is currently above the 95th percentile for her height. In the past two visits, Cindy's mother has brought up weight as a major concern. Cindy's mother, who runs daily and feels that fitness is very important, is angry that her daughter is overweight. Cindy is not allowed to eat sweets or junk food at home, even though her brother is allowed to eat these foods.

Cindy and her mother are meeting with the pediatrician. After an initial welcome, the pediatrician asks in a neutral tone: *How are things going?*

Mother: *Very frustrating. Cindy continues to eat and gain weight. She won't exercise, no matter how much I try to get her to. She just doesn't realize that I "nag" her for her own good.*

Pediatrician: *What concerns you about Cindy's weight?*

Mother: *I am worried that she is being teased—kids can be very mean these days. I am also worried about her health. I don't want her to develop diabetes, which runs in our family. I also want her to be a happy teenager and I know that teens with weight problems are depressed.*

Pediatrician: *Cindy, I am sure that you have heard this from your mother before. Does she know what concerns you have, if any, about your weight?*

Cindy: *I want to look prettier. My mom always says I will if I lose some weight.*

Pediatrician: *So you think you would look prettier if you lose some weight and your mother would be less worried about you being teased and your health? Knowing how hard it is to try to lose weight, I am very impressed that your daughter has even considered it. Cindy, on a scale of 1 to 10, how important is it to you to lose weight?*

Cindy: *Maybe a 5—sometimes I really want to and other times I wish everyone would just leave me alone.*

Pediatrician: *It makes a lot of sense that you might have different feelings at different times. Mom, on that same scale, how important is it to you that Cindy loses weight?*
Mother: *Definitely a 10. I worry all the time about it.*
Pediatrician: *So this is a really big concern for you, so much so that you cannot stop thinking about it. You clearly care for your daughter's well-being. That must make it extremely frustrating that you two do not agree.*

In this first phase of the interview, the pediatrician started to develop rapport and express empathy for both Cindy and her mother. The pediatrician has also evaluated the importance of this issue to both family members and validated both perspectives. In starting to develop discrepancy, the next section addresses the pros/cons of trying to lose weight. A decisional balance was created and can be seen in Table 24.2. Excerpts of a conversation in creating this decisional balance are included in the text.

Pediatrician: *I would like to walk through an exercise with you both. This may help us explore your feelings about your weight and where you are in your thoughts about losing weight. There are no right or wrong answers, and you two do not have to agree on your answers. First, let's brainstorm all the good things about staying at your current weight.*
Cindy: *I could eat anything I wanted.*
Pediatrician: *Great start! What else can we think of?*
Mother: *Although I don't see much good about her current weight, it would be better than gaining more weight. Also, we might not argue as much about food.*

Table 24.2. Cindy's decisional balance

Good Things About Current Weight	Not So Good Things About Current Weight
-maintaining is better than gaining - less arguing - eat anything I want - can watch as much TV as I want	- teasing - no good clothes - no energy - don't like shopping at "fat kid" stores - sad sometimes - don't like eating in front of others at school - lots of fighting with my mom
Good Things About Trying to Lose Weight	**Not So Good Things About Trying to Lose Weight**
- can exercise together (mom and Cindy) - might feel better about herself - less worry about Cindy's health - buy new clothes - mom will stop nagging - healthier - might get picked in gym - more energy - do more fun activities - feel happier	- hard work - have to eat differently than my family - have to do too much exercise - don't like exercise - might disappoint mom - can't have ice cream - might get embarrassed at school

Pediatrician: *Excellent. How about the "not so good things" about Cindy's current weight?*

Mother: *That's easy – she gets teased, she is overweight, she has a hard time finding nice clothes, and she has no energy most of the time.*

Cindy: *Mom! I do not get teased as much as you think. I do wish I could find nicer clothes—I don't like shopping in the "fat kid" stores. I also don't like eating at school in front of the other kids.*

Pediatrician: *So both of you have different ideas of what is good and not so good about Cindy's current weight, but it is impressive that you both were able to come up with ideas. Now, if you decided to try to lose weight, what would be the "not so good things" about trying to lose weight?*

Note here that the pediatrician is not telling Cindy to lose weight. This is an important distinction because the mother in this case is already convinced that Cindy needs to lose weight while Cindy remains ambivalent. A statement directly telling Cindy she needs to lose weight is likely to lead to resistance and further family conflict.

Mother: *Well, I can see that it is hard work. Cindy would have to eat differently than everyone and exercise more.*

Cindy: *It takes too much time. If I tried and then cheated on my diet, my mom would be even more mad. I wouldn't be able to eat ice cream anymore and I wouldn't know what to do at school when they have a party.*

Pediatrician: *It is hard work and does take a lot of time! Both are true! One more question - if you did decide to try to lose weight, what would be the "good things" about losing weight?*

Cindy: *I could get new clothes. And my mom wouldn't always be nagging me.*

Mother: *We could exercise together. Cindy would feel better about herself. I wouldn't worry about her health so much.*

Pediatrician: *So, if I can summarize our exercise, both of you were able to come up with some pros and cons for Cindy staying at the same weight and for Cindy losing weight. While it would be easier to stay the same weight and Cindy worries about making her mother more mad if she cheated on her diet, both of you highlighted that losing weight could lead to new clothes and Cindy feeling better about herself. It might also lead to less conflict around this issue. What I find most interesting is that both of you are saying that there are some clear benefits to trying to lose weight. Cindy, when you have tried to lose weight in the past, what has worked for you?*

Cindy: *Well, I gave up ice cream for a week, but then that's all I wanted and mom got mad. One time I did go for walks with mom and that was kind of nice but then when I ate the ice cream mom told me it was a waste of time to walk with me.*

Pediatrician: *It seems like you are trying very hard to make your mother happy, and even enjoyed the time you walked with your mother. And you were successful in not eating ice cream for a week! That can be very hard, and you showed yourself that you can do it!*

Mother: *She did do a great job that week.*

This section highlighted the use of a decisional balance to help both mother and Cindy look at the pros/cons of losing weight without directly telling Cindy that she must lose weight. The pediatrician was able to summarize each individual's motivation, acknowledging the ambivalence and highlighting the positive aspects of weight loss that each identified. The pediatrician also tried to elicit self-efficacious statements by inquiring about what has been successful for Cindy in the past. In this situation, helping the mother acknowledge any positive steps will go a long way toward helping Cindy feel more motivated to lose weight and increase Cindy's confidence in her ability successfully change her health behaviors. The next step may be to set up a reasonable goal for the family to work on—framed in a supportive manner—that will also promote Cindy's self-efficacy.

Pediatrician: *Given what we have discussed today, it sounds like at times you are both interested in Cindy trying to lose some weight. At other times, only mom is interested. In the past, Cindy has done an excellent job eliminating a high-fat food from her diet for a period of time. She has also been interested in and expressed enjoyment at taking walks with her mother. I wonder if it would be helpful to set just one goal for the next month?*

Cindy: *Like losing weight? What do I have to do?*

Mother: *What do you suggest?*

Pediatrician: *I am open to your suggestions. You both mentioned that you liked walking. I wonder if that is one place to start. You could take time together, which is important to both of you. Cindy, you also mentioned that you have been successful at walking with your mother in the past as part of trying to lose weight.*

Cindy: *I would like to walk with mom a couple times a week if she promises not to argue with me or ask me about what I am eating.*

Mother: *No arguing on walks. I will also promise not to argue about food for the next month.*

With guidance, the family was able to set one goal that met both Cindy and her mother where they were. In this case, the pediatrician might also meet separately with the mother—given that her motivation is highest—and discuss in this same style what the mother can and is willing to do on a family level to support weight loss. For example, the mother might say that it is not fair to stop buying ice cream since her son and husband do not have a weight problem. However, with some empathetic statements intended to define the mother's goals for good health for everyone in the family along with problem solving, the mother might be willing to purchase healthier foods at home for everyone.

Finally, many practitioners will encounter cases when a parent is clearly ambivalent regarding his/her child's weight and is not ready to make any changes for the whole family. This is particularly problematic with younger children, who cannot make many of their own decisions regarding healthy eating and activity. However, this can also be true when a young teenager wants to try to lose weight but the family continues to eat unhealthy meals and snacks while providing little opportunity for exercise. Because pediatric weight management clearly involves several different behaviors that contribute to overweight, it is possible that a MI intervention could be very effective with ambivalent parents. The goal of the MI might be to find one behavior that the parent recognizes as a target for positive behavior change and feels confident about helping to change that specific behavior. Developing rapport with parents, using a decisional balance to help the parent identify the pros/cons of making changes, and increasing self-efficacy in the parent that they are capable making the change and following through, are all examples of how this intervention may apply to ambivalent parents.

CONCLUSION AND FUTURE DIRECTIONS

While originally developed as an intervention for substance abuse, MI and AMIs have demonstrated promise in several areas of health-behavior change, including changing diet and exercise behaviors. Of particular importance to pediatrics is the emerging data demonstrating efficacy with several adolescent populations. When designing interventions for pediatric weight loss, motivation needs to be addressed on several levels, including both the family and the identified patient. The complexity and difficulty of pediatric weight loss make it an ideal area for the application of MI.

While there is solid empirical evidence that family-based cognitive behavioral group intervention is effective for weight loss in younger children (Epstein et al., 1994), this intervention is not always available to patients. Introducing MI techniques may allow providers at many levels to intervene successfully when group-based treatments are not available or desired by the family. For those involved in group treatments, it may be beneficial to add MI or AMI interventions to existing CBT treatments to enhance efficacy and long-term weight management. Furthermore, a brief MI/AMI session subsequent to a CBT intervention may help weight-loss maintenance.

While many more weight-loss interventions are now available for adolescents than for children, a single most effective intervention is yet to be identified. Given the efficacy of AMIs in promoting health-behavior change among adolescents in other areas (e.g., substance abuse, cigarette smoking, enhanced diabetes control), utilizing MI or adding MI components to other treatments shows promise as an intervention for adolescent weight-control problems. Future research, including randomized clinical trials, is clearly needed to evaluate the efficacy of MI for pediatric weight loss. Studies conducted in primary-care settings should also be considered to give direct-care providers effective tools to help families and children with this difficult issue.

REFERENCES

Bandura, A. (1977). *Self-efficacy: The exercise of control.* New York: Freeman.

Berg-Smith, S. M., Stevens, V. J., Brown, K. M., Van Horn, L., Gernhofer, N., Peters, E., et al. (1999). A brief motivational intervention to improve dietary adherence in adolescents. *Health Education Research, 14,* 399–410.

Biddle, S. J., & Fox, K. R. (1998). Motivation for physical activity and weight management. *International Journal of Obesity and Related Metabolic Disorders, 22*, S39–S47.

Bowen, D., Ehret, C., & Pedersen, M. (2002). Results of an adjunct dietary intervention program in the Women's Health Initiative. *Journal of the American Dietetic Association, 102*, 1631–1637.

Britt, E., Hudson, S. M., & Blampied, N. M. (2004). Motivational interviewing in health settings: A review. *Patient Education and Counseling, 53*, 147–155.

Burk, B. L., Arkowitz, H., & Menchola, M. (2003). The efficacy of motivational interviewing: A meta-analysis of controlled clinical trials. *Journal of Consulting and Clinical Psychology, 71*, 843–861.

Burke, B. L., Dunn, C. W., Atkins, D. C., & Phelps, J. S. (2004). The emerging evidence base for motivational interviewing: A meta-analytic and qualitative inquiry. *Journal of Cognitive Psychotherapy: An International Quarterly, 18*, 309–322.

Channon, S., Smith, V. J., & Gregory, J. W. (2003). A pilot study of motivational interviewing in adolescents with diabetes. *Archives of Disease in Childhood, 88*, 680–683.

Colby, S. M., Monti, P. M., Barnett, M. P., Rohsenhow, D. J., Weissman, K., & Spirito, A. (1998). Brief motivational interviewing in a hospital setting for adolescent smoking: A preliminary study. *Journal of Consulting and Clinical Psychology, 66*, 574–578.

Dietz, W. H. (2006). What constitutes successful weight management in adolescents? *Annals of Internal Medicine, 145*, 145–146.

DiLillo, V., Siegfried, H. J., & West, D. S. (2003). Incorporating motivational interviewing into behavioral obesity treatment. *Cognitive and Behavioral Practice, 10*, 120–130.

Dishion, T. J., & Kavanagh, K. (2003). Intervening in adolescent problem behavior: A family centered approach. New York: The Guilford Press.

Dishion, T. J., Nelson, S. E., & Kavanagh, K. (2003). The family check up with high risk young adolescents: Preventing early onset substance use by parent monitoring. *Behavior Therapy, 34*, 553–571.

Dunn, C., Deroo, L., & Rivara, F. P. (2001). The use of brief interventions adapted from motivational interviewing across behavioral domains: A systematic review. *Addiction, 96*, 1725–1742.

Epstein, L. H. (2003). Development of evidence-based treatments for pediatric obesity. In A. E. Kazdin & J. R. Weisz (Eds.), *Evidence-based psychotherapies for children and adolescents* (pp. 374–388). New York: The Guilford Press.

Epstein, L. H., Valoski, A., Wing, R. R., & McCurley, J. (1994). Ten year outcomes of behavioral family-based treatment for childhood obesity. *Health Psychology, 13*, 373–383.

Freedman, D. S., Dietz, W. H., Srinivasan, S. R., & Berenson, G. S. (1999). The relation of overweight to cardiovascular risk factors among children and adolescents: The Bogalusa Heart Study. *Pediatrics, 103*, 1175–1182.

Goldberg, J. H., & Kiernan, M. (2005). Innovative techniques to address retention in a behavioral weight-loss trial. *Health Education Research, 20*, 439–447.

Harland, J., White, M., Drinkwater, C., Chinn, D., Larr, L., & Howel, D. (1999). The Newcastle exercise project: A randomized controlled trial of methods to promote physical activity in primary care. *British Medical Journal, 319*, 828–832.

Jelalian, E., & Saelens, B. E. (1999). Empirically supported treatments in pediatric psychology: Pediatric obesity. *Journal of Pediatric Psychology, 24*, 223–248.

Kirk, S., Scott, B. J., & Daniels, S. R. (2005). Pediatric obesity epidemic: Treatment options. *Research, 105*, S44–S51.

Knight, K. M., Bundy, C., Morris, R., Higgs, J. F., Jameson, R. A., Unsworth, P., et al. (2003). The effects of group motivational interviewing and externalizing conversations for adolescents with Type-1 diabetes. *Psychology, Health & Medicine, 8*, 149–157.

Ludwig, D. S., & Ebbeling, C. B. (2001). Type 2 diabetes mellitus in children: Primary care and public health considerations. *Journal of the American Medical Association, 286*, 1427–1430.

Melnick, G., DeLeon, G., Hawke, J., Jainchill, N., & Kressel, D. (1997). Motivation and readiness for therapeutic community treatment among adolescents and adult substance abusers. *American Journal of Drug and Alcohol Abuse, 23*, 485–506.

Mhurchu, C. N., Margetts, B. M., & Speller, V. (1998). Randomized clinical trial comparing the effectiveness of two dietary interventions for patients with hyperlipidaemia. *Clinical Science*, 95, 479–587.

Miller, W. R., Benefield, R. G., & Tonigan, J. S. (1993). Enhancing motivation for change in problem drinking: A controlled comparison of two therapist styles. *Journal of Consulting and Clinical Psychology*, 61, 455–461.

Miller, W. R., & Rollnick, S. (2002). *Motivational interviewing: Preparing people for change (2nd ed.)*. New York: Guilford Press.

Monti, P. M., Colby, S. M., Barnett, N. P., Spirito, A., Rohsenow, D. J., & Myers, M. (1999). Brief motivational interviewing for harm reduction with alcohol-positive older adolescents in a hospital emergency department. *Journal of Consulting and Clinical Psychology*, 67, 989–994.

Ogden, C. L., Carroll, M. D., Curtin, L. R., McDowell, M. A., Tabak, C. J., & Flegal, K. M. (2006). Prevalence of overweight and obesity in the United States, 1999-2004. *Journal of the American Medical Association*, 295, 1549–1555.

Prochaska, J. O., & DiClemente, C. C. (1982). Transtheoretical therapy: Toward a more integrative model of change. *Psychotherapy: Theory, Research and Practice*, 19, 276–288.

Project MATCH Research Group. (1997). Matching alcoholism treatment to client heterogeneity: Project MATCH posttreatment drinking outcomes. *Journal of Studies on Alcohol*, 58, 7–29.

Resnicow, K., Davis, R., & Rollnick, S. (2006). Motivational interviewing for pediatric obesity: Conceptual issues and evidence review. *Journal of the American Dietetic Association*, 106, 2024–2033.

Resnicow, K., DiIorio, C., Soet, J. E., Borrelli, B., Hecht, J., & Ernst, D. (2002). Motivational interviewing in health promotion: It sounds like something is changing. *Health Psychology*, 21, 444–451.

Resnicow, K., Jackson, A., & Wang, T. (2001). A motivational interviewing intervention to increase fruit and vegetable intake through black churches: Results of the Eat for Life Trial. *American Journal of Public Health*, 91, 1686–1693.

Resnicow, K., Taylor, R., & Baskin, M. (2005). Results of Go Girls: A nutrition and physical activity intervention for overweight African American adolescent females conducted through Black churches. *Obesity Research*, 13, 1739–1748.

Rollnick, S., Mason, P., & Butler, C. (1999). *Health behavior change: A guide for practitioners*. London: Harcourt Brace.

Rubak, S., Sandboek, A., Lauritzen, T., & Christensen, B. (2005). Motivational interviewing: A systematic review and meta-analysis. *British Journal of General Practice*, 55, 305–312.

Sindelar, H. A., Abrantes, A. M., Hart, C., Lewander, W., & Spirito, A. (2004). Motivational interviewing in pediatric practice. *Current Problems in Pediatric and Adolescent Health Care*, 34, 322–339.

Smith, D. E., Heckemeyer, C. M., Dratt, P. P., & Kehryl, M. (1997). Motivational interviewing to improve adherence to a behavioral weight-control program for older obese women with NIDDM: A pilot study. *American Diabetes Association*, 20, 52–54.

Spirito, A., Monti, P. M., Barnett, N. P., Colby, S. M., Sindelar, H., Rohsenow, D. J., et al. (2004). A randomized clinical trial of a brief motivational intervention for alcohol-positive adolescents treated in an emergency department. *The Journal of Pediatrics*, 145, 396–402.

Stephens, R. S., Roffman, R. A., & Curtin, L. (2000). Comparison of extended versus brief treatments for marijuana use. *Journal of Consulting and Clinical Psychology*, 68, 898–908.

Treasure, J. L., Katzman, M., Schmidt, U., Troop, N., Todd, G., & de Silva, P. (1999). Engagement and outcome in the treatment of bulimia nervosa: First phase of a sequential design comparing motivation enhancement therapy and cognitive behavioral therapy. *Behaviour Research and Therapy*, 37, 405–418.

U.S. Department of Health and Human Services. (2000). *Healthy people 2010: Understanding and improving health (2nd ed.)*. Washington, DC: U.S. Government Printing Office.

VanWormer, J. J., & Boucher, J. L. (2004). Motivational interviewing and diet modification: A review of the evidence. *The Diabetes Educator, 30*, 404–419.

Viner, R. M., Christie, D., Taylor, V., & Hey, S. (2003). Motivational/solution-focused intervention improves HbA$_{1c}$ in adolescents with type 1 diabetes: A pilot study. *Diabetic Medicine, 20*, 739–742.

Whitaker, R. C., Wright, J. A., Pepe, M. S., Seidel, K. D., & Dietz, W. H. (1997). Predicting obesity in young adulthood from childhood and parental obesity. *The New England Journal of Medicine, 337*, 869–873.

Williams, G. C., Grow, V. M., Freedman, Z. R., Ryan, R. M., & Deci, E. L. (1996). Motivational predictors of weight loss and weight-loss maintenance. *Journal of Personality and Social Psychology, 70*, 115–126.

Wilson, G. T., & Schlam, T. R. (2004). The transtheoretical model and motivational interviewing in the treatment of eating and weight disorders. *Clinical Psychology Review, 24*, 361–378.

Woollard, J., Beilin, L., Lord, T., Puddey, I., MacAdam, D., & Rouse, I. (1995). A controlled trial of nurse counseling on lifestyle change for hypertensives treated in general practice: Preliminary results. *Clinical and Experimental Pharmacology and Physiology, 22*, 466–468.

25

Treatment of Children and Adolescents with Obesity and Comorbid Psychiatric Conditions

ALAN ZAMETKIN, ALANNA JACOBS, and JESSICA PARRISH

The effective treatment of childhood obesity—a challenge in itself—is complicated further when accompanied by comorbid psychiatric disorders. Weight management has become an important concern in the treatment of psychopathology due to the significant weight gain induced by many psychotropic medications. The objectives of this chapter are to review the literature on the relationship between obesity and psychiatric conditions, examine the utility of current obesity treatments for use in these populations, and elucidate the role of psychopharmacology in the weight status of these children. In doing so, we will highlight areas that merit further investigation in the effort to develop more precisely targeted treatments.

THE RELATIONSHIP BETWEEN OBESITY AND MENTAL HEALTH

There are mixed findings regarding the association between psychiatric conditions and obesity. Many population-based studies have found high rates of psychological disorders in obese children and adolescents—especially in females. Buddeburg-Fisher, Klaghofer, and Reed (1999) found higher

ALAN ZAMETKIN, ALANNA JACOBS, and JESSICA PARRISH • National Institute of Mental Health, Bethesda, MD 20892.

rates of such disorders as somatoform, mood, pain, and anxiety in over-weight Swiss high school girls. They also reported a correlation between poorer body image and increased psychiatric comorbidity. However, in a study of 3,197 adolescent females, Pesa, Syre, and Jones (2000) found that after controlling for body-image dissatisfaction, the difference in psychopathology between nonobese and obese females ages 15–17 was insignificant. Erickson, Robinson, Haydel, and Killen (2000) found similar results in a study of third graders. In another population-based study of 10,000 adolescents, Gortmaker (1993) found no correlation initially or at seven-year follow-up between obesity and psychological comorbidity.

Some research indicates that there is a significant difference in the incidence of psychiatric comorbidity between obese pediatric patients who are clinically referred for obesity and obese children in the general population. Those seeking clinical treatment for obesity have increased levels of depression, anxiety, somatoform, and eating disorders (Britz et al., 2000; Epstein, Klein, & Wisniewski, 1994; Sheslow et al., 1993; Wallace, Sheslow, & Hassink, 1993). One study investigating the prevalence of psychiatric disorders in extremely obese adolescents reported that the rate of bulimia nervosa, eating disorders not otherwise specified (EDNOS), and anorexia nervosa to be six times higher among obese pediatric patients compared to a population-based, control group (Britz et al.).

Within the obese population, 60 percent of females and 35.3 percent of males reported binge-eating episodes in which the quantity of food intake exceeded that of most people under similar circumstances. Wallace et al. (1993) found that 32 percent of obese children had depression, and Seshlow et al. (1993) reported a rate of 50 percent. These data parallel findings that clinically referred obese adults have higher psychiatric comorbidity than population-based obese adults (Britz et al., 2000; Pesa et al., 2000). Spitzer et al. (1993) performed a multisite study of binge-eating disorder (BED) involving 1,785 adult subjects, and found that 29 percent of the subjects in weight-control programs met the criteria for BED. A study by Yanovski, Nelson, Dubbert, and Spitzer (1993) found that 43 percent of the 128 obese adult subjects met the criteria for BED.

Controlling for alternative factors may diminish the incidence of psychological disorders in clinically referred obese patients. Two studies by Epstein et al. (1994) and Epstein, Myers, and Anderson (1996) compared psychopathology in obese patients and controls, covarying mother's psychopathology and child's BMI. Results indicated significant differences between groups in psychological problems, showing "58 percent of boys and 44 percent of girls met criteria on at least one Child Behavior Checklist/4–18 (CBCL) behavioral problem scale" (Achenbach, 1991; Epstein et al., 1996, p. 65). However, after controlling for maternal psychopathology, no significant difference remained in the psychological comorbidity and socioeconomic status of the obese pediatric population.

In population-based studies, a significant difference in behavior (not disorders) is evident between obese and nonobese children. Stradmeijer, Bosch, Koops, and Seidell (2000) used parent and teacher reports on two groups of children—prepubertal (ages 10–13) and adolescent (ages 13–16). They found that mothers and teachers reported significantly more behavior problems in obese children and adolescents than nonobese peers, especially among the prepubertal age group.

In summary, the evidence cited shows behavioral problems in subgroups of obese children, but there is no clear indication of higher rates of psychiatric comorbidity in the general population of obese children. Friedman and Brownell (1995) suggest research to identify protective factors and vulnerabilities influencing the development of psychopathology in obese children.

CAUSE OR CONSEQUENCE?

There is speculation about whether obesity results from currently classified psychiatric disorders. Recent longitudinal studies have shown that obesity in childhood or adolescence predicts obesity in adulthood after controlling for a variety of variables. Goodman and Whitaker (2002) found that depressed mood at baseline independently predicted obesity at follow-up after controlling for race and socioeconomic status. In a nonclinical population, researchers found that females who reported depressive symptoms as children had greater BMI and risk for obesity in middle age than females without depressive symptoms, and males after controlling for family history of weight problems, demographic variables, adult psychopathology, alcohol consumption, and antidepressant use (Hasler et al., 2005). In a longitudinal study of 644 adolescents, Pine, Cohen, Brook, and Coplan (1997) found a significant relationship between adolescent symptoms of conduct disorder and subsequent increased BMI in young adulthood. They also found significant gender differences in psychological comorbidity in adolescents who later became obese young adults. The results showed a positive correlation between obesity and depression in females, but no correlation for males. A lack of BMI data during the subjects' adolescence limits interpretation of the results. Long-term, epidemiological studies similar to Pine et al. and Goodman and Whitaker provide the methodology to examine temporal relationships between onset of obesity and onset of other psychiatric disorders.

Although it is speculated that the relationship between obesity and depression is unidirectional, little research has been done to verify this hypothesis. Given the complex interaction between these two disorders, it is necessary to determine the causal mechanisms that lead from depression to obesity to better target treatment options via psychopharmacology or lifestyle interventions. For instance, a study by Goodman and Whitaker suggested that the probability of becoming obese increased two-fold if the subject was depressed at the beginning of the study. In general, obesity is hard to treat. If a connection between obesity and depression could be established, a successful treatment of one disorder may hinder the development of the other. For example, if in some individuals "depressed mood increases the risk of obesity, treatment of depression may also prevent development of weight gain" (Goodman & Whitaker 2002, p. 502).

In addition, a study by Pine, Goldstein, Wolk, and Weissman (2001) supported a positive correlation between youth depression and obesity in adults. The results indicated that women have a higher risk of developing and maintaining obesity later in life. Depressed female children and adolescents may learn to eat in response to stress, and these patterns of consumption may continue even after the disorder has remitted. Clinicians working with depressed females should carefully assess their weight and eating patterns to identify eating disturbances that may be addressed to prevent the risk of obesity.

Atypical depression—a type of depression in which the core symptoms include overeating, oversleeping, leaden paralysis, and rejection sensitivity—may be an especially potent force driving the findings that depression predicts obesity. The predictors of atypical depression include female gender, young age of onset, and high BMI. This disorder may represent one that merits careful attention with respect to the risk of obesity.

The sleep disturbances that are associated with many psychiatric conditions may play a role in increasing the incidence of obesity in children with mental disorders. Anxiety and depression are both associated with insomnia and impaired sleep, while bipolar disorder is associated with a decreased need for sleep. Insufficient sleep has been linked to increased carbohydrate craving, diminished satiety signal, and increased hunger signals (Spiegel, Knutson, Leproult, Tasali, & Van Cauter, 2005). Research investigating a possible substrate linking sleeping disorders to weight gain is needed. Sleep disturbances may be an important symptom to target when treating youth with psychiatric comorbidity to decrease the risk of weight gain.

Children with psychiatric conditions may be especially vulnerable to social factors that may contribute to obesity. Social factors associated with obesity include neglect, abuse, and generally nonsupportive home environments (Strauss, 1999). Neglected children are nine times more likely than others to become obese (Lissau & Sorensen, 1994). Adults seeking treatment for obesity demonstrate a four-fold increase in the prevalence of childhood sexual abuse, as well as a two-fold increase in nonsexual abuse compared with a control population (Felleti, 1993). One psychosomatic theory of obesity is that food provides comfort and, therefore, eating serves as a compensatory mechanism for children who have survived traumatic experiences or who live in difficult environments (Parsons, Power, Logan, & Summerbell, 1999; Strauss, 1999). Thus, obese children may overeat as a consequence of environmental deprivation or as a result of depression, somatization, or familial abuse (Christoffel & Forsyth, 1989; Fellitti, 1993).

Another factor that may contribute to the high rates of obesity in psychiatric populations is an unhealthy lifestyle. Adults with serious mental illness tend to be more sedentary and less active (Davidson et al., 2001) than the general population. This tendency has yet to be explored in children. Also, the interpersonal deficits experienced by children with psychiatric disorders may perpetuate a less active lifestyle among this population since they may be reluctant to join group activities. Alternatively, they may pursue solitary activities such as playing video games or watching television.

With regard to substance abuse, studies by Neumark-Sztainer et al. (1997), Strauss and Mir (2001), and Wichstrom (1995) all concluded that there was no correlation between adolescent weight and the use of substances that included tobacco, marijuana, and alcohol. However, similar mechanisms in the brain have been used to explain both behaviors. Neural circuitry involved in reward, motivation, and decision-making has been implicated in the craving for both drugs and highly palatable foods (Volkow & Wise, 2005). GABA agonists are beginning to be used to treat addiction, and there is speculation that it may also help curb food binges (Simansky, 2005).

TREATMENT

In working with obese youth with comorbid psychiatric conditions, there is a paucity of evidence available to guide treatment because psychiatric disorders are often exclusion criteria in studies investigating treatments of childhood obesity. Consequently, it is not clear whether treatments that have been demonstrated as efficacious in the general population will be successful in patient populations. Research including patient groups in addition to control groups is required to address this issue.

Psychiatric Assessment

The treatment of mental disorders often supersedes the need for a weight-management program, and the primary goal of treatment is always stabilization. During such times, any change in routine may cause unnecessary distress for the patient. A child with an acute psychiatric episode may not be ready to meet the demands of a weight-loss program, so it is important to perform a psychiatric assessment. No studies exist that compare different methods for psychiatric assessment of obese children. Therefore, our recommendation is to use well-validated instruments previously used in normal and psychiatric populations. There are a variety of tools that exist for conditions most commonly associated with eating disorders. For more information on the different types of screening devices or psychiatric scales, see Zametkin, Zoon, Klein, and Munson (2004).

Readiness to Change

For a weight-management program to succeed, it is essential that the obese patient be ready to change his/her lifestyle. An unsuccessful weight-management program may not only diminish the child's self-esteem, but also impair future weight-loss efforts. Two reliable measures that have been successfully used to assess weight-management program readiness in obese children and adolescents are *The Children's Eating Behavior Inventory* (Archer, Rosenbaum, & Streiner, 1991) and the *Children's Eating Attitude Test* (Braet & Van Strien, 1997; Maloney, McGuire, and Daniels, 1988).

If the patient is a young child, the readiness of the parent overseeing the weight-management program should also be assessed. Signs that the child or his/her family is not ready for change include lack of concern about the child's obesity, belief that the obesity is inevitable, and belief that the child is incapable of losing weight (Barlow & Dietz, 1998). The physician should also be sure that the patient is not regularly using drugs or alcohol, because substance abuse is likely to hinder program adherence.

Risks of Obesity Interventions

Concern that dieting and weight-loss programs prompt both eating disorders and mood disturbances has been expressed. Self-imposed dietary restriction may result in binges and psychological symptoms such as preoccupation with food, increased emotional responsiveness, dysphoria, irritability, and distractibility (Polivy, 1996). According to the dietary restraint model, cognitive control over eating, rather than using physiological cues, increases the risk for uncontrolled eating. Occasionally, the disruptions of cognitive processes can lead to over-consumption (Polivy & Herman, 1985). Dieting may also deplete the body's stores of tryptophan—a precursor in the manufacturing of serotonin. It has been suggested that low tryptophan levels may lead to binge-eating behaviors, especially of foods high in carbohydrates (Kaye, Gendall, & Strober, 1998). It is important that therapists working with children with comorbid obesity and psychological conditions are familiar with the hazards of dieting. For patients with psychiatric disorders, inappropriate dieting may lead to weight gain and worsen their mood.

Recent research has shown that in healthy controls, safe, moderately restrictive weight-loss programs do not produce the same effects (Presnell & Stice, 2003). In a study examining the effect of a weight-maintenance program on bulimic symptoms in adolescent girls, the authors found that the treatment group exhibited decreased bulimic symptoms and negative affect at six-month and one-year follow-ups compared to a control group (Stice, Presnell, Groesz, & Shaw, 2005). These investigations present multiple conclusions—first and foremost that a third variable may be responsible for the association between dieting, binge eating, and negative affect. Or, they may suggest that unhealthy dieting behaviors, such as meal skipping, may be responsible for the bulimic pathology and effects on mood. Excessive caloric restriction, fasting, and extreme levels of dietary restraint often seen in fad diets may pose a risk for exacerbating disturbances in eating and mood.

Due to the greater incidence of eating disorders in adults who were overweight as children (Fairburn, Welch, Doll, Davies, & O'Connor, 1997), there is speculation on whether an integrated approach to the prevention of obesity and eating disorders can be useful. New Moves—an obesity prevention program geared towards adolescent girls—incorporates messages commonly used in eating disorder prevention programs (Neumark-Sztainer, Story, Hannan, & Rex, 2003). The efficacy of this approach has yet to be determined.

Exercise and Mental Health

The effects of exercise on mental health and mood have been widely touted. Several studies have indicated that exercise can reduce the severity of symptoms in depressed patients and lift mood (Dimeo, Bauer, Varahram,

Proest, & Halter, 2005; Lawlor & Hopker, 2001). A meta-analysis also showed that the effects of exercise on depression were similar to those found from other psychotherapeutic interventions, including medication and psychotherapy (Lawlor & Hopker). Similarly, there has been some indication that physical activity can be beneficial for people with generalized anxiety disorder, phobias, panic attacks, or stress disorders (O'Conner, Raglin, & Martinsen, 2000). In individuals with schizophrenia, exercise has also been shown to improve secondary symptoms such as low self-esteem and social withdrawal (Faulkner & Biddle, 1999). The physiological and biochemical changes involving neurotransmitters that occur as a result of exercise are the suspected mechanisms in the emotional effects. The release of B-endorphin and dopamine may produce analgesic effects and exercise may increase the concentration of certain neurotransmitters associated with depression such as serotonin.

Less is known about the effects of exercise on psychiatric symptoms in children. In one recent study on the effects of different types of exercise on depression scores in adolescent girls, the authors found that only aerobic exercise was associated with reduced depressive symptoms, as indicated by lower scores on the Beck Depression Inventory (Stella et al., 2005). This finding needs to be replicated in a clinical population of adolescents, but suggest that high-intensity aerobic exercise can be an important component in treating the physical and emotional well-being of these youths.

A concern that may arise with exercise in this population is adherence. Studies of structured exercise programs found similar retention rates among patients with psychiatric illnesses in comparison to the general population (Martinsen, 1993). However, one study on a lifestyle activity intervention reported significantly lower rates of retention than studies in the general population (Richardson, Avripas, Neal, & Marcus, 2005).

Cognitive-behavioral Therapy (CBT) and Interpersonal Therapy (IPT)

Cognitive-behavioral therapy (CBT) is widely accepted in the treatment of a host of psychiatric conditions in children, and has received empirical support for the treatment of anxiety and depressive disorders in children and adolescents (Compton et al., 2004). CBT uses principles from both behavioral and cognitive therapies to change thoughts and feelings, and, consequently, improve functional behavior. CBT confronts maladaptive cognitions and teaches children to recognize physiological and psychological indicators of psychological distress. Children are also taught appropriate ways to reappraise information and cope with stressful situations.

CBT is also a well-established treatment for binge-eating disorders (Wilfley & Cohen, 1997). For BED, CBT focuses on helping patients identify episodes of over- and under-restriction and encourage normalization of eating patterns. Cognitive restructuring helps patients challenge harsh stereotypical views of overweight, and promotes acceptance of diverse body sizes. Relapse-prevention strategies are learned, such as problem-solving and coping with high risk situations. This suggests that CBT may be effective in treating adolescents with obesity and comorbid psychiatric conditions if the obesity is a result of eating disturbances.

The behavioral modification strategies involved in CBT, such as goal-setting and shaping, may contribute to the success of a weight-management program—especially for those affected by mental illness. However, there is little research on the effectiveness of CBT to address comorbid weight and psychological problems. It has been suggested that motivational interviewing (MI) should be integrated with CBT to improve treatment outcomes for depression and anxiety. MI has been defined as a client-centered directive method for increasing motivation and exploring and resolving ambivalence (Miller & Rollnick, 2002). For more information about MI, see Chapter 24. CBT and behavior therapy are more effective for both weight loss and psychological disorders when parents are involved (Mendelowitz et al., 1999), suggesting that family involvement may be an important component in treating this population.

Another treatment that has been shown to be as efficacious as CBT for the treatment of binge-eating disorder is interpersonal therapy (IPT) (Wilfley et al., 2002). IPT has been used in group formats for both depression and binge-eating disorder among adolescents. IPT focuses on addressing the social and interpersonal deficits among individuals with psychiatric disorders, such as depression and BED, by teaching skilled communication and promoting positive relationships. Despite the lack of focus on weight loss, individuals with BED who ceased to binge tended to lose weight (Wilfley et al., 2002). A model for IPT has been adapted for the prevention of inappropriate weight gain (IPT-WG) (Tanofsky-Kraff et al., 2007).

The above treatments—CBT and IPT—are less effective in the treatment of children. Children may not have the cognitive capacity necessary to benefit from this type of intervention. Therapists should assess the youth's cognitive abilities before embarking on a treatment program, to ensure the individual can meet the dem ands of therapy.

PEDIATRIC PSYCHOPHARMACOLOGY AND OBESITY

There is little doubt that modern pediatric psychopharmacology has highly effective tools for the treatment of a wide range of psychiatric disorders in children and adolescents. However, these agents can be the proverbial double-edged sword for children and adolescents. On the one hand, these drugs are highly effective in treating an array of symptoms such as severe impulsivity, anxiety, depression, mania, mood lability, and psychosis. On the other hand, many of these clearly cause clinically significant weight gain, and some even induce insulin resistance. Alternatively, other psychotropics such as stimulants frequently diminish appetite, and produce weight loss. The exact mechanism of weight gain induced by psychotropic medication is not yet known. Circumstantially, the most likely neurochemical correlate is the modulation of the dopamine neural tract and the reward system of the hypothalamus, given that most antipsychotics are dopamine antagonists, and psychostiumlants—appetite suppressants—block the presynaptic dopamine receptor. The purpose of this section is to concisely spell out the current state of knowledge of the treatment of psychiatric disorders in overweight adolescents and children, and point out where obvious vacuums exist in evidence-based drug clinical decision-making.

Before discussing different classes of medications, a few general principles should be addressed:

- If two therapies have equal efficacy (CBT and medications), and one does not have the side effect of weight gain, the obvious choice is nonpharmacological.
- Our overwhelming bias, although currently not evidence-based, is to treat the documented psychiatric disorder first, before instituting a weight-loss program. It is important to address the most immediate threats to life and safety. Suicidal ideations and severe depression must be alleviated despite the negative impact treatment may have on immediate weight status. If psychiatric symptoms are in the mild to moderate range, concurrent treatments may seem reasonable. The rationale for these practices are drawn by common sense (often empirically proven to be wrong), but given the current dearth of empirical data in this area, clinical consensus and judgment remains the only justification.

Weight loss may prove to be especially difficult because key symptoms of the major treatable psychiatric disorder are potential impediments to compliance in current obesity treatment programs. For example, the low energy, low motivation, weight gain, and hopelessness associated with depression; the impulse control deficits seen in ADHD; the severe impulsivity and poor judgment that characterize bipolar disorder; and the negative symptoms and confusion that are typical in psychosis, may make successful weight-loss extremely difficult.

TREATMENT OF PSYCHOTROPIC DRUG INDUCED WEIGHT GAIN

Antipsychotics

Antipsychotics are a class of psychotropic medications used for the treatment of childhood onset schizophrenia, severely aggressive children and adolescents, and conduct disorder in low-IQ youth (Sikich, Hamer, Bashford, Sheitman, & Lieberman, 2004). Another indication is for the initial stability and occasional long-term therapy for bipolar or manic depressive disorder. Older generation medications (e.g., thioridazine, haloperidol, trifluoperazine) have been largely replaced by newer atypical antipsychotics (e.g., risperidone, clozapine, aripiprazole) because the newer generation medications are not associated with permanent chronic movement disorders known as tardive dyskinesia. Although safer than earlier generation antipsychotics, the newer generation is well-documented to have serious negative effects on weight gain, diabetes mellitus, and the rare development of *metabolic syndrome*. Given that the new atypical antipsychotics have now been on the market long enough to generate data, more informed decisions can be made regarding the risks and benefits. Fortunately, a seminal report appeared in 2005 to guide clinicians, which we will discuss briefly.

The Clinical Trials of Antipsychotic Intervention Effectiveness (CATIE), published in the New England Journal of Medicine, clearly showed—in a comparison of the newer and older antipsychotic medications for schizophrenia—that olanzapine, an atypical newer antipsychotic, was associated with the largest weight gain. In addition, there was a clinically insignificant superior outcome as evidenced by fewer patients prematurely discontinuing the drug (Lieberman et al., 2005). The take home message for clinicians is the older *typical* antipsychotics, such as haloperidol, are associated with less weight gain and similar rates of efficacy. Given that the newer class of antipsychotics currently holds 90 percent of the market share in the United States, and are much more expensive, this landmark study is critical for all psychiatric practitioners to understand.

Figure 25.1 is a critical tool in choosing antipsychotic medication for obese children or adolescents. It should be noted that Figure 25.1 is a meta-analysis of adult studies, so a future direction would be to collect a similar dataset in children and adolescents.

There are a number of important points to be made regarding causation of weight gain in individuals treated with antipsychotics. First,

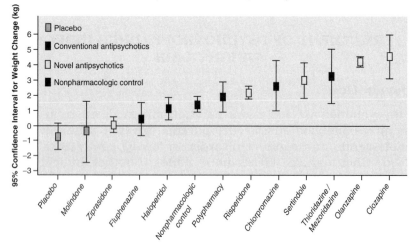

Figure 25.1. Ninety-five percent Confidence Intervals (CIs) for estimated weight change after 10 weeks of treatment with standard drug doses. (Reprinted with permission from the American Journal of Psychiatry, Copyright [1999]. American Psychiatric Association).

untreated schizophrenia is associated with obesity (Allison & Casey, 2001), so factors other than the medication may be responsible for weight gain. Some antipsychotics are associated with more weight gain than others. Initially, olanzapine and risperidone are associated with *extreme weight gain* in adolescents (Ratzoni et al., 2002), followed by a plateau effect at 6–7 weeks. In contrast, haloperidol showed a mild 2 percent weight gain even at 12 weeks. Ratzoni et al. stated that risk factors for weight gain were male gender and low BMI at baseline (2002). Individuals with lower BMI at baseline gained more weight, which is consistent with adult studies (Beasley, Tollefson, & Tran, 1997). Ratzonni et al. also noted that patients' weight gain was positively correlated with paternal weight (2002), which certainly merits further research.

The only other direct evaluation of new atypical antipsychotic medications and older *typical* antipsychotics in adolescents is a comparative study using haloperidol. Researchers reported that "weight gain on atypical antipsychotics was more prevalent and severe than reported in adults" (Sikich et al., 2004, p. 133). Average weight gain on olanzapine, risperidone, and haloperidol was 7.1 kg, 4.5 kg, and 3.5 kg, respectively. Treatment response, although not statistically significant, was 88 percent on olanzapine, 74 percent on resperidone, and 53 percent on haloperidol.

Several important points need to be made regarding antipsychotic use in youth. Because most of the data on antipsychotics comes from adult studies, they need to be replicated in youth. Much of the future research in this field should be directed toward youths and the effects of weight gain and antipsychotic medications in children. In adults, the pattern of weight gain appears to decline with time.

Currently, the primary approach to the treatment of weight gain associated with psychotropic medications should be prevention, and then behavioral modification (e.g., diet and exercise). However, without head-to-head comparisons of behavioral interventions versus pharmacological interventions, clinicians must be guided by individual clinical experience. Obviously, polypharmacy is to be avoided, and the treatment of a side effect of one medication with another can be less then optimal. However, with the low success rates of nonpsychiatrically ill, overweight people in current behavioral treatment programs, one could argue that medicated individuals suffering from mental illness may have less success with weight management programs. With that said, there are many examples in medicine where the side effects of one medication are safely and relatively easily counteracted with another pharmaceutical agent. We would like to briefly review several potential pharmacological interventions for psychotropic-induced weight gain with the full knowledge that no single agent has proven to be highly effective for primary obesity.

In one of the few systematic studies of a pharmacological intervention of antipsychotic/mood stabilizing medication in children and adolescents, Gracious, Krysiak, and Youngstrom (2002) published a case report of eight boys and one girl ages 9–16 who were treated in an open trial of amantadine (100 mg) two or three times per day. Five of the eight actually lost weight, and three appeared to have a slowing of weight gain. In those who lost weight, length of treatment was correlated with weight loss. However, the greatest drawback of this study was the unblinded nature of the trial, and the well-established phenomenon of plateauing of weight gain over time in nontreated individuals. Clearly, a future direction would be a double-blind, placebo, controlled, random assignment design study of amantadine in antipsychotic treated subjects starting early in the course of treatment.

In one of the few placebo-controlled trials of weight loss medication in antipsychotic (olanzapine) treated adult subjects, Cavazzoni, Tanaka, Roychowdhury, Breier, and Allison (2003) used nizatidine (150 or 300 mg) twice daily to attempt to stem weight gain. Although an early nonstatistically significant effect was noted by week 16 of the trial, no significant reduction in weight gain was noted.

Two medications currently under investigation for primary obesity are orlistat and sibutramine. Orlistat is a reversible inhibitor of lipase that acts by inhibiting the absorption of dietary fats in the gastrointestinal tract. Sibutramine inhibits the reuptake of norepinephrine, serotonin, and dopamine. To date, no data exists on the coadministration of these weight-control agents in children or adolescents on psychotropic medications, with the exception of a brief report by Morrison, Cottingham, and Barton (2002).

In 2002, Morrison reported a 12-week open label trial of metformin in 19 patients ages 10–18 who had gained over 10 percent of baseline weight while being treated with olanzapine, risperidone, quetiapine, or valproate. Of the 19 patients, 15 lost weight, three gained 1.6 kg or less, and one had no change. This report is highly encouraging, and the fact that weight was actually lost demonstrates the possibility of a true major effect. Clearly, this work needs to be replicated with a double blind placebo-controlled design. Another future direction would be to start the metformin at the initiation of the psychotropic medication trial to try to prevent the initial 10 percent weight gain.

While these weight-loss agents may be effective in curbing weight gain, the side effects associated with these drugs may well prove to be intolerable for children and adolescents with psychiatric conditions. The most common side effects include flatulence, fecal incontinence, high blood pressure, and increased pulse rate, which may be especially anxiety-invoking for adolescents. To attenuate these side effects requires adherence to a hypocaloric diet, and compliance to such a stringent diet may be particularly difficult for youth with psychiatric disorders. Also, it is important to be aware that the risk of overdose could be serious in the mentally ill. Youth must be carefully monitored when prescribed these medications.

In summary, the use of polypharmacy to combat weight gain induced by psychotropic medications is fought with difficulty. A major goal for this field is the development of a well-tolerated agent with low abuse potential, slow onset of action, high safety profile, and few drug-drug interactions that could be used prophylactically to treat youth with psychiatric disorder who need psychotropic agents. Unfortunately, one set of drugs used in children that produces weight loss—psychostimulants—have abuse potential, are contraindicated in psychosis, and lack data supporting their use in nonpsychiatric patients. An avenue for future research would be to assess their safety and efficacy in adult psychiatric patients on certain psychotropic medications. By some mechanism, they may be more useful in this special population than the general population. However, given they have clear-cut effects on mood, their use might be quite complicated.

For an excellent review of eight concomitant pharmacological approaches to the treatment of weight gain associated with psychotropics, see a complete review written by Werneke, Taylor, and Sanders (2002). They conclude that "the current evidence does not support the general use of pharmacological interventions for overweight patients treated with antipsychotic medication, although individually selected patients may benefit (p. 145)."

Antidepressants and Weight

There is considerable data available about the effects of antidepressant medications on weight gain in adults. It is not yet known whether these data can be extrapolated to children and adolescents, but we do not believe that it would be prudent at this time. With current datasets available as more investigators and manufacturers study psychotropic medication in youth, one should be able to classify antidepressants by propensity for weight gain. Lacking pediatric data, a brief summary of the adult data is currently the only guidance one has in medicating anxious and depressed youth. Another unanswered question is whether weight gain varies for different agents as a function of the underlying psychiatric condition. For example, are youth with generalized anxiety disorders more or less susceptible to weight gain than youth with major depression disorder?

Figure 25.2 is a summary of a review article by Arronne and Segal (2003) on the effects of medication in patients with mood disorders. What becomes clear in head-to-head comparisons between selective serotonin reuptake inhibitors (SSRIs) and older tricyclic antidepressants (TCAs) (i.e.,

Effects of Antidepressants on Body Weight

Marked	Moderate	Mild	No Change	Loss
amitryptyline	paroxetine	phenelzine	fluoxetine	SSRI*
doxepin	mirtazapine		fluvoxamine	
imipramine	desipramine		sertraline	
clomipramine	isocarboxazid		citalopram	
nortryptiline			nefazodone	
			bupropion*	
			venlafaxine	
			tranylcypromine	

* Only first weeks

Figure 25.2. The effects of antidepressant medications on body weight. (From Sporn, A. (2004, October). Presentation to the American Academy of Child and Adolescent Psychiatry.)

imipramine) is that paroxetine is more likely to produce a greater incidence of weight gain larger than 7 percent from baseline than fluoxetine
or sertraline. Also apparent is that the older TCAs—probably due to their
anticholinergic effects—are associated with weight gain, with amitryptyline
producing the most weight gain.

However, all of these studies lack a placebo control group (Fava, 2000),
although historical controls do argue that anywhere from 2.8 percent
(Michelson et al., 1999) to 6.3 percent (Mackle & Kocsis, 1998) of depressed
patients on placebo have *significant* weight gain. There are several atypical antidepressants not associated with weight gain, such as bupropion
(Croft, Houser, & Leadbetter, 2000) and nefazodone (Sussman, Ginsberg,
& Bikoff, 2001), which are off the market. Bupropion may be weight negative (Croft et al.), while nefazodone is relatively weight neutral.

Mood Stabilizers

The exact prevalence of disorders, such as bipolar I or II in children
and adolescents, remains quite controversial. What is not controversial
is that more and more youth with a wide array of behavioral difficulties
ranging from mood dysregulation to chronic to classic mania are requiring
pharmacological therapy with *mood stabilizers*. Little published data exist
on the effects of these medications on weight in children and adolescents.
The current thinking on mood stabilizers in youth is extrapolated from
adults.

Figure 25.3 reflects generally known characteristics for the most commonly used mood stabilizers. Lithium—the mainstay of treatment since
the 1970s—has weight gain as a side effect, occurring in as many as one
third of the patients treated (Arrone & Segal, 2003). Valproate is clearly
known to produce weight gain in a variable proportion of adult patients,
even more so than carbamazepine and phenytoin—other medications used
to treat bipolar behavior (Arrone & Segal).

Effects of Mood Stabilizers on Body Weight

Marked: lithium, valproate

Moderate: carbamazepine

No Change: gabapentin, lamotrigine

Loss: topiramate

Figure 25.3. The effects of mood stabilizers on body weight (From Sporn, A. (2004, October).
Presentation to the American Academy of Child and Adolescent Psychiatry).

Two newer agents—lamotrigine and topiramate (both anti-epileptic medications)—appear to be effective for mood stabilization in adults, and are not associated with weight gain. The major disadvantage of both drugs is the fact that their efficacy in children and adolescents with mood dysregulation and or classic bipolar disorder has not been well-established. On an optimistic note, topiramate seems not only to be weight neutral, but promotes weight loss in patients with either neurological or psychiatric disorders, including binge-eating disorder (Shapira, Goldsmith, & McElroy, 2000).

CONCLUSION

In conclusion, obesity is a complex disease marked by a wide variety of environmental, genetic, and psychological factors. Given the rapid growth of obesity among youth in the United States, psychiatrists should be aware of the association between psychopathology, psychopharmacology, and weight gain. In addition, the BMI of child and adolescent psychiatric patients should be closely monitored because certain medications can induce weight gain.

ACKNOWLEDGEMENTS

This research was supported by the Intramural Program of the National Institute of Mental Health. The authors wish to acknowledge Michelle Gilchrist of the University of Rochester for her assistance with the preparation of this chapter.

REFERENCES

Achenbach, T. M. (1991). *Manual for the Child Behavior Checklist/4–18 and 1991 Profile*. Burlington, VT: University of Vermont.

Allison, D. B., & Casey, D. E. (2001). Antipsychotic-induced weight gain: A review of the literature. *Journal of Clinical Psychiatry, 62*(Suppl. 7), 22–31.

Allison, D. B., Mentore, J. L., Heo, M., Chandler, L. P., Cappelleri, J. C., Infante, M. C., et al. (1999). Antipsychotic-induced weight gain: A comprehensive research synthesis. *American Journal of Psychiatry, 156*, 1686–1696.

Archer, L. A., Rosenbaum, P. L., & Streiner, D.L. (1991). The children's eating behavior inventory: Reliability and validity results. *Journal of Pediatric Psychology, 16*, 629–642.

Aronne, L. J., & Segal, K. R. (2003). Weight gain in the treatment of mood disorders. *Journal of Clinical Psychiatry, 64*(Suppl. 8), 22–29.

Barlow, S. E., & Dietz, W. H. (1998). Obesity evaluation and treatment: Expert Committee recommendations. The Maternal and Child Health Bureau, Health Resources and Services Administration and the Department of Health and Human Services. *Pediatrics, 102*, E29.

Beasley, C. M., Jr., Tollefson, G. D., & Tran, P. V. (1997). Safety of olanzapine. *J Clinical Psychiatry, 58*(Suppl. 10), 13–17.

Braet, C., & Van Strien, T. (1997). Assessment of emotional, externally induced and restrained eating behavior in nine to twelve-year-old obese and non-obese children. *Behaviour Research and Therapy, 35*, 863–873.

Britz, B., Siegfried, W., Ziegler, A., Lamertz, C., Herpertz-Dahlmann, B. M., Remschmidt, H., Wittchen, H. U., & Hebebrand, J. (2000). Rates of psychiatric disorders in a clinical study group of adolescents with extreme obesity and in obese adolescents ascertained via a population based study. *International Journal of Obesity and Related Metabolic Disorders, 24,* 1707–1714.

Buddeburg-Fisher B., Klaghofer, R., & Reed, V. (1999). Associations between body weight, psychiatric disorders and body image in female adolescents. *Psychotherapy and Psychosomatics, 68,* 325–332.

Cavazzoni, P., Tanaka, Y., Roychowdhury, S. M., Breier, A., & Allison, D. B. (2003). Nizatidine for prevention of weight gain with olanzapine: A double-blind placebo-controlled trial. *European Neuropsychopharmacology, 13,* 81–85.

Christoffel, K. K., & Forsyth, B. W. (1989). Mirror image of environmental deprivation: Severe childhood obesity of psychosocial origin. *Child Abuse and Neglect, 13,* 249-256.

Compton, S. N., March, J. S., Brent, D., Albano, A. M., Weersing, R., & Curry, J. (2004). Cognitive-behavioral psychotherapy for anxiety and depressive disorders in children and adolescents: An evidence-based medicine review. *Journal of the American Academy of Child and Adolescent Psychiatry, 43,* 930–959.

Croft, H., Houser, T. L., Jamerson, B. D., Leadbetter, R., Bolden-Watson, C., Donahue, R., et al. (2002). Effect on body weight of bupropion sustained-release in patients with major depression treated for 52 weeks. *Clinical Therapeutics, 24,* 662–672.

Croft, J., Houser, T., Leadbetter, R. et al. (2000). Effects of buproprion on weight in the long term treatment of depression. *Obesity Research, 8,* 10S.

Croft, H., Settle, E., Jr., Houser, T., Batey, S. R., Donahue, R. M., & Ascher, J. A. (1999). A placebo-controlled comparison of the antidepressant efficacy and effects on sexual functioning of sustained-release bupropion and sertraline. *Clinical Therapeutics, 21,* 643–658.

Daniels, J. (2005). Weight and weight concerns: Are they associated with reported depressive symptoms in adolescents? *Journal of Pediatric Health Care, 19,* 33–41.

Davidson, S., Judd, F., Jolley, D., Hocking, B., Thompson, S., & Hyland, B. (2001). Cardiovascular risk factors for people with mental illness. *Australia and New Zealand Journal of Psychiatry, 35,* 196–202.

Deberdt, W., Winokur, A., Cavazzoni, P. A., Trzaskoma, Q. N., Carlson, C. D., Bymaster, F. P., et al. (2005). Amantadine for weight gain associated with olanzapine treatment. *European Neuropsychopharmacology, 15,* 13–21.

Dimeo, F., Bauer, M., Varahram, I., Proest, G., & Halter, U. (2001). Benefits from aerobic exercise in patients with major depression: A pilot study. *British Journal of Sports Medicine, 35,* 114–117.

Epstein, L. H., Klein, K. R., & Wisniewski, L. (1994). Child and parent factors that influence psychological problems in obese children. *International Journal of Eating Disorders, 15,* 151–158.

Epstein, L. H., Myers, M. D., & Anderson, K. (1996). The association of maternal psychopathology and family socioeconomic status with psychological problems in obese children. *Obesity Research, 4,* 65–73.

Erickson, S. J., Robinson, T. N., Haydel, K. F., & Killen, J. D. (2000). Are overweight children unhappy? Body mass index, depressive symptoms, and overweight concerns in elementary school children. *Archives of Pediatric and Adolescent Medicine, 154,* 931–935.

Fairburn, C. G., Welch, S. L., Doll, H. A., Davies, B. A., & O'Connor, M. E. (1997). Risk factors for bulimia nervosa. A community-based case-control study. *Archives of General Psychiatry, 54,* 509–517.

Fava, M. (2000). Weight gain and antidepressants. *Journal of Clinical Psychiatry, 61*(Suppl. 11), 37–41.

Fava, M., Judge, R., Hoog, S. L., Nilsson, M. E., & Koke, S. C. (2000). Fluoxetine versus sertraline and paroxetine in major depressive disorder: Changes in weight with long-term treatment. *Journal of Clinical Psychiatry, 61,* 863–867.

Faulkner, G., & Biddle, S. (1999). Exercise as an adjunct treatment for schizophrenia: A review of the literature. *Journal of Mental Health, 8,* 441–457.

Fellitti, V. J. (1993). Childhood sexual abuse, depression, and family dysfunction in adult obese patients. *Southern Medical Journal, 86,* 732–736.

Friedman, M. A., & Brownell, K. D. (1995). Psychological correlates of obesity: Moving to the next research generation. *Psychological Bulletin, 117,* 3–20.

Goodman, E., & Whitaker, R. C. (2002). A prospective study of the role of depression in the development and persistence of adolescent obesity. *Pediatrics, 110*, 497–504.

Gortmaker, S. L. (1993). Social and economic consequences of overweight in adolescence and young adulthood. *New England Journal of Medicine, 329*, 1008–1012.

Gracious, B. L., Krysiak, T. E., & Youngstrom, E. A. (2002). Amantadine treatment of psychotropic-induced weight gain in children and adolescents: Case series. *Journal of Child and Adolescent Psychopharmacology, 12*, 249–257.

Hasler, G., Pine, D. S., Kleinbaum, D. G., Gamma, A., Luckenbaugh, D., Ajdacic, V., et al. (2005). Depressive symptoms during childhood and adult obesity: The Zurich cohort study. *Molecular Psychiatry, 10*, 842–850.

JKaye, W., Gendall, K., & Strober, M. (1998). Serotonin neuronal function and selective serotonin reuptake inhibitor treatment in anorexia and bulimia nervosa. *Biological Psychiatry, 44*, 825–838.

Lawlor, D. A., & Hopker, S. W. (2001). The effectiveness of exercise as an intervention in the management of depression: Systematic review and meta-regression analysis of randomized controlled trials. *British Medical Journal, 322*, 763–767.

Lieberman, J. A., Stroup, T. S., McEvoy, J. P., Swartz, M. S., Rosenheck, R. A., Perkins, D. O., et al. (2005). Effectiveness of antipsychotic drugs in patients with chronic schizophrenia. *New England Journal of Medicine, 353*, 1209–1223.

Lissau, I., & Sorensen, T. I. A. (1994). Parental neglect during childhood and increased risk of obesity in young adulthood. *Lancet, 343*, 324–327.

Mackle, M, & Kocsis, J. (1998). Effects on body weight of the SSRI citalopram. Presented at the 27th annual meeting of the Am. College of Neuropsychopharmacology, Las Croabas, Puerto Rico.

Maloney, M. J., McGuire, J. B., & Daniels, S. R. (1988). Reliability testing of a children's version of the Eating Attitude Test. *Journal of the American Academy of Child and Adolescent Psychiatry, 27*, 541–543.

Martinsen, E. (1993). Therapeutic implications of exercise for clinically anxious and depressed patients. *International Journal of Sport Psychology, 24*, 185–199.

Mendlowitz, S. L., Manassis, K., Bradley, S., Scapillato, D., Miezitis, S., & Shaw, B. F. (1999). Cognitive-behavioral group treatments in childhood anxiety disorders: The role of parental involvement. *Journal of the American Academy of Child and Adolescent Psychiatry, 38*, 1223–1229.

Michelson, D., Amsterdam, J. D., Quitkin, F. M., Reimherr, F. W., Rosenbaum, J. F., Zajecka, J., et al. (1999). Changes in weight during a 1-year trial of fluoxetine. *American Journal of Psychiatry, 156*, 1170–1176.

Miller, W. R., & Rollnick, S. (2002) *Motivational interviewing: Preparing people for Change*, (2nd ed.). New York: Guilford Press.

Morrison, J. A., Cottingham, E. M., & Barton, B. A. (2002). Metformin for weight loss in pediatric patients taking psychotropic drugs. *American Journal of Psychiatry, 159*, 655–657.

Neumark-Sztainer, D., Story, M., French, S. A., Hannan, P. J., Resnick, M. D., & Blum, R. W. (1997). Psychosocial concerns and health-compromising behaviors among overweight and nonoverweight adolescents. *Obesity Research, 5*, 237–249.

Neumark-Sztainer, D., Story, M., Hannan, P. J., & Rex, J. (2003). New Moves: A school-based obesity prevention program for adolescent girls. *Preventative Medicine, 37*, 41–51.

O'Conner P. J., Raglin J. S., & Martinsen E. W. (2000). Physical activity, anxiety, and anxiety disorders. *International Journal of Sport Psychology 31*, 136–155.

Parsons, T. J., Power, C., Logan, S., & Summerbell, C. D. (1999). Childhood predictors of adult obesity: A systematic review. *International Journal of Obesity and Related Metabolic Disorders, 23*(Suppl. 8), S1–107

Pesa, J. A., Syre, T. S., & Jones, E. (2000). Psychosocial differences associated with body weight among female adolescents: The importance of body image. *Journal of Adolescent Health, 26*, 330–337.

Pine, D. S., Cohen, P., Brook, J., & Coplan, J. D. (1997). Psychiatric symptoms in adolescence as predictors of obesity in early adulthood: A longitudinal study. *American Journal of Public Health, 87*, 1303–1310.

Pine, D. S., Goldstein, R. B., Wolk S, & Weissman M. M. (2001). The association between childhood depression and adulthood body mass index. *Pediatrics, 107,*1049–1056

Polivy, J. (1996). Psychological consequences of food restriction. *Journal of the American Dietetics Association, 96*, 589.

Polivy, J., & Herman, C. P. (1985). Dieting and binging: A causal analysis. *American Psychologist, 40*, 193–201.

Presnell, K., & Stice, E. (2003). An experimental test of the effect of weight-loss dieting on bulimic pathology: Tipping the scales in a different direction. *Journal of Abnormal Psychology, 112*, 166–170.

Ratzoni, G., Gothelf, D., Brand-Gothelf, A., Reidman, J., Kikinzon, L., Gal, G., et al. (2002). Weight gain associated with olanzapine and risperidone in adolescent patients: A comparative prospective study. *Journal of the American Academy of Child and Adolescent Psychiatry, 41*, 337–343.

Richardson, C. R., Avripas, S. A., Neal, D. L., & Marcus, S. M. (2005). Increasing lifestyle physical activity in patients with depression or other serious mental illness. *Journal of Psychiatric Practice, 11*, 379–388.

Shapira, N. A., Goldsmith, T. D., & McElroy, S. L. (2000). Treatment of binge-eating disorder with topiramate: A clinical case series. *Journal of Clinical Psychiatry, 61*, 368–372.

Sheslow, D., Hassink, S., Wallace, W., et al. (1993), The relationship between self-esteem and depression in obese children. *Annals of the New York Academy of Science, 699*, 289–291.

Sikich, L., Hamer, R. M., Bashford, R. A., Sheitman, B. B., & Lieberman, J. A. (2004). A pilot study of risperidone, olanzapine, and haloperidol in psychotic youth: A double-blind, randomized, 8-week trial. *Neuropsychopharmacology, 29*, 133–145.

Simansky, K. J. (2005). NIH symposium series: Ingestive mechanisms in obesity, substance abuse and mental disorders. *Physiology & Behavior, 86*, 1–4.

Spiegel, K., Knutson, K., Leproult, R., Tasali, E., & Van Cauter, E. (2005). Sleep loss: A novel risk factor for insulin resistance and Type 2 diabetes. *Journal of Applied Physiology, 99*, 2008–2019.

Spitzer, R. L., Yanovski, S., Wadden, T., Wing, R., Marcus, M. D., Stunkard, A., et al.(1993). Binge eating disorder: Its further validation in a multisite study. *International Journal of Eating Disorders, 13*, 137–153.

Stella, S. G., Vilar, A. P., Lacroix, C., Fisberg, M., Santos, R. F., Mello, M. T., et al. (2005). Effects of type of physical exercise and leisure activities on the depression scores of obese Brazilian adolescent girls. *Brazilian Journal of Medical and Biological Research, 38*, 1683–1689.

Stice, E., Presnell, K., Groesz, L., & Shaw, H. (2005). Effects of a weight maintenance diet on bulimic symptoms in adolescent girls: An experimental test of the dietary restraint theory. *Health Psychology, 24*, 402–412.

Stradmeijer, M., Bosch, J., Koops, W., & Seidell, J. (2000). Family functioning and psychosocial adjustment in overweight youngsters. *International Journal of Eating Disorders, 27*, 110–114.

Strauss, R. S. (1999). Childhood obesity. *Current Problems in Pediatrics, 29*, 1–2.

Strauss, R. S., & Mir, H. M. (2001). Smoking and weight loss attempts in overweight and normal-weight adolescents. *International Journal of Obesity and Related Metabolic Disorders, 25*, 1381–1385.

Sussman, N., Ginsberg, D. L., & Bikoff, J. (2001). Effects of nefazodone on body weight: A pooled analysis of selective serotonin reuptake inhibitor- and imipramine-controlled trials. *Journal of Clinical Psychiatry, 62*, 256–260.

Tanofsky-Kraff, M., Wilfley, D. E., Young, J. F., Mufson, L., Yanovski, S. Z., Glasofer, D. R., et al. (2007). Preventing excessive weight gain in adolescents: interpersonal psychotherapy for binge eating. *Obesity, 15*, 1345–1355.

Volkow, N. D., & Wise, R. A. (2005). How can drug addiction help us understand obesity? *Natural Neuroscience, 8*, 555–560.

Wallace, W. J., Sheslow, D., & Hassink, S. (1993). Obesity in children: A risk for depression. *Annals of the New York Academy of Science, 699*, 301–303.

Werneke, U., Taylor, D., & Sanders, T. A. (2002). Options for pharmacological management of obesity in patients treated with atypical antipsychotics. *International Clinical Psychopharmacology, 17*, 145–160.

Wichstrom, L. (1995). Social, psychological and physical correlates of eating problems. A study of the general adolescent population in Norway. *Psychological Medicine, 25,* 567–579.

Wilfley, D. E., & Cohen, L. R. (1997). Psychological treatment of bulimia nervosa and binge eating disorder. *Psychopharmacological Bulletin, 33,* 437–454.

Wilfley, D. E., Welch, R. R., Stein, R. I., Spurrell, E. B., Cohen, L. R., Saelens, B. E., et al. (2002). A randomized comparison of group cognitive-behavioral therapy and group interpersonal psychotherapy for the treatment of overweight individuals with binge-eating disorder. *Archives of General Psychiatry, 59,* 713–721.

Yanovski, S. Z., Nelson, J. E., Dubbert, B. K., & Spitzer, R. L. (1993). Association of binge eating disorder and psychiatric comorbidity in obese subjects. *American Journal of Psychiatry,* 150, 1472–1479.

Zametkin, A., Zoon, C. K., Klein, H. W, & Munson, S. (2004). Psychiatric Aspects of Child and Adolescent Obesity: A Review of the Past 10 Years. *Journal of the American Academy of Child and Adolescent Psychiatry,* 43, 134–150.

26

Application of Empirically Supported Treatments to Clinical Settings

CRAIG A. JOHNSTON
and WILLIAM T. DALTON III

Approximately 17 percent of all school-aged children are either classified as at-risk of overweight or as overweight in the United States, and the prevalence of overweight has been increasing for decades (Ogden et al., 2006). Furthermore, more overweight has been seen in children at younger ages over the past two decades (e.g., Ogden et al.). Not only is there an increased prevalence of overweight in children, but overweight children have consistently been getting heavier (Jolliffe, 2004). These rates of overweight in children are not only seen in the United States. Over 22 million children under the age of five are estimated to be overweight worldwide (Deckelbaum & Williams, 2001). In light of the incidence and prevalence of overweight in children (Ogden et al.), and the impact it can have on their lives (e.g., Schwimmer, Burwinkle, & Varni, 2003; Zeller, Roehrig, Modi, Daniels, & Inge, 2006; Zeller, Saelens, Roehrig, Kirk, & Daniels, 2004), the need for successful and feasible treatments is clear.

In terms of treatment of pediatric overweight, numerous studies have been conducted examining weight-management programs for children. Most treatments take a multidisciplinary approach and include strategies for improving eating habits, increasing physical activity, and decreasing sedentary behavior. In terms of empirical support, behaviorally based therapies have consistently reported the best outcomes (e.g., Summerbell et al., 2003). In fact, behavior-based treatments have long been described as the *state-of-the-art* approach for child weight management (Robinson, 1999).

CRAIG A. JOHNSTON and WILLIAM T. DALTON III • USDA/ARS Children's Nutrition Research Center, Baylor College of Medicine, Houston, TX 77030.

Although behavior-based treatments have considerable support in research settings, few of these treatments have been examined in more applied or *real world* settings. Kazdin and Weisz (1998) discuss the importance of not only determining the efficacy of a treatment in a controlled setting, but also of determining its effectiveness when applied in the clinic. Although empirically supported treatments (ESTs) are frequently shown to produce positive treatment effects when compared to no treatment or other treatments, without knowing the clinical significance of these positive effects, the real world significance will be difficult to realize (Kazdin & Weisz).

Specific to the treatment of pediatric overweight, children receiving weight-loss treatment in an applied setting may differ greatly from children in research samples, and these differences could impact the efficacy of treatment. For example, recruited participants in applied studies may not have sought or received treatment independent of the research program provided (e.g., Steele & Roberts, 2003). Other factors, such as incurring fees and motivation of those treated, may significantly differ between participants in research and applied samples. Thus, the characteristics of these samples call into question the applicability of treatment. Specifically, findings from studies with recruited participants in research settings may not generalize to individuals who are self-referred (Chorpita, Barlow, Albano, & Daleidan, 1998).

In addition to the differences in recruitment of participants, the noted limitations of the EST literature include that efficacy studies have utilized restrictive inclusion criteria that may impact the ability to generalize the findings to clinical practice (e.g., Elliot, 1998; Westen, Novotny, & Thompson-Brenner, 2005). For example, it is not uncommon for studies on overweight children to exclude individuals who are very overweight (i.e., more than 100 percent overweight) or participants with comorbid features (e.g., Epstein, Wing, Koeske, Andrasik, & Ossip, 1981; Epstein, Wing, Steranchak, Dickson, & Michelson, 1980). Both of these critiques address an important issue raised by Gaston, Abbott, Rapee, and Neary (2006). Basically, it is possible that studies of ESTs have excluded poor-prognosis patients that have created samples that are unrepresentative of clinical practice. A final possible limitation of using ESTs in clinic settings is that the overall feasibility of providing them is not realistic due to issues such as cost effectiveness (e.g., Elliot).

The noted limitations of ESTs notwithstanding, a wealth of information is available through the EST literature on treating pediatric overweight for clinicians, and we would be remiss if this information was not used to benefit those seeking treatment in applied settings. Additionally, some evidence has been provided that the use of an EST for pediatric overweight in an applied setting has beneficial results (Johnston & Steele, 2007). It is the goal of this chapter to identify the components that have considerable support in treating this problem, and provide examples of how these can be implemented in a clinical setting. In most cases, ESTs for overweight children have many similarities, and these similarities will be listed in an attempt to provide a clinician with multiple components that should be incorporated throughout treatment. This chapter will also provide some limitations and possible adjuncts to ESTs that are being examined.

BEHAVIORAL COMPONENTS

Multiple behavioral strategies are commonly used in weight management for children. Several specific behavioral components have been used successfully in a number of programs that have produced sustained weight loss over time (Epstein et al., 1981; Israel, 1999; McLean, Griffin, Toney, & Hardeman, 2003; Summerbell et al., 2003). Although studies that determine the individual impact each behavioral component has on treatment outcomes (i.e., dismantling studies) have not been conducted with children, using these strategies together has been demonstrated to significantly impact diet and physical activity. In addition to impacting weight-related behaviors, the use of these components has considerable empirical support in terms of actual weight loss (e.g., Epstein, 1996; Golan, Fainaru, & Weizman, 1998; Israel, Silverman, & Solotar, 1988).

Self-monitoring

Self-monitoring can be defined as the systematic observation and recording of specified behaviors (Kanfer, 1970). Simply having individuals observe their behavior can often have the effect of changing the target behavior in the desired direction. Furthermore, this information is invaluable to the clinician who will need to determine future directions for the family to take, and make recommendations for subsequent sessions. Because self-monitoring can be inaccurate with both the child and parent reporting somewhat differently, and with neither appearing to be *more accurate* than the other, it is important that the clinician use the information from both the parent and the child. The treatment provider may choose to discuss discrepancies in reporting between children and parents to determine possible areas of difficulty or misunderstanding.

In the clinic, self-monitoring should take place with any behavior that is a focus in treatment. For example, behaviors associated with the adoption of a healthier lifestyle often include diet, physical activity, and sedentary behavior. As discussed by Epstein et al. (1995), a "habit book" may be beneficial for maintaining records. This provides a treatment provider with information to monitor participant progress across multiple behaviors. For example, older children can be taught to keep a food diary in which they can identify the number of fruits and vegetables as well as junk foods consumed daily/weekly. Children can also be taught to monitor time spent in behaviors such as physical activity or sedentary behaviors (e.g., television viewing, video-game playing).

A final aspect of weight management that should be monitored is the child's actual weight. From a practical standpoint, movements in the child's weight may be some of the most important information the child receives, because this may lead to learning which behaviors lead to weight loss, gain, or maintenance. Several programs that have exhibited significant weight loss require children to weigh themselves on a regular basis and chart their weights (Epstein et al., 1995; Israel, Guile, Baker, & Silverman, 1994). Further support is provided by literature demonstrating associations between daily self-weighing and less weight regain in adults attempting to maintain weight loss (Wing, Tate, Gorin, Raynor, & Fava, 2006).

Clinicians are faced with the difficult task of treating children of varying ages. Because of this variability in ages, several considerations should be given when using self-monitoring in a clinical setting. Although most children can be taught self-monitoring, some young children may have significant difficulty consistently keeping records. In these cases, parents may need to be responsible for completing self-monitoring records—however, depending on each child's ability, children should be given self-monitoring tasks to encourage active participation in their lifestyle change (Israel, Stolmaker, & Andrian, 1985a). For example, a child may be taught to identify and count vegetables during a mealtime. Because maintaining a healthy lifestyle is beneficial throughout one's lifespan, self-monitoring should be taught as a valuable skill for assisting in this endeavor.

Goal-setting

Developing a plan with realistic goals that can be met within a specified time frame are typically important parts of weight-management programs for children. With the use of goals, families can have a specific focus on the changes that should be made for the next session. For goal-setting to be effective, self-monitoring of behaviors is required. In essence, baseline information is needed to structure goals, and continuous self-monitoring is needed to determine if goals have been met. For example, the clinician may review food records and collaborate with the child and/or family to set a goal for improving diet, such as eating one fruit per day for one week. At the end of the week, families can evaluate food records to determine if the goal has been achieved.

For the treatment provider, goals are beneficial in that they provide structure for treatment sessions as well as reinforce change. Specifically, discussing goals provides an opportunity for families to recognize patterns, notice strengths and weaknesses, and determine how to proceed. It is important to make goals specific, manageable, assessable, realistic, and time-specific. Children benefit from concrete and easily achievable goals, especially in the beginning. Ultimately, achieving initial goals may improve children's self-efficacy for change. Goal setting is a learned skill that can aid in health behavior change as well as generalize to other behaviors and settings.

Contingency Management

Contingency management refers to multiple strategies that change behavior by modifying its consequences. One important form of contingency management is positive reinforcement. Positive reinforcement increases the likelihood of a behavior being exhibited in the future by providing the child with something preferred. In the case of weight management, the child is rewarded with something he or she likes when a healthy behavior is exhibited. A powerful form of positive reinforcement is social praise. For example, a parent provides praise (positive attention such as stating "Good Job!" or offering a "high 5") when the child eats vegetables (an exhibited healthy behavior).

Positive reinforcement can also include the use of rewards. This may be most applicable when a child is having difficulty with a specific behavior. A reward can be considered anything that the child prefers that follows the accomplishment of a target behavior. For example, the child gets to play his or her game of choice with a parent after engaging in an hour of physical activity after school. Some rewards incur monetary cost. In these cases, it is important that the cost be kept to a minimum so it does not become burdensome to parents, as well as allow for intrinsic reinforcement for behavior. The most appropriate rewards include parental attention, such as one-on-one parent time playing games or doing other child-chosen activities. In terms of weight loss, appropriate rewards may also include activities that promote further positive change, such as taking family bike rides or going to a park.

Clinicians may choose to teach families another form of contingency management, which is *contracting*. Contracts are basic agreements that outline the consequences of specific behaviors. In making contracts, parents and children are taught how to administer specific rewards when particular behaviors are displayed. For example, parents agree to allow their child to have additional free time when the child successfully increases his or her vegetable consumption by an agreed-upon amount. Reciprocal contracting has also been described as a beneficial strategy to use in the treatment of childhood overweight (Epstein, Valoski, Wing, & McCurley, 1990). In reciprocal contracting, children and parents provide mutually agreed upon rewards for each other when specified behavioral criteria are met. In this case, parents not only reward child behavior, but children also provide rewards for specified parental behavior. For example, parents may be allowed to choose a family activity because they provided vegetables at each meal.

A major consideration for treatment providers when using rewards and reinforcement successfully is the need for individualizing them for each family. Determining individual preferences is critical when identifying appropriate reinforcers. It may be an important first step for clinicians to assist families in initially determining what rewards might be appropriate. The therapist would need to solicit both the parent's and child's thoughts on those things that are motivating and that can be realistically provided by the family. Clinician assessment of the level of motivation of each family is important (Israel, Stolmaker, & Andrian, 1985b) because this may also contribute to the development of an individualized reward system.

Stimulus Control

Stimulus control is a term that is used to describe changes made to an environment to increase the likelihood of behavior change. This has also frequently been called "cue control." Stimulus control in the treatment of child overweight includes having families change their home environment to reduce cues associated with less-healthy behaviors, and increase cues associated with more healthy behaviors. For example, a "cupboard cleaning" typically takes place in which families are instructed to remove less healthy foods from the home and increase the visibility of fruits and vegetables (e.g., Golan et al., 1998). In terms of decreasing sedentary behaviors, families may be encouraged to remove televisions from the children's bedroom or have specified times for playing video games. Families may be instructed to keep toys used to play outside readily accessible to encourage outdoor free play and physical activity.

Despite advantages, several considerations should be made when using stimulus control in clinical settings. First, although children can begin to practice stimulus or cue control, parents are typically in charge of this because they hold primary responsibility for structuring children's food environments, as well as encouraging and providing opportunities for physical activity. Parents typically buy groceries and prepare meals, allowing ample opportunities to use stimulus control. For example, parents determine which foods are presented at meals and which foods are kept out of sight (e.g., high fat or sugar), as well as structure appropriate portion sizes. Next, as is the case with all treatment components, the active participation on the child's part facilitates learning and is always encouraged. Therefore, children may be taught and made responsible for packing a healthy lunch for school or assisting parents in portioning food. Finally, as an important side note, the role of stimulus control for nutrition is to establish a healthy food environment and provide healthy food options. However, parents should typically not restrict the amount (quantity) of food eaten. Restriction of food when attempting weight management with children has been associated with poor outcomes (Johnson & Birch, 1994).

Modeling

Modeling can be defined as a way of learning in which individuals observe others and determine how to act based on this observation. The importance of parents as role models for healthy behaviors is well-supported in the literature (Epstein et al., 1980; Golan & Crow, 2004). Parents should be active participants during treatment, so each target behavior identified for the child should also be considered a target behavior for parents. Modeling allows parents to demonstrate healthy behaviors, which encourages the modification of child behavior accordingly. Reviews of the literature (e.g., Davison & Birch, 2001) provide empirical support for parental influence on development of child eating and activity behaviors, thus suggesting that altering unhealthy parent patterns may significantly impact treatment. Consistent with these ideas, it is vital to have parents participating in (i.e., modeling) healthy changes to ensure that lifestyle changes are attainable for a child.

OVERALL APPROACHES

Multidisciplinary

There is strong evidence for the efficacy of multicomponent treatments (Fulton, McGuire, Caspersen, & Dietz, 2001; Jelalian & Saelens, 1999) that often exceeds changes in studies with adults (Epstein, 1996; Epstein, Valoski, Kalarchian, & McCurley, 1995; Jeffrey et al., 2000; Wilson, 1994). Despite progress, treatment is often marked by small change and substantial relapse (Epstein, Myers, Raynor, & Saelens, 1998; Robinson, 1999). Overall, few beneficial strategies for weight maintenance have been identifed.

As suggested above, most ESTs take a multidisciplinary approach and include individuals such as pediatricians, child psychologists, nutritionists, and "trained therapists" (Braet, Van Winckel, & Van Leeuwen, 1997; Brownell, Kelman, & Stunkard, 1983). In light of the multiple behaviors that are being targeted (physical activity and nutrition) and the numerous comorbidities that may be present (physiological and psychological), the need for multiple professionals with differing backgrounds is evident. Although all of these treatment providers may not be needed for each session, access to these types of professionals throughout treatment is essential. As children become more overweight and suffer the associated consequences of this, the need for a multidisciplinary approach will likely become even more apparent. Clinicians should be aware of local resources in each of these areas and be willing to modify treatment recommendations based on the needs specific to individual families.

Family-based

Family-based interventions focus on the entire family and consider both children and parents as targets of change. Whereas the only comprehensive meta-analysis on pediatric overweight treatment provided mixed findings for including parents (Haddock, Shadish, Klesges, & Stein, 1994), a recent review showed family-based interventions as superior to controls (Kitzmann & Beech, 2006), and the longest-lasting effects for children have been demonstrated with parental involvement (Epstein, McCurley, Wing, & Valoski, 1990; Epstein, Valoski, Wing, & McCurley, 1994). Studies vary in inclusion (e.g., parent and child together, parent and child separately, parent only) and treatment approach (e.g., focusing on parental weight loss, educating parents on nutrition, teaching children and parents behavioral modification strategies for improving diet and activity) (Kitzmann & Beech). In this growing literature, the preponderance of empirical support for treating pediatric overweight is for family-based (including both the child and parent) interventions (e.g., McLean et al., 2003; Summerbell et al., 2003).

The clinician may draw from several studies that have examined parental and family factors impacting treatment. For example, parent psychiatric symptoms as well as distress have been found to influence level of participation and child weight reduction in treatment (Epstein, Paluch, Gordy, Saelens, & Ernst, 2000; Epstein, Paluch, Saelens, Ernst, & Wilfley, 2001; Epstein, Wisniewski, & Weng, 1994; Favaro & Santonastaso, 1995). Similarly, healthier family functioning has been found to be predictive of retention and weight reduction (Kirschenbaum, Harris, & Tomarken, 1984). The importance of families is also demonstrated in that perceptions held by overweight children's parents may influence weight control. Uzark, Becker, Dielman, Rocchini, and Katch (1988) found that a positive parental attitude with regard to child weight loss resulted in the child being less likely to be overweight in the future, and was associated with greater weight loss compliance. Similarly, Nova, Russo, and Sala (2001) found parental self-commitment to treatment as predictive weight loss in their children. In yet another study, overweight youth who perceived an increase in father acceptance after treatment had better changes in percent overweight over 12 months than youth with lower ratings of father acceptance (Stein, Epstein, Raynor, Kilanowski, & Paluch, 2005). Together these findings highlight just how crucial parental and family factors may be in treatment.

Clinicians may also find it beneficial to assess parenting and family factors prior to structuring treatment. For example, a family characterized by frequent parent-child conflict may benefit from children and parents meeting separately and children collaborating more independently on a behavior change plan. On the other hand, indications of parental distress and poor family functioning may warrant a referral to individual or family therapy prior to, or in conjunction with, treatment of overweight. For instance, Flodmark, Ohlsson, Ryden, and Sveger (1993) found that families who received family therapy in conjunction with conventional treatment produced more positive results (i.e., reduced skin-fold, less weight gain, improved physical fitness). It appears equally important for clinicians to assess children and parent's commitment, motivation, and self-efficacy for health behavior change, to provide an understanding of where to begin with families.

CONSIDERATIONS FOR TREATMENT

Ethnicity

Ethnic minorities are among those at greatest risk for overweight (Ogden et al., 2006). Unfortunately, limited culturally tailored interventions have been developed to address the needs of these groups (Nesbitt et al., 2004). Keller, Gonzales, and Fleuriet (2005) recognize the need for culturally specific understanding of issues such as recruitment, adherence, and retention for improving intervention efforts. It is important to note that several interventions with ethnic minority children have shown the importance of taking a family-based approach (e.g., Beech et al., 2003; Johnston et al., in press; Resnicow et al., 2000). Clinicians should specifically consider attitudes and practices, as well as stressors and challenges specific to these groups (Kumanyika & Grier, 2006).

Severe Overweight

Given that overweight children have consistently been getting heavier (Jolliffe, 2004), and more overweight has been seen in children at younger ages for several decades (e.g., Ogden et al., 2006), a significant proportion of children seen in clinic settings are likely to be severely overweight. Though fewer in number when compared to the literature regarding treatment for moderate pediatric overweight, several studies have directly examined the impact of the application of weight management treatments to severely overweight children. For instance, a study by Levine, Ringham, Kalarchian, Wisniewski, and Marcus (2001) tracked weight loss in children aged 8–12 years who were at 160 percent of their ideal body weight. Children who completed the program (approximately two-thirds) lost a significant amount of weight and also exhibited improvements in depressive symptomatology, anxiety, and eating attitudes. Another study by Dao et al. (2004) reported a preservation of lean muscle mass in addition to a mean reduction of total fat mass with a particularly steep decrease in trunk fat among severely overweight adolescents enrolled in a multidisciplinary weight-reduction program that lasted 6–12 months. These results are particularly encouraging because of the volumes of literature underlining the association between visceral fat and the development of life-threatening comorbidities. Despite limited empirical support for treating severe overweight, clinicians may access a plethora of information for treating overweight, as already discussed.

Physiological Comorbidites

It is not uncommon for overweight children with comorbidities to be excluded from a study for having a history of disease other than overweight, or for taking certain medications. Such exclusions limit the ability to generalize research findings to overweight pediatric patients who present at clinics with physiological comorbidities. Several studies have demonstrated that treatments, not necessarily designed for pediatric patients with comorbidities, can improve several physiological dimensions. For example, studies have shown improved physiological outcomes, including decreased blood pressure and cholesterol (e.g., Epstein, Valoski, et al., 1990). Similarly, a study examining whether severity of sleep-disordered breathing determined insulin resistance and altered lipidemia in snoring children and found overweight to be the major determinant (Tauman, O'Brien, Ivanenko, & Gozal, 2005). The authors highlighted the idea that weight-intervention programs will not only treat the problem of overweight, but also improve associated physiological comorbidities.

Because the incidence of type II diabetes is increasing rapidly (e.g., Fagot-Campagna, 2000; Rosenbloom, Joe, Young, & Winter, 1999), the need for interventions to address this issue is becoming more critical. However, a child with diabetes may respond to weight-loss treatment differently than a child free of this disease. A study by Redmon et al. (2003) demonstrated that children with type II diabetes enrolled in a weight-loss program benefited by not only losing weight but by also improving their diabetes control. The authors further concluded that weight loss may be the single most important therapeutic objective for individuals with type II diabetes. Comorbidities are likely for children and families seeking treatment in applied settings. Research shows numerous benefits associated with weight loss that may generalize to other areas of physical health. However, in cases of comorbidity, clinicians should seek information to ensure that treatment recommendations are not contraindicated, as well as determine if other adherence-related issues are important to address.

Psychological Comorbidities

As discussed by Zeller et al. (2004), most studies for pediatric weight-management programs have excluded children and families with significant psychological problems. In the few studies where these children have been treated for their overweight status, the results are promising. For example, a study by Fossati et al. (2004) has shown that enrollment in a weight-management program not only helps these patients lose weight, but also to experience improvements in depression, anxiety, and associated eating disorders. A study by Levine et al. (2001) also demonstrated improvements in mood and eating-disordered behavior after the completion of a weight-management program. Because children who are overweight may have increased psychological symptomatology, it is imperative that treatment providers recognize the significance of psychosocial difficulties as related to a pediatric weight loss intervention. It has been suggested that psychosocial problems play a role in the exacerbation of obesity, even if they are not involved in the initial etiology of the excess weight gain (Tershakovec, 2004).

Clinicians should also be aware that weight gain has been associated with the use of some psychotropic medications, which may further exacerbate the weight problems of the overweight child (Tershakovec, 2004). Healthcare providers should initially assess for psychosocial difficulties and may monitor these issues during treatment. If clinicians are concerned about psychological symptomatology, children and/or families may benefit from being referred to a mental health provider.

MODIFICATIONS/ADJUNCTS TO TREATMENT

Length of Treatment

Because children completing weight-loss programs typically remain overweight, and some significantly so (e.g., Epstein, Valoski et al., 1990; Israel et al., 1985a), adjuncts or modifications to current treatments may be indicated. One such addition may include the length of treatment. Typically, research studies last for approximately 12 months, with few studies seeing and treating children for much longer. Accordingly, there is little information available allowing us to track weight loss of overweight children when the treatment timeline is expanded. Presumably, if most overweight children remain overweight at the end of treatment, it will take a longer period of treatment for these children to reach a healthy weight status.

Providers in applied settings should consider several issues prior to extending treatment. By lengthening the treatment timeline, families may be given additional support in successfully making lifestyle changes associated with a healthier weight. Although the issue of extending the timeline of treatment may appear logical to treat this chronic condition, literature on extended treatment of pediatric overweight is not available. Clinicians should be aware that asking families to commit to a longer treatment may result in higher rates of attrition and lower rates of adherence. In addition, the cost associated with increasing the length of treatment may make such treatments accessible to fewer individuals. This is particularly concerning because lower socioeconomic status is associated with higher rates of overweight (Wang & Zhang, 2006).

Pharmacotherapy

Several studies have demonstrated the efficacy of using pharmacotherapy as a method of weight reduction among severely overweight pediatric patients. A study by Norgren, Danilesson, Jurold, Lotborn, and Marcus (2003) demonstrated successful weight loss in overweight prepurbertal children when treated with a drug that discouraged consumption of high fat-content meals. A few additional studies have evaluated the effects of pharmacotherapy in overweight adolescents and have demonstrated significant weight loss (Berkowitz et al., 2006; Violante-Ortiz et al., 2005). Other positive health outcomes of these studies included improved triglycerides, overall cholesterol, and insulin levels. Additional studies combining pharmacological and behavioral methods are likely forthcoming. With the advent of safer, effective weight management drugs, the number of multicomponent interventions that include pharmacotherapy will likely increase in the near future. Those working in applied settings should stay abreast of the pharmacotherapy literature and refer children and/or families for a medication evaluation when health indicators arise or treatment difficulties persist.

Meal Replacements

Weight-reduction programs featuring meal replacements have also demonstrated significant weight loss in overweight adolescents. A study by Ball and colleagues (2003) found that overweight adolescents on a low glycemic index (GI) meal replacement plan requested additional food later than those adolescents on a high GI meal replacement plan. The authors concluded that the prolonged satiety, as seen with the low GI meal replacements, may be an effective method for reducing caloric intake—important for achieving long-term weight control. This limited research also suggests that meal replacements may prove to be most beneficial for very overweight adolescents. Clinicians may consider this alternative treatment strategy with this population, especially if little success is made with conventional treatment.

CONCLUSIONS

Few studies to date have addressed the issue of what works for child weight-management programs in the real world. Johnston and Steele (2007) began to address this issue by applying a modified version of an EST for child overweight to patients in a clinical setting. The basis of the intervention included all of the components and approaches outlined in this chapter. Children in this study were not excluded based on the presence of comorbidities or weight status (i.e., severely overweight children were included). Results of the study demonstrated that children significantly reduced their standardized BMI by the end of active treatment. Children who were severely overweight, and who had physiological and/or psychological comorbidities, all significantly reduced their standardized BMI. This study should provide treatment providers with a hopeful outlook regarding weight loss in their pediatric patients. However, longer-term follow-up of these children is needed to be able to determine the true impact of the intervention. Possibly more importantly, though, this provides preliminary evidence that such a program can feasibly be provided in an applied setting.

A firm foundation for the behavioral treatment of pediatric overweight has been established. This allows clinicians the opportunity to use this wealth of information to provide informed treatments for children and their families. Clinical practice is fortunate to have greater flexibility, and often demands that empirically supported treatments be modified for the individual patient. More specifically, in the cases that children or families are refractory to the approach being provided, the clinician may modify the treatment approach or provide an adjunct to make the treatment more individualized. If Plato (trans. 2004) was correct in stating "necessity is the mother of invention," much information can be gained from the need for more effective clinical interventions. It is likely that much of this information will come from clinical experiences in treating pediatric overweight. Finally, advances in the treatment of pediatric overweight will result from practitioners and researchers modifying, enhancing, or adding to currently existing treatments for use with diverse groups and with new technologies.

ACKNOWLEDGEMENTS

Preparation of this paper was supported, in part, by a grant from the United States Department of Agriculture (USDA ARS 2533759358). The authors would also like to acknowledge the Peanut Institute for their support.

REFERENCES

Ball, S. D., Keller, K. R., Moyer-Mileur, L. J., Ding, Y., Donaldson, D., & Jackson, W. D. (2003). Prolongation of satiety after low versus moderately high glycemic index meals in obese adolescents. *Pediatrics, 111*, 488–494.

Beech, B. M., Klesges, R. C., Kumanyika, S. K., Murray, D. M., Klesges, L., McClanahan, B., et al. (2003). Child- and parent-targeted interventions: The Memphis GEMS pilot study. *Ethnicity and Disease, 13*(Suppl. 1), 40–53.

Berkowitz, R. I., Fujioka, K., Daniels, S. R., Hoppin, A. G., Owen, S., Perry, A. C., et al. (2006). Effects of Sibutramine treatment in obese adolescents: A randomized trial. *Annals of Internal Medicine, 145*, 81–90.

Braet, C., Van Winckel, M., & Van Leeuwen, K. (1997). Follow-up results of different treatment programs for obese children. *Acta Paediatrica, 86*, 397–402.

Brownell, K. D., Kelman, J. H., & Stunkard, A. J. (1983). Treatment of obese children with and without their mothers: Changes in weight and blood pressure. *Pediatrics, 71*, 515–523.

Chorpita, B. E., Barlow, D. H., Albano, A. M., & Daleidan, E. L., (1998). Methodological strategies in child clinical trials: Advancing the efficacy and effectiveness of psychosocial treatments. *Journal of Abnormal Child Psychology, 26*, 7–16.

Dao, H. H., Frelut, M. L., Oberlin, F., Peres, G., Bourgeois, P., & Navarro, J. (2004). Effects of a multidisciplinary weight loss intervention on body composition in obese adolescents. *International Journal of Obesity, 28*, 290–299.

Davison, K. K., & Birch, L. L. (2001). Childhood overweight: A contextual model and recommendations for future research. *Obesity Reviews, 2*, 159–171.

Deckelbaum, R. J., & Williams, C. L. (2001). Childhood obesity: The health issue. *Obesity Research, 9*, 239s-243s.

Elliot, R. (1998). Editor's introduction: A guide to the empirically supported treatments controversy. *Psychotherapy Research, 8*, 115–125.

Epstein, L. H. (1996). Family-based behavioural intervention for obese children. *International Journal of Obesity, 20*, 14–21.

Epstein, L. H., McCurley, J., Wing, R. R., & Valoski, A. (1990). Five-year follow-up of family-based behavioral treatments for childhood obesity. *Journal of Consulting and Clinical Psychology, 58*, 661–664.

Epstein, L. H., Myers, M. D., Raynor, H. A., & Saelens, B. E. (1998). Treatment of pediatric obesity. *Pediatrics, 101*, 554–570.

Epstein, L. H., Paluch, R. A., Gordy, C. G., Saelens, B. E., & Ernst, M. M. (2000). Problem solving in the treatment of childhood obesity. *Journal of Consulting and Clinical Psychology, 68*, 717–721.

Epstein, L. H., Paluch, R. A., Saelens, B. E., Ernst, M. M., & Wilfley, D. E. (2001). Changes in eating disorder symptoms with pediatric obesity treatment. *The Journal of Pediatrics, 139*, 58–65.

Epstein, L. H., Valoski, A. M., Kalarchian, M. A., & McCurley, J. (1995). Do children lose and maintain weight easier than adults: A comparison of child and parent weight changes from six months to ten years. *Obesity Research, 3*, 411–417.

Epstein, L. H., Valoski, A., Vara, L. S., McCurley, J., Wisniewski, L., Kalarchian, M. A., et al. (1995). Effects of decreasing sedentary behavior and increasing activity on weight change in obese children. *Health Psychology, 14*, 109–115.

Epstein, L. H., Valoski, A., Wing, R. R., & McCurley, J. (1990). Ten-year follow-up of behavioral family-based treatment for obese children. *Journal of the American Medical Association, 264*, 2519–2523.

Epstein, L. H., Valoski, A., Wing, R. R., & McCurley, J. (1994). Ten-year outcomes of behavioral family-based treatment for childhood obesity. *Health Psychology, 13*, 373–383.

Epstein, L. H., Wing, R. R., Koeske, R. R., Andrasik, F. & Ossip, D. (1981). Child and parent weight loss in family-based behavior modification programs. *Journal of Consulting and Clinical Psychology, 49*, 674–685.

Epstein, L. H., Wing, R. R., Steranchak, L., Dickson, B., & Michelson, J. (1980). Comparison of family-based behavior modification and nutrition education for childhood obesity. *Journal of Pediatric Psychology, 5*, 25–37.

Epstein, L. H., Wisniewski, L., & Weng, R. (1994). Child and parent psychological problems influence child weight control. *Obesity Research, 2*, 509–515.

Fagot-Campagna, A. (2000). Emergence of type 2 diabetes mellitus in children: Epidemiological evidence. *Journal of Pediatric Endocrinology and Metabolism, 13*, 1395–1402.

Favaro, A., & Santonastaso, P. (1995). Effects of parents' psychological characteristics and eating behaviour on childhood obesity and dietary compliance. *Journal of Psychosomatic Research, 39*, 145–151.

Flodmark, C., Ohlsson, T., Ryden, O., & Sveger, T. (1993). Prevention of progression to severe obesity in a group of obese schoolchildren treated with family therapy. *Pediatrics, 91*, 880–884.

Fossati, M., Amati, F., Painot, D., Reiner, M., Haenni, C., & Golay, A. (2004). Cognitive-behavioral therapy with simultaneous nutritional and physical activity education in obese patients with binge eating disorder. *Eating and Weight Disorders, 9,* 134–138.

Fulton, J. E., McGuire, M. T., Caspersen, C. J., & Dietz, W. H. (2001). Interventions for weight loss and weight gain prevention among youth. *Sports Medicine, 31,* 153–165.

Gaston, J. E., Abbott, M. J., Rapee, R. M., & Neary, S. A. (2006). Do empirically supported treatments generalize to private practice? A benchmark study of a cognitive-behavioural group treatment programme for social phobia. *British Journal of Clinical Psychology, 45,* 33–48.

Golan, M., & Crow, S. (2004). Parents are key players in the prevention and treatment of weight-related problems. *Nutrition Reviews, 62,* 39–50.

Golan, M., Fainaru, M., & Weizman, A. (1998). Role of behavior modification in the treatment of childhood obesity with the parents as the exclusive agents of change. *International Journal of Obesity, 22,* 1217–1224.

Haddock, C. K., Shadish, W. R., Klesges, R. C., & Stein, R. J. (1994). Treatments for childhood and adolescent obesity. *Annals of Behavioral Medicine, 16,* 235–244.

Israel, A. C. (1999). Commentary: Empirically supported treatments for pediatric obesity: Goals, outcome criteria, and the societal context. *Journal of Pediatric Psychology, 24,* 249–250.

Israel, A. C., Guile, C. A., Baker, J. E., & Silverman, W. K. (1994). An evaluation of enhanced self-regulation training in the treatment of childhood obesity. *Journal of Pediatric Psychology, 19,* 737–749.

Israel, A. C., Silverman, W. K., & Solotar, L. C. (1988). The relationship between adherence and weight loss in a behavioral treatment program for overweight children. *Behavior Therapy, 19,* 25–33.

Israel, A. C., Stolmaker, L., & Andrian, C. A. (1985a). The effects of training parents in general child management skills on a behavioral weight loss program for children. *Behavior Therapy, 16,* 169–180.

Israel, A. C., Stolmaker, L., & Andrian, C. A. (1985b). Thoughts about food and their relationship to obesity and weight control. *International Journal of Eating Disorders, 4,* 549–558.

Jeffrey, R. W., Drewnowski, A., Epstein, L. H., Stunkard, A. J., Wilson, G. T., & Wing, R. R. (2000). Long-term maintenance of weight loss: Current status. *Health Psychology, 19*(Suppl. 1), 5–16.

Jelalian, E., & Saelens, B. E. (1999). Empirically supported treatments in pediatric psychology: Pediatric obesity. *Journal of Pediatric Psychology, 24,* 223–248.

Johnson, S. L., & Birch, L. L. (1994). Parents' and children's adiposity and eating style. *Pediatrics, 94,* 653–661.

Johnston, C. A., & Steele, R. G. (2007). Treatment of pediatric overweight: An examination of feasibility and effectiveness in an applied clinical setting. *Journal of Pediatric Psychology, 32,* 106–110.

Johnston, C. A., Tyler, C., Fullerton, G., Poston, W. S. C., Haddock, K., McFarlin, B., et al. (in press). Results of an intensive school-based weight loss program with overweight Mexican American children. *International Journal of Pediatric Obesity.*

Jolliffe, D. (2004). Extent of overweight among U.S. children and adolescents from 1971 to 2000. *International Journal of Obesity, 28,* 4–9.

Kanfer, F. H. (1970). Self-monitoring: Methodological limitations and clinical applications. *Journal of Consulting and Clinical Psychology, 35,* 148–152.

Kazdin, A. E., & Weisz, J. R. (1998). Identifying and developing empirically supported child and adolescent treatments. *Journal of Consulting and Clinical Psychology, 66,* 19–36.

Keller, C. S., Gonzales, A., & Fleuriet, K. J. (2005). Retention of minority participants in clinical research studies. *Western Journal of Nursing Research, 27,* 292–306.

Kirschenbaum, D. S., Harris, E. S., & Tomarken, A. J. (1984). Effects of parental involvement in behavioral weight loss therapy for preadolescents. *Behavior Therapy, 15,* 485–500.

Kitzmann, K. M., & Beech, B. M. (2006). Family-based interventions for pediatric obesity: Methodological and conceptual challenges from family psychology. *Journal of Family Psychology, 20,* 175–189.

Kumanyika, S., & Grier, S. (2006). Targeting interventions for ethnic minority and low-income populations. *The Future of Children, 16*, 187–207.

Levine, M. D., Ringham, R. M., Kalarchian, M. A., Wisniewski, L., & Marcus, M. D. (2001). Is family-based behavioral weight control appropriate for severe pediatric obesity? *International Journal of Eating Disorders, 30*, 318–328.

McLean, N., Griffin, S., Toney, K., & Hardeman, W. (2003). Family involvement in weight control, weight maintenance and weight loss interventions: A systematic review of randomized trials. *International Journal of Obesity, 27*, 987–1005.

Nesbitt, S. D., Ashaye, M. O., Stettler, N., Sorof, J. M., Goran, M. I., Parekh, R., et al. (2004). Overweight as a risk factor in children: A focus on ethnicity. *Ethnicity and Disease, 14*, 94–110.

Norgren, S., Danilesson, P., Jurold, R., Lotborn, M., & Marcus, C. (2003). Orlistat treatment in obese prepubertal children: A pilot study. *Acta Paediatrica, 92*, 666–670.

Nova, A., Russo, A., & Sala, E. (2001). Long-term management of obesity in paediatric office practice: Experimental evaluation of two different types of intervention. *Ambulatory Child Health, 7*, 239–248.

Ogden, C. L., Carroll, M. D., Curtin, L. R., McDowell, M. A., Tabak, C. A., & Flegal, K. M. (2006). Prevalence of overweight and obesity in the United States, 1999–2004. *Journal of the American Medical Association, 295*, 1549–1555.

Plato (translated 2004). *Republic* (C. D. C. Reeve, Trans.). Indiana: Hackett Publishing.

Redmon, J. B., Raatz, S. K., Reck, K. P., Swanson, J. E., Kwong, C. A., Fan, Q., et al. (2003). One-year outcomes of a combination of weight loss therapies for subjects with type 2 diabetes: A randomized trial. *Diabetes Care, 26*, 2505–2511.

Resnicow, K., Yaroch, A., Davis, A., Wang, D. T., Carter, S., Slaughter, L., et al. (2000). Go girls! Results from a nutritional and physical activity program for low-income, overweight African-American adolescent females. *Health Education Research, 5*, 616–631.

Robinson, T. N. (1999). Behavioral treatment of childhood and adolescent obesity, *International Journal of Obesity, 23*(Suppl. 2), 52–57.

Rosenbloom, A. L., Joe, J. R., Young, R. S., & Winter, W. E. (1999). Emerging epidemic of type 2 diabetes in youth. *Diabetes Care, 22*, 345–354.

Schwimmer, J. B., Burwinkle, T. M., & Varni, J. M. (2003). Health-related quality of life of severely overweight children and adolescents. *Journal of the American Medical Association, 289*, 1813–1819.

Steele, R. G., & Roberts, M. C. (2003). Therapy and interventions research with children and adolescents. In M.C. Roberts & S.S. Ilardi (Eds.), *Methods of Research in Clinical Psychology: A Handbook*. Oxford: Blackwell.

Stein, R. I., Epstein, L. H., Raynor, H. A., Kilanowski, C. K., & Paluch, R. A. (2005). The influence of parenting change in pediatric weight control. *Obesity Research, 13*, 1749–1755.

Summerbell, C. D., Ashton, V., Campbell, K. J., Edmunds, L. D., Kelly, S., & Waters, E. (2003). Interventions for treating obesity in children. *Cochrane Database of Systematic Reviews, 3*, Article CD001872.

Tauman, R., O'Brien, L. M., Ivanenko, A., & Gozal, D. (2005). Obesity rather than severity of sleep-disordered breathing as the major determinant of insulin resistance and altered lipidemia in snoring children. *Pediatrics, 116*, E66-E73.

Tershakovec, A. M. (2004). Psychological considerations in pediatric weight management. *Obesity Research, 12*, 1537–1538.

Uzark, K. C., Becker, M. H., Dielman, T. E., Rocchini, A. P., & Katch, V. (1988). Perceptions held by obese children and their parents: Implications for weight control behaviors. *Health Education Quarterly, 15*, 185–198.

Violante-Ortiz, R., Del-Rio-Navarro, B. E., Lara-Esqueda, A., Perez, P., Fanghanel, G., Madero, A., et al. (2005). Use of sibutramine in obese Hispanic adolescents. *Advances in Therapy, 23*, 506–507.

Wang, Y., & Zhang, Q. (2006). Are American children and adolescents of low socioeconomic status at increased risk of obesity? Changes in the association between overweight and family income between 1971 and 2002. *American Journal of Clinical Nutrition, 84*, 707–716.

Westen, D., Novotny, C. M., & Thompson-Brenner, H. (2005). EBP ≠ EST: Reply to Crits-Christoph et al. (2005) and Weisz et al. (2005). *Psychological Bulletin, 131,* 427–433.

Wilson, G. T. (1994). Behavioral treatment of childhood obesity: Theoretical and practical implications. *Health Psychology, 13,* 371–372.

Wing, R. R., Tate, D. F., Gorin, A. A., Raynor, H. A., & Fava, J. L. (2006). A self-regulation program for maintenance of weight loss. *The New England Journal of Medicine, 355,* 1563–1571.

Zeller, M. H., Roehrig, H., Modi, A. C., Daniels, S. R., & Inge, T. H. (2006). Health-realted quality of life and depressive symptoms in adolescents with extreme obesity presenting for bariatric surgery. *Pediatrics, 117,* 1155–1161.

Zeller, M. H., Saelens, B. E., Roehrig, H., Kirk, S., & Daniels, S. R. (2004). Psychological adjustment of obese youth presenting for weight management treatment. *Obesity Research, 12,* 1576–1586.

27

Future Directions in Pediatric Obesity Prevention and Intervention: Research and Practice

ELISSA JELALIAN, RIC G. STEELE, and CHAD D. JENSEN

Almost before our eyes, pediatric obesity has grown to epidemic proportions in the United States and elsewhere, and is now known to be associated with a number of medical and psychosocial comorbidities that may last a lifetime. Within the span of less than two generations, the number of children and youth with obesity and overweight has more than doubled in some age groups, and has tripled in others (Centers for Disease Control and Prevention [CDC], 2007). If estimates of the trajectory are correct, by 2010 approximately 50 percent of children in North America and 38 percent of children in the European Union will be overweight or obese (Wang & Lobstein, 2006).

The alarming increase in the prevalence of obesity is likely due to a constellation of factors, including biological, behavioral, sociological, and economic. Correspondingly, just as there are multiple etiological factors for the condition, we argue that the solutions to the problem are likely

ELISSA JELALIAN • Warren Alpert Medical School of Brown University, Providence, RI 02912. **RIC G. STEELE and CHAD D. JENSEN** • University of Kansas, Lawrence, KS 66045.

to require changes within multiple and interacting systems within society. These include changes at the individual level, changes in local and regional policy, and perhaps changes in values at the national level.

Consistent with Bronfenbrenner's socioecological model (1979), Kazak, Rourke, and Crump (2003) and Power, Dupaul, Shapiro, and Kazak (2003) proposed a socioecological view of pediatric health and illness that places the child at the center of a number of concentric rings (see Figure 27.1). At the center of the system is the developing child, with the genetic, biological, and behavioral components that propel development. Moving out from the center, *microsystems* comprise the individual relationships in the child's experience that have the most direct influence on development (e.g., relationships with parents, teachers, peers, etc.), as well as parameters of the illness itself that affect development (i.e., how the child responds to the illness or condition). Continuing outward, the *mesosystems* refer to interactions between two or more microsystems (e.g., interactions between caregivers and teachers, or between teachers and health care professionals). Influencing how and where these mesosystemic interactions occur is the *exosystem*—the infrastructure or establishments that allow and facilitate the interaction of systems (e.g., Parent-Teacher Organizations; community centers, etc.). Finally, the model recognizes that a society's cultural values and beliefs (i.e., the *macrosystem*) influence the degree to which exosystems will be established. Similar to other illness conditions, we suggest that this model provides a useful framework for considering the

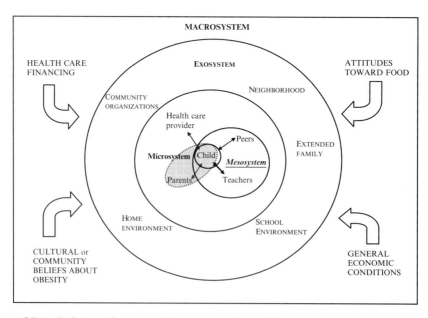

Figure 27.1. Pediatric obesity in the context of Bronfenbrenner's (1979) socioecological model (adapted from Steele, Nelson, & Cole, 2007).

factors that contribute to pediatric obesity, as well as prevention and intervention programs.

Factors at the Individual Level

Research conducted during the past several decades has provided a wealth of knowledge regarding the individual factors that contribute to weight-control problems. In particular, information about the genetic factors predicting risk for obesity has increased exponentially. Although specific genetic markers have not been conclusively identified, research has demonstrated that obesity risk in each child aggregates with general family risk (Mair, Ch. 11). Further, genetic research has provided useful insights into a number of the biological factors related to the physiology of weight management (e.g., satiety and activity level) (Fields, Ch. 8). Information about genetic risk and physiological (biological) variables related to weight regulation has the potential to inform prevention and intervention programs, although the extent to which this potential has been realized is not clear.

Also addressing obesity from an individual perspective, many interventions for obesity designed for children and adolescents focus on altering individual behavior. Interventions that promote changes in physical activity and dietary intake have received evidentiary support from many clinical trials. However, less is known about the most effective delivery methods for such interventions (e.g., primary care or community settings) or techniques to motivate and retain children and adolescents in these interventions so that maximum results can be achieved (Delamater, Ch. 14).

Further, information about the efficacy of intensive interventions, including pharmacological treatments (Han and Yanovski, Ch. 15) and residential treatments (Gately and Cooke, Ch. 16) is emerging. However, research addressing the effectiveness of behavioral or lifestyle treatments for severely overweight (> 100 percent overweight) children is lacking, with many treatment studies excluding severely overweight children (Raynor, Ch. 17). Thus, a number of areas of inquiry that address intra-individual factors in the treatment of pediatric obesity remain important for further study.

Factors within the Microsystem

Our understanding of how the microsystem can have multiple effects on child behavior has increased in recent years. Research has highlighted the importance of a number of microsystem variables in the development of overweight in the preschool and elementary school years, including maternal sensitivity (O'Brien et al., 2007), parenting style (Rhee, Lumeng, Appugliese, Kaciroti, & Bradley, 2006), and opportunities for involvement with stimulating activities (i.e., books and games) at home (O'Brien et al.). Further, we have learned much about the efficacy of interventions for pediatric obesity that target relationships within microsystems. Of particular importance is the knowledge that has accumulated regarding family-based interventions that include education and behavioral components (Epstein, Paluch, Roemmich, & Beecher, 2007; Wilfley et al., 2007).

However, despite recent advances in our knowledge about the effects of the microsystem, there remains a great deal of work left to be done. The current literature is particularly informative with regard to effective treatments for children under the ideal circumstances of a motivated family, moderate level of overweight, and adequate economic and organizational resources. However, even with the information that we currently have, effect sizes remain relatively modest, and have demonstrated relatively little change over the past two decades (Epstein et al., 2007). Similarly, the number of children who remain overweight (despite clinically significant changes in BMI from pre- to post-treatment) remains relatively high, as does the number of youth who *relapse* into obesity or overweight following intervention (Jelalian, Markov Wember, Bungeroth, & Biramer, 2007). Additional clinical and translational research is needed to further explore ways to improve treatment efficacy (e.g., integration of larger systems into family based treatment), as well as examine factors related to weight-loss maintenance.

One of the significant limitations to the treatment literature is a lack of translational research that examines what will work in practice settings and in populations that deviate from those typically examined in randomized clinical trials (Epstein et al., 2007; Jelalian et al., 2007). Although some translational research is emerging (see Eliakim et al., 2002; Johnson & Steele, 2007), much more is needed. Furthermore, most intervention studies have targeted school-age children between the ages of 8 and 12 years. As a result, less is known about the efficacy of treatments for young children (Raynor, Ch. 13) and adolescents (Delamater, Ch 14). Finally, while studies have demonstrated that peer support can impact the effect of weight-loss interventions (Jelalian, Mehlenbeck, Lloyd-Richardson, Birmaher, & Wing, 2006), less is known about the positive effects of normal-weight peers on children and adolescents' weight-loss efforts (Delamater, Ch. 18).

Beyond the Microsystem

While the bulk of the treatment literature remains solidly within the level of the individual or the microsystem, some research is beginning to examine mesosystemic or exosystemic factors as potential targets for improving children's health. For example, several studies demonstrate a relationship between characteristics of the *built environment*, such as access to sidewalks, distance to school, neighborhood safety, and physical activity levels in children (Sallis & Glanz, 2006). A recent study demonstrated a relationship between neighborhood *walkability* and participation in moderate-to-vigorous physical activity in adolescents (Kligerman, Sallis, Ryan, Frank, & Nader, 2007). Future research may focus on demonstrating a link between improving aspects of the built environment and weight status (Sallis & Glanz).

Finally, we know the least about the relationship between cultural values (macrosystem) and pediatric obesity. Values, as reflected by attitudes displayed toward children who are overweight, suggest some degree of intolerance of obesity. For example, Strauss and Pollack (2003) found that while overweight children listed a similar number of friends as their nonoverweight peers, other children were less likely to nominate them as friends. At the same time, it is clear that western culture (American culture, in particular) provides mixed messages with regard to food, nutrition, and health. As a result, intolerance of obesity (and the resulting prejudice against children and individuals who are overweight) coexists with a reluctance to make policy changes necessary to curb the prevalence of overweight.

This juxtaposition of apparently incompatible values was recently driven home to one of the authors at a recent local school district meeting. District representatives were extremely enthusiastic about policy changes designed to increase physical activity during the school day (e.g., taking time to stretch and walk, lesson plans that incorporate physical activity into learning activities). However, many of those who were most in favor of increased activity to help reduce and prevent obesity were vehemently opposed to a proposed policy change to limit (not eliminate) the use of dessert items in classroom celebrations.

Inconsistencies such as the one in the above example are not uncommon, and are a reflection of the ambivalence that still characterizes public views about the causes of, and solutions to, the obesity epidemic. Ultimately, policy changes will be driven by a shift in national values to perception of obesity as a complex condition brought about by interactions among genetic, social, cultural, and environmental circumstances rather than as solely a condition of personal responsibility.

The Future of Interventions and Intervention Research

The ubiquity of overweight among children and adolescents suggests that interventions must reach more of those in need than are currently being served. As noted by Epstein and colleagues (2007), the translation of research-based pediatric obesity interventions into the clinic is "long overdue" (p. 389). Some research suggests that primary-care settings may be a viable treatment setting that would accommodate more children in need of weight-management intervention (Patrick et al., 2001; Saelens et al., 2002). However, additional controlled studies are needed to examine the degree to which currently available treatments can be reliably implemented in primary-care settings.

Saelens and Liu (2007) recently commented on the lack of consistent use in primary care settings of strategies that are known to be effective (e.g., behavior modification). Simply put, many clinicians are not using techniques that have the best evidence for their efficacy. In some cases, clinicians in primary-care settings may lack adequate training in behavioral strategies themselves and may not have easy access to professional staff who are skilled in this area. Alternatively, the differences in practice patterns may reflect differences in attitudes toward obesity and weight management techniques (Jelalian, Boergers, Alday, & Frank, 2003; Moyers, Bugle, & Jackson, 2005; Story et al., 2002). Further research into practice patterns of healthcare providers and service utilization (e.g., service systems research) vis-à-vis pediatric overweight is necessary alongside future research to further explore treatment outcomes (see Steele, Mize Nelson, & Nelson, 2008).

Similarly, the use of technology has been identified as an alternative strategy for reaching a greater number of children and adolescents who would benefit from intervention. Although outcomes were not maintained over time, Williamson and colleagues (2006) demonstrated positive short-term effects using a Web-based intervention for pediatric overweight. Future research should address the need to provide engaging and inter-active programs that will promote continued use of such interventions among youth while including effective behavior change techniques (Hurl-ing, Fairley, & Dias, 2006). Research should also examine the impact of intervention setting (electronic vs. clinic) on attention and adherence to technological treatment approaches (Tate, Ch. 23).

Another question that has been relatively neglected in pediatric inter-vention research is the economic benefit of weight-control interventions. A recent review of child obesity prevention interventions noted that only one study among the many investigations reviewed analyzed the cost effective-ness of treatment (Flodmark, Marcus, & Britton, 2006). Similarly, cost effectiveness has rarely been analyzed in weight-loss intervention studies. This area of research becomes increasingly relevant as obesity prevalence rises and costs for treatment must be managed to provide care to the many youths in need of treatment (Goldfield, Epstein, Kilanowski, Paluch, & Kogut-Bossler, 2001).

As noted by Wilson and Kitzman-Ulrich (Ch. 18), there remain rela-tively few studies targeting pediatric overweight in ethnic minority popu-lations, despite the fact that minority children are at significantly greater risk for obesity than European-American children. Ogden and colleagues (2006) reported that Mexican-American children and African-American female children and adolescents were at particular risk relative to their European-American counterparts. Although several weight-management programs have demonstrated efficacy in clinical studies and field trials, the degree to which ethnicity or culture moderates the efficacy of these interventions is largely unknown. Further, recent research suggests that youth from diverse backgrounds are less likely to attend and benefit from programs designed for and evaluated in primarily European-American samples (e.g., Zeller et al., 2004). Theory-based research examining differ-ences in efficacy across ethnic or cultural groups (and the reasons behind such differences) remains sorely needed.

Prevention Programs

Moving from treatment to prevention, there are some data available regarding the effectiveness of prevention studies targeting pediatric weight control—a significant number of which have been conducted in the school environment. Given the scope of the current epidemic and the challenge of developing effective interventions, reversing the trend may rely on prevention strategies that serve to reduce the initial onset of obesity in children and adolescents (Janicke, Sallinen, & White Plume, Ch. 20).

The majority of school-based prevention efforts have provided broad interventions targeting all students, regardless of weight status. While there are data to support the efficacy of this broad application, less is known about how to reach children who are already overweight in a community setting without stigmatization or labeling. There is also relatively little known about the types of messages that should be used to decrease obesity risk without increasing the risk of children developing unhealthy weight control habits or eating disorders (Neumark-Sztainer, Story, Hannan and Rex, 2003). Researchers have suggested that prevention of overweight should be approached from a life-cycle perspective, addressing the impact of excessive weight gain during pregnancy, infancy, and childhood, as well as early in the onset of puberty (Johnson, Gerstein, Evans, & Woodward-Lopez, 2006). Future studies concerning the impact of these variables will further inform prevention efforts and may eventually lead to a reduction in rates of overweight among children and adolescents.

Consistent with an ecological framework, future intervention and prevention efforts may be most effective by attending to the multiple environments in which children function, with corresponding focus on connecting systems of care across these settings—i.e., family, school, physical environment, primary care, and policy. There are a number of potential mechanisms for increasing continuity across settings. For example, it may be effective for school systems to provide weight-control interventions and/or standard prevention programs, including behavioral specialists, nutritionists, and pediatricians within the school setting. This may be a logical extension of BMI reporting, which has been adopted by the state of Arkansas (CDC, 2006), as well as other school districts throughout the country. One possible model of intervention on multiple levels—both individual and societal—uses the example provided by the intervention to decrease tobacco use. Clinical intervention, education, regulation, economic strategy, and a combination of these strategies have all been critical in decreasing tobacco use in the United States. Researchers have suggested that these lessons are applicable to weight-management treatment, and provide an exemplary approach that combines direct intervention, education, and prevention through public and economic policy (Mercer et al., 2003).

CONCLUSIONS

There has been considerable public attention focused on pediatric obesity during the last decade. However, the extent to which increased public awareness will impact cultural values, policy, and systems of care remains to be seen. As reflected in the chapters in this volume, increased public awareness has been paralleled by enhanced research efforts focused on identifying gene/environment interactions predisposing children to obesity, recognizing individual, family, and environmental level variables related to weight control, and developing effective prevention and intervention strategies. Such efforts, combined with increased focus on policy change related to nutrition and physical activity, may serve to decrease the unprecedented rise in pediatric obesity observed in industrialized countries. While there continues to be significant concern, a number of promising prevention and intervention strategies coupled with recommended policy change offer hope that we are on the threshold of slowing, if not reversing the pediatric obesity epidemic.

REFERENCES

Bronfenbrenner, U. (1979). *The Ecology of Human Development.* Cambridge, MA: Harvard University Press.

Centers for Disease Control and Prevention. (2006). Overweight among students in grades K-12-Arkansansas, 2003–04 and 2004–05 school years. *Morbidity and Mortality Weekly Report, 13,* 5–8.

Centers for Disease Control and Prevention. (2007). *Prevalence of Overweight among Children and Adolescents: United States, 2003–2004.* Rockville, MD: National Center for Health Statistics. Retrieved September 19, 2007 from http://www.cdc.gov/nchs/products/pubs/pubd/hestats/overweight/overwght_child_03.htm#Table%201.

Eliakim, A., Kaven, G., Berger, I., Friedland, O., Wolach, B., & Nemet, D. (2002). The effect of a combined intervention on body mass index and fitness in obese children and adolescents – a clinical experience. *European Journal of Pediatrics, 161,* 449–454.

Epstein, L. H., Paluch, R. A., Roemmich, J. N., & Beecher, M. D. (2007). Family-based obesity treatment, then and now: Twenty-five years of pediatric obesity treatment. *Health Psychology, 26,* 381–391.

Flodmark, C. E., Marcus, E., & Britton, M. (2006). Interventions to prevent obesity in children and adolescents: A systematic literature review. *International Journal of Obesity, 30,* 579–589.

Goldfield, G. S., Epstein, L. H., Kilanowski, C. K., Paluch, R. A., & Kogut-Bossler, B. (2001). Cost-effectiveness of group and mixed family-based treatment for childhood obesity. *International Journal of Obesity, 25,* 1843–1849.

Hurling, R., Fairley, B. W., & Dias M. B. (2006). Internet-based exercise interventions: Are more interactive designs better? *Psychological Health, 21,* 757–772.

Jelalian, E., Boergers, J., Alday, C. S., & Frank, R. (2003). Survey of physician attitudes and practices related to pediatric obesity. *Clinical Pediatrics, 42,* 235–245.

Jelalian, E., Mehlenbeck, R., Lloyd-Richardson, E. E., Birmaher, V., & Wing, R. R., (2006). 'Adventure therapy' combined with cognitive-behavioral treatment for overweight adolescents. *International Journal of Obesity, 30,* 31–39.

Jelalian, E., Wember, Y. M., Bungeroth, H., & Birmaher, V. (2007). Practitioner review: Bridging the gap between research and clinical practice in pediatric obesity. *Journal of Child Psychology and Psychiatry, 48,* 115–127.

Johnson, D. B., Gerstein, D. E., Evans, A. E., & Woodward-Lopez, G. (2006). Preventing obesity: A life cycle perspective. *Journal of the American Dietetic Association, 106,* 97–102.

Johnston, C. A., & Steele, R. G. (2007). Treatment of pediatric obesity: An examination of effectiveness in an applied clinical setting. *Journal of Pediatric Psychology, 32,* 106–110.

Kazak, A. E., Rourke M. T., & Crump, T. A. (2003). Families and other systems in pediatric psychology. In M.C. Roberts (Ed.), *Handbook of Pediatric Psychology,* (3rd ed., pp. 159–175). New York: Guilford.

Kliegerman, M., Sallis, J. F., Ryan, S., Frank, L. D., & Nader, P. R. (2007). Association of neighborhood design and recreation environment variables with physical activity and body mass index in adolescents. *American Journal of Health Promotion, 21,* 274–277.

Mercer, S. L., Green, L. W., Rosenthal, A. C., Husten, C. G., Khan, L. K., & Dietz, W. H. (2003). Possible lessons from the tobacco experience for obesity control. *American Journal of Clinical Nutrition, 77,* 1073S-1082S.

Moyers, P., Bugle, L., & Jackson, E. (2005). Perceptions of school nurses regarding obesity in school-age children. *The Journal of School Nursing, 21,* 86–93.

Neumark-Sztainer, D., Story, M., Hannan, P. J., & Rex, J. (2003). New moves: A school-based obesity prevention program for adolscent girls. *Prevention Medicine, 37,* 41–51.

O'Brien, M., Nader, P. R., Houts, R. M., Bradley, R.,Friedman, S. L., Belsky, J. et al., (2007). The ecology of childhood overweight: A 12-year longitudinal analysis. *International Journal of Obesity, 31,* 1469–1478.

Ogden, C. L., Carroll, M. D., Curtin, L. R., McDowell, M. A., Tabak, C. J., & Flegal, K. M. (2006). Prevalence of overweight and obesity in the United States, 1999–2004. *Journal of the American Medical Association, 295,* 1549–1555.

Patrick, K., Sallis, J. F., Prochaska, J. J., Lydston, D. D., Calfas, K. J., Zabinski, M. F., et al., (2001). A multicomponent program for nutrition and physical activity change in primary care. *Pediatric and Adolescent Medicine, 155,* 940–946.

Power, T., DuPaul, G., Shapiro, E., & Kazak, A. (2003). *Promoting Children's Health: Integrating School, Family, and Community.* New York: Guilford.

Rhee, K. E., Lumeng, J. C., Appugliese, D. P., Kaciroti, N., & Bradley, R. H. (2006). Parenting styles and overweight status in first grade. *Pediatrics, 117,* 2047–2054.

Saelens, B. E., & Liu, L. (2007). Clinician's comment on treatment of childhood overweight meta-analysis. *Health Psychology, 26,* 533–536.

Saelens, B. E., Sallis, J. F., Wilfey, D. E., Patrick, K., Cella, J. A., & Butcha, R. (2002). Behavioral weight control for overweight adolescents initiated in primary care. *Obesity Research, 10,* 22–32.

Sallis, J. F., & Glanz, K. (2006). The role of built environments in physical activity, eating, and obesity in childhood. *Future of Children, 16,* 89–108.

Steele, R. G., Mize Nelson, J. A., & Nelson, T. D. (2008). Methodological issues in the evaluation of therapies. In R.G. Steele, T.D. Elkin, & M.C. Roberts (Eds.) *Handbook of Evidence-Based Therapies for Children and Adolescents.* Berlin Heidelberg New York: Springer.

Steele, R. G., Nelson, T. D., & Cole, B. P. (2007). The psychosocial adjustment of children and adolescents with HIV: Review from a socio-ecological perspective. *Journal of Developmental and Behavioral Pediatrics, 28,* 58–69.

Story, M. T., Neumark-Stzainer, D. R., Sherwood, N. E., Holt, K., Sofka, D., Trowbridge, F. L., et al. (2002). Management of child and adolescent obesity: Attitudes, barrier, skills, and training needs among health care professionals. *Pediatrics, 110,* 210–214.

Strauss, R. S., & Pollack, H. A. (2003). Social marginalization of overweight children. *Archives of Pediatric and Adolescent Medicine, 157,* 746–752.

Wang, Y., & Lobstein, T. (2006). Worldwide trends in childhood overweight and obesity. *International Journal of Pediatric Obesity, 1,* 11–25.

Wilfley, D. E., Tibbs, T. L., Van Buren, D. J., Reach, K. P., Walker, M. S., & Epstein, L. H. (2007). Lifestyle interventions in the treatment of childhood overweight: A meta-analytic review of randomized control trials. *Health Psychology, 26,* 521–532.

Williamson, D. A., Walden, H. M., White, M. A., York-Crowe, E., Newton, Jr., R. L., Alfonso, A., et al., (2006). Two-year internet-based randomized controlled trial for weight loss in African-American girls. *Obesity Research, 14,* 1231–1243.

Zeller, M., Kirk, S., Claytor, R., Khoury, P., Grieme, J., Santangelo, M., & Daniels, S. (2004). Predictors of attrition from a pediatric weight management program. *Journal of Pediatrics, 144,* 466–470.

Name Index

Subject Index

Printed in the United States of America